1985
YEAR BOOK OF
PEDIATRICS®

THE 1985 YEAR BOOKS

The YEAR BOOK series provides in condensed form the essence of the best of the recent international literature in medicine and the allied health professions. The material is selected by distinguished editors who critically review more than 500,000 journal articles each year.

Anesthesia: Drs. Miller, Kirby, Ostheimer, Saidman, and Stoelting

Cancer: Drs. Hickey, Clark, and Cumley

Cardiology: Drs. Harvey, Kirkendall, Kirklin, Nadas, Resnekov, and Sonnenblick

Critical Care Medicine: Drs. Rogers, Booth, Dean, Gioia, McPherson, Michael, and Traystman

Dentistry: Drs. Cohen, Hendler, Johnson, Jordan, Moyers, Robinson, and Silverman

Dermatology: Drs. Sober and Fitzpatrick

Diagnostic Radiology: Drs. Bragg, Keats, Kieffer, Kirkpatrick, Koehler, Sorenson, and White

Digestive Diseases: Drs. Greenberger and Moody

Drug Therapy: Drs. Hollister and Lasagna

Emergency Medicine: Dr. Wagner

Endocrinology: Drs. Schwartz and Ryan

Family Practice: Dr. Rakel

Hand Surgery: Drs. Dobyns and Chase

Infectious Diseases: Drs. Wolff, Gorbach, Keusch, Klempner, and Snydman

Medicine: Drs. Rogers, Des Prez, Cline, Braunwald, Greenberger, Bondy, Epstein, and Malawista

Neurology and Neurosurgery: Drs. De Jong, Sugar, and Currier

Nuclear Medicine: Drs. Hoffer, Gore, Gottschalk, Sostman, and Zaret

Obstetrics and Gynecology: Drs. Pitkin and Zlatnik

Ophthalmology: Dr. Ernest

Orthopedics: Dr. Coventry

Otolaryngology: Drs. Paparella and Bailey

Pathology and Clinical Pathology: Dr. Brinkhous

Pediatrics: Drs. Oski and Stockman

Plastic and Reconstructive Surgery: Drs. McCoy, Brauer, Haynes, Hoehn, Miller, and Whitaker

Podiatric Medicine and Surgery: Dr. Jay

Psychiatry and Applied Mental Health: Drs. Freedman, Lourie, Meltzer, Nemiah, Talbott, and Weiner

Sports Medicine: Drs. Krakauer, Shephard, and Torg, Col. Anderson, and Mr. George

Surgery: Drs. Schwartz, Najarian, Peacock, Shires, Spencer, and Thompson

Urology: Drs. Gillenwater and Howards

1985

The Year Book of PEDIATRICS®

Editors

Frank A. Oski, M.D.
Professor and Chairman, Department of Pediatrics,
State University of New York Upstate Medical Center

James A. Stockman, III, M.D.
Professor and Chairman, Department of Pediatrics,
Northwestern University School of Medicine; Physician in Chief, The
Children's Memorial Hospital, Chicago

Year Book Medical Publishers, Inc.
Chicago

The editor for this book was Roberta A. Mendelson and the production manager was H. E. Nielsen. The Managing Editor for the Year Book series is Caroline Scoulas.

Table of Contents

The material covered in this volume represents literature reviewed up to May 1984.

Journals Represented

Acta Oto-Laryngologica
Acta Paediatrica Scandinavica
Acta Radiologica: Diagnosis
American Journal of Cardiology
American Journal of Clinical Nutrition
American Journal of Clinical Pathology
American Journal of Diseases of Children
American Journal of Gastroenterology
American Journal of Medicine
American Journal of Obstetrics and Gynecology
American Journal of Ophthalmology
American Journal of Pediatric Hematology/Oncology
American Journal of Psychiatry
American Journal of Roentgenology
American Journal of Sports Medicine
American Journal of Surgery
American Review of Respiratory Diseases
Anesthesia and Analgesia
Annales Chirurgiae et Gynecologiae
Annals of Allergy
Annals of Internal Medicine
Annals of Neurology
Annals of Ophthalmology
Annals of Otology, Rhinology and Laryngology
Annals of Rheumatic Diseases
Annals of Surgery
Annals of Thoracic Surgery
Archives of Dermatology
Archives of Disease in Childhood
Archives of Neurology
Archives of Ophthalmology
Archives of Pathology and Laboratory Medicine
ASDC Journal of Dentistry for Children
Australian Paediatric Journal
British Journal of Psychiatry
British Journal of Radiology
British Journal of Urology
British Medical Journal
Cancer
Chest
Circulation
Cleveland Clinic Quarterly
Clinical Allergy
Clinical Pediatrics
Gastroenterology
Hepatology
Hypertension

International Surgery
Investigative Ophthalmology and Visual Science
Journal of Allergy and Clinical Immunology
Journal of the American Academy of Child Psychiatry
Journal of the American Medical Association
Journal of Bone and Joint Surgery (British vol.)
Journal of Laryngology and Otology
Journal of Nervous and Mental Disease
Journal of Neurology, Neurosurgery and Psychiatry
Journal of Pediatric Gastroenterology and Nutrition
Journal of Pediatric Ophthalmology and Strabismus
Journal of Pediatric Surgery
Journal of Pediatrics
Journal of Thoracic and Cardiovascular Surgery
Journal of Urology
Lancet
Laryngoscope
Medicine
Medicine and Science in Sports and Exercise
Neurology
Neuropediatrics
New England Journal of Medicine
Obstetrics and Gynecology
Ophthalmologica
Ophthalmology
Oral Surgery, Oral Medicine, Oral Pathology
Pediatric Infectious Disease
Pediatrics
Physician and Sports Medicine
Psychoneuroendocrinology
Public Health Reports
Science
Southern Medical Journal
Spine
Thorax
Transfusion
Western Journal of Medicine
Zeitschrift fur Kinderchirurgie

Publisher's Preface

Publication of the 1985 YEAR BOOKS marks the eighty-fifth anniversary of the original PRACTICAL MEDICINE YEAR BOOKS. To mark this milestone, the YEAR BOOKS are being issued with a more contemporary cover design, and the format for the contents has been modified to identify the article titles, authors' names, and journal citations more readily. The substance of the YEAR BOOK—the abstracts of scholarly articles with substantive editorial comments—is unchanged. What is new is the isolation of the reference information as a discrete block of copy. Other, less-visible changes will continue to be made as we strive to make the YEAR BOOKS the very best they can be.

The YEAR BOOK OF PEDIATRICS is a proud member of the original series of PRACTICAL MEDICINE YEAR BOOKS. From 1901 through 1923, pediatrics was combined with orthopedic surgery in one YEAR BOOK, but the YEAR BOOK OF PEDIATRICS has been a separate book since 1924. We are proud to hail the longevity of this outstanding member of the YEAR BOOK series.

1 The Newborn

Relationship of Cerebral Intraventricular Hemorrhage and Early Childhood Neurologic Handicaps
Lu-Ann Papile, Ginny Musick-Bruno, and Anne Schaefer (Univ. of New Mexico, Albuquerque)
J. Pediatr. 103:273–277, August 1983   1–1

To determine whether cerebral intraventricular hemorrhage (CVH) is associated with early developmental or neuromotor handicaps, a comparison was made of the outcome in 198 surviving infants with very low birth weight (VLBW) (less than 1,501 gm) with and without CVH, as determined by computed tomography scans.

Developmental assessment was normal in 61 of the infants without CVH, suspect in 43, and abnormal in 11. Neuromotor and developmental testing of these 116 infants showed that 57 were normal, 46 had a minor handicap, and 12 had a major handicap. Seven of the 12 were multihandicapped (Table 1).

Among 33 of 39 infants with a grade 1 CVH who were alive at age 1 year, 16 were not handicapped, 14 had a minor handicap, and 3 had a major handicap. Two of the last 3 were multihandicapped. Nine of 18 infants with a grade 2 CVH had no handicap, 7 had a minor handicap, and 2 had a major handicap. No child in this group was multihandicapped. Evaluation of 14 infants with a grade 3 CVH showed that 2 were normal, 7 had a minor handicap, 5 had a major handicap, and 4 were multihandicapped. Of the 17 infants with a grade 4 CVH, 2 had no handicap, 2 had a minor handicap, 13 had a major handicap, and 10 were multihandicapped.

TABLE 1.—NEURODEVELOPMENTAL OUTCOME OF INFANTS
WITH VLBW RELATED TO CVH GRADE

	None	Grade 1	Grade 2	Grade 3	Grade 4
Infants (n)	147	48	23	20	22
Alive at 1 year	138	39	21	16	18
Evaluated	116*	33	18	14	17
Birth weight (kg)	1.18	1.07	1.12	1.14	1.06
Gestational age (wk)	30.2	29.2	29.4	28.9	29.1
Outcome					
Normal	57	16	9	2	2
Minor handicap	46	14	7	7	2
Major handicap	12	3	2	5	13
Multiple handicaps	7	2	0	4	10

*One infant untestable.
(Courtesy of Papile, L.-A., et al.: J. Pediatr. 103:273–277, August 1983.)

TABLE 2.—Neurodevelopmental Outcome of Infants With Grades 3 and 4
CVH Related to Development of Posthemorrhagic Hydrocephalus

Clinical status	Number of patients	Grade 3 CVH		Grade 4 CVH	
		Hydrocephalus	No hydrocephalus	Hydrocephalus	No hydrocephalus
Alive at 1 year	34	8	8	10	8
Evaluated	31	8	6	9	8
Normal	4	1	1	0	2
Minor handicap	9	4	3	2	0
Major handicap	18	3	2	7	6
Multiple handicaps	14	3	1	7	3

(Courtesy of Papile, L.-A., et al.: J. Pediatr. 103:273–277, August 1983.)

Posthemorrhagic hydrocephalus developed in 22 infants with CVH (Table 2). All had a grade 3 or grade 4 CVH. Ten of these 22 infants had a major handicap and 10 were multihandicapped. The incidence of major handicaps in these infants was similar to that in comparable infants without posthemorrhagic hydrocephalus.

Infants with VLBW who have grades 1 and 2 CVH do not have a higher incidence of major handicaps in early childhood than comparable infants without CVH. However, there is a direct relationship between grades 3 and 4 CVH and major handicaps. Posthemorrhagic hydrocephalus does not increase the risk for major handicaps, but does influence the incidence of multihandicaps.

▶ It has become traditional to solicit a comment from Dr. Joseph Volpe on the subject of cerebral hemorrhage in the low birth weight infant. Doctor Volpe, Professor of Developmental Neurology, Pediatrics, Neurology, and Biological Chemistry, Washington University School of Medicine, always provides an incisive analysis. I couldn't think of a better way to start this book than with the following remarks from Doctor Volpe:

"This report by Papile et al. is addressed to the neurologic outcome of premature infants with intraventricular hemorrhage (IVH). The authors conclude that infants with the smallest hemorrhages do not exhibit an increased incidence of subsequent neurologic deficits, whereas those with the largest hemorrhages do. However, a simple relationship between the quantity of intraventricular blood and neurologic outcome is not apparent. This large series confirms data obtained from previously reported smaller series. The lack of a linear relationship between the severity of intraventricular bleeding and the neurologic outcome has provoked debate and confusion in the medical literature, but we believe that there is no need for either. The critical determinant of neurologic outcome with IVH is the severity of the associated *cerebral* abnormality, and the relationship between this critical parenchymal involvement and the amount of intraventricular blood is by no means clear. Our task in predicting and understanding outcome in these infants is assessment of the severity of the *cerebral* involvement. In the following discussion, let us consider the major determinants of the cerebral injury in infants with IVH, the current means of assessing this injury, and our understanding of the cause(s) of the parenchymal injury.

"First, regarding the major determinants of the cerebral injury in infants with IVH, we can identify six major factors: (1) preceding or concurrent hypoxic-ischemic insult(s), (2) increased intracranial pressure with decreased cerebral perfusion, (3) destruction of periventricular white matter by intraparenchymal blood, (4) destruction of glial precursors in the germinal matrix, (5) focal cerebral ischemia secondary to vasospasm, and (6) posthemorrhagic hydrocephalus. Concerning these factors, preceding or concurrent hypoxic-ischemic insults are not uncommon in infants with major IVH. Such insults are especially likely to cause periventricular leukomalacia, i.e., injury to periventricular white matter. Infants with severe IVH may exhibit increased intracranial pressure and, because cerebral perfusion is related to arterial blood pressure minus intracranial pressure and because arterial blood pressure may fall in infants with major IVH, impairment of cerebral perfusion may occur and cause ischemic injury to brain. Destruction of periventricular white matter by intraparenchymal blood previously has been considered the cause of the brain injury observed in infants with so-called grade IV IVH, i.e., IVH with intraparenchymal "extension." We now believe that simple intraparenchymal extension of blood from the lateral ventricle or germinal matrix into previously normal white matter is uncommon and that prior or concurrent injury to white matter is necessary to cause the intraparenchymal bleeding (see below). Destruction of the germinal matrix, of course, is a uniform feature of IVH, which emanates from this structure, the source of the glial cells that subsequently will migrate to cerebral white matter and lead to myelination. Does destruction of these glial precursors impair subsequent brain development? We can't answer this question yet, but the possibility is real. Focal cerebral ischemia, secondary to vasospasm, analogous to the vasospasm observed in older patients with subarachnoid hemorrhage, is a theoretical possibility. This possibility is supported by one study of cerebral blood velocity (Bada et al.: *J. Pediatr.* 95:775, 1979). The frequency and importance of this complication remain unclear. Finally, posthemorrhagic hydrocephalus certainly can complicate severe IVH, as shown in the article by Papile et al. Although the precise relationship between posthemorrhagic hydrocephalus and neurologic outcome is unknown, rapidly progressive hydrocephalus that is not promptly treated clearly can contribute to the brain injury in these infants.

"Second, regarding the current means of assessing the critical cerebral injury in the newborn with IVH, real-time cranial ultrasonography has been useful. The largest study of infants with IVH reported to date (McMenamin et al.: *Ann. Neurol.* 15:285, 1984) described the outcome as a function of cerebral involvement, identified on cranial ultrasonography as periventricular echodense lesions. Thus, of 177 infants with IVH, 64 had periventricular echodense lesions, and of the latter, 33 had large, unilateral, globular lesions (large IPE) and 31 had small, bilateral, linear lesions (small IPE). The outcome differed markedly in these two groups. Of the 33 infants with IVH and large IPE (grade IV IVH in most classifications), 76% died in the neonatal period and *all* of the survivors had subsequent moderate or severe neurologic deficits. Of the 31 infants with small IPE, 29% died and only 14% had subsequent moderate neurologic deficits (none had severe neurologic deficits). The periventricular echodensities were considered to represent white matter injury, perhaps hypoxic-ischemic in basic nature and perhaps in part reversible in the infants with small IPE. Clearly, this study showed that the most critical determinant of severe parenchymal involvement and poor neurologic outcome in the infant with IVH is the presence of large IPE.

"The nature of the large intraparenchymal lesion observed on cranial ultrasonography was defined recently in a study of regional cerebral blood flow by positron emission tomography (PET) in 6 infants with this critical lesion (for reference). Thus, it was possible to adapt to the newborn the remarkably powerful technique of PET to measure regional cerebral blood flow. The essential finding was an impairment of cerebral blood flow in infants with large IPE that was much more extensive than could be accounted for by the locus of the intraparenchymal blood. The marked decrease in cerebral blood flow involved all of the cerebral white matter, although the IPE on cranial ultrasonography appeared to involve only anterior cerebral white matter. The decrease in cerebral blood flow indicated that the cerebral white matter had sustained extensive injury. Neuropathologic observations corroborated this conclusion. The topography of the cerebral involvement defined in the 6 patients by PET suggested that the intracerebral injury is ischemic in basic nature, because the lesion resided especially in those periventricular regions known to be vulnerable in the premature infant to impairment of cerebral perfusion. When and how this ischemic lesion occurs remain to be defined. It is most probable that the cerebral lesion occurs prior to the IVH and that the secondary hemorrhage into the anterior portion of the cerebral lesion occurs at the time of or shortly after the IVH. (It is of interest in this regard that 4 of the 6 infants studied by PET had sustained prior perinatal asphyxia.) The essential point is that the critical intracerebral lesion in infants with IVH and large IPE, the subset of infants that accounts for the large majority of neurologic morbidity observed with IVH, in general, is an extensive infarction, the anterior portion of which is hemorrhagic. What remains for us to accomplish is definition of the cause of this infarction, so that we can proceed to the most important goal, i.e., prevention."

Intracranial Hemorrhage in the Term Newborn
Gerald M. Fenichel, David L. Webster, and Walter K. T. Wong (Vanderbilt Univ.)
Arch. Neurol. 41:30–34, January 1984   1–2

The findings in 22 term newborn infants seen in a 5-year period with intracranial hemorrhage on computed tomography (CT) examination were reviewed. Ultrasonography also was used in the later cases. The study was partly prospective. Where both intraventricular hemorrhage (IVH) and subarachnoid hemorrhage (SAH) were present, it was assumed that the IVH was primary and was followed by extravasation of blood into the subarachnoid space.

Primary SAH was the most common form of hemorrhage in this series

(Table 1). Eight of the 10 infants had diffuse SAH, mainly supratentorial, and 2 had focal bleeding over an area of hemispheric infarction. Half the infants in this group were products of prolonged labors and traumatic deliveries and had suffered intrauterine asphyxia. Three other infants had severe intrauterine asphyxia with syndromes of hypoxic-ischemic encephalopathy immediately after birth. Eight infants had IVH (Table 2). Several of them would have been diagnosed as having primary SAH had CT not been carried out. Five of the infants had had very difficult deliveries. Four infants (Table 3) had intracerebral hemorrhage. Three of them were products of normal pregnancies, labors and deliveries and appeared normal at birth. The infant with cerebellar hemorrhage was apneic and hypotonic shortly after birth by vacuum extraction.

Primary SAH may be either diffuse or focal in nature. All infants in the present study with diffuse SAH had seizures on the first day of life. Most infants with IVH were products of difficult deliveries and had experienced some degree of intrauterine asphyxia. Infants with intracerebral hemor-

TABLE 1.—SUBARACHNOID HEMORRHAGE*

Patient/ Gestational Age, wk/Sex	Birth Weight, kg	CT Scan Diagnosis	Pregnancy, Labor, and Delivery	Apgar Score, 1-5-10 min	Postnatal Course	CSF	EEG	Outcome
1/41/M	3.3	SAH	G1 P0; Difficult forceps delivery; umbilical cord around neck ×3	5-8-...	Bruising and molding of head; left focal seizures and apneic spells 8 hr post partum	Normal	Background attenuation, multifocal discharges	Mental retardation, cortical blindness
2/41/M	3.4	SAH	G2 P0; abruptio placenta; difficult forceps delivery	4-8-...	Resuscitation for 4 min; bruising and molding of head; L facial palsy; seemed well until age 2 days, then eye rolling and opisthotonos	Bloody	Lack of variability	Normal at 3 yr
3/40/M	3.8	SAH	G3 P1; difficult forceps delivery	6-8-...	Multiple skull fractures; L leg seizures at 24 hr; generalized seizures	...	Lack of variability	Normal at 8 mo
4/40/F	3.0	SAH	G1 P0; cephalopelvic disproportion; prolonged labor; decelerations; meconium staining; umbilical cord around neck ×4; intrauterine hyperextension of neck; cesarean section	5-7-...	Lip smacking and arching of back at 12 hr; focal seizures of L arm	Normal	...	Normal at 6 mo
5/41/F	3.2	SAH	G4 P3; breech with difficult delivery of head	4-6-...	Resuscitation required; tense fontanelle at birth; multifocal seizures at 6 hr	Bloody	L central spikes	Mild motor delay at 1 yr
6/42/M	3.7	SAH	G1 P0; sustained fetal bradycardia; meconium stained; vertex forceps	...	Encephalopathic from birth; apneic and multifocal seizures at 12 hr	Normal	Burst-suppression multifocal discharges	Mental retardation; cerebral palsy; epilepsy
7/44/M	3.5	SAH	G1 P0; sustained fetal bradycardia; meconium stained; vertex forceps	0-3-5	Encephalopathic from birth; apneic and multifocal seizures at 6 hr	Normal	...	Mental retardation; cerebral palsy
8/40/M	2.5	SAH	G1 P0; one of twins, the other stillborn; sustained fetal bradycardia; meconium stained; cesarean section	1-2-6	Encephalopathic from birth; apneic and tonic seizures at 12 hr	...	Suppression multifocal discharges	Died
9/41/M	3.2	SAH; L parietal infarct	G1 P0; Difficult forceps rotation; sustained fetal bradycardia	4-4-9	Appeared well until day 7, then multifocal seizures	Normal	Normal background; multifocal sharp waves	Mild weakness of R hand at 1 yr
10/40/F	3.4	SAH; R parietal infarct	G3 P2; Uncomplicated vaginal vertex delivery	7-9-...	Appeared well until day 2, then L focal seizures	...	Lack of variability	Normal at 3 yr

*CT indicates computed tomography; SAH, subarachnoid hemorrhage; G, gravida; and P, para.
(Courtesy of Fenichel, G.M., et al.: Arch. Neurol. 41:30–34, January 1984; copyright 1984, American Medical Association.)

TABLE 2.—INTRAVENTRICULAR HEMORRHAGE*

Patient/ Gestational Age, wk/Sex	Birth Weight, kg	CT Scan Diagnosis	Pregnancy, Labor, and Delivery	Apgar Score, 1-5-10 min	Postnatal Course	CSF	EEG	Outcome
11/40/M	3.0	IVH, 4th ventricle; SAH	G4 P3; breech with difficult delivery of head	1-3-5	Bruising of feet and buttocks; resuscitation required; appeared to improve for 24 hr, then seizures developed	Bloody	...	Normal at 5 mo
12/40/M	3.3	IVH, fourth ventricle	G2 P0; breech with difficult delivery of head	3-6-...	Resuscitation required; tense fontanelle at birth; multifocal seizures at 6 hr	Bloody	...	Mental retardation
13/38/M	3.0	IVH, grade 3	G2 P1; unexpected 2nd twin; transverse lie; difficult forceps rotation; breech extraction	X-5-...	Resuscitation required; floppy at birth; opisthotonos at 8 hr	Bloody	Background attenuation	Normal at 1 yr
14/40/F	3.1	IVH, grade 3; SAH	G2 P0; difficult forceps delivery	9-......	Bruising and molding of head; L facial palsy; appeared well until day 2, then multifocal seizures	...	...	Mental retardation; cerebral palsy
15/42/M	3.1	IVH, L lateral horn	G1 P0; cephalopelvic disproportion	5-7-...	Marked bruising and molding of head; cephalohematoma; appeared well until day 2, then multifocal seizures	Bloody	Normal	...
16/40/F	3.4	IVH, grade 3; SAH	G1 P0; maternal urinary tract infection; vaginal vertex	7-9-...	Apnea, cyanosis, and multifocal seizures at 2 hr	Bloody	Burst-suppression multifocal discharge	Normal at 10 mo
17/39/M	3.5	IVH, grade 3; L lateral and 3rd ventricle	G4 P3; vaginal vertex	9-9-...	Apnea and cyanosis shortly after birth	Bloody	...	Progressive hydrocephalus
18/40/M	3.0	IVH, grade 4	G1 P0; elective low forceps	8-9-...	Appeared well at birth; seizures at 8 hr	Bloody	Frequent spike discharges on L temporal lobe	Progressive hydrocephalus

*CT indicates computed tomography; IVH, intraventricular hemorrhage; G, gravida; and P, para.
(Courtesy of Fenichel, G.M., et al.: Arch. Neurol. 41:30–34, January 1984; copyright 1984, American Medical Association.)

rhage are nearly always products of difficult labors and deliveries. No subdural hematomas were detected during a 4-year period of CT surveillance.

▶ Another pleasant tradition is a commentary by James Schwartz, Professor of Neurology at Emory University School of Medicine. Doctor Schwartz writes:
"In recent years, numerous studies have provided a wealth of information about the incidence, pathophysiologic basis, clinical presentation, natural history and outcome of periventricular and intraventricular hemorrhage (IVH) in the preterm infant, but little attention has been directed to the various types of intracranial hemorrhage in the term infant. Fenichel et al. present their findings in 22 term newborns with subarachnoid hemorrhage (SAH), IVH, and intracerebral hemorrhage (ICH) diagnosed by CT or cranial ultrasound (US) during a 5-year time period. The frequency of occurrence of these hemorrhages is unclear from this report, because this was not a prospective serial study; no denominator figures are available for computing incidence or assessing risk factors. This would be important information because we need to know which term infants are "at risk," i.e., which infants should have US or CT. Fenichel et al.

TABLE 3.—Intracerebral Hemorrhage*

Patient/ Gestational Age, wk/Sex	Birth Weight, kg	CT Scan Diagnosis	Pregnancy, Labor, and Delivery	Apgar Score, 1-5-10 min	Postnatal Course	CSF	EEG	Outcome
19/42/M	3.0	ICH, R parietal and post-temporal	G2 P1; maternal hypertension and urinary tract infection; vaginal vertex	6-9- . . .	Appeared well for 24 hr, then apnea and multifocal seizures	Bloody	L temporal discharge; multifocal sharp waves	Mental retardation; cerebral palsy
20/40/M	4.0	ICH, L parietal and occipital	G2 P1; maternal urinary tract infection; vaginal vertex	8-9- . . .	Appeared well until day 7, then focal seizures of face	Normal	Spike focus L parietooccipital	Mental retardation; cerebral palsy
21/38/M	3.5	ICH, R putamen and internal capsule	G1 P0; vaginal vertex	9-10- . . .	Appeared well until day 2, then tonic seizures	Bloody	Amplitude attenuation of R	L hemiplegia at 1 yr
22/42/M	3.2	ICH, cerebellar	G3 P0 A3; minimum variability on fetal monitor, delivered by vacuum extraction	3-4- . . .	Apneic spells and hypotonia shortly after birth	Bloody	Burst suppression	Died at 3 wk

*CT indicates compound tomography; ICH, intracerebral hemorrhage; G, gravida; P, para; and A, abortus.
(Courtesy of Fenichel, G.M., et al.: Arch. Neurol. 41:30–34, January 1984; copyright 1984, American Medical Association.)

performed these tests on the basis of four criteria: prolonged labor (not clear is how long is "prolonged"), traumatic delivery, perinatal asphyxia, and neonatal seizures. These appear to be reasonable criteria, but it would be of interest to know how many term infants with similar perinatal histories had no evidence of SAH, IVH, or ICH.

"Birth trauma as a cause of neonatal intracranial bleeding is thought to be a rare problem today. It is disheartening to learn that traumatic deliveries with intracranial hemorrhages still occur, although it may be impossible to distinguish the separate effects of trauma and asphyxia. Of the 22 infants in this report, which comes from a tertiary center, 19 were born in other hospitals, implying, not surprisingly, that infants born in outlying hospitals with lower-level neonatal units are at greater risk of having more problems, or lesser degrees of good obstetric care, than those infants born in secondary or tertiary centers. Again, denominator figures would be of interest.

"Computed tomography and US studies by Pape, Fitzhardinge, and Harwood-Nash on hypoxic-ischemic encephalopathy have directed attention to focal or multifocal areas of hypodensity with or without areas of cerebral infarction as important findings in the asphyxiated full-term infant. The present paper provides evidence of focal or diffuse areas of SAH as additional lesions after asphyxia. Trauma was the main cause of IVH in 5 of 8 infants with IVH, with asphyxia as a contributory cause. However, 3 full-term infants with IVH had neither trauma nor asphyxia, leaving the problem of full-term IVH as one requiring much further study. Finally, there are 3 infants with ICH that was totally unexplained as to cause.

"This study reiterates the point that perinatal asphyxia is the neurologic insult of paramount importance in the full-term infant and that the consequences of this insult may include intracranial hemorrhage, although, importantly, even the presence of such a hemorrhage does not preclude a good outcome. Finally, the authors point out the observation that seizures in the first week of life are an important sign of cerebral injury, which may be associated with a variety of types of intracranial bleeding, as well as with hypoxic-ischemic injury, and that neonatal seizures are a strong indication for diagnostic US, although not to be overlooked is the importance of diagnostic lumbar puncture and other well-established laboratory tests."

Myelomeningocele Newborn Management: Time for Parental Decision
E. B. Charney, L. N. Sutton, D. A. Bruce, and L. B. Schut (Univ. of Pennsylvania)
Z. Kinderchir. 38(Suppl. 2):90–93, 1983   1–3

Both patient selecting and timing have been problems in the management of neonates with myelomeningocele. One hundred ten consecutive newborn infants referred with myelomeningocele in the past 5 years. High lumbar or thoracic paralysis was present in 45% of cases, midlumbar paralysis in 18%, and low lumbar or sacral paralysis in 37%. Twenty infants had congenital hydrocephalus. Eight had congenital kyphoscoliosis, and 5 had other gross congenital defects. Closure was done in the first 2 days of life in 47% of cases, whereas 29% of patients had "delayed" closure within 3–7 days, and 11% had "late" surgery after the first week of life. The time of surgery is related to the clinical picture in Figure 1–1. Fourteen patients never had surgery.

Survival is related to the time of surgery in Figure 1–2. Over 90% of the patients having early or delayed surgery and all those having late surgery were alive at 10 months. No patient survived past this age without surgery. Deterioration of motor function could not be related to the timing

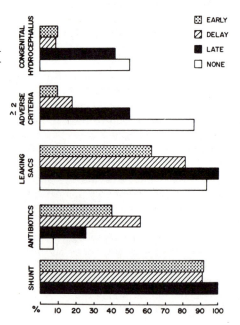

Fig 1–1.—Time of surgery and other variables. (Courtesy of Charney, E.B., et al.: Z. Kinderchir. 38(Suppl. 2):90–93, 1983.)

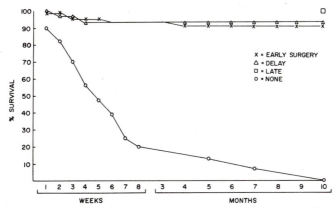

Fig 1–2.—Time of surgery and survival. (Courtesy of Charney, E.B., et al.: Z. Kinderchir. 38(Suppl. 2):90–93, 1983.)

of surgery. Ventriculitis developed in 10% of patients who were operated on; it could not be related to the time of operation. Developmental delay was observed in 36% of 74 children evaluated at age 1 year or later. Severe delay was present in 3 cases. Developmental delay also could not be related to the timing of surgery.

There would appear to be no urgency in operating on newborn infants with myelomeningocele. Time can be taken to thoroughly discuss the situation with the parents and obtain adequate informed consent for surgery. A 1-week interval seems reasonable, during which time broad-spectrum antibiotic therapy can be given to reduce the risk of infection. Mortality is increased beyond 1 week, and parents must recognize that there is not an indefinite time for delaying surgery.

▶ The authors have provided us with a valuable lesson by sharing their experience. With all of the "Baby Doe hysteria" that stalks our nurseries, this kind of level-headed and unhurried approach is most welcome. The authors' own words, in their closing paragraph, say it best. They write, "Some may argue that an additional 6 or 7 days cannot alleviate the shock or grief experienced by parents of a defective newborn. Others point out that all newborns have the right to live and that there really is no need for a time for decision since surgical intervention is the only avenue of action, irrespective of parental wishes. Respectful of both points of view, we nevertheless propose that there is a 'better' time for parents to be actively involved in a decision process that will affect their child, themselves, and their entire family for many years to come. Such a decision process is best handled in an atmosphere wherein feelings of emergency or urgency are minimized and time for parental discussion is maximized. Recognition and appreciation of the need for this process can help health professionals counsel parents in a more understanding and informative manner. Through such counseling, a relationship of trust and confidence may be established."—F.A.O.

Temperature Measurement in Term and Preterm Neonates

Steven R. Mayfield, Jatinder Bhatia, Kenneth T. Nakamura, Gladys R. Rios, and Edward F. Bell (Univ. of Iowa)
J. Pediatr. 104:271–275, February 1984   1–4

Different methods of temperature measurement were compared in 99 term and 44 preterm neonates aged 1 month and younger. Core temperature was measured 5 cm beyond the anus with an electronic telethermometer and rectal temperature was measured at 2 cm with a mercury-in-glass thermometer. Axillary and skin-mattress temperatures also were recorded. This study was done because various differences in axillary and rectal temperatures have been reported in newborn infants, and measurement techniques have not been standardized.

Temperatures measured at the four sites agreed closely in this group of largely normothermic infants (Table 1). Stabilization times at all sites were 3–5 minutes in term infants and 4–4½ minutes in preterm infants (Table 2). Five of the 7 term infants with core temperatures more than 1.5 SD below or above the mean would have been considered to be normothermic by all the other measurement methods. The preterm infants had lower temperatures that varied less with the site of measurement, indicating a smaller core-surface temperature gradient due to a relative lack of thermal insulation by body fat. Axillary temperature readings were as reliable as rectal measurements, and skin-mattress temperatures were nearly as accurate as the others. All but 10% of measurements were within 0.1 C of the final reading within 5 minutes for all measurement sites and both types of thermometer.

Axillary temperature appears to be as useful as rectal temperature when measured in the usual way with a mercury thermometer, and skin-mattress temperatures are nearly as accurate as the other methods. A reasonable goal in caring for neonates is to keep the body temperature within 1 SD of the mean. This would imply that the axillary temperatures be kept at 36.7–37.2 C in term infants and at 36.4–37.1 C in preterm infants. Mercury-in-glass thermometers should be kept in place for 5 minutes at any site before being read.

▶ Axillary temperature was measured by placing the thermometer in the axilla with the bulb at the apex and halfway between the anterior and posterior mar-

TABLE 1.—STABILIZATION TEMPERATURES IN DEGREES CENTIGRADE

Measurement site	Term			Preterm			
	Mean	SD	Range	Mean	SD	Range	P*
Core (deep rectum)	37.04	0.33	36.3 to 38.1	36.76	0.35	35.4 to 37.4	<0.001
Rectum	36.96	0.33	36.1 to 37.7	36.66	0.38	35.5 to 37.7	<0.001
Axilla	36.94	0.28	36.1 to 37.6	36.76	0.36	35.4 to 37.4	<0.005
Skin-mattress	36.82	0.33	35.9 to 37.8	36.76	0.38	35.5 to 37.7	>0.200

*Level of statistical significance by two-tailed t test.
(Courtesy of Mayfield, S.R., et al.: J. Pediatr. 104:271–275, February 1984.)

TABLE 2.—STABILIZATION TIMES IN MINUTES

	Term			Preterm		
Measurement site	*Mean*	*SD*	*Range*	*Mean*	*SD*	*Range*
Core (deep rectum)	3.0	1.8	1 to 8	3.9	2.4	1 to 10
Rectum	4.1	2.2	1 to 10	4.4	2.1	1 to 10
Axilla	4.8	1.9	2 to 10	3.8	1.1	2 to 6
Skin-mattress	5.1	1.9	2 to 10	4.2	1.5	1 to 8

(Courtesy of Mayfield, S.R., et al.: J. Pediatr. 104:271–275, February 1984.)

gins of the axilla, which is the warmest point in the axilla. The arm then was held at the infant's side so that the axilla was closed. Skin-mattress temperature was measured by placing the thermometer underneath the infant between the skin and the surface of the mattress, between the levels of the fourth and tenth thoracic vertebrae.

Perhaps the best site to measure temperature is in the ear. The aural, *not oral,* temperature correlates well with the rectal temperature (see 1979 YEAR BOOK, pp. 72–73; and Mayfield and this same group of authors in *Early Hum. Dev.* 9:241, 1984). The aural temperature may prove to be a measure of cerebral metabolism.

Please note that I refrained from making the comment, "When you're hot, you're hot, and when you're not, you're not." That would have been a cheap shot.—F.A.O.

Direct Hyperbilirubinemia Complicating ABO Hemolytic Disease of the Newborn

Yakon Sivan, Paul Merlob, Jacob Nutman, and Salomon H. Reisner
Clin. Pediatr. (Phila.) 22:537–538, August 1983   1–5

Hemolytic disease of the newborn (HDN) may be complicated by elevated levels of direct-reacting bilirubin. This complication was reported in up to 8% of infants with HDN caused by Rh incompatibility. A few reports suggest the possibility of direct hyperbilirubinemia resulting from HDN caused by ABO incompatibility, but the incidence of this complication is unknown. The authors retrospectively assessed the incidence and diagnostic implications of conjugated hyperbilirubinemia complicating ABO hemolytic disease of the newborn in a review of the records of 27,623 liveborn infants observed between April 1, 1973, and March 31, 1981 at the Beilinson Medical Center in Petah Tigva, Israel.

Hemolytic disease of the newborn attributable to ABO incompatibility was diagnosed in 264 infants, 8 of whom also had elevated levels of conjugated bilirubin. All 8 infants, 7 of whom were female, were born at term of uncomplicated pregnancies. Four of the infants were first deliveries and 4 represented two pairs of siblings. Four had O/A incompatibility and 4 had O/B incompatibility. Hemoglobin concentrations ranged from 14.3

gm/dl to 16.9 gm/dl during the first 24 hours. In all infants, jaundice developed during the first 24 hours of life, and direct bilirubin was usually evident within 24–48 hours. The mean maximal total bilirubin concentration was 17 mg/dl, with direct-reacting bilirubin accounting for a mean of 34% of the total. Exchange transfusion was performed in 3 infants. The duration of conjugated hyperbilirubinemia was short, lasting for more than 2 weeks in only 2 infants.

The findings suggest that conjugated hyperbilirubinemia is a benign complication of ABO-HDN that resolves within a month.

▶ We haven't heard much about the "inspissated bile syndrome" in the past decade. A consensus has never been achieved with respect to its etiology. Hepatic necrosis, giant cell transformation, and extramedullary hematopoiesis obstructing intrahepatic canaliculi have all been proposed as mechanisms for the increase in conjugated bilirubin seen in about 3% of infants with hemolytic disease. Sacrez and associates first described this finding in ABO disease in 1962 (*Ann. Pediatr.* 38:317, 1962) and described 7 infants in whom conjugated hyperbilirubinemia first was detected between the second and fifth day of life, the conjugated fraction ranged from 15% to 35% of the total bilirubin concentration, and the total bilirubin concentration reached 8 to 24 mg/dl.

The take-home lesson is an old one. At least one bilirubin determination should involve the measurement of both conjugated and unconjugated fractions.—F.A.O.

Relationship of Breast-Feeding and Weight Loss to Jaundice in the Newborn Period: Review of the Literature and Results of a Study
Diane A. Butler and Julia P. MacMillan (Cleveland Clinic)
Cleve. Clin. Q. 50:263–268, Fall 1983   1–6

The relation of breast-feeding to neonatal jaundice is of increasing importance as more women nurse their infants. The authors examined this relationship in a series of 588 consecutive infants born at a community hospital, excluding any infant with a potential risk for jaundice. The characteristics of the infants remaining in the study are given in Table 1 and the causes of elimination from the study are given in Table 2. The breast-fed and formula-fed groups were similar in sex distribution and cesarean delivery rates, but more formula-fed infants were delivered by repeat cesarean section, and more breast-fed infants were delivered by primary cesarean section. The mean birth weight was slightly greater for the formula-fed group.

Serum bilirubin levels above 10 mg/dl were significantly more frequent in the breast-fed group. The use of phototherapy was comparable in both groups, but 5 other breast-fed infants who required phototherapy were eliminated from the study because of formula supplementation. The two groups are compared in Table 3. The breast-fed infants had greater weight losses than the formula-fed group. Differences in serum bilirubin were less significant when adjusted for weight loss, suggesting that weight loss may

TABLE 1.—Characteristics of Total Infant
Population

	Present study	Comparative studies*
Mean birth weight (g)	3403	3457[1]
		3358[2]
Sex ratio (% males)	51.4	51.4[3]
		51.0[†]
Breast milk fed (%)	52.2	43.4[4]
		54.0[5]
		55.0[6]
		82.0[7]
Cesarean delivery (%)	24.1	15.8[†]
		15.2[†]
		16.2[†]

*Personal communication: Anderson F. Cleveland Metropolitan General Hospital Neonatal Statistical Report, 1979; 1980 and 1981 Annual Report of the Department of Gynecology; 1982 MacDonald House Statistics.

(Courtesy of Butler, D.A., and MacMillan, J.P.: Cleve. Clin. Q. 50:263–268, Fall 1983.)

contribute to the higher bilirubin levels seen in breast-fed infants in the first week of life.

The prolonged jaundice occasionally observed in breast-fed infants appears to result from consumption of an inhibitor of glucoronyl transferase in breast milk. A significant minority of breast-fed infants exhibit an ex-

TABLE 2.—Factors Resulting in Elimination
From Study Group

	Breast milk fed (Number)	Formula fed (Number)
Total number of infants eliminated	123	105
Reasons for elimination*		
Maternal risk factors[†]	7	7
Fetal distress	8	6
Apgar score < 7[‡]	4	5
Prematurity[§]	13	12
Birth weight ≥4000 g, ≤2500 g	41	39
Sickness[‖]	7	5
Positive Coombs' test[¶]	4	8
Formula-supplemented breast milk fed infants	36	0
Laboratory data incomplete	41	49

*Groups not mutually exclusive.
†Gestational diabetes, severe preeclampsia, placenta previa.
‡One- or 5-minute Apgar scores.
§<38 weeks' gestation by date of examination.
‖Respiratory distress syndrome, suspected sepsis, meconium aspiration, or any congenital condition requiring emergency transfer to a level III nursery.
¶Direct Coombs' test (performed routinely on all infants of Rh negative or type O mothers, or when indicated).
(Courtesy of Butler, D.A., and MacMillan, J.P.: Cleve. Clin. Q. 50:263–268, Fall 1983.)

TABLE 3.—COMPARISON OF STUDY GROUP INFANTS

	Breast milk fed	Formula fed
Number of infants (%)	183 (51.1%)	175 (48.9%)
Mean birth weight (g)	3406	3314
Sex ratio (% males)	46.4	52
Cesarean delivery (%)	21.9	17.7
Primary	11.5	4.6
Repeat	10.4	13.1
Number of infants with:		
Peak bilirubin >10 mg (%)*	73 (39.8)	28 (16)
Peak bilirubin >15 mg (%)*	8 (4.4)	0 (0)
Phototherapy (%)†	7 (3.8)	1 (0.6)

*Chi-square test $P < .01$.
†Fisher's exact test $P = .08$.
(Courtesy of Butler, D.A., and MacMillan, J.P.: Cleve. Clin. Q. 50:263–268, Fall 1983.)

aggerated physiologic jaundice in the first week of life. Many previous reports probably include cases of both forms of neonatal jaundice. Further studies are needed to determine whether the early and late forms of breast milk-related jaundice are qualitatively or only quantitatively different.

▶ The conclusion that the degree of weight loss bears a relationship to the degree of jaundice in the breast-fed infants is contrary to previously published reports (see 1974 YEAR BOOK, pp. 28–33), but is supported by the paper by Lucy Osborn and co-workers (*Pediatrics* 73:520, 1974).

What sense can we make out of all of this? There is a significant association between breast-feeding and the incidence of hyperbilirubinemia (bilirubin values in excess of 12 mg/dl in the term infant). This association may be observed as early as the third day of life, but is more pronounced by the fourth day (Maisels, M. J., et al.: *Am. J. Dis. Child.* 137:561, 1983; and Osborn, L. M., et al.: *Pediatrics* 73:520, 1974). The majority of infants in whom hyperbilirubinemia without apparent cause occurs are breast-fed. Look aggressively for a cause for hyperbilirubinemia in the non-breast-fed infant.

The earlier, and the more frequently, you allow an infant to be nursed by the mother, the less likely you are to encounter hyperbilirubinemia (De-Carvalho, M., et al.: *Am. J. Dis. Child.* 136:737, 1982). Until evidence to the contrary is provided, the presence of uncomplicated hyperbilirubinemia ("uncomplicated" means no associated hemolytic disease or other pathologic process) in the breast-fed infant should be viewed as harmless and the infant should not be subjected to frequent bilirubin determinations or phototherapy.

Is there a bilirubin value in the breast-fed term infant at which intervention should take place? Yes. Here is a useful rule: The bilirubin value, multiplied by the number of maternal breasts, should not exceed 28 mg/100 ml.—F.A.O.

Neonatal Polycythemia: I. Early Diagnosis and Incidence Relating to Time of Sampling

Mordechai Shohat, Paul Merlob, and Salomon H. Reisner (Sackler School of Medicine, Tel Aviv)
Pediatrics 73:7–10, January 1984   1–7

Neonatal polycythemia (NP), defined as a central venous hematocrit of 65% or greater, may be associated with life-threatening disorders and neurologic impairment, but the best time for screening of newborn infants remains unclear. The authors measured venous hematocrit and blood viscosity longitudinally in 50 healthy term infants of 38–42 weeks' gestational age in the first 18 hours of life, following early clamping of the umbilical cord. Antecubital venous blood samples were taken at ages 15 minutes, 2 and 6 hours, and 12–18 hours.

The mean hematocrit rose from 53% in cord blood to 60% at age 2 hours (Fig 1–3). A significant decrease was noted at age 6 hours, and a further reduction occurred at 12–18 hours when the mean value was 52%. Blood viscosity showed a similar trend at all shear rates. Neonatal polycythemia was present in 20% of infants at age 2 hours and in 12% by age 6 hours. Only 1 infant remained polycythemic at 12–18 hours. The only infant with a hematocrit above 70% at age 6 hours underwent partial exchange transfusion. A linear correlation was noted between the umbilical cord hematocrit and the peripheral venous hematocrit at 2 hours (Fig 1–4). The time of cord clamping did not correlate significantly with the hematocrit at age 2 hours (table).

Significant changes occur in both hematocrit and blood viscosity in the first hours of life. The cord blood hematocrit correlates well with the hematocrit at 2 hours and can be used to screen for NP in term infants with birth weight appropriate to gestational age.

▶ Here is a subject that drives reasonable people to become unreasonable.

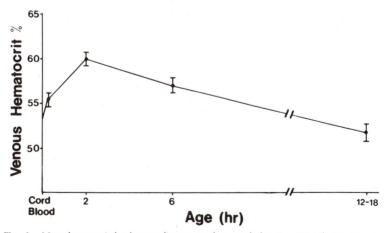

Fig –3.—Mean hematocrit levels according to age from cord clamping (50 infants). (Courtesy of Shohat, M., et al.: Pediatrics 73:7–10, January 1984. Copyright American Academy of Pediatrics 1984.)

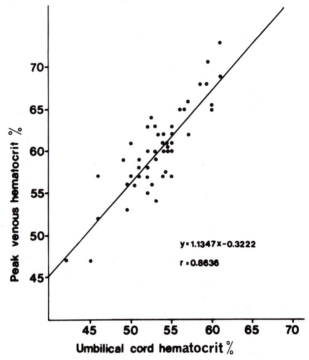

$y = 1.1347x - 0.3222$

$r = 0.8636$

Fig 1–4.—Correlation between umbilical cord hematocrit levels and venous levels at age 2 hours. (Courtesy of Shohat, M., et al.: Pediatrics 73:7–10, January 1984. Copyright American Academy of Pediatrics 1984.)

And who gets left holding the catheter? It is the practitioner who is being pressured to make therapeutic decisions.

Neonatal polycythemia (see 1984 YEAR BOOK, pp. 24–25) fits perfectly two of Murphy's laws. They are:

1. Just because your doctor has a name for your condition doesn't mean he knows what it is.

MEAN INCREASE IN HEMATOCRIT AT TWO
HOURS ACCORDING TO TIME OF CORD
CLAMPING

Time of Cord Clamping (s)	No. of Infants	Mean Increase in Hct at 2 h (%)
10	17	6.8 ± 3.2
11–20	20	6.7 ± 2.1
21–30	13	7.5 ± 2.3

(Courtesy of Shohat, M., et al.: Pediatrics 73:7–10, January 1984. Copyright American Academy of Pediatrics 1984.)

2. Before ordering a test, decide what you will do if it is (A) positive or (B) negative. If both answers are the same, don't do the test.

This study by Shohat and associates illustrates the importance of timing in the interpretation of a laboratory value. Is the infant born with polycythemia at greater risk than the infant who develops polycythemia as a consequence of a large placental, maternal-to-fetal, or twin-to-twin transfusion? It has long been known that the hemoglobin and hematocrit values rise in the hours after delivery and that the increase is proportional to the volume of placental transfusion that the infant received.

All prospective studies dealing with polycythemia must scrupulously standardize the timing of blood sampling and must distinguish between the many causes of polycythemia before judgments are made regarding long-term prognosis and the need for treatment.

Elizabeth Thilo and associates (*Pediatrics* 73:476, 1984) reported that the incidence of polycythemia was increased among infants who developed necrotizing enterocolitis during the first 24 hours of life. These same infants, however, had a higher incidence of umbilical catheters and exchange transfusions. The insertion of umbilical catheters is known to increase the risk of necrotizing enterocolitis (Thangavel, M., et al.: ibid. 69:799, 1982). This is another example of where the treatment may be worse than the disease.

For another view of the problem of neonatal polycythemia, please read the commentary by William Hathaway (ibid. 72:567, 1983).—F.A.O.

Collection and Preservation of Human Placental Blood

J. M. Brandes, E. F. Roth, Jr., P. D. Berk, E. Bottone, C. T. Milano, L. Sarkozi, and C. G. Zaroulis (Mt. Sinai School of Medicine)
Transfusion 23:325–327, July–Aug. 1983 1–8

The authors evaluated the possibility of using autologous blood from the placenta for high-risk premature infants who require red blood cell transfusions for anemia. Placental blood can be collected in a sterile manner in citrate-phosphate-dextrose (CPD) solution and stored at 4 C. Blood is collected very rapidly after either vaginal delivery or cesarean section. The red blood cell content of adenosine triphosphate remained normal over 8 days of blood storage. The 2,3-diphosphoglycerate level fell sharply, and the P50 of the oxyhemoglobin dissociation curve declined to 24 torr. An exchange of extracellular sodium and potassium occurred, but there was no change in glutathione content. Hemolysis remained less than 1%. Bacteriologic and fungal cultures of 33 consecutive blood samples were negative.

Placental blood stored in CPD solution is not oxidatively stressed, and it would appear to be a suitable red blood cell source for use in neonates. It remains to be determined whether sufficient blood for multiple transfusions can be collected from a placenta and whether the blood is sterile. Like homologous blood, placental blood should be transfused into infants with low birth weight within a week of its collection.

Free Erythrocyte Protoporphyrin as an Index of Perinatal Iron Status

S. K. F. Chong, M. J. Thompson, J. E. H. Shaw, and D. Barltrop (Westminster Med. School, London)
J. Pediatr. Gastroenterol. Nutr. 3:224–229, March 1984   1–9

Iron deficiency anemia is common in infants after the third month of life. It is related to the iron stores present at birth, but fetal iron stores have been difficult to assess in vivo. The authors examined the relation between free erythrocyte protoporphyrin (FEP) values and conventional indices of iron status in 49 mother-infant pairs. White women aged 22 to 25 years with parity greater than 1 participated in the study. Thirty-four matched maternal and umbilical cord blood specimens were obtained at delivery. All mothers received vitamins and iron supplements at 34 weeks' pregnancy, but only 22 were still taking iron at delivery. All infants were delivered normally at term. Fifteen were breast-fed throughout the study period. No infant was clinically anemic at age 6 weeks.

The findings are given in the table. Cord FEP values correlated negatively with maternal ferritin concentrations at 34 weeks' gestation and at delivery and with transferrin saturation at delivery. Infant hemoglobin concentrations at age 6 weeks correlated negatively with maternal FEP values at 34 weeks' pregnancy and at delivery. Cord FEP values did not correlate with birth weight or gestational age.

The cord FEP value is an index of maternal iron status in the last trimester of pregnancy, and the maternal FEP value in the last trimester predicts the degree of physiologic anemia present in the infant at age 6

MEANS ± SD OF FEP, HEMOGLOBIN, SERUM FERRITIN, SERUM IRON, AND TOTAL IRON-BINDING CAPACITY (TIBC) VALUES OF MATERNAL (6 WEEKS BEFORE DELIVERY AND AT DELIVERY), CORD, AND INFANTS' BLOOD

	Maternal (6 weeks predelivery)	Maternal (at delivery)	Cord	Baby (6 weeks old)
FEP (μg/100 ml/RBC)				
Mean ± SD	34.4 ± 9.3	35.1 ± 11.1	56.0 ± 13.8	34.8 ± 7.7
Range	22.1–73.9	21.1–60.2	27.7–88.3	22.2–50.8
Number	49	34	34	19
Haemoglobin (g/dl)				
Mean ± SD	11.8 ± 0.9	13.1 ± 1.9	15.8 ± 2.1	12.3 ± 1.2
Range	10.1–14.4	10.8–18.5	12.1–19.2	10.0–13.9
Number	49	32	30	21
Ferritin (ng/ml)				
Mean ± SD	10.9 ± 14.1	32.9 ± 67.7	94.4 ± 75.0	184.0 ± 95.0
Range	0.5–80.4	0.5–309.8	0.5–303.5	38.3–379.4
Number	40	25	28	16
Iron (μg/100 ml)				
Mean ± SD	108.6 ± 48.6	111.1 ± 59.3	229.3 ± 147.1	94 ± 34.8
Range	36.0–242.0	29–295	49–689	32–170
Number	37	18	20	13
TIBC (μg/100 ml)				
Mean ± SD	456.5 ± 64.1	430.7 ± 91.7	357.9 ± 146.2	227.8 ± 44.3
Range	364–681	225–567	201–724	135–312
Number	37	18	20	13

(Courtesy of Chong, S.K.F., et al.: J. Pediatr. Gastroenterol. Nutr. 3:224–229, March 1984.)

weeks. Perinatal measurement of FEP permits assessment of the iron stores of the fetus in utero. Poor correlation between cord FEP values and maternal iron concentrations may be due to wide serum iron fluctuations related to hormonal factors.

▶ The findings in this study challenge the conventional wisdom that holds that there is little or no relationship between the iron status of the pregnant woman and the hematologic status of her infant. In the 1980 YEAR BOOK (pp. 33–35), studies were cited from India and the Ivory Coast of Africa that demonstrated that when maternal iron deficiency anemia was severe, with hemoglobin levels less than 6 gm/dl, infants were born anemic. Mothers with hemoglobin values of less than 6.0 gm/dl gave birth to infants who had a mean cord blood hemoglobin of 12.7 gm/dl; when the maternal hemoglobin was between 6.1 and 8.5 gm/dl, the cord blood hemoglobin averaged 14.7 gm/dl, as contrasted with a mean hemoglobin of 18.7 gm/dl in those infants born to mothers whose hemoglobin was more than 11.0 gm/dl at the time of delivery (Singla, P. N., et al.: *Acta Paediatr. Scand.* 67:645, 1978).

Increased concentrations of erythrocyte protoporphyrin in cord blood samples may be produced by intense erythropoiesis or intrauterine lead exposure as well as by the lack of maternal iron stores. Of particular interest is the authors' observation that mothers with the highest free erythrocyte protoporphyrin concentrations at the time of delivery had infants with the lowest hemoglobin levels at 6 weeks of age. This bears repeating.—F.A.O.

The Effect of Lumbar Puncture Position in Sick Neonates
Leonard E. Weisman (Walter Reed Army Med. Center), Gerald B. Merenstein, and John R. Steenbarger (Fitzsimons Army Med. Center, Aurora, Colo.)
Am. J. Dis. Child. 137:1077–1079, November 1983   1–10

Clinical deterioration has been observed in sick neonates during lumbar puncture. The authors attempted to determine if hypoxemia occurred during lumbar puncture, if hypoxemia was position dependent, if transcutaneous Po_2 ($TcPo_2$) monitoring affected hypoxemia, and what mechanisms were involved. Twenty-six neonates received lumbar punctures in a standard lateral knees-to-chest position, sitting position, or modified lateral position without knees to chest. Care was taken not to extend or flex the neck.

Birth weight, gestational age, postnatal age, and need for ventilator support prior to lumbar puncture were not different in the three groups. Mean $TcPo_2$ in the standard lateral position was significantly lower than in the sitting or modified lateral positions during lumbar puncture. The time the $TcPo_2$ was under 50 mm Hg (Table 1) was significantly greater in the standard lateral position than in the sitting or modified lateral positions during the procedure. In the standard lateral position only, the time the $TcPo_2$ was less than 50 mm Hg decreased from 4.9 minutes without $TcPo_2$ monitoring to 0.6 minutes with $TcPo_2$ monitoring during the lumbar puncture period only. Significant preductal and postductal

TABLE 1.—Transcutaneous Po₂ Data for Different Lumbar
Puncture Positions*

Variable and Time	Position		
	Standard Lateral	Sitting	Modified Lateral
TcPo₂, mm Hg			
Baseline	68.8 (9.1)†	70.2 (7)	69.3 (8.6)
Transition	71.7 (11.7)	73.7 (9)	74.0 (9.4)
Lumbar puncture	60.5 (16.3)	70.2 (12)‡	76.0 (12.2)§
Baseline	74.3 (10.0)	73.6 (11)	76.0 (9.3)
Time TcPo₂<50 mm Hg, min			
Baseline	0.4 (0.9)‖	1.5 (4.7)	0.6 (1.3)
Transition	0.2 (0.3)	0.3 (0.3)	0.1 (0.2)
Lumbar puncture	3.0 (1.5)	1.5 (1.2)¶	0.7 (0.5)‖
Baseline	0.2 (0.4)	0.2 (0.6)	0.1 (0.3)
Time TcPo₂ >80 mm Hg, min			
Baseline	2.7 (4.7)	3.3 (4.7)	1.5 (1.1)
Transition	1.7 (2.4)	1.5 (2.0)	1.3 (1.6)
Lumbar puncture	1.3 (2.7)	1.3 (2.4)	2.3 (3.1)
Baseline	2.3 (3.8)	2.3 (3.0)	3.0 (5.0)
Total time, min			
Baseline	10.9 (5.6)	10.2 (3.4)	10.8 (4.4)
Transition	0.5 (0.3)	0.6 (0.5)	0.3 (0.3)
Lumbar puncture	10.8 (9.4)	8.8 (6.2)	9.8 (6.4)
Baseline	10.8 (4.7)	9.6 (3.8)	11.5 (3.5)

*TcPo₂ indicates transcutaneous Po₂. Values are expressed as mean (SD).
†$P < .03.$
‡$P < .02.$
§$P < .01.$
‖$P < .001.$
¶$P < .05.$
(Courtesy of Weisman, L.E., et al.: Am. J. Dis. Child. 137:1077–1079, November, 1983;
copyright 1983, American Medical Association.)

TcPo₂ differences (Table 2) were not observed between positions or between baseline and lumbar puncture periods for each position. Mean intraesophageal pressure (IEP) during lumbar puncture was significantly higher for the standard lateral position than for the sitting or modified lateral position. During lumbar puncture, mean IEP was significantly greater than the baseline for the standard lateral position only.

The authors conclude that hypoxemia occurs during lumbar puncture in the sick neonate. However, right-to-left shunting through the ductus arteriosus, as indicated by preductal and postductal TcPo₂ measurement differences, could not be demonstrated as a mechanism of hypoxemia during lumbar puncture in the standard lateral knees-to-chest position. Patients who had lumbar punctures in this position appeared to have an association of increased IEP with hypoxemia. Hypoxemia in this setting may be due to increasing ventilation-perfusion mismatch.

▶ A previous report anticipated these findings. Christine Gleason and associates (*Pediatrics* 71:31, 1983) monitored preterm infants in a variety of positions while performing sham lumbar punctures and concluded that the traditional flexed position for the performance of spinal taps carried the greatest

TABLE 2.—Physiologic Data for Different Lumbar Puncture Positions*

	Position		
Item and Time	**Standard Lateral (n = 4)**	**Sitting (n = 4)**	**Modified Lateral (n = 4)**
Intraesophageal pressure, cm H_2O			
Baseline	3.0 (1.2)	3.0 (1.3)	2.8 (1.0)
Lumbar puncture	7.3 (2.8)†	2.8 (1.2)	2.6 (1.2)
Baseline	3.2 (0.6)	3.1 (0.4)	3.0 (0.7)
Preductal-postductal $TcPo_2$ difference, mm Hg‡			
Baseline	3.8 (3.0)	4.1 (3.8)	2.9 (1.8)
Lumbar puncture	4.0 (3.5)	3.6 (3.2)	3.5 (2.9)
Baseline	3.5 (3.3)	3.7 (4.0)	3.3 (3.0)

*Values are expressed as mean (SD).
†$P < .01$.
‡$TcPo_2$ indicates transcutaneous Po_2.
(Courtesy of Weisman, L.E., et al.: Am. J. Dis. Child. 137:1077–1079, November 1983; copyright 1983, American Medical Association.)

risk of potential morbidity. They recommended that spinal taps be performed with the infant in the upright position or, when they were performed in the lateral position, that the infant have the neck extended rather than flexed. The same cautions should be exercised on the rare occasion when a bone marrow aspiration from the iliac crest is performed in a low birth weight infant.

Position is everything. Head position also influences intracranial pressure in the neonate. When the neck is turned, pressure rises from reduced venous return, probably due to venous congestion (Goldberg, R. N., et al.: *Crit. Care Med.* 11:428, 1983).—F.A.O.

The Effect of Educational Intervention on the Rate of Neonatal Circumcision
Cynthia S. Rand, Carol-Ann Emmons, and John W. C. Johnson
Obstet. Gynecol. 62:64–67, July 1983   1–11

Despite the absence of medical justification, some 80% of all male neonates are circumcised. An attempt made in 1978 to reduce elective circumcisions by having parents read an explicit and clearly worded consent form surprisingly did not reduce the circumcision rate. The authors studied the reasons for this failure, specifically whether the educational procedure was appropriate for the population covered and whether there were other unrecognized reasons accounting for the persistently high circumcision rate.

Studies were conducted with women who had no religious reasons for newborn circumcision and who were predominantly black and had poor reading skills and little medical sophistication; all were receiving public assistance (Table 1). Only about 25% of the women had a clear understanding of the nature of circumcision. Control women received only the usual hospital circumcision consent form from the nursing staff after delivery. For study subjects, the interviewer explained how a circumcision is performed, using illustrations of the operation, explained the information contained in the consent form, and answered questions.

The rate of circumcision was lower among the infants of mothers who received educational intervention than among those of control mothers (Table 2). In addition to reasons given for electing circumcision (Table 3), the circumcision status of the father was a key factor. Noncircumcision

TABLE 1.—CHARACTERISTICS OF SUBJECTS*

	Study cases (N = 54)	Control (N = 59)
Race—black	80%	76%
Mean age (yr)	20.4	20.8
Mean education (yr)	10.7	11.3
Mean parity	0.43	0.64

*There were no significant differences between groups.
(Courtesy of Rand, C.S., et al.: Obstet. Gynecol. 62:64–67, July 1983. Reprinted with permission from the American College of Obstetricians and Gynecologists.)

TABLE 2.—RATE AND RELATIVE RISK OF NONCIRCUMCISION

Group	No. of infants not circumcised	Total no. of infants	Rate	Relative risk of noncircumcision
Control	3	59	5.1%	1.0
Study	15	54	28.0%	5.5*

*$P < .002$; 95% confidence interval, 1.9–21.
(Courtesy of Rand, C.S., et al.: Obstet. Gynecol. 62:64–67, July 1983. Reprinted with permission from the American College of Obstetricians and Gynecologists.)

TABLE 3.—REASONS GIVEN BY MOTHERS FOR ELECTING CIRCUMCISION*

Reason	Study Frequency	Study Percent	Control Frequency	Control Percent
Cleanliness	9	23	12	21
Parents' desire	9	23	5	9
Health reasons	7	18	3	5
Better done when young	6	15	16	29
Prevents infection or disease	5	13	10	18
No reason	2	5	3	5
Later problems	0	0	3	6
Other	1	3	3	7
Total	39	100.0	55	100.0

*(Courtesy of Rand, C.S., et al.: Obstet. Gynecol. 62:64–67, July 1983. Reprinted with permission from the American College of Obstetricians and Gynecologists.)

was elected by only 7% of study mothers who knew that the father was circumcised but by 48% of mothers who knew that the father was not circumcised or were uncertain about his circumcision status ($P<.01$). The importance of social variables in the decision to circumcise was shown by the many women who did not know why circumcision is performed, yet nevertheless had a predilection for circumcising their sons. Many women apparently believe that circumcision is as natural and necessary as cutting the umbilical cord.

When obstetric patients are told of the risks and potential advantages of circumcision, many choose not to circumcise their sons. A direct recommendation might further reduce the circumcision rate. The intervention used in this study was simple and short and easily could be included in the usual prenatal and postpartum information exchange between patient and physician. Inclusion of the fathers in these discussions might further decrease the circumcision rate.

▶ Probably the most effective means of reducing the number of circumcisions is to reduce the economic reward for their performance. The procedure should be defined as cosmetic surgery and the insurance companies will stop paying for them. This is another form of educational strategy, and obstetricians are capable, under unusual circumstances, of learning fast.

Speaking of circumcision, 18 healthy male newborns were subjects in a study of the effects of a pacifier on their behavioral and adrenocortical responses to circumcision (Gunnar, M. R., et al.: *J. Am. Acad. Child. Psychiatry* 23:34, 1984). Providing the pacifier reduced crying by about 40% but have no effect on the adrenal response. Cortisol levels rose in response to the pain. How does that grab you? For more on the use of a topical anesthetic to reduce the pain of circumcision, see the 1984 YEAR BOOK, pages 9–11.—F.A.O.

Disseminated Fungal Infections in Very Low Birth Weight Infants: Clinical Manifestations and Epidemiology
Jill E. Baley, Robert M. Kliegman, and Avroy A. Fanaroff (Case Western Reserve Univ.)
Pediatrics 73:144–152, February 1984   1–12

Sepsis, including fungal sepsis, is an important cause of morbidity and mortality in very low birth weight infants. The authors noticed an apparent increase in disseminated fungal infections in such infants in 1979 and 1980. Ten clinically diagnosed and 4 autopsy-diagnosed cases of systemic fungal infection in infants weighing less than 1,500 gm at birth were encountered in these 2 years. The clinical group represented 2.7% of very low birth weight infants seen in this period. Mean birth weight was 788 gm, and mean gestational age was 28 weeks. The clinical data are given in Table 1 and predisposing factors in Table 2. All infants but 1 had an umbilical or radial arterial line in place. All the infants had received broad-spectrum antibiotics, and 7 had received four to six different antibiotics.

Mean age at onset of the systemic fungal infection was 33 days. Nine infants were infected by *Candida albicans* and 1 by *Pityrosporum orbi-*

TABLE 1.—DATA ON INFANTS WITH DISSEMINATED FUNGOUS
INFECTIONS*

Infant No.	Birth Weight (g)	Gestational Age (wk)	Neonatal Problems	Other Infections
Clinically diagnosed				
1	890	28	RDS	Abscess
2	600	27	RDS, BPD, PDA-ligation, IVH	*Staphylococcus aureus* sepsis
3	710	26	RDS, PDA-ligation, ↑ Bili-3 exchange transfusions	*Escherichia coli* sepsis
4	1,060	27	RDS, ↑ Bili-8 exchange transfusions, RLF-grade 3	Cytomegalovirus infection
5	740	34	RDS, BPD, PDA	*Pseudomonas* and *S epidermidis* sepsis, cellulitis
6	830	30	RDS, BPD, PDA, IVH, RLF-grade 2	*E coli* sepsis, *Serratia marcescens* and *S aureus* abscesses
7	770	26	RDS, PDA-indomethacin	Cellulitis and abscess
8	630	24–26	RDS, PDA, ↑ Bili-5 exchange transfusions, RLF-grade 4	Omphalitis
9	950	29	RDS, BPD, PDA, IVH, RLF-grade 2	*S epidermidis* sepsis, pneumonia
10	700	26	RDS, BPD, PDA	None
Autopsy diagnosed				
11	700	24	RDS, PBD, PDA-ligation, IVH	None
12	1,120	27	RDS, BPD, PDA	None
13	740	28	RDS, BPD, PDA	None
14	890	28	RDS, BPD, PDA-ligation, triplet A, IVH-grade 4	*Klebsiella pneumoniae* sepsis

*RDS, respiratory distress syndrome; BPD, bronchopulmonary dysplasia; PDA, patent ductus arteriosus; IVH, intraventricular hemorrhage; ↑ Bili, hyperbilirubinemia; RLF, retrolental fibroplasia.

(Courtesy of Baley, J.E., et al.: Pediatrics 73:144–152, February 1984. Copyright American Academy of Pediatrics 1984.)

culare. Presenting features are listed in Table 3. Seven infants were carbohydrate intolerant at the onset. Seven infants had intermittently positive fungal cultures before treatment (Table 4). Candidal endophthalmitis was present in 4 infants and candidal meningitis in 3. The 4 autopsy cases represented 4% of autopsies done on very low birth weight infants during

TABLE 2.—PREDISPOSING FACTORS*

Infant No.	Site	Presentation Duration (d)	Status at Presentation	Age at Presentation (d)	Before Amphotericin Antibiotics Drugs	Duration (d)
1	UAC	15	Out (5 d)	20	A, G, O, C	29
2	UAC	12	In	12	A, G, O	13
3	UAC	20	In	16	A, G, C, M	23
4	RAD	5	Out	45	A, G, M	17
	SVC	33	In			
5	UAC	15	Out	42	A, G, O, C	29
	SVC	25	In			
6	None	...	...	99	A, G, O, C, M, T	83
7	UAC	5	Out (10 d)	15	A, G, O, M, CHL	19
8	UAC	11	In	11	A, O, C	21
9	UAC	33	Out	53	A, G, O, V	39
	SVC	32	In			
10	UAC	10	Out (8 d)	18	A, G	13

*UAC, umbilical arterial catheter; RAD, radial artery catheter; SVC, superior vena cava catheter; A, ampicillin; G, gentamicin; O, oxacillin; C, carbenicillin; M, methicillin; T, tobramycin; CHL, chloramphenicol; V, vancomycin.

(Courtesy of Baley, J.E., et al.: Pediatrics 73:144–152, February 1984. Copyright American Academy of Pediatrics 1984.)

TABLE 3.—PRESENTING FEATURES OF SYSTEMIC FUNGOUS INFECTION-CLINICAL DIAGNOSIS

Presenting Feature	Infant No.										Sum %
	1	2	3	4	5	6	7	8	9	10	
Temperature instability	+					+	+	+	+	+	60
Hyperglycemia	+	+	+			+	+	+		+	70
Apneas/bradycardias	+	+	+	+	+	+	+	+	*	+	90
Respiratory deterioration	+	+	+	+	+	+	+	+	+	+	100
Intubation required	+	+	+	CPAP	+	CPAP	+	+	*	+	70
Abdominal distension		+	+		+	+	+	+	+		70
Guaiac positive stools		+	+		+	+	+	+			60
Hypotension				+	+						20

*Already intubated. CPAP, continuous positive airway pressure.

(Courtesy of Baley, J.E., et al.: Pediatrics 73:144–152, February 1984. Copyright American Academy of Pediatrics 1984.)

TABLE 4.—NATURE OF FUNGOUS INFECTION IN INFANTS WITH CLINICALLY DIAGNOSED DISSEMINATED FUNGOUS INFECTIONS

Infant No.		Positive Cultures*			Abscess	Others	Positive Urinalysis	Eye Examination	Presence of Rash
	Type	Blood	CSF	Urine					
1	I	+	++	+	Leg, ++		+	+	+
2	I	+	+	++			+	+	+
3	I	++	+				+	Not done	
4	N						+	−	+
5	N					Lung biopsy	−		
6	A	++++		++++	Scalp, ++++ leg, +++ arm, +	Rectal, ++ penile, ++		−	+
7	I	+		+				−	
8	I	+					+	+	+
9	I			+	Forehead, +		+	−	
10	I	+		+	Arm, + Forehead, +		+	+	+

*I, intermittently positive cultures; A, constantly positive cultures; N, always negative cultures; +, no. of positive cultures.

(Courtesy of Baley, J.E., et al.: Pediatrics 73:144–152, February 1984. Copyright American Academy of Pediatrics 1984.)

the 2-year period. All 4 infants had systemic *C. albicans* infection with multiple organ involvement. All the infants had umbilical arterial catheters in place. Three had received ampicillin and gentamicin from birth.

Systemic fungal infections have occurred in very low birth weight infants receiving parenteral alimentation via a central line. The infants also have had multiple bacterial infections and have received broad-spectrum antibiotics. These infections may be increasing in prevalence in intensive care nurseries. Antifungal therapy should be started when the first positive culture is obtained in a clinically ill infant. Retinoscopy or tissue biopsy may be useful in evaluating culture-negative patients.

► This is just one more thing to worry about. Some of these infants of extremely low birth weight remain in the nursery so long is it any wonder that they become moldy?

On a more serious note, Raymond Redline and Beverly Dahms describe an unusual fungal infection in an infant who received long-term intralipid therapy (*N. Engl. J. Med.* 305:1395, 1984). The infant was found to have an infection caused by *Malassezia furfur,* formerly termed *"Pityrosporon orbiculare."* This is a fungus of low pathogenicity known to cause infections of the skin. Members of the genus *Malassezia* lack the capacity to synthesize medium-chain and long-chain fatty acids and require an external source of fatty acids for their growth. The skin is rich in such lipids, and, as a result, this fungus may cause superficial infections such as tinea versicolor, blepharitis, and dacrocystitis. An infant with a birth weight of 740 gm had *M. furfur* identified in an open lung biopsy that revealed vasculitis of small pulmonary arteries and bronchopneumonia. It was hypothesized that the unusual location of this organism in the vasculature of the lung was probably a result of pulmonary artery deposits of lipid associated with the prolonged parenteral nutrition.

A lipid emulsion was incriminated in an outbreak of polymicrobial bacteremia in a neonatal intensive care unit (Jarvis, W. R., et al.: *Pediatr. Infect. Dis.* 2:202, 1983). *Klebsiella pneumoniae* and *Enterobacter cloacae* were isolated from the infants and the lipid emulsion bottle. The bottle was being used repeatedly to dispense intravenous emulsions to a number of infants.

Be on the lookout for fungal infections—particularly in those infants with prolonged intravenous lines or other equipment that breaches their natural barriers.—F.A.O.

Sepsis With Coagulase-Negative Staphylococci in Critically Ill Newborns
Stephen Baumgart, Susan E. Hall, Joseph M. Campos, and Richard A. Polin (Children's Hosp. of Philadelphia)
Am. J. Dis. Child. 137:461–463, May 1983   1–13

Coagulase-negative *Staphylococcus* is increasingly being recognized as a common cause of life-threatening nosocomial infections in high-risk neonates. The authors assessed the incidence of serious coagulase-negative staphylococcal infections in infants and describe the clinical signs, predisposing factors, and treatment in 416 infants admitted to an infant intensive care unit between January 1978 and January 1979.

Coagulase-negative staphylococci were isolated in blood cultures from 50 (12%) of the 416 infants. Of these 50, 13 (26%) had had 14 episodes of coagulase-negative staphylococcal bacteremia that met the criteria for infection (pure growth of the organism in one or more blood cultures exhibiting identical antibiotic sensitivities). Nine of the 13 infants also showed coagulase-negative staphylococci with identical antibiotic sensitivity patterns to the blood culture isolates from other body sites.

Mean birth weight of the infants was 1.91 kg and mean gestational age was 34 weeks (Table 1). Mean age at diagnosis was 49 days (range, 2 to 253 days).

Review of perinatal risk factors showed no incidence of maternal fever, 2 mothers with rupture of membranes longer than 24 hours, and 3 infants with birth asphyxia. Invasive procedures at the time of diagnosis included ventilatory assistance by endotracheal tube (6 infants) and indwelling central venous or arterial catheters, or both (7 infants). All infants but 1 had one or more clinical signs of sepsis (Table 2). Peripheral white blood cell counts were significantly abnormal and were suggestive of bacterial infection in 7 infants. Results of the disk diffusion susceptibility test revealed

TABLE 1.—Characteristics of Infants With Coagulase-Negative
Staphylococcal Sepsis

Infant	Birth Weight, kg	Gestation, wk	Sex/Age, Days	Initial Diagnosis*	Invasive Procedures at Time of Bacteremia			
					Assisted Ventilation	Umbilical Catheters	Central Venous Catheters	Surgery
1	0.55	29	F/19	IUGR	–	–	–	–
2	0.90	27	M/15, 55†	RDS	+	–	+	–
3	0.93	26	M/21	RDS	+	+	–	–
4	1.00	29	F/74	RDS	–	–	–	–
5	1.20	30	F/12	RDS	+	+	–	–
6	1.40	34	F/41	NEC	+	–	+	+
7	1.45	33	M/16	RDS	+	+	–	–
8	1.48	30	M/57	RDS	+	–	–	–
9	2.60	40	M/57	Sepsis	–	–	+	–
10	2.75	37	M/21	JS	–	–	–	–
11	2.95	39	F/253	Gastroschisis	–	–	–	–
12	3.70	40	M/2	TTN	–	–	–	–
13	3.92	40	M/46	CHD	–	–	+	–
Mean	1.91	34	8 M/49	...	...	...	...	...
SD	1.13	6	5 F/62	...	...	...	...	...

*IUGR, intrauterine growth retardation; RDS, respiratory distress syndrome; NEC, necrotizing enterocolitis; JS, jejunal stenosis; TTN, transient tachypnea of newborn; and CHD, congenital heart defect.
†Two separate episodes of sepsis.
(Courtesy of Baumgart, S., et al.: Am. J. Dis. Child. 137:461–463, May 1983; copyright 1983, American Medical Association.)

that all but one of the coagulase-negative staphylococci were resistant to penicillin. Eight of 14 isolates were resistant to semisynthetic penicillinase-resistant penicillins, but all were sensitive to cephalothin and vancomycin hydrochloride. Two infants died, 1 at 10 days and 1 at 2 weeks after the onset of sepsis.

Coagulase-negative staphylococci are currently the most frequently en-

TABLE 2.—Clinical Signs and WBC Counts of
Patients With Coagulase-Negative
Staphylococcal Sepsis

Infant	Clinical Signs	Total WBC Count/cu mm	TN* Count/cu mm	IN* Count/cu mm	IN-TN Ratio
1	Apnea/bradycardia	8,300	4,648	498	0.11
2†	Apnea/bradycardia,	10,100	6,262	707‡	0.11
	stool test positive for occult blood (Hematest)	19,400	12,416	0	0
3	Apnea/bradycardia, feeding intolerance	11,000	7,150	1,100‡	0.15‡
4	Apnea/bradycardia	16,000	5,920	0	0
5	Lethargy, poor perfusion	12,500	7,125	125	0.01
6	Abdominal distention	10,800	2,428	0	0
7	Irritable, poor perfusion	25,100	15,813	3,012‡	0.19‡
8	Apnea/bradycardia, lethargy	6,300	2,583	756‡	0.29‡
9	Abdominal distention	13,900	7,645	0	0
10	Vomiting, hyperbilirubinemia	13,900	1,529‡	278	0.18‡
11	No signs demonstrated	4,500	1,710‡	135	0.08
12	Lethargy, feeding introlerance	9,000	6,750	1,080‡	0.16‡
13	Vomiting, diarrhea	12,800	6,016	0	0

*TN, total neutrophil; IN, immature neutrophil.
†Two separate episodes of sepsis.
‡Significantly abnormal, suggestive of bacterial infection.
(Courtesy of Baumgart, S., et al.: Am. J. Dis. Child. 137:461–463, May 1983; copyright 1983, American Medical Association.)

countered nosocomial pathogens in this intensive care unit. In this series these pathogens caused symptomatic bacteremia in 3% of all infants admitted to the unit. Coagulase-negative staphylococci recovered from blood culture should not be considered as a contaminant. In such cases the patient should be examined carefully for clinical signs of sepsis. Chronically ill infants who are receiving parenteral alimentation by central catheter are at greatest risk. Therapy for patients with suspected sepsis caused by coagulase-negative staphylococci should include vancomycin hydrochloride.

▶ Sheldon Korones, Professor of Pediatrics and Obstetrics and Gynecology, University of Tennessee College of Medicine, and Director of the Newborn Center, Memphis City Hospital, comments:

"We are not at the inception of a new era in the agonized history of nosocomial infections; we are in the midst of it. The authors describe an epidemiologic experience that occurred in 1978. Coagulase-negative staphylococci have been producing serious disease for a long time, but with considerably increased frequency in the past few years. One surmises, without documentation, that they are more invasive. There is no doubt that they now have acquired resistance to most antibiotics; this much is well documented. In the past, disease states due to the coagulase-negative staphylococci have most often been associated with implanted foreign bodies such as indwelling catheters and ventriculoperitoneal shunts. Now they seem to be a threat inherent in any of the invasive procedures that comprise intensive care.

"Recent realization of the pathogenic capacity of these staphylococci recalls the saga of *Serratia marcescens*. It was used as a harmless marker in numerous experiments, some as late as the 1960s, only to be identified as a frequent life-threatening pathogen in epidemics during the 1970s. While they are of less nosocomial significance, one is also reminded of group B streptococci. They were reported as the most frequent cause of neonatal septicemia in 1966, after several isolated reports during the preceding years. A preexisting concensus held that these streptococci were a problem for the veterinarian because they were so frequently implicated in bovine mastitis. Through 3 to 4 decades we have witnessed similar changes in the roles of several bacterial species, and each event has exerted a major impact on the mortality and morbidity of neonates in nurseries. The gram-negative enteric organisms assumed a leading role about 40 years ago only after the introduction of penicillin, and they have been with us every since. Reminiscences are incomplete without allusion to the worldwide pandemic of *Staphylococcus aureus* during the late 1950s. These organisms, too, developed resistance to the antibiotics then in use, yet the cryptic cause of their recession several years later was apparently unrelated to the use of more effective antibiotics.

"These onslaughts by particular bacterial species have regularly precipitated intensive exercises in self-assessment among nursery personnel, especially concerning nursery technique. The *S. aureus* experience stimulated volumes of writings on every aspect of nursery demeanor, ranging from measurement of organism concentration in the air to the use of masks, gowns, and assiduous handwashing. We emerged from that era with concensus about one single fact of nursery technique, namely, that handwashing was the most important component of clean behavior and that in its absence, disease inevitably spreads. We also learned, and then forgot, that excessive use of antibiotics promoted these periodic epidemics.

"The coagulase-negative staphylococci are more dangerous today than they were in the past. This is not because they are more ubiquitous, nor is it a function of increased performance of invasive procedures. The capstone of contemporary considerations is the development of resistance to antibiotics. This unquestionably is related to a persistent misconception that every severely ill infant must be treated for or protected from bacterial disease by the administration of antibiotics. We will continue to pay the piper unnecessarily until we learn how to limit the use of antibiotics in neonatal intensive care facilities. The paper from Baumgart et al. is a big red flag."

Low-Flow Oxygen Therapy in Infants

A. N. Campbell, Y. Zarfin, M. Groenveld, and M. H. Bryan (Hosp. for Sick Children, Toronto)
Arch. Dis. Child. 58:795–798, October 1983   1–14

Fifty-one infants who were oxygen dependent after treatment for neonatal respiratory disease were entered in a program in which 100% oxygen was delivered at low flow through a nasal catheter after they were transferred from the level III neonatal intensive care unit to a level II intermediate care unit. Use of this method was possible when oxygen requirement was less than 55% and the infant weighed more than 1,500 gm.

A feeding catheter (8 F) was inserted 1 to 2 cm into one naris and secured by tape; oxygen was delivered from a wall source via a low-flow meter. Actual inspired oxygen concentration was unknown because the infant was also breathing room air. Nasal catheter changes were done by using alternate nostrils every 3 days. For infants weighing more than 2,500 gm who required oxygen and were medically stable, consideration was given to discharge on low-flow oxygen.

Over a 3-year period ending in June 1982, 51 infants were discharged on 100% low-flow oxygen ranging from 0.05 to 0.5 L per minute. Thirty-five infants went home, 7 went to the local children's convalescent hospital, and 9 went to their peripheral referral hospital. Table 1 lists the respiratory diagnoses, gestational ages, birth weights and lengths, and types of respiratory support before introduction of 100% low-flow oxygen. Table 2 shows the age at discharge and cessation of oxygen therapy. Mean duration of 100% low-flow oxygen therapy for the 35 infants treated at home was 14.1 weeks. Thirty-four of the 35 were weaned from 100% low-flow oxygen and 32 survive. Eight infants required readmission during home therapy for management of upper respiratory infections on 12 separate occasions, representing 146 days of additional hospital treatment. All infants of less than 36 weeks' gestation had their fundi examined monthly for retrolental fibroplasia (RLF) during their initial illness and subsequently on readmission. No infant developed RLF. Parents were carefully instructed in the symptoms of hypoxia before discharge of the infants and

TABLE 1.—CLINICAL DATA FOR 51 INFANTS TREATED WITH LOW-FLOW OXYGEN

Diagnosis	No	Gestational age (wks)	Birthweight (kg)	Days on IPPV	Days on CPAP	Days in head box
Bronchopulmonary dysplasia	38	30·2 (24–37)	1·28 (0·6–2·3)	16 (2–76)	7 (0–30)	44 (2–134)
Wilson-Mikity syndrome	8	28·3 (27–31)	1·17 (0·7–1·5)	2 (0–7)	4 (0–17)	43 (21–68)
Hypoplastic lungs	2	32 (28–36)	1·54 (1·1–1·9)	14 (0–28)	3 (0–6)	37 (11–64)
Other*	3	35 (32–40)	1·7 (1·2–4·2)	3 (0–6)	7 (0–21)	33 (18–52)

Values are mean (range). IPPV, intermittent positive-pressure ventilation; CPAP, continuous positive airway pressure.
*Meconium aspiration (2), eventration of diaphragm (1).
(Courtesy of Campbell, A.N., et al.: Arch. Dis. Child. 58:795–798, October 1983.)

were advised to seek immediate medical advice for admission if any of these signs occurred.

It is believed that 100% low-flow oxygen therapy at home allows normal interpersonal relationships to develop between the infant and the family, perhaps enhancing infant growth and development. For the same reasons, this therapy is beneficial in the hospital and insures a more constant oxygen delivery than conventional methods.

TABLE 2.—Treatment of 51 Infants on Low-Flow Oxygen*

Diagnosis	No	Age discharged on LFO₂ Mean (range) (wks)	Age when LFO₂ ceased Mean (range) (wks)
Bronchopulmonary dysplasia	38	18·1 (5–59)	29·9 (9–75)
Wilson-Mikity syndrome	8	15·3 (9–25)	29·3 (15–45)
Hypoplastic lungs	2	8 (5–11)	22·5 (20–23)
Other	3	15·6 (3–25)	21·6 (10–32)

*LFO₂, low-flow oxygen.
(Courtesy of Campbell, A.N., et al.: Arch. Dis. Child. 58:795–798, October 1983.)

Diuresis and Pulmonary Function in Premature Infants With Respiratory Distress Syndrome

Thomas P. Green, Theodore R. Thompson, Dana E. Johnson, and James E. Lock (Univ. of Minnesota)
J. Pediatr. 103:618–623, October 1983   1–15

In a prospective study of 99 premature infants, the effects of furosemide and chlorothiazide on the incidence of patent ductus arteriosus (PDA) were compared in patients with respiratory distress syndrome (RDS). Results were analyzed to examine the relationships of diuretic administration and diuresis to survival and to the duration and degree of mechanical ventilatory support.

If a patient had not initiated the expected spontaneous diuresis (urine output greater than fluid intake for at least 8 hours), furosemide (1 mg/ml) or chlorothiazide (20 mg/ml) was administered in an initial dose of 1 ml/kg. Thirty-three infants received furosemide, 33 received chlorothiazide, and 33 received no diuretic. Incidence of PDA was 18 in the furosemide group and 8 in the clorothiazide group. Furosemide was the most important factor related to the appearance of PDA, whereas chlorothiazide was not related to PDA.

Fluid intake was restricted (60 to 80 ml/kg/day) as long as mechanical ventilation was required. Diagnosis of PDA was based on an infant having the characteristic murmur on 2 consecutive days or having ductal ligation. Diagnosis of bronchopulmonary dysplasia was based on continued requirement for supplemental oxygen after 2 weeks of life in the presence of typical radiologic findings.

Infants given furosemide experienced postnatal weight loss nearly identical to that in infants deemed not to need a diuretic, whereas infants given chlorothiazide lost weight more slowly and had significantly greater body weight on postnatal days 4 and 5. Survival was independently correlated with high birth weight, low initial airway pressure, absence of intraventricular hemorrhage, and use of furosemide. Use of furosemide was associated with a 15% improvement in survival rate, whereas the presence of intraventricular hemorrhage was associated with a 23% decrease in survival. Ventilator mean airway pressure on day 7 and duration of mechanical ventilation were both related to diuresis.

As a group, patients given furosemide did not have a higher incidence of mortality and morbidity than might be expected to accompany PDA. This finding may depend on the early ductal ligation performed during this study.

Importance of water homeostasis in determining the course of RDS in premature infants is shown in this study, which indicates that administration of furosemide is beneficial when spontaneous diuresis does not occur; it may be particularly effective when combined with early closure of the ductus arteriosus.

▶ Green and his co-workers previously demonstrated that furosemide appears to increase the incidence of patent ductus arteriosus in premature infants with respiratory distress syndrome (see 1984 YEAR BOOK, pp. 211–213). This furosemide-associated increase in the incidence of patent ductus is believed to be mediated by prostaglandin E_2, a potent ductal smooth muscle dilator that is produced by the kidney in response to the administration of the drug. Despite this observation, the authors now feel that its benefits outweigh the risks.

Another vote for aggressive medical management and early surgical closure of the ductus, rather than indomethacin, for the low birth weight infant with severe respiratory distress syndrome was provided by J. T. Zerella and associates (J. Pediatr. Surg. 18:835, 1983). The conclusion was prompted by a retrospective analysis of their experience.

Even surgery cannot always be trusted. S. R. Daniels and co-workers (Pediatrics 73:56, 1984) describe two premature infants who developed recurrence of patent ductus arteriosus after surgical closure. Both infants initially did well and then again developed congestive heart failure. Both infants displayed echocardiographic evidence of recurrence. One of the infants had a second operation. Preterm infants should be monitored for the return of clinical signs of a patent ductus even after surgical treatment. I have come to expect recurrences for hernias, but a recurrence of patent ductus—this is ridiculous.—F.A.O.

The Presence or Absence of Fetal Breathing Movements Predicts the Outcome of Preterm Labor

Bruce M. Castle and A. C. Turnbull (Univ. of Oxford)
Lancet 2:471–472, Aug. 27, 1983   1–16

Contractions subside spontaneously and pregnancy continues in at least 50% of women in apparently established preterm labor. To establish if the presence or absence of fetal breathing movements (FBM) might predict whether or not preterm labor would progress, 54 patients who were admitted in preterm labor before the 34th week of gestation were investigated by real-time ultrasound scanning.

Fetal breathing was considered present if sustained for 20 seconds or more and was considered absent if no sustained movements could be detected during at least 45 minutes. Presence or absence of fetal breathing movements in relation to outcome of preterm labor is shown in the table. Fetal breathing was absent in 19 of 25 patients who delivered within 48 hours, whereas in 25 of 34 with fetal breathing on admission, pregnancy continued for a week or more. Of the remaining 9 pregnancies that proceeded to delivery within 1 week despite fetal breathing detectable on admission, spontaneous rupture of the membranes occurred in 6.

Predictive value of the presence or absence of FBM on admission was assessed according to whether pregnancy ended within 48 hours or within 1 week of admission. In 24 patients admitted with painful uterine contractions only, fetal breathing was detected in 19, of whom 1 delivered within 48 hours and another within 1 week. Of 5 patients admitted with contractions only but no detectable FBM, all delivered within 48 hours (table).

Comparison of patients with or without FBM on admission showed average birth weights of 2,640 gm (± 761 gm) versus 1,462 gm (± 396 gm) and average gestation on delivery of 252 days (± 27) versus 208 days (± 17).

Differences in FBM between fetuses and daily variations in FBM in

Clinical presentation	Outcome	FBM present	FBM absent	Total
PRESENCE OR ABSENCE OF FETAL BREATHING MOVEMENTS IN RELATION TO OUTCOME OF PRETERM LABOR*				
Painful uterine contractions alone	Continued >1 wk	17	0	17
	Delivered <1 wk	2 (1)	5 (5)	7 (6)
	All	19	5	24
Spontaneous rupture of membranes	Continued >1 wk	1	0	1
	Delivered <1 wk	6 (4)	10 (10)	16 (14)
	All	7	10	17
Antepartum haemorrhage	Continued >1 wk	5	1	6
	Delivered <1 wk	1 (1)	2 (2)	3 (3)
	All	6	3	9
Multiple pregnancy	Continued >1 wk	2	0	2
	Delivered <1 wk	0	2 (2)	2 (2)
	All	2	2	4
Total	Continued >1 wk	25	1	26
	Delivered <1 wk	9 (6)	19 (19)	28 (25)
	All	34	20	54

*Number delivered within 48 hours in parentheses.
(Courtesy of Castle, B.M., and Turnbull, A.C.: Lancet 2:471–472, Aug. 27, 1983.)

individual fetuses are so great that FBM were simply assessed as "present" or "absent." The link between labor and FBM may be fetal prostaglandin E_2 (PGE_2). The level of PGE_2 in fetal blood increases during labor, apparently coming from the placenta, because the concentration is higher in blood from the umbilical vein than in blood from the artery. In laboratory animals, PGE_2 can inhibit fetal breathing as well as stimulate uterine contractility.

In preterm labor with intact membranes, presence of FBM seems to indicate that pregnancy will continue, while absence foreshadows early delivery. The predictive power of FBM, if confirmed by further studies, should increase greatly the precision of obstetric diagnosis, facilitate objective assessment of the value of treatment, and lead to logical and effective management of preterm labor.

▶ This is a nice little predictor if the authors' experience can be reproduced by others. Fetal movements, as contrasted with fetal breathing movements, previously have been reported to be a helpful prognostic sign (Mathews, D. D.: *Br. Med. J.* 1:439, 1972; and Sadovsky, E., et al.: *Obstet. Gynecol.* 41:845, 1973). It has been shown to be of practical use as a clinical routine. A total of 3,111 pregnant women participated in a prospective clinical trial of fetal movement in Denmark. One half of the group received detailed instructions regarding the significance of fetal movements, while the rest served as controls. In the control group, 12 fetuses that weighed more than 1,500 gm and had no major congenital malformations died, compared to 3 in the treatment group. During the study, 62 women followed the instructions to contact the clinic to report that they felt less fetal movement; 36 were sent home after a careful examination by a midwife, whereas 26 were examined with ultrasound and 10 underwent emergency cesarean section because of abnormally low fetal activity (Neldam, S.: *Dan. Med. Bull. 30:274, 1983)*. Lives presumably were saved.—F.A.O.

Controlled Trial of Dexamethasone Therapy in Infants With Bronchopulmonary Dysplasia
Mark C. Mammel, Dana E. Johnson, Thomas P. Green, and Theodore R. Thompson (Univ. of Minnesota Hosp., Minneapolis)
Lancet 1:1356–1358, June 18, 1983   1–17

The acute effects of dexamethasone on pulmonary function were assessed in a double-blind, placebo-controlled, randomized crossover study of 6 infants with severe bronchopulmonary dysplasia who had required mechanical ventilation for at least 4 weeks despite treatment with diuretics, methylxanthines, bronchodilators, fluid restriction, nutritional supplementation, and ligation of the patent ductus arteriosus when indicated.

Mean gestational age was 28.7 weeks (range, 27 to 33 weeks) and mean birth weight was 1,049 gm (range, 800 to 1,730 gm) (Table 1). Three infants had mild or moderate and 1 had severe intraventricular hemorrhage. At admission to the study, mean inspired oxygen concentration was

TABLE 1.—Patient Characteristics

Patient	Birth weight (g)	Gestational age (wk)	Entry age (days)	Patent ductus arteriosus*	Intraventricular haemorrhage
1	900	28	31	L	. .
2	825	28	31	L	Mild
3	1000	28	30	L	Moderate
4	800	27	36	L	Mild
5	1730	33	34	L	. .
6	1040	28	35	. .	Severe
Mean	1049	28·7	32·8	—	—

*L, ligation (surgical) of patent ductus arteriosus.
(Courtesy of Mammel, M.C., et al.: Lancet 1:1356–1358, June 18, 1983.)

0.49, mean respiratory rate was 19.3 breaths per minute, mean peak inspiratory pressure was 26.2 cm H_2O, mean end expiratory pressure was 3.5 cm H_2O, and mean alveolar arterial oxygen gradient was 235.5 torr (Table 2).

Treatment with dexamethasone (0.5 mg/kg/day) produced significant decreases in all these ventilator variables except for end-expiratory pressure (Table 3). Placebo treatment did not significantly change baseline values. Dexamethasone was continued at the same dose in 4 infants and at a reduced dose in 2. When 1 who received the reduced dose deteriorated and the other showed no additional improvement after 48 hours, they were switched to the higher dose. All infants continued to improve while receiving the higher dose, and all 6 were successfully weaned from the mechanical ventilator and extubated at a mean of 7.4 days after dexamethasone therapy was initiated. Three of the 6 infants survived and 3 died (Table 4). All 3 who survived and 2 of the infants who died developed infections, among other complications, while receiving steroids.

Dexamethasone may decrease exposure to mechanical ventilation and

TABLE 2.—Ventilator Settings for Individual Patients on Admission to Study

Patient	Inspired oxygen concentration	Resp rate (breaths/min)	Peak inspiratory pressure (cm H_2O)	End expiratory pressure (cm H_2O)	AaDO$_2$*
1	0·60	14	40	4	313 *(41·73)*
2	0·60	20	26	5	301 *(40·13)*
3	0·60	40	24	2	313 *(41·73)*
4	0·38	14	26	4	168 *(22·40)*
5	0·40	13	22	3	177 *(23·59)*
6	0·34	15	19	3	141 *(18·80)*
Mean	0·49	19·3	26·2	3·5	235·5 *(31·40)*

*AaDO$_2$, alveolar-arterial oxygen gradient in torr, calculated from alveolar gas equation; numbers in parentheses are values in kPa.
(Courtesy of Mammel, M.C., et al.: Lancet 1:1356–1358, June 18, 1983.)

TABLE 3.—Effect of Dexamethasone and Placebo on
Pulmonary Function in Patients With
Bronchopulmonary Dysplasia

	Respiratory rate	Peak inspiratory pressure (cm H_2O)	End expiratory pressure (cm H_2O)	Fractional inspired oxygen concentration	AaDO$_2$†
Pretreatment baseline	19±10	26± 7	3·5±1	0·49±0·13	236±183 (31·46±24·40)
Dexamethasone	5± 7*	14±15*	2·7±1·5	0·31±0·06*	159±55* (21·20±7·33*)
Placebo	17±15	23±13	3·3±0·8	0·49±0·25	271±183 (36·13±24·40)

*P < .05 compared with baseline values.
†AaDO$_2$, alveolar-arterial oxygen gradient in torr; numbers in parentheses are values in kPa.
(Courtesy of Mammel, M.C., et al.: Lancet 1:1356–1358, June 18, 1983.)

TABLE 4.—Outcome

Patient	Extubation	Duration of therapy (wk)	Survived	Cause of death	Complications*
1	Day 10	9	Yes	..	Septicaemia
2	Day 7	4	Yes	..	SBE, RLF, (stage II)
3	Day 12	4	No	SIDS	RLF, (stage II)
4	Day 3	16	No	Pneumonia	Septicaemia
5	Day 9	16	No	Pneumonia	Septicaemia, CMV excretion
6	Day 3	8	Yes	..	Septicaemia, CMV excretion RLF (stage II)

*SBE, subacute bacterial endocarditis; RLF, retrolental fibroplasia; SIDS, sudden infant death syndrome; CMV, cytomegalovirus.
(Courtesy of Mammel, M.C., et al.: Lancet 1:1356–1358, June 18, 1983.)

oxygen therapy in infants with bronchopulmonary dysplasia, but the risk of substantial morbidity is high. However, further studies of patient selection, dose schedules, short- and long-term side effects, and the mechanisms of action of this agent are needed before treatment with dexamethasone can be recommended.

▶ Doctor Victor Chernick, Professor of Pediatrics, University of Manitoba, comments as follows:
"This is a small series in which moderately encouraging results were ob-

tained. Infection is a potential problem. I don't believe that neonatologists should join this bandwagon until larger, more convincing, carefully controlled series are published in which less subjective criteria are used for assessment of pulmonary improvement. Previous attempts at prevention (vitamin E) have resulted in initial encouraging results, followed by more careful studies indicating no benefit. Bronchopulmonary dysplasia (BPD) continues to be a serious and vexing complication of artificial ventilation of the preterm infant. The disorder is being studied from many aspects at the present time, including pathogenesis prevention, therapy, and long-term management. To my mind, the key is in understanding the pathogenesis more fully. There is something different about the response of the preterm lung to excess oxygen. Interestingly, some 17 abstracts devoted to BPD were in the 1984 APS/SPR program, one which suggested the efficacy of bovine superoxide dismitase in preventing the disorder. Hopefully, this degree of attention by capable investigators will unravel the mystery. I have one further thought. Will the use of artificial surfactant (surfactant replacement therapy) prevent or greatly reduce the incidence of BPD? I'm certain we will hear more about this possibility within the near future."

Factors Associated With Pulmonary Air Leak in Premature Infants Receiving Mechanical Ventilation

R. A. Primhak (Univ. of Sheffield Children's Hosp., Sheffield, England)
J. Pediatr. 102:764–768, May 1983   1–18

Pneumothorax or other pulmonary air leak develops in 15% to 48% of infants who receive intermittent positive-pressure ventilation (IPPV) for hyaline membrane disease. It is likely that this complication contributes to intraventricular hemorrhage. The clinical data and ventilator flow rates and pressures were studied retrospectively in 57 infants, 30 of whom had pulmonary air leak and required IPPV for respiratory failure or intractable hypoxia that complicated respiratory distress. These 57 were among 373 infants admitted to a neonatal intensive care unit during 1981.

All 57 were delivered between 26 and 34 weeks' gestation. There were no significant differences between groups with regard to mean birth weight, gestational age, 1- or 5-minute Apgar scores, or age at initiation of IPPV. Mean age at which air leak occurred was 23.5 hours (range, 2 to 66.5 hours), when the infants had been ventilated for a mean of 17.9 hours.

Mean maximum positive end-expiratory pressure, peak inspiratory pressure (PIP), mean airway pressure (MAP), mean maximum and minimum Pa_{CO_2} values, and mean alveolar-arterial oxygen difference at age 6 hours did not differ significantly between infants with pulmonary air leak and those without air leak (table). However, mean maximum inspiratory time was significantly prolonged in infants who subsequently developed air leak, although mean minimum expiratory time did not differ significantly between groups.

In infants with air leak, PIP and MAP were significantly higher for 8 hours prior to the occurrence of air leak. However, inspiratory time in

VENTILATOR SETTINGS PRIOR TO AIR LEAK

	Air leak (n = 28)	Controls (n = 26)	P
Highest PIP (mbar)	22.7 ± 5.7 (16 to 35)	22.1 ± 5.2 (15 to 35)	NS
Highest PEEP (mbar)	3.4 ± 1.3 (2 to 6)	4.1 ± 1.3 (2 to 7)	NS
Highest MAP (mbar)	14.7 ± 5.0 (7 to 26)	14.2 ± 4.6 (7 to 25)	NS
Longest T_{insp} (sec)	1.27 ± 0.32 (1 to 2)	1.10 ± 0.17 (1 to 1.5)	< 0.05 (Wilcoxon rank sum)
Shortest T_{exp} (sec)	0.84 ± 0.28 (0.5 to 2)	0.87 ± 0.30 (0.5 to 2)	NS
Highest Pa_{CO_2} (mm Hg)	60.8 ± 18.8 (40.5 to 132.8) (n = 26)	73.5 ± 29.3 (39.8 to 150)	NS
Lowest Pa_{CO_2} (mm Hg)	33.0 ± 12.8 (18.0 to 69) (n = 26)	29.3 ± 9.8 (12.0 to 54)	NS
A-a$DO_2$6 (mm Hg)	454.5 ± 169 (n = 22)	393.0 ± 161 (n = 21)	NS

Values are mean ± SD; range is given in parentheses.
(Courtesy of Primhak, R.A.: J. Pediatr. 102:764–768, May 1983.)

these patients was highly prolonged for 16 hours prior to air leak and was the most significant of all observed changes. Expiratory time was shorter during the period from 4 to 12 hours prior to air leak, but the significance of this finding was much less than that for inspiratory time.

Prolonged inspiratory time in infants receiving IPPV may be a significant factor in the pathogenesis of pulmonary air leak.

► Leo Stern, Professor of Pediatrics, and Chairman, Department of Pediatrics, Brown University, writes the following:

"Although it is theoretically possible that pulmonary air leak syndromes (pneumothorax, pneumomediastinum, etc.) can result as a direct consequence of excess respirator pressures, the very large gradient between the inspiratory pressure applied, as measured at the entrance to the airway, and the actual effective intra-alveolar pressure that results would make such an etiology *alone* rather unlikely. Pathophysiologically, such air leaks, which are not an uncommon occurrence in the course of neonatal respiratory disease in the absence of respirator management, occur as a consequence of the presence of one or more areas in which there is a partially fixed obstruction to a bronchus. Accordingly, it would appear more appropriate that the assignation of responsibility for the occurrence of air leaks in infants treated with a mechanical ventilator account not only for the use of the ventilator and its settings, but also for the contribution of the nature and severity of the underlying disease.

"The study reported by Doctor Primhak tends to implicate the ventilator alone and suggests that responsibility should be placed on a prolongation of the inspiratory time. The conclusion is based on a retrospective comparison of two groups of infants, both of which were ventilated but only one of which developed air leaks. Aside from the difficulties inherent in retrospective studies, such a comparison that seeks to implicate the ventilator as the responsible factor would need initially to compare the incidence of occurrence of the air leak syndrome in infants treated with, as opposed to without, a respirator for a similar degree of respiratory difficulty. Having first established that such a difference does occur, it would then be a next step to attempt to implicate differences in the respirator settings or other performance factors of the equipment utilized.

"This study unfortunately does not specify either the rationale for or the degree of respiratory impairment involved that necessitated 'the need for IPPV,' nor is their any indication as to what governed the selection of a particular inspiratory time setting for any individual infant. This latter feature would be critical, because prolonging the inspiratory time is an acceptable and effective technique for achieving better oxygenation, and it may, therefore, well be that those infants who were treated with prolonged inspiratory time settings were 'sicker' than those who were not and required prolongation of the inspiratory time in order to be able to achieve adequate oxygenation as a consequence of their disease.

"The study gives cause for reflection, but it would be unfortunate if it were used as a rationale for decrying the advantages of a prolonged inspiratory phase in the use of positive-pressure respirators in newborn infants. Not only is it possible generally to achieve better oxygenation (as a function of the optimal time of transfer of oxygen across the alveoli), but it is frequently possible to achieve desired arterial P_{O_2} levels at a reduced $F_{I_{O_2}}$ as a consequence of the maneuver. There is the additional possibility that with prolongation of the inspiratory time, there is an increase in the mean pressure attained for the duration of the inspiratory pressure curve, which thereby reduces the peak pressures that might otherwise be necessary with a shorter inspiratory phase. The apparent reduction in resultant barotrauma, which appears to be associated with a reduction in chronic ventilator lung disease (Reynolds, E. O. R., and Taghizade, A.: Arch. Dis. Child. 49:505, 1974), is a positive feature to such usage which should not be readily abandoned even though it is possible that a higher incidence of air leak syndrome may result from it."

Postural Effects on Gas Exchange in Infants
D. P. Heaf, P. Helms, I. Gordon, and H. M. Turner (Hosp. for Sick Children, London)
N. Engl. J. Med. 308:1505–1508, June 23, 1983   1–19

Gas exchange in adults with unilateral lung disease can be improved by positioning the patient so that the good lung is dependent. However, because infants and very young children breathe at lower lung volumes than adults do because of reduced support to the lungs given by their floppy chest walls, the influence of gravity could have a different effect on gas exchange in very young age groups. The authors assessed the effects of body position on gas exchange in 10 infants with unilateral lung disease by measuring transcutaneous oxygen and carbon dioxide pressures in the supine and right and left lateral positions. Regional ventilation was assessed by krypton-81m lung scans, and changes in thoracic gas volume were measured in 4 infants.

Measurement of changes in transcutaneous oxygen and carbon dioxide pressures showed that optimal oxygenation occurred when the good lung was uppermost and the sick lung was dependent (table). In this position, the mean transcutaneous oxygen pressure was 82 mm Hg, compared with 78 mm Hg in the supine position and 73 mm Hg when the good lung was dependent. The mean transcutaneous carbon dioxide pressure of 38 mm Hg did not change with changes in position. Krypton ventilation scans showed that ventilation was distributed preferentially to the uppermost lung in both the left and right lateral decubitus positions (Fig 1–5). The opposite is seen in adults, with ventilation being distributed preferentially to the dependent lung. The mean proportion of ventilation to the good lung when it was in the dependent position was 46%. This increased significantly to 59% ($P < .02$) when the infants were in the supine position, increasing further to 64% when the good lung was uppermost and the sick lung dependent. Thoracic gas volume, tidal volume, and dynamic lung compliance measurements did not change significantly with changes in position.

In contrast to what is observed in adults, the findings indicate that oxygenation in infants with unilateral lung disease is best when the good lung is uppermost and the diseased lung dependent. Further study is nec-

CLINICAL CHARACTERISTICS AND TRANSCUTANEOUS OXYGEN AND CARBON DIOXIDE PRESSURES IN 10 INFANTS WITH UNILATERAL LUNG DISEASE*

INFANT No.	AGE	WEIGHT	RESPIRATORY SUPPORT	FIO2	TRANSCUTANEOUS PO2/PCO2		
					GOOD LUNG DEPENDENT	SUPINE	GOOD LUNG UPPERMOST
	days	*kg*					
1	9	2.95	—	0.21	70/37	73/38	75/39
2	2	3.25	CPAP	0.28	95/38	96/37	96/39
3	240	5.45	IPPV	0.60	55/32	67/34	80/32
4	60	4.40	—	0.21	67/29	72/29	72/29
5	4	2.50	—	0.21	64/41	69/40	72/42
6	2	2.86	IPPV	0.45	103/31	113/30	125/31
7	2	3.08	CPAP	0.35	71/42	70/41	72/39
8	30	2.80	—	0.21	41/43	43/43	46/43
9	5	3.60	IPPV	0.40	109/35	117/35	116/34
10	21	1.52	—	0.40	55/54	60/56	63/56

Mean±S.E.: 73±7/38±2.3   78±7/38±2.4   82±7/38±2.5

*FIO2, fractional inspired oxygen concentration; PO2, partial pressure of oxygen; PCO2, partial pressure of carbon dioxide; CPAP, constant positive airway pressure of 4–6 cm of water; IPPV, intermittent positive-pressure ventilation.

(Courtesy of Heaf, D.P., et al.: N. Engl. J. Med. 308:1505–1508, June 23, 1983. Reprinted by permission of the New England Journal of Medicine.)

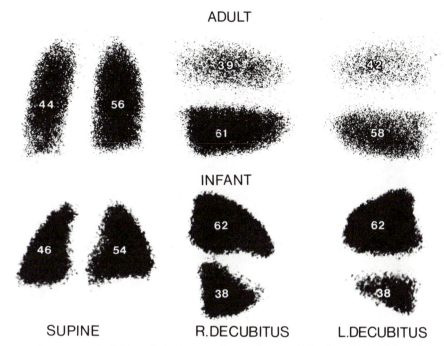

Fig 1–5.—Posterior [81m]Kr ventilation lung scans in normal man aged 31 and in a child aged 2 months after repair of a right congenital diaphragmatic hernia. Note in the adult that ventilation is preferentially distributed to the dependent lung, whereas in the infant the reverse occurs, ventilation being greater in the uppermost lung. Ventilation to each lung is expressed as a percentage of the total to both lungs. (Courtesy of Heaf, D.P., et al.: N. Engl. J. Med. 308:1505–1508, June 23, 1983. Reprinted by permission of the New England Journal of Medicine.)

essary to determine the age at which the adult pattern of optimal oxygenation is adopted.

▶ Mary Ellen Avery, Professor of Pediatrics, and Chairman, Department of Pediatrics, Harvard Medical School, supplied the following comment:

"The observations by Heaf et al. are puzzling and probably not generalizable. The 10 infants studied included 8 seen after repair of diaphragmatic hernia. Changes in the pulmonary vessels of these hypoplastic lungs may alter the distribution of perfusion with postural changes. Moreover, the differences in oxygen tensions between subjects with the good lung uppermost or dependent were only 9 torr on the average, which is probably not of great clinical significance.

"The question of optimal position for an infant with localized lung disease is nonetheless of importance. Careful studies of regional pleural surface expansile forces in intact dogs (Hoffman, E. A., et al.: J. Appl. Physiol. 55:1523–1529, 1983) show that distending pressures are greatest in the uppermost regions. These observations would suggest that if the therapeutic aim were to overcome atelectasis, the atelectatic area should be uppermost. If, on the other hand, the aim were to maximize gas exchange in the presence of a hypoplastic lung, the normal lung should be uppermost.

"Since patients differ with respect to the nature and extent of pulmonary parenchymal and vascular disease and with respect to size and postnatal age, which affect lung and chest wall compliance, individualization of position would be appropriate. Heaf et al. have shown that transcutaneous oxygen measurements are reasonable ways to assess optimal oxygenation. They have not established a general principle for management of infants with unilateral lung disease."

Evaluation of a Protocol for Postmortem Examination of Stillbirths

Robert F. Mueller, Virginia P. Sybert, Jennifer Johnson, Zane A. Bown, and Wei-Jen Chen (Univ. of Washington)
N. Engl. J. Med. 309:586–590, Sept. 8, 1983   1–20

The purpose of a careful examination of stillbirths and neonatal deaths is to determine the cause of the pregnancy loss or infant death and the likelihood of recurrence. The authors studied the relative usefulness of gross and microscopic autopsy, photography, radiography, bacterial cultures, and chromosome studies in 71 stillbirths and 53 neonatal deaths.

Gross autopsy alone was the basis for separation of subjects into normal and abnormal cases. In 25 of the stillbirths (35%) and 19 of the neonatal deaths (36%) the infants were abnormal (Tables 1–3). The single most useful tool for establishing a specific diagnosis was the gross postmortem examination. Microscopic examinations were essential to establish a specific diagnosis in 8 subjects found to be abnormal on gross examination, but in none of the normal subjects. Radiographs were essential in 3 abnormal cases and bacterial cultures were informative in 7. Chromosome

TABLE 1.—CHROMOSOMAL ABNORMALITIES AMONG 124
CASES OF STILLBIRTH AND NEONATAL DEATH

ABNORMALITY	NO. OF CASES	RECURRENCE RISK (%)	TYPE OF CASE
47,XY,+13	1	≤1	Neonatal death
47,XX,+18	1	≤1	Stillbirth
47,XY,+21	1	≤1	Stillbirth
45,X	1	0	Stillbirth
69,XXX	1	0	Stillbirth
Translocation			
+13 [(46,XX,−13,+t(13;13)]	1	2–15	Neonatal death
46,XY,t(14;20) (14qter→cen→ 20pter;20qter→cen→14pter) *	1	?	Stillbirth
Total	7		

*Whether this apparently balanced translocation was related to multiple congenital anomalies in stillbirth is not known.

(Courtesy of Mueller, R.F., et al.: N. Engl. J. Med. 309:586–590, Sept. 8, 1983. Reprinted by permission of the New England Journal of Medicine.)

TABLE 2.—CASES OF SINGLE-GENE DISORDERS

DISORDER	NO. OF CASES	TYPE OF DISORDER	RECURRENCE RISK (%)	TYPE OF CASE
Thanatophoric dwarfism	2	Autosomal dominant or autosomal recessive	0–25	Neonatal death
Erythroblastosis fetalis	2	Autosomal dominant	66	Stillbirth
Polycystic kidneys	2	Autosomal recessive	25	1 stillbirth, 1 neonatal death
Spondylocostal dysplasia	1	Autosomal dominant or autosomal recessive	0–50	Neonatal death
Hydrocephalus with aque-ductal stenosis	1	X-linked recessive	0–25	Neonatal death
Postaxial polydactyly	1	Autosomal dominant	0–50	Stillbirth
Total	9			

(Courtesy of Mueller, R.F., et al.: N. Engl. J. Med. 309:586–590, Sept. 8, 1983. Reprinted by permission of the New England Journal of Medicine.)

TABLE 3.—POLYGENIC, MULTIFACTORIAL, SPORADIC, AND UNDETERMINED DISORDERS

DISORDER	NO. OF CASES	RECURRENCE RISK (%)	TYPE OF CASE
Polygenic/multifactorial			
Anencephaly *			
Isolated	2	2–3	1 stillbirth, 1 neonatal death
With gastroschisis	1	3–5?	Neonatal death
With postaxial polydactyly †	1	2–25	Stillbirth
In twinning	1	3–5?	Neonatal death
Potter's syndrome			
With urethral valves *†	1	0–25	Neonatal death
With bilateral renal agenesis *†	4	3–25	Neonatal death
Unilateral renal agenesis *†	2	0–25	1 stillbirth, 1 neonatal death
Nonimmunologic hydrops fetalis	5 (2 *)	0–50	Stillbirth
Gastroschisis	1	0?	Stillbirth
Cleft lip or palate	1	3–5	Neonatal death
Sporadic			
Cyllosomus	2	0	1 stillbirth, 1 neonatal death
Acardiac twin	1	0.01	Stillbirth
Undetermined			
Suspected trisomy 13	2 (1 *)	?	Stillbirth
Suspected triploidy *	1	?	Neonatal death
Multiple congenital anomalies *	3	?	Stillbirth
Total	28		

*Chromosomes either were normal or failed to grow.
†Possibly single gene.
(Courtesy of Mueller, R.F., et al.: N. Engl. J. Med. 309:586–590, Sept. 8, 1983. Reprinted by permission of the New England Journal of Medicine.)

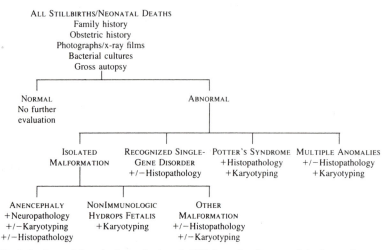

ALL STILLBIRTHS/NEONATAL DEATHS
Family history
Obstetric history
Photographs/x-ray films
Bacterial cultures
Gross autopsy

NORMAL
No further
evaluation

ABNORMAL

ISOLATED
MALFORMATION

RECOGNIZED SINGLE-
GENE DISORDER
+/−Histopathology

POTTER'S SYNDROME
+Histopathology
+Karyotyping

MULTIPLE ANOMALIES
+/−Histopathology
+Karyotyping

ANENCEPHALY
+Neuropathology
+/−Karyotyping
+/−Histopathology

NONIMMUNOLOGIC
HYDROPS FETALIS
+Karyotyping

OTHER
MALFORMATION
+/−Histopathology
+/−Karyotyping

Fig 1–6.—Protocol for selective evaluation of stillbirths and early neonatal deaths; + denotes recommended examination and +/− denotes examination to be performed at discretion of examiner, depending on results of autopsy. (Courtesy of Mueller, R.F., et al.: N. Engl. J. Med. 309:586–590, Sept. 8, 1983. Reprinted by permission of the New England Journal of Medicine.)

studies were indicated in 66% of abnormal cases but in only 23% of all 124 cases.

These findings suggest that the protocol for evaluation of stillbirths and neonatal deaths can be abbreviated (Fig 1–6). Gross postmortem examination, including evaluation of the placenta, should always be performed. Tissue samples should be obtained for karyotypic and histopathologic examinations; these should be discarded or processed as indicated by autopsy. Postmortem photography and radiography are low-cost procedures that are valuable as permanent records and may aid in clarification of some diagnoses, i.e., skeletal dysplasia. It is suggested that karyotyping not be done routinely, but be reserved for cases involving multiple abnormalities or growth retardation, unless a specific single-gene or sporadic disorder is recognized. Family history of abnormal children or an obstetric history of recurrent pregnancy loss are also indications for karyotyping. Indications for histopathologic evaluation (Potter's syndrome, polycystic kidneys or other renal abnormalities, anencephaly) should be evident at gross autospy.

In some instances, accurate diagnosis and prediction of risk of recurrence will be possible only with completion of the entire protocol, i.e., the anencephaly and polydactyly seen in 1 case. In most cases with a specific abnormality, there is an increased risk of recurrence of only that disorder, and risk of loss or other abnormalities in subsequent pregnancies should not be increased.

Careful evaluation of stillbirths and early neonatal deaths is indicated to establish accurate diagnosis and predict risk of recurrence; an appropriate approach will minimize use of low-yield procedures and reduce costs.

Retrolental Fibroplasia and Vitamin E in the Preterm Infant: Comparison of Oral Versus Intramuscular-Oral Administration

Helen M. Hittner, Michael E. Speer, Arnold J. Rudolph, Cindy Blifeld, Prabhujeet Chadda, M. E. Blair Holbein, Louis B. Godio, and Frank L. Kretzer (Baylor College of Medicine)
Pediatrics 73:238–249, February 1984   1–21

The authors evaluated the efficacy of four early intramuscular injections of vitamin E, given in addition to continuous minimal oral supplementation, to suppress the occurrence of severe retrolental fibroplasia (RLF) in a double-masked study of 168 infants weighing 1,500 gm and less at birth. All required supplemental oxygen for respiratory distress. All the infants received oral vitamin E therapy in a dosage of 100 mg/kg daily (Table 1) until retinal vascularization was complete. Seventy-nine infants also received injections of 15, 10, 10, and 10 mg/kg on days 1, 2, 4, and 6, respectively (Table 2).

The results are shown in Figure 1–7. Multivariate analysis of infants who survived for 10 weeks or longer indicated no significant difference in the occurrence of severe RLF in the two treatment groups. Plasma vitamin E concentrations never exceeded a mean of 3.3 mg/dl, and no toxicity was observed. Ultrastructural studies showed identical kinetics of gap junction formation between adjacent spindle cells in the eyes of infants in the two treatment groups.

It is recommended that three early intramuscular vitamin E injections be given starting on the first day of life, using the best available preparation, and that continuous oral supplementation be continued until retinal vascularization is complete. Injections should also be given if oral feedings

TABLE 1.—Oral Preparations

Hoffmann-La Roche (1980 Study)	Aquasol E (1981 Study)	Texas Children's Hospital Preparation (1982 Study)
dl-α-tocopherol	*dl*-α-tocopheryl acetate	*dl*-α-tocopheryl acetate (26.8 g)*
Tween 80	Tween 80	Polysorbate 80 (2.8 g = 2.6 mL)
Propylene glycol	Propylene glycol	MCT (medium chain triglycerides) oil (60 g = 63.6 mL)
Distilled water	Distilled water	Distilled water (90 mL)
	Sorbitol	
	Oil of anise	
	Sodium saccharin	
	Imitation butterscotch flavor	
Osmolality: 3,000 mosm	Osmolality: 3,000 mosm	Osmolality: 150 mosm
pH: 6.5	pH: 5.7	pH: 5.4

*Hoffmann-La Roche investigational drug containing 500 IU of vitamin E per gm compounded with gelatin and 3% silicon dioxide, 0.2% sorbic acid, and 0.1% sodium benzoate. Prepared as described, emulsion contains 100 IU/1.5 ml with total volume of 201 ml. It is stable if refrigerated and protected from light for at least 6 wk.

(Courtesy of Hittner, H.M., et al.: Pediatrics 73:238–249, February 1984. Copyright American Academy of Pediatrics 1984.)

TABLE 2.—Intramuscular Preparations

E-ferol (O'Neal, Jones & Feldman, Commercially Available)	Ephynal (Hoffmann-La Roche)* (1982 Study)
dl-α-tocopheryl acetate, 200 mg/mL	dl-α-tocopherol, 55 mg/mL
Benzyl alcohol, 20 mg/ mL	Benzyl alcohol, 0.01 mL/mL
Sesame oil, USP, sufficient quantity (qs), 1.0 mL	Propylene glycol, 0.1 mL/ mL
	Ethyl alcohol (200 proof), 0.1 mL/mL
	Emulphor E1-620 0.1 mL/ mL
	Sodium acetate trihydrate, 0.3 mg/mL
	Glacial acetic acid, 2.5 mg/ mL
	Sodium chloride, 9.0 mg/mL
	Disodium edetate, 0.1 mg/ mL
	Water, qs, 1.0 mL
	Osmolality: 3,600 mosm
	pH: 4.0

*Placebo injections used same components without the dl-α-tocopherol.
(Courtesy of Hittner, H.M., et al.: Pediatrics 73:238–249, February 1984. Copyright American Academy of Pediatrics 1984.)

are interrupted or transfusions reduce the plasma vitamin E concentration. A plasma vitamin E concentration of 3.5 mg/dl should not be exceeded. Retinal screening should be done at age 8 weeks and later as necessary depending on the findings. If severe RLF does develop, cryoretinopexy should be applied to the avascular retina before detachment occurs.

▶ Poor vitamin E! Just when carefully collected, objective evidence demonstrates a role for this antioxidant in reducing the severity of retrolental fibroplasia, it gets involved in a scandal—a scandal occasioned by slipshod practices on the part of the manufacturer and the Food and Drug Administration. As of this writing, all the facts have not been made public, but it would appear that the deaths that occurred as a result of the intravenous administration of vitamin E to low birth weight infants were a probable result of the suspending vehicle and not the vitamin E itself. Hittner and co-workers observed no toxicity from the vitamin. They gave it either by mouth or by the intramuscular route. When the vitamin is used for the prevention of severe degrees of cicatricial retrolental fibroplasia, the serum concentration of tocopherol should be kept in the 1.5 to 2.5 mg/dl range. Vitamin E was once termed "the shady lady of human nutrition" by Dr. Harry Gordon. It is difficult to overcome a bad reputation.

Vehicles can kill—and not just motor vehicles, either. Remember the "gasp-

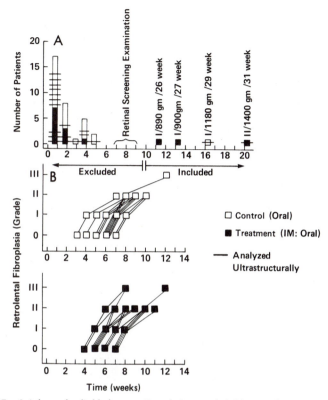

Fig 1–7.—**A,** infants who died before age 10 weeks were excluded from analysis as maximal clinical manifestation of RLF at these time points has not developed. Analysis includes 4 infants who died at ages 11, 13, 16, and 20 weeks, i.e., after adequate time to develop RLF (RLF grade per birth weight in grams per gestational age in weeks is given for these 4 infants). Control infants (oral vitamin E therapy) are indicated by open boxes, and treated infants (intramuscular plus oral vitamin E therapy) are indicated by solid boxes; horizontal line through box indicates that eyes were studied ultrastructurally. **B,** RLF grades plotted against time in 28 infants (13 control and 15 treated) who developed RLF ≥ grade II; RLF ≥ grade II developed only after sixth week. Control infants are indicated by open squares, and treated infants are indicated by solid squares. Lines connect time of last normal retinal examination to first examination showing grade I, to first examination showing grade II, and to first examination showing grade III. (Courtesy of Hittner, H.M., et al.: Pediatrics 73:238–249, February 1984. Copyright American Academy of Pediatrics 1984.)

ing syndrome" and its relationship to benzyl alcohol poisoning? The benzyl alcohol was present in the bacteriostatic sodium chloride and bacteriostatic water used to flush the catheters of small infants (1984 YEAR BOOK, pp. 442–443).

For more on the role of vitamin E and retrolental fibroplasia see the study of N. N. Finer and associates (*Ophthalmology* 90:428, 1983).—F.A.O.

2 Infectious Disease and Immunity

Rifampin Prophylaxis Versus Placebo for Household Contacts of Children With *Hemophilus influenzae* Type b Disease
Trudy V. Murphy, Dale F. Chrane, George H. McCracken, Jr., and John D. Nelson (Univ. of Texas, Dallas)
Am. J. Dis. Child. 137:627–632, July 1983   2–1

The incidence of secondary infection with *Hemophilus influenzae* type b is greatest among household contacts aged 2 years or younger of children with the disease. The authors studied the efficacy of rifampin prophylaxis (20 mg/kg/day in 2 doses for 4 days) in eliminating pharyngeal *H. influenzae* type b from household contacts of 38 patients with invasive *Hemophilus* disease under placebo-controlled conditions.

Index patients ranged in age from 2 to 67 months; 66% were male, 37% were black, and 53% attended a child-care facility. Thirty-four (89%) had meningitis, 3 (8%) had cellulitis, and 1 (3%) had pneumonia. The contact unit comprised 312 persons who were randomly assigned to rifampin or placebo; 22% of the contacts were carriers of *H. influenzae* type b, and 94% were colonized with the same biotype as the index case. No carriers were identified in infants aged 6 months or younger, whereas the rate in children aged 1–4 years was 61%.

At the end of treatment, rifampin efficacy was 91% in subjects younger than age 5 years and 100% in those older than age 5. The carrier rate for *H. influenzae* type b among rifampin-treated subjects was significantly smaller than that of placebo-treated subjects 1 month after prophylaxis. Based on cultures obtained 1–4 weeks after prophylaxis, 22%–25% of rifampin-treated carriers younger than age 5 years were colonized with *H. influenzae* type b, but 75% of placebo-treated carriers were still positive at this time.

Failure of rifampin to eradicate *H. influenzae* type b organisms may result from inexact dosage due to loss of rifampin during preparation of suspension, reduced absorption when rifampin is given with food, individual variation in absorption or metabolism of rifampin, temporary suppression of *H. influenzae* type b without eradication, or reacquisition of the organism after treatment. In one *H. influenzae* type b strain, resistance to rifampin developed during the present study.

The Committee on Infectious Diseases of the American Academy of Pediatrics has issued recommendations for rifampin prophylaxis of *H. influenzae* type b disease for all index patients, adult and pediatric household contacts in the presence of a child younger than age 4 years, and children and adult workers in day-care centers in which there has been an index case. The practice of giving rifampin to index patients without including other members of the household and nonresident contacts younger than age 4 years is questionable. In the present study there were 16 contacts, on the average, per index case. It remains to be determined whether rifampin prophylaxis will bring with it a reduction in *H. influenzae* type b disease significant and sustained enough to justify the cost ($10 per 4-day course) and other problems inherent in its widespread use.

▶ We start off this section with a tough problem. Fortunately, we have good help. Ralph Feigin, J. S. Abercrombie Professor of Pediatrics, and Chairman, Department of Pediatrics, Baylor College of Medicine, comments as follows:

"This article brings into sharp focus the continuing controversy and concern with regard to rifampin prophylaxis of *Hemophilus influenzae* infection in both household and day-care center contacts of an index case.

"The most comprehensive study that has examined the spread of *Hemophilus* infection among household contacts was coordinated by the Centers for Disease Control (*N. Engl. J. Med.* 301:122–126, 1979), in which they analyzed data collected prospectively from 19 states. *Hemophilus influenzae* meningitis was reported in 1,403 patients. Eighty-two percent of exposed families were investigated for the occurrence of *H. influenzae* invasive disease within 30 days of its onset in the index patient. In 9 of 1,687 contacts (0.5%) who were younger than age 6 years, systemic disease due to *H. influenzae* type b developed. The risk in children younger than age 1 year was 6%; the risk in patients less than age 4 years was 2.1%. In the 30 days after the onset of meningitis in the index case, the risk of secondary infection of household contacts proved to be 585 times greater than the age-adjusted risk in the general population and was similar to the risk of secondary meningococcal disease in household contacts. This nationwide study provided the impetus for finding a chemoprophylactic regimen that could prevent secondary infection in households.

"Between 1978 and 1984, a number of regimens were studied, including the use of ampicillin, cefaclor, erythromycin-sulfa and trimethoprim-sulfamethoxazole. None of these drugs or drug combinations reliably eradicated the carriage of *H. influenzae* from the nasopharynx of children.

"A number of studies have appeared between 1978 and the present time in which investigators have utilized rifampin to determine if it was efficacious in eradicating nasopharyngeal carriage of *H. influenzae* type b organisms. Some of these studies were retrospective, others prospective, some randomized, and others nonrandomized. Regardless of the study design, a 20-mg/kg dose provided once each day for 4 days proved to be far superior in eradicating nasopharyngeal carriage of *H. influenzae* than was a 10-mg/kg dose once a day or a 10-mg/kg dose given twice each day (*Pediatrics* 67:430–433, 1981; *Br. Med. J.* 2:899–901, 1980; *Pediatrics* 63:397–401, 1979; *J. Pediatr.* 97:854–860, 1980; ibid. 92:713–717, 1978; and ibid. 98:485–491, 1981).

"On the basis of an analysis of these data, the Infectious Disease Committee of the American Academy of Pediatrics recommended that rifampin be provided orally once each day for 4 days in a 20-mg/kg dose (maximum dose, 600 mg/day) to all household contacts (children and adults) in households where there are children (other than the index case) younger than age 4 years. An implicit portion of the American Academy of Pediatrics recommendation is the statement, *often overlooked,* that exposed children who develop a febrile illness should receive prompt medical evaluation and, if indicated, antimicrobial therapy appropriate for *H. influenzae* invasive disease whether or not they are already receiving rifampin prophylaxis. Although the Infectious Disease Committee of the American Academy of Pediatrics also made a similar recommendation for nursery school and day-care center contacts, they have reconsidered this latter recommendation recently and no longer insist on its use when only a single case has been reported in a day-care center. It should be emphasized that there is no information to document the safety of rifampin during pregnancy. Therefore, prophylaxis with rifampin is not recommended for pregnant women who are contacts of affected infants or who are known carriers of *H. influenzae* type b.

"The recommendations for rifampin prophylaxis of household contacts have been made following a detailed consideration of the cost of the drug, its possible nonavailability in certain communities, the possibility that resistance to rifampin might develop among selected isolates of *H. influenzae* type b, the difficulties that might be encountered because rifampin is formulated as a capsule, and the possibility that prophylaxis may eradicate carriage from some children in whom the carriage of *H. influenzae* type b might subsequently elicit an antibody response that could protect them from invasive disease.

"Although the cost of providing rifampin often is raised as a particularly important issue, a cost-benefit analysis reveals the following: (1) the cost of rifampin to treat a family of 6 would average $55–$60; (2) the cost to society to prevent 1 case of *H. influenzae* disease, based on a secondary attack rate of 2% and estimating the efficacy of rifampin in eliminating nasopharyngeal carriage at 90%, is $2,500; and (3) the cost of 1 case of *H. influenzae* disease (acute care costs only) is $10,000. Clearly, the cost of rifampin cannot be a serious consideration when related to the cost of *H. influenzae* invasive disease to either the family or to society.

"Children with invasive disease frequently continue to carry *H. influenzae* type b in the nasopharynx despite optimal systemic therapy for their disease. For this reason, prior to discharge from the hospital, all children with invasive *H. influenzae* infection who are returning to a household in which another child younger than age 4 years resides should receive rifampin therapy (once daily for 4 days in a 20-mg/kg dose; maximum dose, 600 mg/day) to avoid reintroduction of the organism into their household.

"The more elusive issue is to determine whether or not the use of rifampin prophylaxis not only is effective in eliminating nasopharyngeal carriage but actually is efficacious in preventing secondary disease. A nationwide collaborative prospective study was organized by the Centers for Disease Control several years ago. This was a multicenter prospective placebo-controlled trial among household (children younger than age 6 years) and day-care center contacts of persons with invasive *H. influenzae* type b disease. Three hundred twenty-five index patients constituted the study population. There were 1,365 household contacts and 584 day-care center contacts of the index patients. Rifampin was provided during this study in a 10-mg/kg dose for 2–4 days or a 20-mg/kg dose for 4 days or a placebo was provided. The 20-mg/kg dose for 4 days was given after previous studies (see above) documented the superiority of that regimen to the 10-mg/kg/dose regimen. Because a change in recommendation was made during the course of this prospective study and incorporated within the study design after the study was under way, it is difficult to analyze the study results. Nevertheless, at the time this study was terminated, 4 of 839 (0.5%) placebo-treated contacts developed secondary invasive *H. influenzae* disease compared to 0 of 1,101 rifampin-treated contacts. This difference was statistically significant at $P = .03$. To date, the study has been presented only in abstract form (abstract 17, read before the 21st Interscience Conference on Antimicrobial Agents and Chemotherapy, Chicago, Ill., Nov. 4–6, 1981). It should be noted that if 1 patient from the placebo-treated group is moved to the rifampin-treated group, the difference is not statistically significant. It also should be pointed out that the authors of this study analyzed the data by lumping together both household and day-care center contacts. When a separate analysis of the data is made for each of these groups of contacts separately, no significance is achieved for day-care center contacts of persons with *H. influenzae* infection.

"It is indeed unfortunate that the only prospective national study was terminated prior to a time where the question with regard to efficacy of this regimen could be answered conclusively. It is unlikely that a similar study will ever be repeated because of the high frequency of secondary cases in household contacts and the efficacy of rifampin, 20 mg/kg once daily for 4 days, in eliminating nasopharyngeal carriage. Thus, it is unlikely that recommendations with regard to chemoprophylaxis of household contacts will change in the foreseeable future.

"Ultimately, the answer to prevention of all cases of invasive *H. influenzae* disease awaits the development of an effective vaccine that not only elicits an antibody response reliably in children as young as 3 months of age but also proves to be effective in the prevention of *H. influenzae* invasive disease."

Treatment of Occult Bacteremia: A Prospective Randomized Clinical Trial
William L. Carroll, Michael K. Farrell, Jonathan I. Singer, Mary Anne Jackson, Jeffrey S. Lobel and Edward D. Lewis (Univ. of Cincinnati)
Pediatrics 72:608–612, November 1983   2–2

Antibiotic therapy for children without foci of infection and at risk for bacteremia is controversial. The authors conducted a prospective randomized clinical trial using expectant antibiotic therapy in children at risk for bacteremia. A total of 96 children, aged 6–24 months, with temperatures of more than 40 C, no identifiable source of infection, and a leukocyte count $\geq 15,000/\mu l$ or sedimentation rate ≥ 30, or both, were enrolled. All children had blood culture, chest roentgenogram, urinalysis, and urine culture performed. A lumbar puncture was performed if a child was aged 12 months or younger. Patients were randomized to receive either no antibiotic therapy or Bicillin C-R, 50,000 units/kg intramuscularly, followed by penicillin V, 100 mg/kg per day, orally 4 times a day for 3 days.

Patients were examined at 24 and 72 hours. Fifty were treated expectantly and 46 received no antibiotic.

Results showed that 10 of the 96 patients were bacteremic (10.4%), 5 from each study group. *Streptococcus pneumoniae* was cultured in 9, and *Hemophilus influenzae* type b in 1. Table 1 shows there were no differences in mean age, initial temperature, white blood cell (WBC) count, or erythrocyte sedimentation rate between the treated and untreated children. Bacteremic children had a significantly higher WBC count than nonbacteremic children (Table 2). Lumbar punctures were performed in 8 of the bacteremic children; 4 from each group. The outcome of bacteremia is shown in Table 3. The final diagnosis of the nonbacteremic children was similar

TABLE 1.—CLINICAL AND LABORATORY FEATURES OF PATIENTS: EXPECTANT THERAPY VS. NO EXPECTANT THERAPY*

	Age (mo)	Temperature (°C)	WBC Count (/μL)	ESR (mm/h)
Expectant therapy (n = 50)	13.3 ± 0.74	39.9 ± 0.1	19,046 ± 789	32.8 ± 2.2
No expectant therapy (n = 46)	13.6 ± 0.75	39.9 ± 0.1	20,022 ± 867	31.6 ± 1.9

*Values are means ± SEM.
(Courtesy of Carroll, W.L., et al.: Pediatrics 72:608–612, November 1983. Copyright American Academy of Pediatrics 1983.)

TABLE 2.—CLINICAL AND LABORATORY FEATURES OF PATIENTS: NONBACTEREMIC VS. BACTEREMIC CASES*

	Age (mo)	Temperature (°C)	WBC Count (/μL)	ESR (mm/h)
Nonbacteremic (n = 86)	13.2 ± 1.7	39.9 ± 0.2	19,000 ± 1,647†	32.6 ± 4.4
Bacteremic (n = 10)	12.4 ± 0.5	40.1 ± 0.1	23,790 ± 870	27.3 ± 1.7
Expectant therapy (n = 5)	12.8 ± 2.4	40.0 ± 0.3	24,180 ± 3,263	29.4 ± 8.9
No expectant therapy (n = 5)	12.0 ± 1.6	40.1 ± 0.2	23,400 ± 4,083	24.8 ± 5.1

*Values are means ± SEM.
†Significantly less than counts for bacteremic children ($P < .02$, Student's t test).
(Courtesy of Carroll, W.L., et al.: Pediatrics 72:608–612, November 1983. Copyright American Academy of Pediatrics 1983.)

TABLE 3.—OUTCOME OF PATIENTS WITH OCCULT BACTEREMIA

	Expectant Therapy	No Expectant Therapy
Improved*	4	0
Unimproved	1	5†
Persistant fever with no focus	1	1
Otitis media	0	2
Meningitis	0	2

*Afebrile with no identifiable focus and negative follow-up blood culture at 48 hours.
†$P < .05$ Fisher exact test.
(Courtesy of Carroll, W.L., et al.: Pediatrics 72:608–612, November 1983. Copyright American Academy of Pediatrics 1983.)

TABLE 4.—FINAL DIAGNOSIS OF NONBACTEREMIC
CHILDREN

	Expectant Therapy	No Expectant Therapy
Nonspecific illness	38	34
Identifiable illness		
Aseptic meningitis	0	1
Otitis media	3	2
Pharyngitis (Group A *Streptococcus*)	0	2*
Pneumonia	1	2
Salmonella	1	1*
Urinary tract infection	2	0
Total	45	41

*One patient with salmonellosis and streptococcal pharyngitis.
(Courtesy of Carroll, W.L., et al.: Pediatrics 72:608–612, November 1983. Copyright American Academy of Pediatrics 1983.)

whether or not they received expectant therapy (Table 4). All children were specifically monitored for allergic reactions.

Based on these results, the authors recommend expectant antibiotic therapy for children who have no obvious source of infection and who have the clinical characteristics associated with occult bacteremia. Because this group of children is at risk for developing serious illness, close clinical follow-up is mandatory.

▶ Here is another tricky area that is surrounded with controversy. Help comes from Paul McCarthy, Professor of Pediatrics, Yale University School of Medicine, who supplies the following:

"The study by Carroll et al. is one of several reports that has addressed the issue of expectant antibiotic therapy for febrile children at risk of bacteremia and is one of two *prospective* studies regarding expectant antibiotics. Carroll et al. found that significantly more bacteremic children were unimproved at follow-up when no antibiotics were used than when expectant antibiotics were used (Table 3). The follow-up assessments, however, were not blinded as to study group. Significant differences in the proportion of unimproved children among treated versus untreated patients would not persist if otitis media were excluded from the analysis. Jaffe et al. (*Abstracts, Ambulatory Pediatric Association,* Washington, D.C., p. 28, 1983), in a randomized double-blind trial of expectant outpatient oral amoxicillin versus placebo for presumptive bacteremia, have enrolled 475 children aged 3–36 months with fever >39.0 C and no apparent focus of infection. Among the 19 bacteremic children, there was no significant difference in the occurrence of *serious* complications (persisting bacteremia or focal complications *other than otitis media*) among those treated with placebo (N = 6) versus amoxicillin (N = 13). Even though the study now encompasses 1,000 patients, 27 of whom were bacteremic (Gary Fleisher, Grand Rounds, Yale-New Haven Hospital, Apr. 25, 1984), and no differences in the frequency of serious complications have been seen between placebo- and amoxicillin-treated patients, the number of bacteremic children studied has been insufficient to state that, in fact, there is no difference in serious complications between those treated and untreated, that is, the power of their study is not of sufficient magnitude to accept the null hypothesis.

"Two retrospective studies (Teele et al.: *Pediatr. Clin North Am.* 26:773, 1979; and Wood et al.: *Abstracts, Ambulatory Pediatric Association,* Washington, D.C., p. 25, 1983) have accumulated larger numbers of bacteremic children, and both reports note fewer complications in antibiotic-treated children. For example, Woods et al. note that of 194 bacteremias in outpatients that were caused by *S. pneumoniae,* 85 were untreated and 109 were treated. Twelve percent of untreated children developed a major complication (2, meningitis; 1, periorbital cellulitis; 5, pneumonias; and 1, adenitis), whereas only 2.8% of treated children developed a major complication (3, pneumonias). The difference in major complications at follow-up between treated and untreated children is significant, $P < .025$. There are, however, many methodologic problems that make it difficult to answer questions about drug efficacy from retrospective analysis, the most important being the lack of comparability of those who are treated versus those who are not treated.

"Thus, 3 of 4 available studies support expectant antibiotic therapy for presumptive bacteremia but do have major methodologic flaws. The largest and most carefully designed prospective study has insufficient statistical power to resolve this issue.

"Perhaps in the near future sufficient numbers of prospectively studied patients will be accumulated to answer this question more definitively. In the interim, my own bias is to use expectant oral amoxicillin therapy for children ≤24 months who are at increased risk for bacteremia, that is, for children with fever ≥39.0 C, WBC ≥15,000, and with either no focus of infection or otitis media. If a child meets these criteria but also appears ill, then inpatient intravenous antibiotic therapy is warranted."

Which Children With Febrile Seizures Need Lumbar Puncture?: A Decision Analysis Approach
Alain Joffe, Marie McCormick, and Catherine DeAngelis
Am. J. Dis. Child. 137:1153–1156, December 1983   2–3

Whether or not all children brought to the emergency room with a first seizure and fever require lumbar puncture (LP) remains controversial. The authors reviewed the emergency room records of 241 children aged 6 months to 6 years who had this clinical picture when brought to the emergency room at Sinai Hospital or Johns Hopkins Hospital, Baltimore, in 1978 through 1980 and sought to identify factors that could serve as a screening test for meningitis and as a guide in selecting patients warranting LP.

Although a total of 254 patients were eligible for this study, only the 241 who had LP were included. Of these 241, 228 (94.6%) did not have meningitis (group 1). Thirteen (5.4%) had pleocytosis of the cerebrospinal fluid (CSF) and were hospitalized (group 2). Eleven of the 13 had positive bacterial cultures of CSF.

Five items in the history and physical examination discriminated significantly between children who had meningitis and those who did not: (1) a visit to a physician in the 48 hours prior to seizure, (2) seizure on arrival at the emergency room, (3) type of seizure (focal versus generalized), (4) suspicious findings on physical examination, and (5) abnormal findings on neurologic examination.

Results of the analysis are shown in Table 1. The sensitivity, specificity, and positive and negative predictive value (PV) of each of the five items are shown in Table 2. Abnormal findings on neurologic examination proved to be the most sensitive factor for detecting meningitis and also had the highest negative PV. Results of combining some of these factors are shown in Table 3. Selecting children who had had either a prior visit to a physician or abnormal findings on neurologic examination, or both, would have identified all children with meningitis who required inpatient therapy and would have spared 144 children the need for LP. If LP was performed only on a child who had one or more risk factors, 137 children (62% without meningitis) would not have undergone LP.

It is concluded that routine LP is not warranted if the five risk factors

TABLE 1.—CHARACTERISTICS OF STUDY GROUPS

	Group*		
Characteristic	1	2	P
n	228	13	...
Mean age, mo	23	22	NS
% male	63	46	NS
% nonwhite	74	46	NS
% who saw physician within 48 hr before seizure	16.2	46.2	<.01
% who had seizure on arrival at emergency room	3.9	23.0	<.05
% with focal seizure	8.8	38.5	<.01
% with suspicious physical findings	4.4	23.1	<.05
% with abnormal neurologic findings	16.3	92.3	<.001

*Group 1 had febrile seizures; group 2 had meningitis.
(Courtesy of Joffe, A., et al.: Am. J. Dis. Child. 137:1153–1156, December 1983; copyright 1983, American Medical Association.)

TABLE 2.—SENSITIVITY, SPECIFICITY, AND POSITIVE AND NEGATIVE PREDICTIVE VALUES OF RISK FACTORS AS SCREENING TESTS FOR MENINGITIS*

	Sensitivity	Specificity	+PV†	−PV
Sought care	0.46	0.84	0.14	0.96
Had seizure at emergency room	0.23	0.96	0.27	0.95
Focal seizure	0.38	0.91	0.20	0.96
Suspicious physical findings	0.23	0.97	0.23	0.96
Abnormal neurologic findings	0.92	0.84	0.26	0.99

*Group 1 versus group 2.
PV, predictive value.
(Courtesy of Joffe, A., et al.: Am. J. Dis. Child. 137:1153–1156, December 1983; copyright 1983, American Medical Association.)

TABLE 3.—Sensitivity, Specificity, and Positive and Negative
Predictive Values of Risk Factors Used in Combination

	Sensitivity	Specificity	+PV*	−PV
Sought care or focal seizure	0.69	0.78	0.16	0.98
Sought care or abnormal neurologic findings	1.00	0.71	0.16	1.00
Sought care or had seizure at emergency room	0.54	0.82	0.15	0.97
Focal seizure or suspicious physical findings	0.46	0.89	0.20	0.97
Focal seizure or abnormal neurologic findings	0.92	0.82	0.24	0.99
Any of 5 above	1.00	0.62	0.13	1.00

*PV, predictive value.
(Courtesy of Joffe, A., et al.: Am. J. Dis. Child. 137:1153–1156, December 1983; copyright 1983, American Medical Association.)

are lacking. In reaching this conclusion the authors assume that a careful history and physical examination have been performed and that immediate follow-up for children not receiving an LP is available. If these assumptions are not met, LP may still be warranted.

▶ The authors base their recommendations on two very important assumptions, i.e., that a careful history and physical examination have been performed and that immediate follow-up is available for those patients not receiving a lumbar puncture. By the way, suspicious findings on physical examination included rash or petechiae, cyanosis, hypotension, and grunting respirations—nothing very subtle. Abnormal findings on neurologic examination included stiff neck, increased tone, deviated eyes, ataxia, no response to voice, inability to fix and follow, no response to painful stimuli, positive doll's eye sign, floppy muscle tone, nystagmus, and bulging to tense fontanelle— again, nothing subtle. The authors had a 5% rate of abnormal cerebrospinal fluid findings. Is that too high or too low? For more on seizures and fever, please look at the following article.—F.A.O.

Convulsions in Shigellosis: Evaluation of Possible Risk Factors
Shai Ashkenazi, Gabriel Dinari, Raphael Weitz, and Menachem Nitzan (Tel Aviv Univ.)
Am. J. Dis. Child. 137:985–987, October 1983   2–4

Convulsions occur more often in children with shigellosis than in those with other common febrile infections. The authors studied risk factors for development of convulsions in 158 children with shigellosis.

Of the 158 children, 37 (23.4%) had convulsions. The convulsions were generalized and all lasted less than 10 minutes. One child had postictal coma lasting 24 hours, and 2 others had two or three recurrent convulsive episodes. No child had clinical or cerebrospinal fluid evidence of meningitis. Of the historical, clinical, and laboratory data compared between

POSSIBLE RISK FACTORS FOR CONVULSIONS IN 158 CHILDREN WITH
SHIGELLOSIS

Factor	Children With Convulsions	Children Without Convulsions	P
Age, yr	3.79 ± 2.35*	5.77 ± 3.27	<.005
Family history of convulsions, %	15.2	1.1	<.01
Individual history of febrile convulsions, %	15.2	3.3	NS
M:F ratio	1.5:1	1.2:1	NS
Temperature peak, °C	39.6 ± 0.6	39.2 ± 0.8	<.01
Bloody or mucous stool, %	38.9	37.7	NS
Hematocrit level, %	36.7 ± 4.2	36.6 ± 3.5	NS
Leukocyte count, 10⁹/L	8.66 ± 2.62	8.84 ± 2.70	NS
Absolute band count, 10⁹/L	1.91 ± 1.31	2.01 ± 1.41	NS
Glucose level, mmole/L	6.7 ± 2.3	6.3 ± 1.9	NS
Calcium level, mmole/L	2.3 ± 0.3	2.3 ± 0.2	NS
Serum urea nitrogen level, mmole/L	3.5 ± 1.8	4.3 ± 1.7	NS
Sodium level, mmole/L	133.7 ± 3.6	134.2 ± 3.8	NS
Potassium level, mmole/L	3.9 ± 0.6	3.9 ± 0.5	NS
pH	7.34 ± 0.68	7.39 ± 0.05	NS
Base excess, mmole/L	−7.8 ± 2.8	−5.0 ± 3.6	<.005
Standard bicarbonate, mmole/L	16.9 ± 2.8	17.5 ± 3.0	NS

*Mean ± SD.
(Courtesy of Ashkenazi, S., et al.: Am. J. Dis. Child. 137:985–987, October 1983; copyright 1983, American Medical Association.)

children with and without convulsions (table), only age, family history of convulsions, peak temperature, and base deficit differed significantly. Of children with convulsions, 73% were between 0.5 and 4 years of age; the oldest was 11 years. Multivariate analysis showed that age, temperature peak, and family history of convulsive disorders independently influenced the risk of seizures. The incidence of seizures was slightly, but not significantly, higher in *Shigella flexneri* infections than in *S. sonnei, S. boydii,* or *S. dysenteriae* infections.

In a child with shigellosis, young age, a high peak temperature, and a family history of seizures should alert the physician to the possibility of a convulsive episode.

Simultaneous Determination of Cerebrospinal Fluid Glucose and Blood Glucose Concentrations in the Diagnosis of Bacterial Meningitis

Peter R. Donald, Christina Malan, and Adri van der Walt (Tygerberg, South Africa)

J. Pediatr. 103:413–415, September 1983

2–5

Evaluation of glucose concentration in cerebrospinal fluid (CSF) is of greatest importance in children with possible bacterial meningitis. Simultaneous determination of glucose concentration in CSF and in blood was done in 119 of 201 children with bacterial meningitis seen at a pediatric emergency room over a 2-year period. Determinations were made at admission, prior to initiation of therapy. Causative organisms encountered were *Neisseria meningitidis* (101 patients), *Streptococcus pneumoniae* (10), *Hemophilus influenzae* (5), *Escherichia coli* (1), *Staphylococcus aureus* (1), and *Salmonella* group B (1). Predominance of *N. meningitidis* resulted from an epidemic of meningococcal disease at the time. Mean age of patients was 28.7 months.

Results obtained in these patients were compared with those for 97 children seen during the same period with aseptic meningitis and 133 children with no meningitis. In the group with aseptic meningitis the CSF contained more than 5 leukocytes/cu mm. Gram's stain revealed no organisms and no bacteria were grown from CSF or blood. Viral culture of CSF was positive in 24 cases; most demonstrated enteroviruses. In the group with no meningitis both CSF and blood were sterile on culture.

Absolute glucose values in CSF and CSF-blood glucose ratios of the three groups are compared in Figures 2–1 and 2–2. Greatest specificity (100%) was reached with a CSF-blood glucose ratio of 0.30; sensitivity of the test at this level was only 69.75%. A ratio of 0.40 achieved a sensitivity of 79.83% and a specificity of 97.73%, but a ratio of 0.50 had a sensitivity of 86.55% and a specificity of 85.91%. Absolute glucose concentration in CSF of 2.2 mmol/L achieved a sensitivity of 72.27% and a specificity of 99.10%.

Glucose concentration in CSF is dependent on that in blood. Glucose concentration in blood of acutely ill children in whom meningitis is suspected may not be constant; neither may be the relationship of glucose in blood to glucose in CSF. Experience suggests that a CSF-blood glucose ratio of 0.40 or an absolute glucose concentration in CSF of 2.2 mmol/L provides realistic lower "limits" of "normal." Values below these limits are highly specific for bacterial meningitis. Whatever the level chosen, a

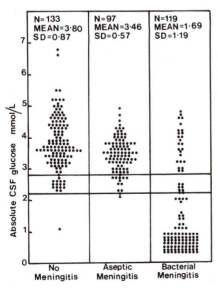

Fig 2–1.—Absolute CSF glucose values in three study groups. Multiplication factor for conversion of blood and CSF glucose SI units to traditional units, 18. (Courtesy of Donald, P.R., et al.: J. Pediatr. 103:413–415, September 1983.)

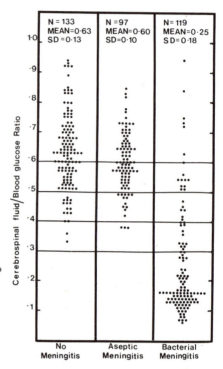

Fig 2–2.—The CSF-blood glucose ratios in three study groups. (Mean blood glucose value: no meningitis 6.142 mmol/l, SD = 1.505; aseptic meningitis 5.860 mmol/l, SD = 0.976; bacterial meningitis 7.069 mmol/l, SD = 2.543.) (Courtesy of Donald, P.R., et al.: J. Pediatr. 103:413–415, September 1983.)

large percentage of patients with bacterial meningitis (from 13.5% to 21% in this series) will have normal glucose concentrations in CSF.

▶ Leonard Weiner, Associate Professor of Pediatrics, and Chief, Division of Infectious Disease, State University of New York Upstate Medical Center, comments:

"This article carefully underscores the variability of CSF glucose values encountered in patients with bacterial meningitis. Considering the adequate sample size and appropriate age matching of the three patient subpopulations in this study, the results are most convincing. Despite the 100% specificity associated with a CSF-blood glucose ratio of 0.30, the sensitivity was only 69.75%. As the authors point out, 'whatever the level chosen, there will be a large percentage of patients with bacterial meningitis, from 13.5% to 21% in our series, with a normal CSF glucose concentration.'

"It is unfortunate for the pediatric practitioner that no CSF parameter exists that allows for the clear-cut definition of bacterial from nonbacterial meningitis. Because meningeal and brain inflammation underlie the CSF changes associated with all of these infections, it is not surprising that various etiologic agents stimulate overlapping CSF findings. The inflammatory process per se and not the infecting agent is responsible for the disturbance in central nervous system glucose transport. For example, some patients with viral meningitis due to mumps, enteroviruses, and herpes simplex virus have CSF glucose levels of less than 40 mg/dl. Other investigators have shown that CSF total white blood cells, percent polymorphonuclear leukocytes, or mononuclear cell counts, lactic dehydrogenase, lactic acid, and pH determinations fail to differentiate etiologies of meningitis completely. Many children with enteroviral meningitis, especially young infants, have initial CSF findings with greater than 200 white blood cells/cu mm or polymorphonuclear leukocyte predominance, or both.

"Of the 119 patients in this study with bacterial meningitis, 101 had *N. meningitidis* meningitis. This is not the usual distribution encountered in the United States. *Neisseria meningitidis* tends to produce less in the way of CSF inflammatory changes than either *H. influenzae* or *S. pneumoniae*. An increased frequency of normal CSF lactic dehydrogenase values in meningococcal meningitis has been noted previously. It would be interesting to know how many of the 33 patients with bacterial meningitis and CSF glucose levels greater that 40 mg/dl in this study had *N. meningitidis* as the causative organism."

Prospective Comparative Trial of Moxalactam Versus Ampicillin or Chloramphenicol for Treatment of *Hemophilus influenzae* Type b Meningitis in Children

Sheldon L. Kaplan, Edward O. Mason, Jr., Sally K. Mason, Francis I. Catlin, Rita T. Lee, Mary Murphy, and Ralph D. Feigin (Baylor College of Medicine)
J. Pediatr. 104:447–453, March 1984   2–6

Isolates of *Hemophilus influenzae* b (HIB) are resistant to both ampicillin and chloramphenicol. Moxalactam is highly active in vitro against HIB and is effective in the treatment of non-CNS infections caused by HIB in children. The efficacy of moxalactam was compared with that of ampicillin and chloramphenicol in children at least as old as 2 months with bacterial meningitis caused by HIB. Forty-four children received moxalactam, 100 mg/kg, followed by 200 mg/kg daily, intravenously; 47 received ampicillin, 300 mg/kg daily after a loading dose of 100 mg/kg, or chloramphenicol in a dose of 100 mg/kg daily. Chloramphenicol treatment was discontinued if the HIB isolate was found to be sensitive to ampicillin.

The cerebrospinal fluid (CSF) findings were similar in the two treatment groups. More of the ampicillin-chloramphenicol group received previous oral antibiotic therapy. The hospital course was similar in the two groups (Table 1). Adverse effects of treatment are shown in Table 2. Half of the children in each group were followed up for at least a year after discharge. Five survivors (6%) had severe to profound bilateral hearing loss as a result of HIB meningitis (Table 3). Hearing loss was related to a lower initial CSF glucose level, but not to duration of illness before admission. Higher levels of polyribosephosphate in the CSF also were related to hearing loss.

Moxalactam appears to be as effective as ampicillin or chloramphenicol is in the treatment of children with HIB meningitis. Ampicillin still is recommended for use in susceptible patients, however. Moxalactam is considered for use in treating meningitis caused by HIB that is resistant

TABLE 1.—Selected Laboratory and Clinical Features of Hospital Course in Study Children

	Ampicillin-chloramphenicol		Moxalactam	
	$\overline{X} \pm 1\ SD$	Range	$\overline{X} \pm 1\ SD$	Range
Initial peripheral WBC count ($\times 10^{-3}$/mm³)	13.6 ± 7.2	2.4 to 35.4	13.5 ± 8.4	3.5 to 36.2
Initial serum sodium (mEq/L)	134 ± 4	118 to 140	135 ± 4	124 to 147
Number <135 mEq/L	26 (55%)		19 (43%)	
Lowest serum sodium (mEq/L)	132 ± 3	118 to 139	133 ± 4	124 to 147
Duration of hyponatremia (hr)	18.5 ± 28.3	0 to 144	16.6 ± 38.4	0 to 240
Duration of fever (days)	5.0 ± 3.6	0 to 16	5.3 ± 4.6	0 to 20
Afebrile after 5 days	68%		67%	
Afebrile after 8 days	80%		84%	
Seizures in hospital	13 (28%)		10 (23%)	
Duration of antibiotic therapy (days)	10.8 ± 1.7	10 to 16	10.7 ± 1.7	10 to 17
>10 days	9/44		6/42	

(Courtesy of Kaplan, S.L., et al.: J. Pediatr. 104:447–453, March 1984.)

TABLE 2.—Adverse Effects of Antibiotics in Study Children

	Ampicillin-chloramphenicol (n = 35)		Moxalactam (n = 41)	
	n	%	n	%
Neutropenia				
<1500/mm³	4	11.4	9	22.0
<1000/mm³	2	5.7	3	7.3
Eosinophilia >700/mm³	5	14.3	6	14.6
Thrombocytosis	3	8.6	11	26.8
Thrombocytopenia	1	2.9	1	2.4
Diarrhea	4	11.4	11	26.8
Mild elevation in transaminases*	ND		7	

ND = not done.
*Less than twice normal values.
(Courtesy of Kaplan, S.L., et al.: J. Pediatr. 104:447–453, March 1984.)

TABLE 3.—Selected Characteristics of Children With Profound Sensorineural Hearing Loss

Age at onset (yr)	Duration of illness prior to admission	Seizures	CSF cell count (/mm³)	CSF glucose (mg/dl)	Quantitative PRP determination in CSF (gm/ml)	Prolonged fever (days)	Therapy
$^{11}/_{12}$	36 hr	−	3,039	4	5.12	9	Chloramphenicol
$^{9}/_{12}$	48 hr	+	Clumped	2	5.12	−	Ampicillin
$2^{5}/_{12}$	3 day	−	3,800	15	0.64	−	Moxalactam
$^{11}/_{12}$	5 days	+	42,500	<10	5.12	−	Moxalactam
$1^{5}/_{12}$	6 days	+	38,160	5	10.24	11	Chloramphenicol

(Courtesy of Kaplan, S.L., et al.: J. Pediatr. 104:447–453, March 1984.)

to both ampicillin and chloramphenicol. Cefotaxime and ceftriaxone also hold promise for the treatment of HIB meningitis.

▶ Moxalactam is a semisynthetic oxa-β-lactam antibiotic that is highly effective in vitro against both β-lactamase-positive and β-lactamase-negative strains of *H. influenzae* type b, including strains that are now recognized to be resistant to chloramphenicol. In contrast to previously produced cephalosporins, moxalactam gets into the cerebrospinal fluid of children with meningitis in very adequate concentrations. It previously has been shown to be effective and safe in children with a variety of non-central nervous system infections. S. A. Chartrand and co-workers (*J. Pediatr.* 104:454, 1984), in a study similar to the one described above, involving 34 children with *H. influenzae* meningitis, also demonstrated that it was as effective as the combination of ampicillin and chloramphenicol. For another effective alternative for the treatment of bacterial meningitis in children, see the following pair of articles.—F.A.O.

Ceftriaxone Versus Ampicillin and Chloramphenicol for Treatment of Bacterial Meningitis in Children
Maria de los A. del Rio, Dale Chrane, Sharon Shelton, George H. McCracken, Jr., and John D. Nelson (Univ. of Texas Health Science Center, Dallas)
Lancet 1:1241–1244, June 4, 1983   2–7

Seventy-eight patients with bacterial meningitis were evaluated in a prospective, randomized study. The groups were comparable in age, sex, days of illness prior to admission, and bacterial colony counts in cerebrospinal fluid (CSF).

Thirty-nine patients treated with ceftriaxone received an intravenous loading dose of 75 mg/kg followed by 50 mg/kg twice daily. Ampicillin (200 mg/kg/day in 4 equal doses) and chloramphenicol (100 mg/kg/day in 4 equal doses) were given to 39 patients by intravenous infusion. Duration of treatment was 10 days, but patients with meningococcal meningitis were treated for 7 days. Cultures and routine examination of blood and CSF were done on hospital admission. Pathogens were *Hemophilus influenzae* (54), streptococci (9), meningococci (9), or unknown (6).

In the ceftriaxone group, 21 patients had repeat lumbar punctures 4–12 hours after the first dose; of the 9 positive cultures, 8 were *H. influenzae* (Table 1) with mean colony counts of 8.8×10^6/ml. Mean decrease in CSF colony count was $4.7 \log_{10}$ colony-forming units/ml. In the comparative group, 19 patients had repeat lumbar puncture 5–12 hours after the first dose of antibiotics; 11 of 16 patients with *H. influenzae* infection had positive cultures with mean colony counts of 2.3×10^4/ml. Mean decrease in CSF colony count was $5.0 \log_{10}$ colony-forming units/ml (Fig 2–3). Minimal bactericidal concentrations were lower for ceftriaxone than for ampicillin in all CSF isolates except group B streptococci and pneumococci (Table 2).

There were no deaths, but 1 patient in each group had devastating

TABLE 1.—Culture Results of First Follow-up CSF
Specimens

	Number positive/number tested (%)	
Treatment	CSF at 4–12 h	CSF at >12 h
Ceftriaxone:		
All patients	9/21 (43)	1/19 (5)
Haemophilus patients	8/16 (50)	0/6
Ampicillin/chloramphenicol:		
All patients	11/19 (58)	1/20 (5)
Haemophilus patients	11/16 (69)	1/16 (6)

(Courtesy of del Rio, M. A., et al.: Lancet 1:1241–1244, June 4, 1983.)

neurologic sequelae. Numbers of patients with transient or permanent sequelae were similar for both groups. Auditory brain stem evoked response testing 1–5 months after completion of therapy showed abnormal responses (loss greater than 30 dB) in one or both ears in 39% of 57 patients tested, and 7% had conductive hearing loss due to middle ear disease. It is recommended that all children who have had bacterial meningitis have hearing tests.

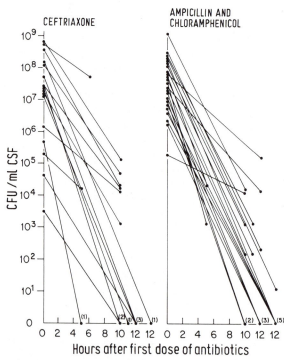

Fig 2–3.—Results of quantitative cultures of CSF before therapy and at the indicated hours after the first dose of antibiotics. Numbers in parentheses indicate number of specimens sterile; *CFU*, colony-forming units. (Courtesy of del Rio, M.A., et al.: Lancet 1:1241–1244, June 4, 1983.)

TABLE 2.—MINIMAL BACTERICIDAL CONCENTRATIONS OF
AMPICILLIN AND CEFTRIAXONE FOR ISOLATES RECOVERED
FROM CSF

Isolate	Number of strains	Range of MBC in μg/ml (median)	
		Ceftriaxone	Ampicillin
H influenzae			
Beta-lactamase negative	39	$\leqslant0\cdot001-0\cdot0312$ (0·002)	0·01−2·0 (0·125)
Beta-lactamase positive	15	$\leqslant0\cdot001-0\cdot008$ ($\leqslant0\cdot004$)	2·5>8 (>8)
N meningitidis	8	$\leqslant0\cdot001$	0·0156−0·08 (0·0156)
Strep pneumoniae	6	0·008−0·0312 (0·0156)	$\leqslant0\cdot008-0\cdot0312$ (0·0312)
Group B streptococcus	2	0·25	0·0625

(Courtesy of del Rio, M.A., et al.: Lancet 1:1241–1244, June 4, 1983.)

Diarrhea occurred more frequently in the ceftriaxone than in the control group; in most cases it was mild and did not require a change in medication. Mean bactericidal titer in CSF was significantly greater in patients receiving ceftriaxone, and there was a trend toward more rapid sterilization of CSF in that group. Bacterial growth was detected only after dilutions were made for quantifying growth, as a specimen containing 10^5 colony-forming units/ml had no growth on plates inoculated with undiluted, $1:10$, and $1:10^2$ dilutions; it showed light growth with a $1:10^3$ dilution and full growth at $1:10^4$ dilution. It is recommended that future studies use dilutions of CSF specimens to unmask viable organisms not detected by routine culture.

Ceftriaxone proved safe and effective for meningitis in this trial. It has the potential advantages over conventional therapy of greater bactericidal activity in CSF and a trend toward more rapid sterilization.

▶ This study and the following one are in agreement and make it clear that ceftriaxone is a suitable one-drug treatment of bacterial meningitis in the infant aged 6 weeks or older. These studies, and article 2–6 describing the efficacy of moxalactam, underscore another far more important point. No matter how effective the drug, the morbidity from meningitis is unacceptably high. In the study of del Rio and associates, 2.5% of the patients had "devastating neurologic sequelae" and 39% had abnormal auditory brain stem evoked potentials, and Steele and Bradsher reported neurologic sequelae in 16% of their group.

It is obvious from all of this that the prevention of meningitis is our best hope. Right now, a vaccine employed in Finland has been reported to be safe and, when used in children older than age 18 months, prevents 90% of cases of invasive *H. influenzae* type b disease (Peltola, H., et al.: *N. Engl. J. Med.* 310:1561, 1984). For more on the status of vaccine, particularly for the child younger than age 2 years, please see two excellent editorials (Lepow, M. L., and Gold, R.: ibid. 308:1158, 1984; and Denny, F. W., Jr.: ibid., p. 1595).

On the lighter side, Bruce Rubin has described a new fourth-generation cephalosporin, which he calls "cephalomacia obfuscate" (*Pediatr. Infect. Dis.* 2:424, 1983). The drug, tentatively named "killacillin," differs from all other cephalosporins in that it is designed to produce pain in the bacteria instead of merely killing it. It belongs to a new class of drug, the bacteropathic antibiotic. Good luck, Doctor Rubin.—F.A.O.

Comparison of Ceftriaxone With Standard Therapy for Bacterial Meningitis
Russell W. Steele and Robert W. Bradsher
J. Pediatr. 103:138–141, July 1983   2–8

The newer β-lactam antibiotics have several unique features that make them particularly attractive in the treatment of bacterial meningitis. These include extremely high in vitro activity against common pathogens, excellent penetration into cerebrospinal fluid (CSF), a broad spectrum of bactericidal activity, and relatively rare toxic effects. Ceftriaxone, a new cephalosporin, has additional advantages through its increased activity against group B *Streptococcus* and its relatively long half-life of 5 to 8 hours.

The therapeutic effects of ceftriaxone (100 mg/kg/day in 2 divided doses) were compared with those of standard therapy (ampicillin, 200 to 400 mg/kg/day, plus chloramphenicol, 100 mg/kg/day, in 4 divided doses) in 30 pediatric patients with bacterial meningitis who were seen at Arkansas Children's Hospital. Four of the patients were aged 14 to 28 days, 22 were infants, and 4 were older than age 2 years.

Hemophilus influenzae was the most frequently isolated organism, followed by *Streptococcus pneumoniae,* group B *Streptococcus, Neisseria meningitidis,* and *Escherichia coli* (table). All organisms were sensitive to ceftriaxone at concentrations of 0.06 µg/ml or less and were susceptible to ampicillin or chloramphenicol at the lowest dilution tested (0.25 µg/ml). Two hours after intravenous infusion of ceftriaxone, concentrations in CSF and plasma in the 15 patients treated with this antibiotic averaged

CEFTRIAXONE SENSITIVITIES FOR ORGANISMS RECOVERED FROM 30 PATIENTS WITH BACTERIAL MENINGITIS

| | Treatment group | | Sensitivity to |
Organism	Ceftriaxone	Standard therapy	ceftriaxone (MIC) (µg/ml)
H. influenzae	6	9	≤0.06
S. pneumoniae	5	3	≤0.06
Group B streptococcus	1	2	≤0.06
N. meningitidis	1	1	≤0.03
E. coli	2	0	≤0.03

(Courtesy of Steele, R.W., and Bradsher, R.W.: J. Pediatr. 103:138–141, July 1983.)

11.0 μg/ml and 128.2 μg/ml, respectively. Thus, average penetration into CSF was 8.6% of plasma concentrations. All samples of CSF were sterile within 24 to 48 hours and other CSF values returned to normal at equivalent rates in the two treatment groups. Patients who received ceftriaxone showed a more rapid return to normal temperature than those who received standard therapy (average, 3.7 versus 5.1 days). However, this difference was not statistically significant in patients with *H. influenzae* (average 4.5 versus 5.3 days). Resolution of other clinical findings did not differ between groups.

No patient died, but 5 developed moderate neurologic sequelae. Three of the 5 had received standard therapy. Four patients, 3 of whom had received ceftriaxone, developed mild diarrhea. There were no local or systemic reactions to ceftriaxone therapy. Six patients who received ceftriaxone and 7 who received standard therapy developed anemia, but this was interpreted as secondary to meningitis, particularly in patients with *H. influenzae.*

In this series there were no clinical or laboratory findings to indicate the therapeutic superiority of ceftriaxone over standard therapy. However, as ceftriaxone penetrates CSF at levels 100 times the minimal inhibitory concentration of the usual pathogens that cause meningitis, ceftriaxone therapy consisting of a 50 mg/kg dose given intravenously every 12 hours compares favorably with standard therapy for patients with bacterial meningitis.

Apparent Meningococcemia: Clinical Features of Disease Due to *Hemophilus influenzae* and *Neisseria meningitidis*

Richard F. Jacobs, Steven Hsi, Christopher B. Wilson, Denis Benjamin, Arnold L. Smith, and Robert Morrow (Univ. of Washington, Seattle)
Pediatrics 72:469–472, October 1983 2–9

Sepsis with coagulopathy, purpura, or adrenal hemorrhage (Waterhouse-Friderichsen syndrome) with or without shock is usually caused by *N. meningitidis* but may also be caused by *H. influenzae* type b. The clinical and laboratory features of 30 cases of apparent meningococcemia caused by *N. meningitidis* were compared with those of 12 cases caused by *H. influenzae.* The 42 cases were seen over a 12-year period.

Compared with patients with disease caused by *H. influenzae,* patients with meningococcal disease were older, more often male, more often became ill in winter or spring, and had a longer duration of antecedent symptoms, but none of these differences was significant. All patients were febrile and appeared to be suffering from toxemia. Similar proportions in each group had shock and disseminated intravascular coagulation on admission (Table 1). Compared with patients with meningococcal disease, those with *H. influenzae* infection were more often lethargic or comatose on admission, had a higher death rate, and had a shorter interval between symptom onset and death. Meningococcal infection was appropriately suspected in some cases from results of Gram-staining procedures (Table

TABLE 1.—CLINICAL PRESENTATION AND OUTCOME

	Neisseria meningitidis (n = 30)	Haemophilus influenzae (n = 12)
Fever (≥38°C)	30	12
Irritable but alert	15	2
Lethargy or coma	15*	10
Vomiting	14	4
Headache	6	1
Rash	30/30	10/12
Petechial	2	4
Purpuric	3	4
Both	25†	2
Maculopapular	1‡	2§
None	0	2
Shock	11	6
Disseminated intravascular coagulation	12	5
Adrenal hemorrhage	2/3‖	5/9
Death	3/30¶	9/12#
Time to death (h) (mean ± SE)	120 ± 74.4*	20.7 ± 4.0

*$P < .05$, compared with *H. influenzae* cases.
†Six children required skin grafts.
‡Petechiae were also present.
§Both were also purpuric.
‖Denominator is no. of patients examined post mortem.
¶$P < .005$, compared with *H. influenzae*; 1 of 14 with meningitis; 2 of 16 without meningitis.
#Six of 9 with meningitis, 3 of 3 without meningitis.
(Courtesy of Jacobs, R.F., et al.: Pediatrics 72:469–472, October 1983. Copyright American Academy of Pediatrics 1983.)

TABLE 2.—LABORATORY FINDINGS AND THERAPY

	Neisseria meningitidis (n = 30)	Haemophilus influenzae (n = 12)
Microbiology		
Blood culture	22	6
Gram stain*	5/9	ND†
CSF culture	14‡	9‡
Gram stain	10/14	7/8
Skin lesion culture	3/13	ND
Gram stain	8/13	ND
Secondary sites of involvement		
Meningitis	14	9
Myocarditis	6	2
Other	Pneumonia, 2; otitis media, 1; osteomyelitis, 1; panophthalmitis, 1	Pneumonia, 2; otitis media, 2; osteomyelitis, 1; septic arthritis, 1; pericarditis, 1
Initial therapy	Penicillin, 11; ampicillin, 19	Penicillin, 5; ampicillin, 7
Complications	Seizures, 2; postmeningitic hydrocephalus, 1; renal failure, dialysis-dependent, 1	Pulmonary hemorrhage, 1

*Buffy-coat Gram's stain.
†ND, not done.
‡Includes patients with sterile blood cultures.
(Courtesy of Jacobs, R.F., et al.: Pediatrics 72:469–472, October 1983. Copyright American Academy of Pediatrics 1983.)

2). In all cases, the organisms were sensitive to penicillin *(N. meningitidis)* or ampicillin *(N. meningitidis* and *H. influenzae)* therapy.

The initial signs, symptoms, foci of infection, or complications do not allow clear distinction between disease caused by these two organisms. Gram stains of the cerebrospinal fluid, skin scrapings from purpuric lesions, and buffy-coat smears are useful in identifying the meningococcus as the causative agent; these techniques should be applied in all such cases. The use of counterimmunoelectrophoresis for meningococcal antigen detection and latex particle agglutination for *H. influenzae* type b antigen detection should improve the determination of the cause of overwhelming sepsis in previously healthy infants. Until the specific agent is identified, such infants should be presumed to have disease caused by either organism and should be treated with chloramphenicol, in addition to penicillin or ampicillin.

▶ Patients with acute meningococcal infections generally fall into three distinct groups based on inspection of the skin; 11% display large purpuric or ecchymotic lesions, 14% have no skin lesions, and 75% have erythematous, macular, or petechial lesions, or some combination of these, on the trunk and extremities (Toews, W. H., and Bass, J. W.: *Am. J. Dis. Child.* 127:173, 1974). As Jacobs and associates emphasize, other infections may produce the same clinical picture. What percent of children presenting with fever and petechiae do, in fact, have a bacterial infection? Q. Van Nguyen and co-workers provide us with an answer to that question (*Pediatrics* 74:77, 1984). The records of 129 patients admitted to the hospital with the findings of fever and petechiae were reviewed to determine the incidence of invasive bacterial disease. From this group, 20.2% had culture-proved bacterial infections. Half of the infections were caused by *N. meningitidis* and 30% were secondary to *H. influenzae,* whereas *Streptococcus pneumoniae, Staphylococcus aureus* and *Escherichia coli* all were found to mimic the clinical picture of presumed meningococcemia.

Maybe *Mycoplasma* infections were missed. Read on.—F.A.O.

Mycoplasma Infection Simulating Acute Meningococcemia

Anselma C. Ramilo, Mildred R. Jackson, Ronald D. Wise, and Aditya Kaul (Illinois Masonic Med. Center, Chicago)
Arch. Dermatol. 119:786–788, September 1983   2–10

Mycoplasma pneumoniae is an important cause of acute respiratory disease that may be associated with various skin lesions, but it rarely causes petechial skin lesions. The authors report a case of *Mycoplasma* infection occurring in a child with a dramatic illness characterized by the sudden onset of fever and purpuric and petechial eruptions that resembled acute menincococcemia. The case suggests that *M. pneumoniae* should be looked for in patients with unexplained exanthems in association with respiratory involvement.

Boy, 9, had an acute illness that began as a generalized erythematous eruption on the trunk and back. The next morning, fever and malaise developed. The eruptions spread to involve the face, arms, and legs. The patient vomited several times but had no cough or respiratory difficulty. On examination, he was conscious but lethargic. The temperature was 40.5 C, pulse rate was 124 beats per minute, respirations were 36 per minute, and blood pressure was 100/50 mm Hg. Purpuric, petechial, and maculopapular lesions were present on the face, trunk, neck, and extremities. They did not blanch on pressure and no target lesions were seen. The chest appeared normal and the lungs were clear to auscultation.

A provisional diagnosis of acute meningococcemia was made. Specimens of blood, cerebrospinal fluid, throat secretions, and fluid from punctured petechial lesions were obtained for bacterial culture. Therapy was started with intravenous administration of chloramphenicol sodium succinate (75 mg/kg/day) because the patient had a history suggesting penicillin hypersensitivity. The boy became afebrile within 8 hours, and the clinical signs and symptoms resolved rapidly during the next 24 hours. On the second hospital day, no new skin lesions were seen and the old ones had not enlarged. The patient now complained of several episodes of shooting pain in the back, each lasting a few minutes. There were no new physical findings and the lungs remained clear to auscultation. A chest roentgenogram showed consolidation of the superior segment of the left lower lobe and lateral segment of the right middle lobe. No bacterial or viral growth was detected in cultures. The patient's condition improved gradually during the next several days, and antibiotic therapy was discontinued after 7 days. In view of the negative bacterial cultures and unexpected finding of pulmonary infiltrates, serum cold agglutinins were obtained and found to be present at a titer of 1:256. A chest roentgenogram on the fifth day showed notable clearing of the pneumonic infiltrates. The patient was discharged on the seventh day with almost complete resolution of the skin lesions. The acute and convalescent *M. pneumoniae* complement-fixing antibody titers, obtained at an interval of 14 days, were 1:4 and 1:128, respectively. A serum specimen obtained 10 months later was negative for cold agglutinins and had a complement fixation antibody titer of 1:32.

▶ Dermatologic involvement in *Mycoplasma pneumoniae* infections have been noted previously. H. M. Foy et al., in a prospective study, found that 17% of patients have exanthems (*JAMA* 214:1666, 1970). J. D. Cherry and associates (*J. Pediatr.* 87:369, 1975) found that the most common lesions seen were erythematous, maculopapular, and vesicular and were distributed primarily on the trunk, arms, and legs. Stomatitis and conjunctivitis were also common.

Everything mimics meningococcemia. The meningococcus never gets a chance to play actor. One of these days I expect to see a title "Meningococcemia simulating *Mycoplasma* infection."—F.A.O.

▶ Jerome O. Klein, Professor of Pediatrics, Boston University, supplied the following comment:

"Respiratory infection due to *Mycoplasma pneumoniae* is frequently accompanied by signs and symptoms in other systems, including the central nervous system by aseptic meningitis, Guillain-Barré syndrome, radiculitis, and acute hemiparesis; the blood by hemolytic anemia, and thrombocytopenia; and the heart by mycocarditis and pericarditis. In some cases, the signs suggest other diseases. A recent report describes five children with febrile illnesses, respiratory signs, and polyarthritis simulating acute rheumatic fever but associated with *M. pneumoniae* because of a rise in the level of complement fixing (CF) antibody (Berant, M., et al.: *Helv. Paediatr. Acta* 36:567, 1982). Another report identifies *M. pneumoniae* as the cause of fever of unknown origin in a young adult (Lam, K., and Bayer, A. S.: *Arch. Intern. Med.* 142:2312, 1982). This report by Ramilo and colleagues presents another diagnostic puzzle with *Mycoplasma* infection presenting in a 9-year-old boy with purpuric rash suggesting meningococcemia. Of importance in most of these cases is the presence of pneumonia or other significant signs of respiratory disease concurrent with signs of disease in other systems.

"Lesions of the skin associated with infection due to *M. pneumoniae* have included maculopapular rashes, erythema nodosum, and erythema multiforme bullosum (Stevens-Johnson syndrome) and petechiae and purpura as in this case report. The pathogenesis of these manifestations is not clear. The most likely cause of the skin eruption is an immune complex of circulating antibody and complement bound to *Mycoplasma.*

"The diagnosis of infection due to *M. pneumoniae* was made by the presence of cold agglutinins and the rise in the level of specific CF antibody. Cold agglutinins were present at a titer of 1:256. Acute and convalescent titers for CF antibody were 1:4 and 1:128. Ten months later, the titer for CF antibody was 1:32. Neither serologic assay is specific for infection due to *M. pneumoniae,* raising some questions about diagnosis based on serology alone. The crude lipid antigen used in the CF test occurs in plants, bacteria, and human brain tissue; thus, the test may reflect antibodies to a cross-reactive glycolipid rather than mycoplasmal protein antigens. This concern is discussed by Kleemola and Kayhty, who found an increase in titers of CF antibodies to *M. pneumoniae* in 40% of patients with bacterial meningitis proved by culture and who doubted that this proportion of patients with meningitis had antecedent or concurrent *Mycoplasma* infection (*J. Infect. Dis.* 146:284, 1982). Although this case of purpuric skin lesions is most likely due to *M. pneumoniae,* it is possible that we may learn more about the CF antibody response in the near future to clarify the issue of specificity."

Treatment of Salmonella Gastroenteritis in Infants: Significance of Bacteremia

Harold S. Raucher, Andrew H. Eichenfield, and Horace L. Hodes (Mount Sinai School of Medicine, New York)
Clin. Pediatr. (Phila.) 22:601–604, September 1983   2–11

Many authors do not recommend using antibiotics to treat nontyphoid *Salmonella* gastroenteritis (NTSalGE) in children with normal immune defenses, but others point to a 7% to 41% incidence of bacteremia in such infants and question the practice of withholding antimicrobial therapy.

During 1981, 20 infants aged 24 months or younger were treated for NTSalGE at the authors' institution. Blood cultures were positive for *Salmonella* in 8 of the 17 patients studied (47%), and in 7 of the 13 (54%) who were aged 3 to 24 months. There was no difference in incidence of bacteremia between very sick and mildly ill children (table). Blood samples were drawn on various days after the onset of illness, but there was no

RELATIONSHIP BETWEEN SEVERITY OF ILLNESS AND *Salmonella* BACTEREMIA

Blood Culture Result

Clinical Condition	Positive	Negative	Not Done
Severely ill, toxic	3	4	0
Mildly ill, not toxic	5	5	3

(Courtesy of Raucher, H.S., et al.: Clin. Pediatr. (Phila.) 22:601–604, September 1983.)

difference in this regard between the culture-positive and culture-negative groups.

When initially seen, 1 bacteremic child was given ampicillin parenterally (she had dehydration and a high white blood cell count), and the other 7 were not treated with antibiotics. When the blood culture results were known, 3 children were afebrile and no longer bacteremic, 1 was still febrile but not bacteremic, and 3 were still febrile and bacteremic; antibiotic therapy (usually a 7- to 10-day course of ampicillin) was begun in these 3 children, 1 of whom appeared to have septicemia. All 20 infants recovered. No focal infectious complications occurred.

In NTSalGe, bacteremia is commonly found when searched for. Serious complications are seen infrequently, yet bacteremia may lead to spread of infection to organs beyond the gastrointestinal tract in some children. Therefore, all infants younger than age 3 months with NTSalGE should have blood cultures performed and receive antibiotic therapy at least until the culture is shown to be negative. Blood cultures should be performed in all children aged 3 to 24 months who have NTSalGE if they are sufficiently ill. A child aged 3 to 24 months whose blood culture is positive should be reexamined and the blood culture repeated. If the child has toxemia, is febrile, or shows signs of infection in organs other than the intestine, antibiotic therapy should be started while awaiting the result of the second culture. Although most children older than age 3 months who have positive blood cultures but appear well on reexamination do well without antimicrobial therapy, bacteremia may persist. Therefore, if the second culture also is positive, antibiotic treatment should be given even if the child does not have evidence of systemic disease.

▶ A YEAR BOOK would never be complete without an article by, and a commentary from, John D. Nelson, Professor of Pediatrics, The University of Texas Health Science Center at Dallas. Here is the comment:

"The report by Raucher, Eichenfield, and Hodes stimulated me to review our experience with bacteremia in infants with *Salmonella* gastroenteritis. From 1981 through 1983 there were 51 patients with a positive stool culture for *Salmonella* species at Children's Medical Center, Dallas. A blood culture was obtained in 22 cases (43%) and was positive in 4 (18%) of the 22. The bacteremic infants were aged 16 days, 4 months, 10 months, and 21 months, respectively; however, only 8 patients were older than age 24 months, and blood cultures were done in only 2 of those. Thus, of the 20 infants younger than age 2 years in whom a blood culture was done, 4 (20%) were positive.

"The mean ages of infants in whom a blood culture was or was not done were 11.3 months and 11.2 months, respectively. If young age was not a factor in prompting a resident to take a blood specimen for culture from an infant with diarrhea, what was? I polled several of our residents and they were uniform in saying that high fever and toxic appearance were the compelling factors. In addition, some residents routinely take blood cultures if an infant has bloody diarrhea.

"The report by Raucher et al. indicates that this may not be an appropriate *modus operandi,* at least in the case of *Salmonella* bacteremia. Mildly ill children were as likely to be bacteremic as those who appeared toxic or severely ill.

"Because some infants spontaneously clear *Salmonella* bacteremia, the erroneous conclusion has been reached by some people that bacteremia complicating gastroenteritis does not require antibiotic therapy and that only focal *Salmonella* infection requires therapy. This is not true.

"There are three possible courses of untreated *Salmonella* bacteremia: (1) prompt, spontaneous resolution; (2) continued bacteremia, with or without focal complications such as meningitis, osteomyelitis, etc.; and (3) spontaneous resolution of bacteremia but development of focal infection. Our 16-day-old infant is an example of the last in that he initially improved rapidly but 10 days later was hospitalized for treatment of *Salmonella* shoulder joint infection.

"To my mind, the situation of *Salmonella* bacteremia in infants is exactly analogous to pneumococcal bacteremia in that age group, and both situations can be managed similarly. If one discovers that an infant not receiving antibiotics effective against *Salmonella* has a positive blood culture, the patient should be reexamined. If he is afebrile and has no evidence of focal disease, a repeat blood culture and continued observation are a satisfactory course of action. If he is still febrile, hospitalization and antibiotic therapy are my preferred course of action. If the child was treated with an antibiotic effective against *Salmonella* (such as aminopenicillins or trimethoprim-sulfamethoxazole) at the time the initial blood culture was taken, all bets are off in terms of reevaluation. I recommend continuing the antibiotic therapy for 7 to 10 days. A longer course of therapy would be necessary for focal disease.

"Raucher et al. recommend that all infants who have *Salmonella* isolated from a stool culture should be recalled to have a blood culture taken, regardless of the mildness or severity of their symptoms. I am not ready to buy that piece of advice as yet, based on their experience with only 8 bacteremic babies. But I am willing to try it until someone accumulates a much larger experience."

Effect of Penicillin Therapy on Symptoms and Signs of Streptococcal Pharyngitis
John D. Nelson (Univ. of Texas, Dallas)
Pediatr. Infect. Dis. 3:10–13, January 1984   2–12

No placebo-controlled study of the effect of antibiotic therapy on the course of streptococcal pharyngitis in children has been reported previ-

TABLE 1.—Response of Signs of Streptococcal Pharyngitis to Penicillin or Placebo

Sign	Total	No. of Patients with Sign <48 hours	>48 hours	Statistical Analysis (P)
Duration after first examination				
Exudate				
Control	15	3	12	0.095
Treated	14	7	7	
Tender cervical lymph node				
Control	15	3	12	0.012
Treated	13	9	4	
Fever				
Control	18	15	3	0.136
Treated	16	16	0	
Injection of pharynx				
Control	18	2	16	0.010
Treated	17	9	8	
Total duration of fever				
Control	18	5	13	0.020
Treated	16	11	5	

(Courtesy of Nelson, J.D.: Pediatr. Infect. Dis. 3:10–13, January 1984.)

ously. Thirty-five children aged 5 and older who had acute pharyngitis without rhinorrhea or cough were included in a study comparing the clinical response when penicillin was given for 48 hours with that when specific treatment was withheld for 2 days. Seventeen received 300,000 units of penicillin G intramuscularly, and the other 18 received a placebo syrup orally. Group A streptococci were isolated from throat cultures of all the children. The two groups were demographically and clinically comparable. After 48 hours, penicillin was given all the patients.

Objective responses were compared in Table 1. Total duration of fever

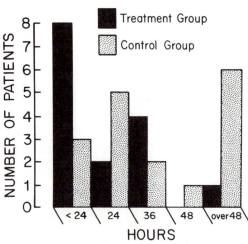

Fig 2–5.—Duration of sore throat after first examination in treated and control patients. (Courtesy of Nelson, J.D.: Pediatr. Infect. Dis. 3:10–13, January 1984.)

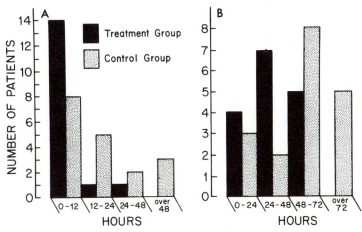

Fig 2–6.—Hours after first examination until child was afebrile (**A**) and total duration of fever (**B**) based on body temperature measurements made by parents in treated and control patients. (Courtesy of Nelson, J.D.: Pediatr. Infect. Dis. 3:10–13, January 1984.)

was significantly less in penicillin-treated patients (Fig 2–5). The durations of sore throat are compared in Figure 2–6, and responses of symptoms to penicillin and placebo are compared in Table 2. The parents felt that their children were completely well significantly sooner when given penicillin than when given placebo. The injections consistently caused local soreness, but no serious adverse reactions occurred.

These findings confirm the clinical impression that specific antibiotic therapy promptly relieves symptoms in most children with streptococcal pharyngitis. Prompt treatment of patients with "classic" cases could pro-

TABLE 2.—Response of Symptoms of Streptococcal
Pharyngitis to Penicillin or Placebo

Symptom	No. of Patients with Symptom			Statistical Analysis (P)
	Total	<48 hours	>48 hours	
Duration after first examination				
Sore throat				
Control	17	10	7	0.030
Treated	15	14	1	
Until improved*				
Control	18	8	10	0.008
Treated	17	15	2	
Until well*a*				
Control	17	0	17	0.022
Treated	17	5	12	
Total duration of sore throat				
Control	17	1	16	0.011
Treated	15	7	8	

(Courtesy of Nelson, J.D.: Pediatr. Infect. Dis. 3:10–13, January 1984.)

vide rapid symptomatic relief and might reduce the likelihood of suppurative complications.

▶ Doctor Nelson reached into his warehouse of unpublished work and brought forth this welcome study. For something old, something borrowed, Caroline Hall and Burtis Breese, in a manuscript entitled "Does Penicillin Make Johnny's Strep Throat Better?" (*Pediatr. Infect. Dis.* 3:7, 1984), wrote the following, "We hope that this settles the issue, for the beneficial effects of penicillin on symptoms and signs during the first 2 days are clearly demonstrated. The value of this head start of even a couple of days should not be underestimated. Obviously, it is important not only to the child, but also to the increasing numbers of working mothers."—F.A.O.

Bacterial Periorbital and Orbital Cellulitis in Childhood

Avery Weiss, David Friendly, Kathy Eglin, Morgan Chang, and Bess Gold
Ophthalmology (Rochester) 90:195–203, March 1983   2–13

Records of all 158 patients admitted between 1976 and 1980 with a diagnosis of periorbital or orbital cellulitis to Children's National Medical Center were reviewed. Lack of involvement of soft tissues of the orbit distinguishes periorbital from orbital cellulitis. Limited ocular motility and proptosis are the most reliable clinical indicators of orbital involvement.

Nasopharyngeal, oropharyngeal, and conjunctival cultures were obtained, blood cultures for aerobes and anaerobes were drawn from all patients, and aspiration of the leading edge of an eyelid cellulitis or infectious wound was performed in most patients. Paranasal sinus roentgenograms were taken on 92 patients. Fourteen patients were selected for computed tomographic (CT) scan on the basis of uncertain clinical signs

TABLE 1.—PREDISPOSING FACTORS IN PATIENTS
WITH PERIORBITAL CELLULITIS

	Age Groups		
	0–2 Mos	2 Mos–5 Yrs	>5 Yrs
Eyelid trauma/infection	9*	44†	14‡
URI §	1	50	13
Unidentified, factors	1	5	0
Total patients	11	99	27

*Includes 5 patients with neonatal conjunctivitis, 3 with dacryocystitis, and 1 with secondary infection after eyelid trauma.
†Includes 4 patients with secondary infection complicating impetigo, 5 with eczema, 2 with varicella, 32 with periorbital trauma, and 1 with dacryocystitis.
‡Includes 2 patients with hordeolum, 1 with chalazion, 1 with staphylococcal pustulosis, 8 with secondary infection complicating periorbital trauma, 1 with contact dermatitis, and 1 with dacryocystitis.
§URI = upper respiratory infection.
(Courtesy of Weiss, A., et al.: Ophthalmology (Rochester) 90:195–203, March 1983.)

of orbital involvement. Intravenous ampicillin (150 mg/kg/day) and oxacillin (100–200 mg/kg/day) was the most common antibiotic combination used.

Periorbital cellulitis was present in 80% of children younger than age 5, whereas 81% of children with orbital cellulitis were older than age 5. Coexisting disease was absent in most cases, except upper respiratory infection. Patients with periorbital cellulitis were divided into groups according to age and antecedent history (Table 1). Trauma to the periorbital structures, rather than eyelid infection prior to onset of periorbital cellulitis, was more common among the older groups. Dermatitis, with secondary pyoderma, hordeolum, and chalazion were the most common eyelid infections among the older children. Fever occurred equally often with orbital and periorbital disease (Table 2). White blood cell counts were mildly elevated in both diseases. Sinus involvement was evident on x-ray films in 90% of patients with orbital cellulitis but only 63% of patients with periorbital cellulitis.

Blood cultures were positive in 23 patients with periorbital cellulitis and only one patient with orbital cellulitis (Table 3). Cultures of a cellulitis edge or wound aspirate were positive in 29 of 93 selected patients (Table 4). Twenty-five of the positive cultures were from patients with periorbital cellulitis related to prior eyelid trauma or infection. Bacteria were rarely

TABLE 2.—RESULTS OF LABORATORY
INVESTIGATIONS

	Periorbital cellulitis	Orbital cellulitis
Temp ≥ 38°	61%	66%
White blood count mean	13,664	13,370
Positive sinus x-rays	63%*	90.4%

*Antecedent upper respiratory infection.
(Courtesy of Weiss, A., et al.: Ophthalmology (Rochester) 90:195–203, March 1983.)

TABLE 3.—POSITIVE BLOOD CULTURES IN
CHILDREN WITH CELLULITIS*

	Age Groups		
	0–2 Mos	2 Mos–5 Yrs	>5 Yrs
Periorbital cellulitis			
Eyelid trauma/infection	1/3	15/34	9/12
URI*	0	3/37	0
Orbital cellulitis			
Sinusitis	—	1/5	0/2

*Five patients with posterior cellulitis had no identifiable predisposing factor, and blood cultures were negative.
†URI = upper respiratory infection.
(Courtesy of Weiss, A., et al.: Ophthalmology (Rochester) 90:195–203, March 1983.)

TABLE 4.—POSITIVE CULTURES OF CELLULITIS
ASPIRATES

	0–2 Mos	2 Mos–5 Yrs	>5 Yrs
Periorbital cellulitis			
Eyelid trauma/infection	0/2	1/44	0/14
URI†	0/9	21/50	1/13
Orbital cellulitis			
Sinusitis	—	0/5	1/16

*URI = upper respiratory infection.
(Courtesy of Weiss, A., et al.: Ophthalmology (Rochester) 90:195–203, March 1983.)

TABLE 5.—BACTERIA ISOLATED FROM
CELLULITIS ASPIRATES

Periorbital cellulitis
  S. aureus (15)
  Streptococcus species (14)
  H. influenzae (2)
  Moraxella species (1)
  E. aerogenes (1)
  E. coli (1)
  Bacteroides species (1)

Orbital cellulitis
  S. aureus (1)

(Courtesy of Weiss, A., et al.: Ophthalmology (Rochester) 90:195–203, March 1983.)

TABLE 6.—BACTERIAL ISOLATES FROM
ETHMOID OR MAXILLARY SINUSES OR
BOTH*

Periorbital cellulitis	
Aerobes	*Staphylococcus aureus* (1)
	Streptococcus species (2)
Anaerobes	Peptostreptococcus (4)
	Fusobacterium nucleatum (1)
	Bacteroides species (2)
Orbital cellulitis	
Aerobes	*Staphylococcus aureus* (2)
	Streptococcus species (4)
Anaerobes	Propionibacterium acnes (2)
	Fusobacterium lentum (2)
	Bacteroides species (2)
	Peptostreptococcus (1)

*Numbers in parentheses indicate number of patients in whom organism was isolated.
(Courtesy of Weiss, A., et al.: Ophthalmology (Rochester) 90:195–203, March 1983.)

isolated from percutaneous aspirates of patients who had periorbital cellulitis with antecedent upper respiratory infection or from patients who had orbital cellulitis (Table 5).

Microbiologic cultures of the paranasal sinuses were obtained only from the 12 patients who had sinus surgery (Table 6). No atypical bacteria, fungi, or parasites were identified.

Hemophilus influenzae and one of the streptococcal species were the only bacterial pathogens isolated from blood; both are invested with polysaccharide capsules. It has been suggested that immunologic responsivity of young children to polysaccharide antigens is defective. Inadequate humoral antibody response to polysaccharide encapsulated bacteria may allow for blood-borne infection. Children with prior eyelid trauma or infection, unlike those with prior upper respiratory infection, tended to have positive percutaneous skin aspirates (51%) and negative blood cultures (99%).

▶ Ellen Wald, Associate Professor of Pediatrics, University of Pittsburgh School of Medicine, and an expert in anything in, or near, the sinuses, wrote the following:

"The child with a swollen eye commonly confronts the pediatrician. In many patients the cause of the eye swelling will be immediately apparent, for example, (1) penetrating trauma to the skin about the eye with secondary bacterial cellulitis, (2) a hordeolum or chalazion with diffuse eye swelling, (3) inflammatory conjunctivitis with reactive thickening of the lids, (4) allergic or contact dermatitis, or (5) dacryocystitis.

"On other occasions, the child with a swollen eye is a diagnostic dilemma—orbital infection must be differentiated from other serious conditions. The most important first step is a careful physical examination of the eye. It is critical to assess whether there is displacement of the globe, complete extraocular eye movements, chemosis, or impairment of visual acuity. If there is proptosis or impaired extraocular eye movements, then orbital infection must be strongly considered; the possibilities include subperiosteal abscess, orbital abscess, or orbital cellulitis (Chandler, J. R., et al.: *Laryngoscope* 80:1414, 1970). The usual risk factors for true orbital infection in children are sinusitis or penetrating eye trauma. A computed tomography scan should be performed to determine if a drainage procedure is required.

"If examination of the globe is normal, then orbital infection is ruled out; however, another important differential is between acute hematogenous infection *(Hemophilus influenzae type b* or *Streptococcus pneumoniae)* causing bacterial periorbital cellulitis and passive venous congestion or inflammatory edema secondary to acute sinusitis (Shapiro, E. D., et al.: *Pediatr. Infect. Dis.* 1:91, 1982). Both of these conditions are examples of preseptal cellulitis. The former is characterized clinically by the abrupt onset of high fever and eye swelling in a young child (usually younger than age 18 months) with a several-day history of upper respiratory infection. The periorbital skin is usually markedly inflamed—often described as violaceous or hemorrhagic—the lids are swollen shut; there is tenderness and induration. Cultures of the blood and tissue aspirate are usually positive. Parenteral antibiotics appropriate for *H. influenzae* are essential in this bacteremic infection of infancy. Most important, as a distinguishing characteristic, is the rapidity of progression of eye swelling from onset to virtually complete eye closure in hours. Inflammatory edema, on the other hand, is a clinical condition with gradual onset of eye swelling (over days) in an older child (usually older than age 2 years) with a several-day history of upper respiratory infection. Although the eye may be dramatically red and swollen, there is usually neither tenderness nor induration, and fever is generally absent or at most low grade. The primary site of infection is in the paranasal sinuses, ethmoid, or maxillary. The venous drainage of the lids is impaired when the ethmoid sinus is fluid or pus-filled; consequently, inflammatory edema or passive venous congestion ensues. Cultures of the blood and tissue aspirate are negative. While this infection is more serious than the ordinary case of sinusitis unaccompanied by eye swelling, it is not a true orbital complication. The primary site of infection is within the sinuses; many physicians will prefer to hospitalize these children and treat with parenterally administered antimicrobials although, in general, these patients may appear only mildly ill apart from the eye swelling. The route of administration of antimicrobials must be individualized and a very diligent follow-up mandated if outpatient management is elected in the mildly ill child with only modest eye swelling."

Urinary Tract Infection in Infants With Unexplained Fever: Collaborative Study
Kenneth B. Roberts, Evan Charney, Ronald J. Sweren, Vincent I. Ahonkhai, David A. Bergman, Molly P. Coulter, Gerald M. Fendrick, Barry S. Lachman, Michael R. Lawless, Robert H. Pantell, and Martin T. Stein
J. Pediatr. 103:864–867, December 1983   2–14

Urine cultures were obtained from 505 febrile and afebrile children up to age 2 years participating in a nine-center study to determine the incidence of urinary tract infection in infants with unexplained fever and whether the incidence is higher among febrile infants than among asymptomatic infants and whether the findings justify doing urine cultures in febrile infants.

Urinary tract infection was confirmed in 0.3% of 312 asymptomatic infants; all of the infections were in girls, for a rate of 0.7% (table). The incidence of confirmed urinary tract infection in the 193 febrile infants was 4.1%. Again, all infections were in girls, for a rate of 7.4%, which was significantly higher than the rate in asymptomatic infants ($P < .01$).

| | \multicolumn{8}{c}{RATE OF CONFIRMED URINARY TRACT INFECTION} |
| | \multicolumn{4}{c}{*Asymptomatic infants*} | \multicolumn{4}{c}{*Febrile infants*} |

	n	UTI	%	Confidence limits* (%)	*n*	UTI	%	Confidence limits* (%)
Boys	178	0	0	0 to 2.1	85	0	0	0 to 4.3
Girls	134	1	0.7†	0 to 4.1	108	8	7.4†	3.2 to 13.9
Overall	312	1	0.3†	0 to 1.8	193	8	4.1†	1.8 to 8.1

*Ninety-five percent.
†Asymptomatic vs. febrile infants, $P < .01$.
(Courtesy of Roberts, K.B., et al.: J. Pediatr. 103:864–867, December 1983.)

The incidence of unconfirmed urinary tract infection was also higher in febrile children (4.1%) than in asymptomatic children (2.5%). *Escherichia coli* was the causative organism in each case. When questioned regarding what yield would be required to warrant performing a urine culture in febrile infants, academicians and pediatricians generally agreed that less than 1% was a "low yield" and that more than 5% was a "high yield." Also, 86% of the responding practitioners stated that they would perform an intravenous pyelography (IVP) on a febrile male infant, but only 39% would perform an IVP on a febrile female infant. The results strongly support the advisability of obtaining urine cultures in febrile female infants with no obvious source of infection.

▶ Charles Ginsburg, Professor of Pediatrics, University of Texas Health Science Center at Dallas, and Medical Director, Children's Medical Center, prepared the following:

"Identifying the infant or toddler with a urinary tract infection (UTI) can be an onerous task for the physician, the patient, and the parents. Additionally, it also can be expensive. This nine-center collaborative study provides data that support the concept that the physician should "rule out" a urinary tract infection in febrile young children who have no readily identifiable source of infection to explain their fever. Additionally, it confirms previous observations that the incidence of UTIs in asymptomatic otherwise healthy infants and toddlers is small. The absence of confirmed infection in male patients in the study undoubtedly relates to the relatively small study population and to the small incidence of infection in this group. It should not, however, dissuade the clinician from evaluating boys, particulary those younger than age 6 months, for UTIs. A retrospective study of UTIs in infants from our institution showed that male infants accounted for the majority of infections in the first 3 months of life, but female patients predominated thereafter. Whether or not uncircumcised males have a larger rate of infection than do those who have been circumcised is unknown, but continues to intrigue us.

"The collaborative project was designed only to assess the incidence of infection in febrile children and in those who were receiving preventive health care. Unfortunately, not all infants with UTIs "signal" us by manifesting fever. Approximately one third of young children with UTIs may have temperatures less than 38 C. Most of these latter infants do, however, have nonspecific constitutional symptoms that should alert one to the possibility that an infection is present.

"It is somewhat discouraging to learn that only 86% and 39% of respondents to the authors' survey would obtain an intravenous myelogram on female and male infants, respectively, who have a confirmed UTI. Whether this sample is representative of practitioners is unknown; however, in my mind, there should be little controversy over whom to workup. Radiographic evaluation should be obtained on all boys regardless of age and on all girls who are 4 years of age or younger who have their first episode of infection and on all girls after two or more episodes after an initial UTI. The only issues are when to do it and which of the various diagnostic procedures (intravenous pyelogram, voiding cystourethrogram, sonography, nuclear scan) provides the most information at the lowest cost and with the least radiation exposure."

Cat-Scratch Disease: A Bacterial Infection

Douglas J. Wear, Andrew M. Margileth, Ted L. Hadfield, Gerald W. Fischer, Charles J. Schlagel, and Frank M. King

Science 221:1403–1405, Sept. 30, 1983   2–15

Even though there have been at least 750 reported cases of cat-scratch disease (CSD) in nearly 4 decades, the etiologic agent has yet to be identified. The clinical diagnosis of CSD requires that three of four criteria be met: a history of animal contact with the presence of a scratch or a primary dermal or eye lesion; a positive CSD skin test result; negative laboratory findings for other causes of lymphadenopathy; and characteristic histopathology of a biopsied lymph node. However, a definitive diagnosis cannot be made until the causative agent is isolated. The authors report the histopathologic findings in lymph nodes obtained from 39 patients meeting the clinical and pathologic criteria for CSD. The specimens were examined at the Armed Forces Institute of Pathology in Washington.

Thirty-seven of the 39 patients had a single cluster of enlarged nodes. Delicate pleomorphic gram-negative bacilli were demonstrated in 34 of the 39 nodes. These bacilli were found in the walls of capillaries and in macrophages lining the sinuses in or near germinal centers (Fig 2–7, A and B). The bacilli were also present in thrombosed vessels and in necrotic foci where they clustered in histiocytes, thus giving the appearance of intracellular multiplication (Fig 2–7, C). The bacilli were best demonstrated by the Warthin-Starry silver impregnation stain. Bacilli in lymph node sections exposed to convalescent serum from 3 patients with CSD and to immunoperoxidase stained with equal intensity in all three samples. The bacilli did not react with hyperimmune serums to *Legionella pneumophilia* nor to several species of *Rickettsia*.

Because the bacteria were morphologically identical among nodes, were found in tissue and were limited to areas of reaction, were intracellular, and increased in number as lesions developed and decreased as lesions resolved, they fulfill the criteria for a pathogenic organism. On the basis of the clinical and histopathologic findings, it appears that the observed bacilli are the cause of CSD.

▶ This is exciting news. I wrote to Doctor Andrew Margileth for an update. Doctor Margileth, Professor and Vice Chairman, Department of Pediatrics, Uniformed Services University of the Health Sciences, Bethesda, Maryland, responded as follows:

"Since publication of this article in *Science* in September 1983, D. J. Wear and Armed Forces Institute of Pathology associates have found the bacilli in biopsied lymph nodes from over 150 patients with cat-scratch disease (CSD). A cat-scratch skin test was positive in all subjects tested. Cat-scratch disease bacilli also were detected in primary skin lesions (Margileth A. M., et al.: *JAMA* 1984, in press) and in conjunctiva lesions of patients with Parinaud's oculoglandular syndrome.

"Doctors T. L. Hadfield and D. J. Wear at the Armed Forces Institute of Pathology have continued efforts to isolate the CDS bacillus in collaboration

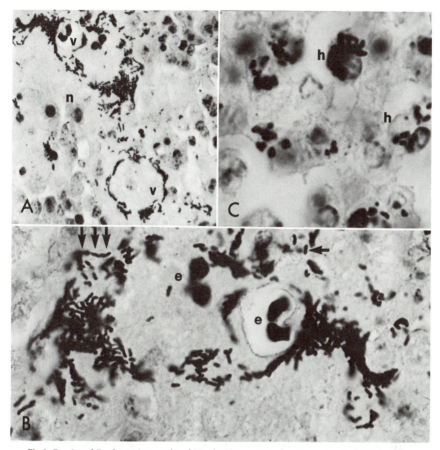

Fig 2–7.—**A** and **B,** photomicrographs of Warthin-Starry-stained sections of an inguinal lymph node from a patient with a positive skin test result for cat-scratch disease. Bacilli at (**A**) low and (**B**) high power in vessel wall *(v).* Cell boundaries are not visible in these photographs. Nuclei *(n),* erythrocytes *(e),* and organisms stain black. **A,** parallel tissue sections stained with hematoxylin-eosin showed a single tortuous blood vessel with cross sections in upper left and lower right, and a tangential cut through the vessel wall between the cross sections; ×500. **B,** upper part of **A,** showing bacilli *(arrows),* singly and in chains, outlining the vessel; ×1,260. **C,** photomicrograph of axillary lymph node obtained from a patient with a primary cat-scratch inoculation pupule and a positive skin test result for cat-scratch disease. Bacilli are seen in small histiocytes *(h),* filling the cytoplasm in one; ×2,000. (Courtesy of Wear, D.J., et al.: *Science* 221:1403–1405, Sept. 30, 1983; Copyright 1983 by the American Association for the Advancement of Science.)

with J. L. Sever and W. T. London at the National Institutes of Health. As of June 1984, they have been unable to isolate the bacillus from 10 lymph nodes known to contain the bacteria. They have used various artificial mediums, tissue culture, and inoculation of animals (mice, guinea pigs, monkeys, and chick embryos).

"In 1983, 101 new patients with CSD were observed, a 40% increase over 1982. About 9% of the 807 patients seen during 26 years (1957 to January 1984) had atypical CSD (Margileth, A. M., et al.: *Am. Fam. Physician,* 1984, in press).

"Management of CSD consists of analgesics for pain, follow-up examination to reassure the patient that the adenopathy is benign, and node aspiration if suppuration occurs. Lack of response to the common antimicrobials is the rule. In most subjects the illness is so mild that no treatment is required.

"In the rare patient having severe disease with marked malaise, fever, headache, and lymphadenitis, a broad-spectrum antibiotic such as trimethoprim-sulfamethoxazole might be tried. Excisional biopsy of the node may be necessary in older patients because of persistent pain or for diagnostic purposes. In children, aspiration of pus relieves painful adenopathy and usually allows the patient to become symptom free within 24 to 48 hours. If fluid recurs, reaspiration may be necessary."

Cat-Scratch Disease Associated With an Osteolytic Lesion
Hugh A. Carithers (Univ. of Florida, Jacksonville)
Am. J. Dis. Child. 137:968–970, October 1983   2–16

Lytic bone involvement accompanying cat-scratch disease has been described in only 3 patients. Carithers describes a fourth patient with this condition—probably the first in whom extension from an involved lymph node to a bone was direct.

Boy, 2½, had a 3-week history of a red papule on the lower right side of the chest and a 3-day history of a second swelling on the chest. The initial lesion measured 1.5 cm in diameter. The other lesion measured 2.5 × 3.5 cm and was movable, firm, slightly tender, and located just lateral to the border of the sternum at the level of the 7th rib, about 4 cm above and medial to the original lesion. The boy had had only a slight fever, did not appear ill, and lived with cats. Roentgenograms showed increasing thickening of the retrosternal soft tissues with two nodular components. The lower two sternal segments showed blurring of the surface, osteoporotic subperiosteal absorption of bone, and a small lytic spot. A bone scan gave normal results. The tumor mass on the chest rapidly increased in size and inflammation and became fluctuant. On day 7, 2 ml of thick, yellow pus was aspirated. Bacterial cultures of it were negative. During the 9-day hospital stay, the initial lesion became smaller and macular. The tumor disappeared after aspiration. No antibiotics were given.

This case was similar in some respects to the 3 previous cases (Table 1). The patient met all the criteria for diagnosis of cat-scratch disease: lymphadenopathy, history of intimate exposure to a cat, positive skin test, identified inoculation site, absence of other disease, and mildness of illness. However, the location of the inoculation site and involved lymph nodes was unusual; of 1,000 patients with cat-scratch disease seen in 1955–1980, none had involvement of parasternal or retrosternal nodes (Table 2). The other 3 patients with osteolytic bone involvement associated with cat-scratch disease had bone lesions distant from the inoculation sites and enlarged lymph nodes, whereas in this patient, it is likely that the causative agent extended directly to the bone from the involved lymph nodes.

▶ Hugh Carithers has seen over 1,000 patients with cat-scratch disease in his own private pediatric practice since 1955. This is the first of his patients with

TABLE 1.—ASSOCIATED OSTEOLYTIC LESIONS IN FOUR PATIENTS WITH CAT-SCRATCH DISEASE*

	Source, yr			
	Adams and Hindman, 1954	Collipp and Koch, 1959	Carithers et al, 1969	Present Study
Sex	M	M	F	M
Age, yr	5	4	6	2½
Exposure	Own cat	Own cat	Neighbor's cat	Own kittens
Involved node	Cervical	Cervical	Axillary	Parasternal and retrosternal
Skin test	Positive	Positive	Positive	Positive
Time of node and bone involvement	3 wk between lymphadenopathy and bone pain	Almost simultaneously	Almost simultaneously	Almost simultaneously
General signs and symptoms	Low temperature, did not become ill before node pain	Low temperature, not very ill	No temperature >32.7 °C, never toxic	One day of fever, maximum temperature of 38.4 °C
Blood count	WBCs, 10,000/cu mm; 55% polymorphonuclear leukocytes, 4% basophils, 27% lymphocytes, 6% lymphocytes, and 5% eosinophils; ESR, 18 mm/hr	WBCs, 15,000/cu mm; 53% polymorphonuclear leukocytes, 23% band forms, 21% lymphocytes, and 3% monocytes; ESR, 61 mm/hr	WBCs, 7,000/cu mm; 34% polymorphonuclear leukocytes, 1% band forms, 58% lymphocytes, 7% monocytes, and 4% eosinophils	WBCs, 9,400/cu mm; 30% polymorphonuclear leukocytes, 4% band forms, 55% lymphocytes, 8% monocytes, 2% eosinophils, and 1% basophils; ESR, 57 mm/hr
Tuberculosis test	Negative	Negative	Negative	Negative
Bone involved	Osteolytic, right ilium, 13×17 mm	Femur	Metatarsal	Sternum
Treatment	Surgical, no antibiotics	Tetracycline, 2 wk without apparent benefit	Erythromycin, 15 days; chloramphenicol, 10 days, without apparent benefit	No antibiotics
Fate of bone	Healed, <9 mo	Healed, after 5 mo	Healed, approximately 2 mo	Unavailable for follow-up
Pathologic condition	Node, granulomatous changes, chronic osteolytic with granulomatous foci	Granulomatous bone with central necrosis	No biopsy	No biopsy

(Courtesy of Carithers, H.A.: Am. J. Dis. Child. 137:968–970, October 1983; copyright 1983, American Medical Association.)

TABLE 2.—LOCATION OF
LYMPHADENOPATHY IN 1,000 PATIENTS
WITH CAT-SCRATCH DISEASE*

Location	Area No. (%)
Axillary	494 (42.2)
Subtotal area	**289 (24.7)**
Cervical	163 (13.9)
Submandibular	83 (7.1)
Submental	43 (3.7)
Subtotal area	**286 (24.4)**
Inguinal	108 (9.2)
Femoral	178 (15.2)
Preauricular	74 (6.3)
Clavicular	27 (1.9)
Scapula	1 (0.8)

*Patients were seen in author's private practice in 1955–1980. Area number totals 1,171 because some patients had lymphadenopathy in more than one location.
(Courtesy of Carithers, H.A.: Am. J. Dis. Child. 137:968–970, October 1983. Copyright 1983, American Medical Association.)

an osteolytic lesion. His more unusual complications have included Parinaud's oculoglandular syndrome (24 cases), erythema nodosum (4 cases), encephalitis (2), thrombocytopenic purpura (1), and erythema marginatum (1).

Others can give you 100 things to do with a dead cat—Carithers can provide us with 1,000 reasons for having a dead cat. If you are looking for reason 1,001, how about the fact that Bubonic plague was transmitted to a 10-year-old girl in Oregon by a scratch wound inflicted by a domestic cat (Weniger, B. G., et al.: *JAMA* 251:927, 1984)? A survey of the 1970s indicated that 82% of human plague cases in the United States were transmitted by the bites of fleas from infected wild animals, 15% by exposure to the tissues of wild animals during skinning or handling, and 3% by contact with domestic cats (Kaufman, A. F., et al.: *J. Infect. Dis.* 141:522, 1980). The contact does not have to be intimate—intimate contact with a cat sounds like some form of perversion anyway. A scratch will do, thank you.

Should patients be placed on prophylactic antibiotics after a cat bite? A prospective, double-blind, placebo-controlled study examined the value of oxacillin on the frequency of infection in cat bite wounds. Adults were evaluated. Only 11 patients completed the study. A wound infection developed in 4 of the 6 patients receiving placebo, but none of the 5 patients receiving oxacillin. Material obtained from 3 of the patients with wound infections proved to be *Pasteurella multocida* (Elenbaas, R. M. et al.: *Ann. Emerg. Med.* 13:155, 1984).—F.A.O.

Variant Strain of *Propionibacterium Acnes:* A Clue to the Etiology of Kawasaki Disease

Hirohisa Kato, Tamotsu Fujimoto, Osamu Inoue, Masaharu Kondo, Yuko Koga, Shigeru Yamamoto, Masahisa Shingu, Kaoru Tominaga, and Yasuyuki Sasaguri (Kurume Univ.)
Lancet 2:1383–1388, Dec. 17, 1983   2–17

Kawasaki disease is an acute febrile illness with mucocutaneous involvement that occurs mainly in young children and produces sudden death from coronary arteritis and its complications. The disease occurs all year round, is prevalent in Japan, and is appearing increasingly in North America and Europe. The authors attempted to determine whether an organism in the house-dust mite has a causative role in Kawasaki disease. Anaerobic cultures were maintained for 3–4 weeks in an effort to obtain isolates from a node biopsy specimen of a boy aged 6 years with typical symptoms in a second recurrence of Kawasaki disease and from blood samples from 38 patients, 23 of whom were studied within a week of the onset of illness. The mean patient age was 16 months.

A variant strain of *P. acnes* was isolated from the node biopsy specimen, from the blood of 5 of 23 patients studied within a week of onset of the disease, and from 1 of 15 blood samples of patients studied later in the course of illness. No anaerobes were isolated from 60 age-matched control patients with various disorders. The same serotype was isolated from house-dust mites in 6 patients' homes. *Staphylococcus epidermidis, Bacillus subtilis,* and *Pseudomonas* species also were isolated from mites. Study patients had significantly higher serum agglutination titers to *P. acnes* than did the control subjects (table). Inoculation of 3 guinea pigs with the lymph node strain of *P. acnes* variably produced inflammatory lesions of reticuloendothelial organs and, in 1 instance, coronary arteritis, focal myocarditis and endocarditis. *Propionibacterium acnes* was isolated from the spinal cord of this animal. Inoculation of human embryo liver cells produced cytoplasmic inclusion bodies of varying size in up to a third of the liver cells.

AGGLUTINATION TITERS OF SERUM SAMPLES FROM 30
PATIENTS AND 30 CONTROLS AGAINST STRAINS OF
Propionibacterium acnes

Strains	Number of subjects with titres						
	≤4	8	16	32	64	128	≥256
From lymph-node							
Controls	14	7	3	3	0	2	1
Patients	0	0	1	4	7	9	9
From blood							
Controls	12	5	4	4	3	2	0
Patients	0	0	1	1	10	9	9
From house-dust mite							
Controls	17	6	6	0	1	0	0
Patients	0	0	3	5	6	10	6
ATCC 11827							
Controls	17	5	3	3	0	1	1
Patients	0	0	2	3	7	11	7

(Courtesy of Kato, H., et al.: Lancet 2:1383–1388, Dec. 17, 1983.)

A variant strain of *P. acnes* may have a causative role in Kawasaki disease, with house-dust mites acting as a vector. In Japan, where Kawasaki disease is most prevalent, the numbers of house-dust mites have increased with changes in housing styles.

▶ This is a provocative lead that deserves further study. It just *mite* be the answer. Kawasaki disease is now being reported in British children (Goel, K. M., et al.: *Lancet* 1:1440, 1983). Of the 4 children described in this report, 2 had been exposed to shampooed carpets and 2 of the patients had increased antimite-specific IgE titers during their illness.

The *Lancet* published a titillating letter describing an apparently effective, albeit unorthodox, treatment for this disease. Fourteen patients with Kawasaki disease received intravenous infusions of human γ-globulin, 400 mg/kg daily for 5 days. The treatment was started within 7 days of illness in 13 of the patients. The controls were 40 patients, who also were treated within 7 days of their illness, by orally administered aspirin, 10–30 mg/kg daily for at least 3 months. Of these controls, 34 were "historical" and only 6 were concurrent. Fever after the start of treatment lasted 2.4 ± 1.9 days in the γ-globulin group and 4.5 ± 3.1 days in the controls. The duration of positive C-reactive protein values after the start of therapy was significantly shorter in the γ-globulin group. Most importantly, selective coronary angiography was done up to the 50th day of illness, and aneurysm formation was recognized in 17% of controls but in none of the γ-globulin group (Furusho, K., et al.: ibid. 2:1359, 1983). We should be hearing more about this—we need more details before anyone should adopt this form of therapy.—F.A.O.

Grade I Reye's Syndrome: Frequent Cause of Vomiting and Liver Dysfunction After Varicella and Upper Respiratory Tract Infection
Philip K. Lichtenstein, James E. Heubi, Cynthia C. Daugherty, Michael K. Farrell, Ronald J. Sokol, Robert J. Rothbaum, Frederick J. Suchy, and William F. Balistreri (Children's Hosp. Med. Center, Cincinnati)
N. Engl. J. Med. 309:133–139, July 21, 1983   2–18

Reye's syndrome is perceived as an illness generally associated with neurologic deterioration and death, but some have suggested that mild, nonprogressing cases exist and are diagnosable clinically and histologically. The authors prospectively examined the hypothesis that vomiting and threefold or greater elevation of serum aspartate or alanine aminotransferase, when preceded by either a viral upper respiratory tract infection or varicella, are manifestations of mild Reye's syndrome.

Of 31 children presenting at the emergency room during 1981 with the above findings, and without jaundice or cerebrospinal fluid infection, 25 had what appeared to be grade I disease (Fig 2–8). Liver biopsies were performed in 19 of them: 10 boys and 9 girls, aged 6 months to 13½ years (average, 6½ years).

Of the 19 biopsy specimens, 14 (74%) were diagnostic of Reye's syndrome according to rigorous light and electron microscopic and histo-

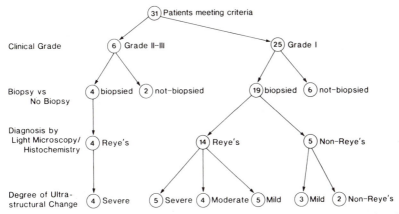

Fig 2–8.—Findings on light and electron microscopy in biopsy specimens from patients clinically diagnosed as having Reye's syndrome. (Courtesy of Lichtenstein, P.K., et al.: N. Engl. J. Med. 309:133–139, July 21, 1983. Reprinted by permission of the New England Journal of Medicine.)

chemical criteria. None of the specimens contained evidence of other acute pathologic processes, including hepatitis. A wide spectrum of mitochondrial alterations existed at the ultrastructural level, ranging from mild to severe lesions that were indistinguishable from those seen in comatose patients with Reye's syndrome. No correlation was observed between the severity of the ultrastructural lesion and the duration of illness and vomiting before hospital admission or the admission levels of serum aspartate aminotransferase, serum salicylate, ammonia, uric acid, or creatine kinase (table). The level of serum alanine aminotransferase was higher in patients with moderate ultrastructural changes than in those with severe ($P < .05$) changes but did not differ from those with mild changes. None of the biopsy-proved cases progressed clinically to more advanced disease.

The incidence of Reye's syndrome was estimated to be at least 3.5 cases per 100,000 children younger than age 17 years (2.7 cases of grade I illness and 0.8 cases of grade II or higher illness). This figure is 11-fold higher than that calculated by the Centers for Disease Control for the same period.

▶ Doctor Michael Barrett, Medical Epidemiologist, Reye's Syndrome Unit, Division of Viral Diseases, Center for Infectious Diseases, Centers for Disease Control, provided the following unofficial comment:

"In 1972, Shubert et al., at the Cincinnati Children's Hospital, developed a clinical classification scheme for Reye's syndrome (RS) consisting of five grades of encephalopathy. Grade 1 was described as "unusually quiet or mildly lethargic." Lichtenstein et al. studied 31 patients meeting a standardized case definition for presumed RS; 25 (80%) presented with what appeared to be grade 1 disease. These, in turn, came from an estimated pool of roughly 100 patients presenting with a prodromal infection and recurrent vomiting (*N. Engl. J.Med.* 310:129, Jan. 12, 1984; correspondence). An aggressive attempt to biopsy the 25 patients was undertaken, and three fourths of the 19 biopsies performed were diagnostic of RS. Although the reported percentage varies

Correlation Between Severity of Hepatic Ultrastructural Involvement and Various Clinical and Chemical Indexes in Patients With Grade I Reye's Syndrome*

Hepatic Ultrastructural Involvement (no. of patients)	Prodromal URI: Varicella	Duration of Illness	Duration of Vomiting	SGOT†	SGPT‡	Ammonia	Serum Salicylate	Uric Acid
	no. of patients	days	hr	IU		µg/dl	mg/dl	mg/dl
Mild (5)	2:3	8 (5–11)	39 (12–48)	744±214 (266–1466)	726±151 (236–1174)	23.5±5.4 (11.2–42)	2.2±0.7 (0–4.4)	7.4±1.1 (5.2–10.5)
Moderate (4)	4:0	8.8 (5–12)	36 (30–48)	1156±317 (364–1912)	1242±366 § (308–1692)	36.5±13.7 (13.2–74)	2.2±0.1 (1.9–2.5)	8.7±0.4 (7.5–8.9)
Severe (5)	3:2	6 (4–7)	30 (17–48)	666±134 (338–976)	526±89 (330–824)	39.2±8.6 (19.6–61.6)	6.8±2.1 (1.9–14.0)	6.4±1.5 (2.6–10.7)

*Plus-minus values are ± SEM. Figures in parentheses are ranges. URI, upper respiratory tract infection. To convert values for ammonia to micromoles per liter, multiply by 0.5872. To convert values for salicylate to millimoles per liter, multiply by 0.07240.
†SGOT, serum aspartate aminotransferase.
‡SGPT, serum alanine aminotransferase.
§P < .05, as compared with severe involvement.
(Courtesy of Lichtenstein, P.K., et al.: N. Engl. J. Med. 133–139, July 21, 1983. Reprinted by permission of the New England Journal of Medicine.)

widely depending on the method of case ascertainment, some patients with grade 1 Reye's syndrome will progress to coma. Consequently, the message to the practicing physician is becoming increasingly clear: any child with the acute onset of recurrent vomiting occurring 2 to 7 days following onset of a viral upper respiratory infection or varicella infection deserves clinical evaluation and measurement of serum aminotransferase levels even in the presence of a paucity of neurologic findings. In lieu of a biopsy, a serum NH_3 determination is presently the most useful single test to aid in the diagnosis of RS.

"Once again, the issue of varicella hepatitis versus nonencephalopathic RS surfaces. Which is more common? How does one distinguish between the two? Lichtenstein et al. report that 8 of their biopsied patients had a varicella prodrome; of these, none had evidence of hepatitis. One of the best discussions of this issue comes from Shope (*Yale J. Biol. Med.* 55:321–327, 1982), who states, 'The presence of elevated liver enzymes without other evidence of hepatocellular damage, and especially without evidence of inflammation or cellular damage consistent with varicella virus replication, cannot be viewed as hepatitis. The condition is more appropriately viewed as hepatopathy . . . .' His characterization of hepatopathy (elevated liver enzyme levels, normal concentrations of bilirubin and alkaline phosphatase, and signs of possible cerebral origin permitted including lethargy, headache, and irritability) is essentially the same as that for grade 1 RS. Shope points out that varicella hepatitis among immunocompetent patients is infrequent, and he goes on to state that, in any patient, hepatitis is accompanied by dissemination to other organs, frequently including the lungs. In the immunocompetent patient convalescing from varicella with the isolated finding of serologic hepatic dysfunction, one should be hesitant to diagnose varicella hepatitis without a liver biopsy demonstrating focal necrosis and intranuclear inclusions.

"Finally, the comparison of Lichtenstein et al. of incidence based on two markedly different techniques (Centers for Disease Control voluntary national surveillance vs. active regional surveillance) is misleading. Their reported 3.5 cases per 100,000 children younger than age 17 years in Cincinnati is less than twice the upper range of the estimated average annual incidence of RS in the United States as reported by the Centers for Disease Control, rather than the suggested 11 times higher. For more on this matter, see the correspondence in the *New England Journal of Medicine,* Jan. 12, 1984, page 128."

Varicella in Immunocompromised Children: Incidence of Abdominal Pain and Organ Involvement
Elaine R. Morgan and Lisa A. Smalley (Northwestern Univ.)
Am. J. Dis. Child. 137:883–885, September 1983   2–19

Two previously unreported manifestations of progressive varicella that may occur in immunocompromised children are severe abdominal or back pain, or both, and inappropriate antidiuretic hormone (ADH) syndrome.

Review of the records of some 600 children who received immunosuppressant therapy between 1975 and 1982 showed 31 who had varicella infections. Of these, 16 had uncomplicated courses with fever, rash, and, in some cases, transient elevation of serum transaminase levels.

The other 15, aged 4 to 13 years, had progressive varicella and required hospitalization. Of these 15, 13 had been receiving chemotherapy for acute leukemia (12 were in remission), 1 had been receiving prednisone for Fanconi's anemia, and 1 had been receiving chemotherapy for metastatic rhabdomyosarcoma. All 15 had rash, fever, hepatitis, and pneumonitis. Eleven had severe multisystem involvement, including severe, cramplike abdominal pain requiring narcotic analgesia in all 11, encephalopathy in 10, coagulopathy in 10, inappropriate ADH syndrome in 10, back pain or myalgia in 5, and myocarditis in 1; 4 of these 11 children died. The other 4 children with disseminated varicella had relatively mild clinical courses with liver and lung involvement only; none died. No survivor had permanent sequelae.

The sequence of symptom appearance was somewhat predictable. Fever, rash, and abdominal or back pain were always the initial complaints. Intense pain invariably heralded severe organ involvement. Elevation of serum transaminase levels was always the next sign. Encephalitis, inappropriate ADH syndrome, coagulopathy, and pneumonitis occurred in random sequence, but were generally apparent within 2 to 4 days after the first signs of progression of infection. The earliest signs of improvement in survivors were stabilization and a subsequent fall in serum transaminase levels. The overall course of varicella infection was about 7 to 10 days.

The ability to predict severe involvement by the onset of intense pain allows for early institution of systemic antiviral therapy with vidarabine or acyclovir, or both. In addition, the relative predictability of the sequence of organ involvement permits anticipatory surveillance and early, aggressive intervention.

▶ Anne Gershon, Professor of Pediatrics, New York University, and one who has done much to develop an effective varicella vaccine, writes as follows:

"Morgan and Smalley have reported an important clinical observation, that disseminated varicella is often heralded by severe abdominal pain. The clinician may find it extremely difficult to decide whether or not varicella is severe enough to initiate antiviral chemotherapy, particularly in immunocompromised patients. In patients who eventually have fatal progressive varicella, the disease may seem to be benign for as long as 1 week after onset. When the need for specific therapy is obvious in these patients, it is often too late to expect antiviral agents to be effective. Past studies have emphasized the requirement to begin antiviral agents within 3 days of onset of varicella. Based on the current study, one significant clinical sign warranting institution of antiviral therapy is persistent abdominal pain.

"There are currently two available means for prevention of severe varicella in immunocompromised patients. One is passive immunization with varicella zoster immune globulin (VZIG). Varicella zoster immune globulin is now licensed and available for varicella-susceptible children with recognized close exposures to varicella or zoster. It should be administered within 3 days after exposure. The other prophylactic, available on a research basis only, is live attenuated varicella vaccine, developed by Takahashi about 10 years ago. Currently, there are a number of ongoing studies of this vaccine in the United States and Canada. The vaccine appears to protect most patients against severe varicella; occasional breakthrough cases of chickenpox in immunocompromised patients have been mild. It is expected that this vaccine will become commercially available within the next few years.

"Antiviral drugs used to treat severe varicella include acyclovir and vidarabine. Because the antiviral drug acyclovir is so well tolerated, most infectious disease experts nowadays choose to treat *all* immunocompromised patients who develop varicella before the illness has become life-threatening. Patients with varicella who have received VZIG under appropriate circumstances or who have been immunized with live vaccine and who develop varicella, however, do not usually require therapy. Acyclovir should be used at a dosage of 1,500 mg/sq m/day in three divided doses, intravenously, for 7 to 10 days. Vidarabine has been shown to be effective in treating severe chickenpox, but it seems to be more toxic than acyclovir.

"There are no data as yet comparing the efficacy of acyclovir and vidarabine for severe varicella, but some data indicate that acyclovir is effective for treatment of severe varicella. Toxicity from vidarabine includes rash, nausea, vomiting, tremors, and hallucinations. Toxicity from acyclovir for patients with varicella appears to be negligible and consists mainly of phlebitis. It is unknown whether vidarabine and acyclovir administered together are helpful for treatment of severe chickenpox."

Sequelae of Maternally Derived Cytomegalovirus Infections in Premature Infants

Anne S. Yeager, Paul E. Palumbo, Natalie Malachowski, Ronald L. Ariagno, and David K. Stevenson (Stanford Univ.)
J. Pediatr. 102:918–922, June 1983   2–20

Acquisition of cytomegalovirus (CMV) in the perinatal period is relatively common; there is no practical way of eliminating infections acquired during the birth process. The authors attempted to determine whether CMV infection acquired from maternal sources results in symptomatic infection in small premature infants. Surveillance for acquired CMV infection was begun at age 1 month. Infants in an intensive care nursery who had received red blood cell transfusions were studied.

CORRELATION OF OXYGEN REQUIREMENT WITH CMV EXCRETION AND BIRTH WEIGHT

Oxygen requirement >7 wk/total (%)

| | Weight (gm) | | |
	759 to 999	*1000 to 1249*	*1250 to 1499*
CMV excretors	3/4 (75)	0/6 (0)	3/8 (37.5)
Nonexcretors	5/23 (21.7)	8/33 (24.2)	2/32 (6.3)

(Courtesy of Yeager, A.S., et al.: J. Pediatr. 102:918–922, June 1983.)

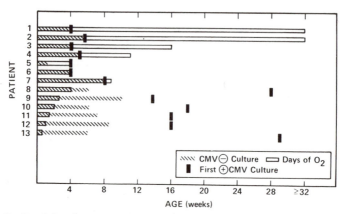

Fig 2–9.—Correlation of oxygen requirements with age at onset of viral excretion. (Courtesy of Yeager, A.S., et al.: J. Pediatr. 102:918–922, June 1983.)

None of 165 infants of seronegative mothers who received red blood cells only from seronegative donors became infected. Banked milk was not an apparent source of infection. Infection occurred in 19% of 231 infants who were born to seropositive mothers and who received red blood cells only from seronegative donors. Eighteen of 106 infants weighing less than 1,500 gm at birth (17%) acquired CMV infection. Most evaluable infants began excreting CMV at age 4–6 weeks. Oxygen requirements in CMV excretors and other infants are compared in the table. Infants who excreted CMV before age 7 weeks had longer oxygen requirements than those excreting virus at an older age (Fig 2–9). Maternal antibody to CMV fell more rapidly in the first months of life in the sick premature infants than would be expected in term infants. Five of 6 infected premature infants had no detectable antibody at the time CMV excretion began.

Both loss of passively acquired antibody to CMV and early excretion of the virus appear to be associated with symptomatic CMV infection in premature infants of seropositive mothers. Some of the present infants had hepatosplenomegaly and hematologic findings of CMV infection. Factors predisposing to symptomatic CMV infection must be identified so that surveillance can be maintained and means can be found for preventing or treating infection.

Cytomegalovirus Infection in Pregnancy: Preliminary Findings From A Prospective Study

Catherine S. Peckham, John C. Coleman, Rosalinde Hurley, Kong Shin Chin, Kathy Henderson, and Philip M. Preece (Charing Cross Hosp., London)
Lancet 1:1352–1355, June 18, 1983   2–21

Of the congenital infections, cytomegalovirus (CMV) infection is the most common and is an important cause of handicap. Estimates of its incidence vary widely, ranging from 0.2% to 2.3% of all births (Table 1).

TABLE 1.—INCIDENCE OF CONGENITAL CYTOMEGALOVIRUS
IN DIFFERENT POPULATIONS

Country	Infants screened	% with congenital infection
USA	2147	1·2
USA	1963	1·0
USA	1412	2·2
Canada	15212	0·4
West Africa	2032	1·4
Denmark	3060	0·4
Sweden	4421	0·4
England	9233	0·4*
England	4259	0·4

*Number of infants screened included an excess of infants in special care units, but when the figures are adjusted to take account of this, the overall infection rate was 0.24%.

(Courtesy of Peckham, C.S., et al.: Lancet 1:1352–1355, June 18, 1983.)

About 90% of infected infants are free of symptoms at birth, fewer than 2% have severe disease with neurologic involvement, and 8% have evidence of extraneural infection, predominantly hepatosplenomegaly, thrombocytopenic purpura, jaundice, or pneumonitis. However, defects develop in some infants who are symptom free at birth.

The risk of acquisition of CMV infection was assessed in a prospective study of 14,789 pregnant women screened for CMV antibodies by complement fixation from September 1979 through August 1982. Screening at the first antenatal visit found that 8,278 of the women (56%) had CMV antibodies at a dilution of 1 : 10 or greater (Table 2). Analysis of the first 2,000 patients showed that more than 90% of Asian women were seropositive, as were 54% of the white women. Forty-two (0.3%) of the 14,200 neonates screened were congenitally infected. Of these, 28 (67%) were born to mothers who had a primary infection (16 confirmed, 12 presumed) (Fig 2–10). It was calculated that infection occurred in the first trimester in 5, in the second trimester in 4, and in the third trimester in 3. Evidence of recurrent infection was observed in 7 women, and, in 7 others it was not possible to determine whether the infection was primary or recurrent. At the most recent follow-up examination, 28 of the congenitally infected children were older than age 1 year and 14 were older than age 2 years. Five (12%) were of low birth weight for gestational age, and 2 of these had other abnormalities attributable to CMV infection (Table 3). As of

TABLE 2.—FREQUENCY OF ANTIBODY IN PREGNANT
WOMEN AT THEIR FIRST ANTENATAL ATTENDANCE

—	No tested	No positive	% positive
Hospital 1	3805	2669	70·1
Hospital 2	6255	3116	49·8
Hospital 3	4729	2493	52·7
Total	14 789	8278	56·0

(Courtesy of Peckham, C.S., et al.: Lancet 1:1352–1355, June 18, 1983.)

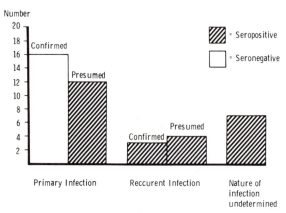

Fig 2–10.—Initial serologic status and type of maternal infection in mothers of 42 children who had congenital cytomegalovirus infections. (Courtesy of Peckham, C.S., et al.: Lancet 1:1352–1355, June 18, 1983.)

the most recent examination, 3 (7%) children with congenital CMV infection have a serious handicap, 14 (33%) have minor or transient problems, and 25 (60%) have no problems as yet.

These findings indicate that routine screening of pregnant women for evidence of primary CMV infection, as a basis for recommending termination of pregnancy because of the risk of congenital handicap, is of limited value.

▶ James Barry Hanshaw, Professor and Chairman, Department of Pediatrics, University of Massachusetts Medical School, and a lifelong student of CMV, comments:

TABLE 3.—FINDINGS IN 42 CHILDREN WITH
CONGENITAL CYTOMEGALOVIRUS INFECTION

Birth-weight	Birth status	Follow-up status (number of children)
Light for gestational age (5 infants)	No problems (3 infants)	Microcephaly, spastic quadriplegia, bilateral sensorineural deafness (1); mild sensorineural hearing-loss (1); conductive hearing-loss (1)
	Immediate problems (2 infants)	Microcephaly, spastic quadriplegia, optic atrophy, severe psychomotor retardation, bilateral hearing-loss (1); failure to thrive, pneumonitis, hepatosplenomegaly at 3 months, small ventricular septal defect (1)
Normal weight for gestational age (37 infants)	No problems (37 infants)	Hepatosplenomegaly and rash (1); pneumonitis (5);* conductive hearing-loss (4);* serous otitis media with normal hearing (3); mild sensorineural hearing-loss (1); no abnormality (24)

*One child had pneumonitis and conductive hearing loss.
(Courtesy of Peckham, C.S., et al.: Lancet 1:1352–1355, June 18, 1983.)

"Doctor Catherine Peckham and her associates in London have provided some useful information bearing on the advisability of screening pregnant women for CMV infection.

"Of 14,789 women screened for CMV antibody seroconversions by complement fixation tests, only 28 were found to have *primary* CMV infection. This is the group most likely to have damaged infants. Of a total of 42 congenitally infected infants, 3 had serious handicaps and only 1 would have been identified antenatally. This infant, however, was not identified until 28 weeks' gestation. A second infected infant was born to a mother with a presumptive recurrent infection, and the type of maternal infection in the third infant could not be determined because of the late gestational age at presentation.

"The above data confirm and support the notion that routine prenatal screening of paired serums is not useful. Practical means are not yet available for detecting primary maternal infection by *single serum testing,* although this may be possible in the future with cytotoxic CMV antibody testing as described by Betts et al. in Rochester. Cytotoxic CMV antibody is an IgM immunoglobulin and, when present in the serum of a pregnant woman, is strong presumptive evidence of primary infection. It apparently does not appear during reactivated infection. Radioimmunoassay, ELISA, and immunofluorescent methods are also capable of detecting specific CMV IgM antibody, but these tests are not practical at this time for large-scale testing during pregnancy.

"There are other good reasons for not embarking on routine screening. Once one gets a high CMV titer, there is often difficulty in interpretation, which may be a source of anxiety to the patient (and the physician). Sometimes the titer is obtained because the pregnant woman is a nurse or a physician who has come in contact with an infected infant. We know from the recent studies of Dworsky and his associates (*N. Engl. J. Med.* 309:950, 1983) that CMV in nurseries is not transmitted to health care workers any more often than to women living in the community. We also know that a health care worker delivering an infected infant may have a strain of CMV totally unrelated to the index case. This kind of molecular epidemiology is now made possible by the use of restriction endonuclease analyses that permit the identification of strain-specific viral DNA.

"It should be emphasized that the identification of the 3 infants who later developed serious handicaps would not have led to termination of the pregnancy. State laboratories now doing routine 'TORCH titers' prenatally should reassess what they are doing. The idea of doing 'TORCH titers' has always been somewhat of a misguided effort. The acronym may be useful in reminding clinicians of some nonbacterial agents that can infect the fetus and the neonate, but it is not a guide to the intelligent use of the laboratory either before or after birth."

Occupational Risk for Primary Cytomegalovirus Infection Among Pediatric Health Care Workers
Meyer E. Dworksy, Kathryn Welch, George Cassady, and Sergio Stagno (Univ. of Alabama, Birmingham)
N. Engl. J. Med. 309:950–953, Oct. 20, 1983   2–22

Pediatric health care workers often are exposed to asymptomatic infants with cytomegalovirus (CMV) infection, who may excrete large amounts of virus into the urine and saliva, and their risk of acquiring CMV infection is a concern. A cross-sectional seroepidemiologic survey was undertaken of the prevalence of CMV antibody in 179 nurses working in newborn nurseries, 159 medical students, 64 pediatric interns and residents, 40 pediatricians, and physicians doing research and caring for patients with CMV infection. The control populations included 3,733 women from a private obstetric practice and 14 private obstetricians.

Cytomegalovirus was shed in the urine or saliva of 1.6% of newborn infants, 13% of premature infants hospitalized for a month or longer, and 5% of older infants seen as outpatients. The serologic findings in the various exposed and control groups are given in Table 1. Blacks had the highest rates of seropositivity. Occupational differences were not significant. Rates of primary infection in the groups at risk are given in Table 2. Annual attack rates in the medical students, house staff, and nurses were no higher than those in young women in the community. None of the CMV research physicians showed seroconversion.

These findings suggest that although pediatric health care workers often unknowingly care for infants who shed CMV, this contact confers no greater risk than that faced by young women in the general population. It is doubtful whether the risk of medical personnel acquiring primary CMV infection is great enough to warrant the imposition of isolation procedures for infants known to be infected. Such infants also need not be denied admission to schools or institutions, because asymptomatic infected children are already present and far outnumber the infants known to be infected. Intimate and possibly prolonged contact with CMV may be the chief determinant in horizontal transmission of infection.

TABLE 1.—DEMOGRAPHIC AND SEROLOGIC
CHARACTERISTICS OF THE POPULATIONS STUDIED

Group	No. of Subjects	Mean Age	% Female	% White	% Seropositive
Exposed to infants					
Nurses	179	29	99	77	59
Medical students	159	25	23	96	32
House staff	64	27	40	95	30
Community pediatricians	40	42	20	90	60
CMV research physicians	10	32	10	100	30
Not exposed to infants					
Middle-class mothers					
During pregnancy	3733	27	100	85	58
Between pregnancies	720	25	100	91	48
Community obstetricians	14	47	0	100	64

(Courtesy of Dworsky, M.E., et al.: N. Engl. J. Med. 309:950–953, Oct. 20, 1983. Reprinted by permission of the New England Journal of Medicine.)

TABLE 2.—Rates of Primary Infection in
Populations at Risk

Group	No. Suscep-tible	Mean Sampling Interval	% Serocon-version/ Year
		mo	
Medical students	89	22	0.6
House staff	25	18	2.7
Nurses	61	24	3.3
Middle-class mothers			
During pregnancy	1549	7.8	2.3
Between pregnancies	372	21	5.5

(Courtesy of Dworsky, M.E., et al.: N. Engl. J. Med. 309:950–953, Oct. 20, 1983. Reprinted by permission of the New England Journal of Medicine.)

▶ This study should help reduce anxiety among health workers. It should, but it probably won't. One of Murphy's laws (Hanggi's law actually) states: "The more trivial your research, the more people will read it and agree. The more vital your research, the less people will understand it."—F.A.O.

Cytomegalovirus Infection of Breast Milk and Transmission in Infancy
Meyer Dworsky, Martha Yow, Sergio Stagno, Robert F. Pass, and Charles Alford (Univ. of Alabama, Birmingham)
Pediatrics 72:295–299, September 1983   2–23

Cytomegalovirus (CMV) infection occurs during the first year of life in 10% to 60% of infants. The authors studied the possibility that infected breast milk is the most important source of such infection.

Prospective longitudinal studies were conducted in 58 unselected pairs of postpartum mothers and their breast-fed infants. The women were aged 15 to 37 years (mean, 24.5 years); 60% were black, 53% were married, and 83% were high school graduates. At enrollment, 17 (29%) were seronegative and 41 (71%) were seropositive for CMV antibody.

None of the seronegative women shed CMV from breast milk, vagina, urine, or saliva at any time during the study. Of the 41 seropositive women, 39% reactivated CMV at some site and 32% shed CMV into breast milk (Table 1); 4 women shed virus into more than one site. In all cases viral shedding was intermittent. Cytomegalovirus was shed into breast milk most frequently between 2 and 12 weeks post partum.

Cytomegalovirus infection before the age of 8 months occurred in no infant born to seronegative mothers, in 12 of 41 (30%) born to seropositive mothers, and in 9 of 13 (69%) born to mothers who shed virus into breast milk (Table 2). In contrast, CMV infection developed in none of 3 infants breast-fed by mothers who shed CMV from other sites and in 3 of 25 breast-fed by mothers with no demonstrable viral excretion. There was

TABLE 1.—Cytomegalovirus Shedding by
Site in 41 Seropositive Postpartum Women

Sample	Mean No. of Cultures/ Woman	No. of Women with Excretion
Breast milk	2.7	13* (32%)
Vagina	4.5	4 (10%)
Urine	4.4	3 (7%)
Saliva	4.5	1 (2%)

(Courtesy of Dworsky, M., et al.: Pediatrics 72:295–299, September 1983. Copyright American Academy of Pediatrics 1983.)

TABLE 2.—Relation Between Breast-Feeding
and Infant Cytomegalovirus (CMV) Infection

Maternal Status	No. of Women	No. of Infants Infected	P Value
Seronegative	17	0	
Seropositive:	41	12 (30%)	.006
Breast-fed <1 mo	10	0	
Breast-fed ≥1 mo	31	12 (39%)	.015
CMV milk excretion	13	9 (69%)	
No CMV milk excretion	28	3 (10%)	.0007

(Courtesy of Dworsky, M., et al.: Pediatrics 72:295–299, September 1983.)

TABLE 3.—Relation of Milk Cytomegalovirus (CMV) Neutralizing
Substance and Immunofluorescent (IF) Antibodies to Maternal Viral
Excretion and Acquisition of Infection by Infant

Maternal Status	Neutralizing Substance	IgM	IgG	IgA	Any IF Antibodies
Seronegative	2/14	0/8	0/8	0/8	0/8
Seropositive:	11/24	2/11	4/11	6/11	9/11*
CMV milk excretion	4/12	1/6	2/6	2/6	4/6
No CMV milk excretion	7/12	1/5	2/5	4/5	5/5
Infants infected	5/11	1/5	2/5	2/5	4/5
Infants uninfected	6/13	2/6	2/6	4/6	5/6

*Versus neutralizing substance (P = .04, Fisher exact test).
(Courtesy of Dworsky, M., et al.: Pediatrics 72:295–299, September 1983. Copyright American Academy of Pediatrics 1983.)

some milk secretory immune response to CMV, but it did not prevent viral shedding or viral transmission (Table 3).

All infected infants chronically shed CMV, but none has yet shown chronic sequelae. Two preterm infants had a significant acute problem (i.e., pneumonitis) that resolved. The possiblity that an unnecessary and perhaps severe illness might occur in low birth weight seronegative infants fed banked human milk from sources other than the mother is disturbing and needs resolution.

▶ This study should give pause to the advocates of pooled-banked human milk for the low birth weight infant. No one would advocate pooling blood for administration. It seems just as primitive to try and get away with pooling milk. History repeats itself. That's one of the things wrong with history. Milk for the premature infant should come from the infant's mother whenever possible. If that is not possible, then its safety should be ascertained before it is administered.—F.A.O.

Aerosolized Ribavirin Treatment of Infants With Respiratory Syncytial Viral Infection: A Randomized Double-Blind Study
Caroline Breese Hall, John T. McBride, Edward E. Walsh, David M. Bell, Christine L. Gala, Stephen Hildreth, Lawrence G. Ten Eyck, and William J. Hall (Univ. of Rochester, Rochester, New York)
N. Engl. J. Med. 308:1443–1447, June 16, 1983   2–24

Ribavirin (1-β-D-ribofuranosyl-1,2,4-triazole-3-carboxamide), a synthetic nucleoside that has antiviral properties in vitro against both RNA and DNA viruses, can ameliorate the course of both influenza A and influenza B infections in adults, especially when administered by small-particle aerosol.

The authors evaluated the efficacy of ribavirin aerosol therapy in the treatment of lower respiratory tract disease caused by respiratory syncytial virus (RSV) in a randomized, placebo-controlled, double-blind study of 33 infants treated continuously for 3–6 days. All infants were ill enough to require hospitalization for at least 3 days.

The severity of illness at the time of hospitalization did not differ significantly between the placebo group and the ribavirin group. However, when therapy was initiated (an average of 1.5 days after admission), the infants in the placebo group had a significantly lower severity of illness score than did infants randomized to receive ribavirin. Even so, improvement after the first day of therapy was greater in the ribavirin group, and the illness severity score was significantly lower in this group by the fourth day of therapy ($P < .01$) (Fig 2–11). In addition, the mean increment of improvement between day 1 and the end of therapy was significantly greater in infants receiving ribavirin ($P < .01$). Except for wheezing, the change or degree of improvement in lower respiratory tract signs was significantly greater in infants randomized to receive ribavirin, although the change in temperature and upper respiratory tract signs did not differ significantly between groups (Table 1). All infants received supplemental oxygen. By the end of therapy, those given ribavirin had significant improvement in mean oxygen tension ($P < .01$); improvement in the placebo group, though significant ($P < .05$), was not as pronounced (Fig 2–12). The increment of improvement from day 1 to the end of therapy averaged

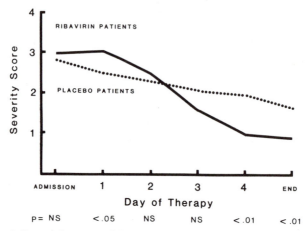

Fig 2–11.—Daily scores for severity of illness (means), with 0 representing normal and 4, most severe. Therapy lasted for an average of 4.7 days in the placebo group and for an average of 4.9 days in the ribavirin group. (Courtesy of Hall, C.B., et al.: N. Engl. J. Med. 308:1443–1447, June 16, 1983. Reprinted by permission of the New England Journal of Medicine.)

13 mm Hg in the ribavirin group and 4 mm Hg in the placebo group ($P < 0.001$). Although similar initially, RSV titers in nasal washes at the end of therapy were significantly lower in the ribavirin group than in those given placebo (Table 2). Isolates of RSV obtained from the infants over the course of therapy showed no appreciable change in sensitivity to ribavirin. No side effects or toxic effects were observed.

The results demonstrate that ribavirin aerosol therapy produces significant improvement in infants with lower respiratory tract infection from RSV. This improvement was associated with improved levels of arterial

TABLE 1.—MEAN SEVERITY SCORE FOR SIGN OR
SYMPTOM AT START AND END OF TREATMENT

	RIBAVIRIN GROUP		PLACEBO GROUP		P VALUE * FOR CHANGE IN SCORE
	START	END	START	END	
Temperature (°C)	37.9	37.2	37.9	37.4	NS
Nasal congestion and discharge	1.8	0.6	2.2	1.0	NS
Cough	2.3	0.9	1.8	1.6	<0.01
Rales	2.2	0.5	1.6	1.4	<0.01
Wheezing	1.1	0.2	1.3	0.8	NS
Retractions	2.2	0.2	1.5	1.0	<0.01
Lethargy	2.3	0.2	2.0	1.2	<0.01

*P value for unit change in score from start to end of therapy for placebo group vs. ribavirin group (Mann-Whitney U test and nonpaired t test). NS means not significant. (Courtesy of Hall, C.B., et al.: N. Engl. J. Med. 308:1443–1447, June 16, 1983. Reprinted by permission of the New England Journal of Medicine.)

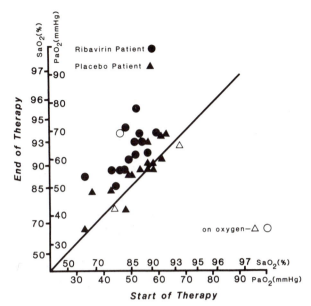

Fig 2–12.—Arterial blood-gas levels initially and at the end of treatment with ribavirin *(solid circle)* or placebo *(solid triangle)*. Diagonal represents line of identity, i.e., no change in values over the course of treatment. *SaO₂*, arterial oxygen saturation; *PaO₂*, arterial oxygen tension. All infants breathed room air, except for the 3 indicated by open symbols. (Courtesy of Hall, C.B., et al.: N. Engl. J. Med. 308:1443–1447, June 16, 1983. Reprinted by permission of the New England Journal of Medicine.)

oxygen saturation and diminished viral shedding. The drug may be particularly beneficial for children at risk for severe and often fatal RSV infection, e.g., infants with congenital heart disease.

▶ I asked Caroline Hall, the senior author of this exciting article, to provide us with an overview and an update. Doctor Hall, Professor of Pediatrics, University of Rochester, responded with the following:

TABLE 2.—TITERS OF RESPIRATORY SYNCYTIAL
VIRUS IN NASAL-WASH ISOLATES

GROUP (No.)	TITER ($\log_{10}$ TCID$_{50}$/ml)		
	BEFORE TREATMENT	AT DAY 3	AT END OF TREATMENT
Ribavirin (12)	7		
Mean	2.1 *	1.2 *	0.3 †
Range	0.4–5.7	0–4.2	0–1.7
Placebo (13)			
Mean	3.0	2.1	1.3
Range	0.4–5.9	0–4.2	0–4.2

*Not significantly different from value for placebo group.
†Significantly different from value for placebo group ($P < .03$ Mann-Whitney U test and Student's t test).
(Courtesy of Hall, C.B., et al.: N. Engl. J. Med. 308:1443–1447, June 16, 1983. Reprinted by permission of the New England Journal of Medicine.)

"Ribavirin at this time remains as an investigational drug in the United States. Although the drug was discovered over a decade ago, clinical trials using the oral form of the drug were initiated only more recently. Knight and colleagues at Baylor University were the first to administer ribavirin as a small-particle aerosol in the successful treatment of college students with influenza A infections (Knight, V., et al.: *Lancet* 2:945, 1981) and subsequently those with influenza B infections (McClung, H. W., et al.: *JAMA* 249:2671, 1983). The first RSV 'patients' to receive aerosolized ribavirin were cotton rats, followed by adult volunteers with experimental RSV infections in whom serial sensitive pulmonary function tests demonstrated no untoward effects of the aerosolized drug (Hall, C. B., et al.: ibid. 249:2666, 1983). Ribavirin for the treatment of infants with RSV infection was evaluated concurrently at Baylor University and the University of Rochester and appeared beneficial in both studies, although the infants at Baylor all had bronchiolitis, were generally less ill, and were treated for shorter periods than at Rochester (Taber, L. H., et al.: *Pediatrics* 72:618, 1983). Also of interest is the report of Gelfand and co-workers (*Lancet* 2:732, 1983) of the treatment of two infants with severe combined immunodeficiency disease and overwhelming RSV and parainfluenza type 3 pneumonia. In these patients the virologic and clinical response to ribavirin delivered by small-particle aerosol was dramatic.

"Ongoing studies of aerosolized ribavirin in several centers should better define the role of ribavirin in the treatment of RSV infections in other types of patients. We recently have been evaluating ribavirin therapy for infants with underlying cardiopulmonary disease, who are perhaps most at risk for severe RSV infection. The results thus far are encouraging, and the drug appears to be well tolerated in these small babies. Currently, ribavirin therapy by small-particle aerosol is only feasible and warranted for hospitalized infants. However, future studies of different dosing schedules and development of new aerosol delivery systems could make outpatient therapy possible.

"At the moment, the charisma of ribavirin appears to me to be its singular character: (1) its relative lack of toxicity, (2) its refusal thus far to provoke viral resistance, and (3) its broad-spectrum activity against both RNA and DNA viruses, which may allow us to prophesize that it shall be the progenitor of potential 'third-generation antivirals.' "

Croup: An 11-Year Study in a Pediatric Practice
Floyd W. Denny, Thomas F. Murphy, Wallace A. Clyde, Jr., Albert M. Collier, and Frederick W. Henderson (Univ. of North Carolina, Chapel Hill)
Pediatrics 71:871–876, June 1983   2–25

Croup, one of the common manifestations of lower respiratory tract infection (LRI) in children, is a syndrome of inspiratory stridor, cough, and hoarseness resulting from obstruction in the region of the larynx. The authors studied the etiology and epidemiology of croup during 1964–1975.

Croup was diagnosed in 951 of 6,165 pediatric cases of LRI. Croup was the sole diagnosis in 93.7% of the 951 cases; 18 children (1.9%) had associated tracheobronchitis, 29 (3.0%) also had wheezing, and 13 (1.4%)

had pneumonia. The incidence of LRI was highest during the first year of life. However, the attack rate for croup was highest in the second year of life, 4.7/100 children, having risen from 2.4/100 children during the first 6 months. After the second year, the rate decreased; after age 6 years it was only 0.46/100 children per year.

Croup was seen predominantly in boys, with those aged 6–12 months having a risk 1.73 times that of girls of the same age (Table 1). Overall, boys were 1.43 times more likely to develop croup than girls. A total of 360 microbes were recovered from 358 patients (Table 2). The overall isolation rate was 37.6% and varied somewhat by age. Parainfluenza viruses accounted for 74.2% of all isolates and were the predominant agents at all ages (Table 3). Respiratory syncytial virus (RSV) caused croup in children younger than age 5 years but not in older children, whereas influenza viruses A and B, and *Mycoplasma pneumoniae* were significant causes of croup only in children older than aged 5 or 6 years. The propensity of the various agents to cause croup was analyzed by patient age (Table 4). Although RSV and *M. pneumoniae* were common causes of LRI, they were relatively unimportant causes of croup.

TABLE 1.—INCIDENCE OF CROUP BY
PATIENT AGE AND SEX, CHAPEL HILL,
N.C., 1964–1975

Age (yr)	Incidence/100 Children/yr (M/F)	Incidence by Sex (M÷F)
0–½	2.76/2.01	1.37
½–1	4.95/2.86	1.73
1–2	5.60/3.66	1.53
2–3	3.55/2.63	1.35
3–4	2.55/1.60	1.59
4–5	1.69/1.16	1.46
5–6	1.15/0.92	1.25
>6	0.47/0.44	1.07
All ages	1.82/1.27	1.43

(Courtesy of Denny, F.W., et al.: Pediatrics 71:871–876, June 1983. Copyright American Academy of Pediatrics 1983.)

TABLE 2.—ETIOLOGIC AGENTS RECOVERED
FROM CHILDREN WITH CROUP, CHAPEL
HILL, N.C., 1964–1975

	No.	% Total
Parainfluenza virus type 1	173	48.1
Parainfluenza virus type 3	63	17.5
Respiratory syncytial virus	36	10.0
Parainfluenza virus type 2	31	8.6
Influenza virus type A	13	3.6
Mycoplasma pneumoniae	13	3.6
Influenza virus type B	12	3.3
Miscellaneous viruses	19	5.3
Total	360	100

(Courtesy of Denny, F.W., et al.: Pediatrics 71:871–876, June 1983. Copyright American Academy of Pediatrics 1983.)

TABLE 3.—DISTRIBUTION OF PRINCIPAL AGENTS RECOVERED FROM CHILDREN
WITH CROUP

Patient Age (yr)	Total Cases of Croup	Cases of Croup with Isolates	Parainfluenza Virus*			Respiratory Syncytial Virus*	Influenza Viruses A and B*	Mycoplasma pneumoniae*
			Type 1	Type 2	Type 3			
0–1	169	53	24 (45)	4 (8)	6 (11)	9 (17)	4 (8)	1 (2)
1–2	251	91	34 (37)	7 (8)	24 (26)	6 (7)	5 (5)	5 (5)
2–3	162	72	44 (61)	2 (3)	14 (19)	11 (15)	0	1 (1)
3–4	114	51	29 (57)	4 (8)	6 (12)	6 (12)	3 (6)	1 (2)
4–5	71	29	15 (52)	6 (21)	3 (10)	4 (14)	1 (3)	0
5–6	48	24	10 (42)	4 (17)	7 (29)	0	3 (13)	0
>6	136	40	17 (43)	4 (10)	3 (8)	0	9 (23)	5 (13)
All ages	951	360	173 (48)	31 (9)	63 (18)	36 (10)	25 (7)	13 (4)

*Values are number of isolates; percent of cases of croup with isolates is shown in parentheses.
(Courtesy of Denny, F.W., et al.: Pediatrics 71:871–876, June 1983. Copyright American Academy of Pediatrics 1983.)

TABLE 4.—OCCURRENCE OF CROUP IN CHILDREN WITH LOWER RESPIRATORY ILLNESSES
DUE TO CERTAIN AGENTS, CHAPEL HILL, N.C., 1964–1975*

	Parainfluenza Virus						Respiratory Syncytial Virus		Influenza Viruses A and B		Mycoplasma pneumoniae	
	Type 1		Type 2		Type 3							
Patient Age (yr)	No.	%	No.	%	No.	%	No.	%	No.	%	No.	%
0–1	42	57	6	66	47	13	91	10	13	31	5	20
1–2	55	62	9	78	47	51	79	8	11	45	12	42
2–3	65	68	6	33	36	39	71	15	10	0	12	8
3–4	44	66	8	50	22	27	42	14	18	17	17	6
4–5	30	50	7	86	21	15	30	13	11	9	15	0
5–6	16	63	5	80	19	37	15	0	18	22	19	0
>6	49	35	11	36	26	12	27	0	78	12	162	3
All ages	301	58	52	60	218	29	355	10	159	16	242	5

*Values are number of total lower respiratory tract illnesses due to agent and percent of illnesses associated with croup.
(Courtesy of Denny, F.W., et al.: Pediatrics 71:871–876, June 1983.)

Croup in this general pediatric population occurred predominantly in late fall and early winter, times when the parainfluenza viruses, especially type 1, occurred most often. That the epidemiology of croup differs from that of bronchiolitis, pneumonia, and tracheobronchitis should be helpful to those caring for children with LRI.

Corticosteroid Treatment of Laryngotracheitis vs. Spasmodic Croup in Children

Gideon Koren, Mira Frand, Zohar Barzilay, and Stuart M. MacLeod
Am. J. Dis. Child. 137:941–944, October 1983
2–26

The efficacy of high-dose corticosteroid therapy for laryngotracheitis (LT) was compared with its efficacy in spasmodic croup (SC), using a double-blind, randomized protocol and objective means for measurement of results.

The trial was conducted with 78 children, aged 8 months to 8 years (mean, 2½), hospitalized with croup, dyspnea, inspiratory stridor, sub-

---

DIAGNOSTIC CRITERIA*

LT (Insidious-Onset Croup)	SC (Acute-Onset Croup)
Signs of URTI preceding croup	No/minimal signs of URTI preceding croup
Often fever	Seldom fever
Insidious appearance of croup (24-72 hr after beginning of URTI)	Sudden onset of croup
May appear by day or night	Onset at evening or night
Generally single attack	Recurrences in part of patients

*Abbreviations: LT, laryngotracheitis; SC, spasmodic croup; URTI, upper respiratory tract infection.

(Courtesy of Koren, G., et al.: Am. J. Dis. Child. 137:941–944, October 1983; copyright 1983, American Medical Association.)

---

costal or suprasternal retraction or both, and a barking cough. None had associated bronchitis, bronchopneumonia, or acute epiglottiditis. Of the 78 children, 49 had LT, 23 had SC, and in 6 LT could not be differentiated from SC by the criteria used (table).

All children were sedated with chloral hydrate (75 mg/kg of body weight, given rectally), and their respirations were recorded hourly for 6 hours. Each was then given a single intramuscular dose of dexamethasone sodium phosphate (0.6 mg/kg) or placebo and placed in a cool mist tent for at least 6 hours. No bronchodilators, racemic epinephrine, or antibiotics were administered. The respirations during sleep were measured hourly for 6 hours.

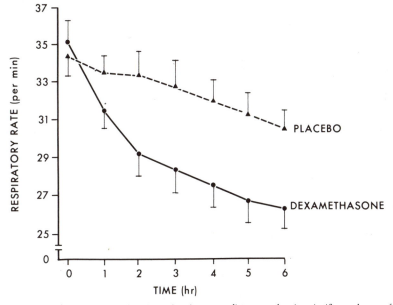

Fig 2–13.—Change in respirations over time in spasmodic croup, showing significant change after dexamethasone sodium phosphate therapy, as compared with placebo. Results are presented as mean ± SE. (Courtesy of Koren, G., et al.: Am. J. Dis. Child. 137:941–944, October 1983; copyright 1983, American Medical Association.)

Dexamethasone administration did not change the respiratory rate in patients with LT, but it caused a significant decrease in respirations in those with SC (Fig 2–13). It is usually possible to differentiate between LT and SC at admission by history and clinical signs. Steroid therapy should be avoided in cases of LT, but it may be of benefit in some cases of SC, such as severe cases that do not improve spontaneously.

▶ Walter Tunnessen, Jr., Professor of Pediatrics and Vice Chairman, State University of New York, Upstate Medical Center, comments:

"The croup story marches on. A half decade ago, Leipzig et al. (J. Pediatr. 94:194–196, 1979) reported a significant response to dexamethasone in children with croup. Unfortunately, that study, as many in the past with similar or dissimilar viewpoints, had a few methodologic problems in design that raised questions about the applicability of the results. One of the concerns centered on the efficacy of steroids in spasmodic croup (SC) versus laryngotracheitis (LT) rather than on the lump sum (undifferentiated croup). Koren et al. have tried carefully to dissect out the meat of this problem. Careful attention was given to avoid the methodologic errors of the past. As suspected clinically by many observers, and in support of the work of Urquhart et al. (Br. Med. J. 1604:1, 1979) who suggested SC was an immune-mediated illness following prior sensitization with a paramyxovirus, those with SC responded to steroids while those who had LT did not.

"One might quibble with the outcome event that these authors chose to reflect the efficacy of steroids. Does a reduction in the respiratory rate correspond with an improvement in the severity of croup? Certainly the rate is numerical and objective, rather than subjective, such as the criteria stridor, cyanosis, and sternal retractions, which were used in past studies. If, as the authors state, none of their patients was in the second stage of respiratory insufficiency during which a patient may tire and the respiratory rate may therefore not reflect the severity of respiratory obstruction, the results appear significant.

"Since SC is self-limited and generally not as severe as LT, steroids are not mandatory treatment but should be reserved for only the most severe cases of apparent SC. I'm sure we have not heard the end of the story, but an end seems in sight!"

Prevention of Perinatally Transmitted Hepatitis B Virus Infections With Hepatitis B Immune Globulin and Hepatitis B Vaccine
R. Palmer Beasley, Lu-yu Hwang, George Chin-yun Lee, Chung-chi Lan, Cheng-hsiung Roan, Fu-yuan Huang, and Chiung-lin Chen (Taipei, Taiwan)
Lancet 2:1099–1102, Nov. 12, 1983   2–27

There are about 200 million hepatitis B virus (HBV) carriers worldwide, and perhaps one-fourth die of cirrhosis, hepatocellular cancer, or both. Mother-to-infant transmission is the usual reason for high carrier rates. Transmission during labor and delivery is frequent, and infection in early life generally leads to carrier status. A blind trial was undertaken of various

Group	Outcome			
	Number persistent HBsAg pos (%)	Number anti-HBs pos (%)	Both negative (%)	Efficacy
HBIG plus vaccine				
Schedule A (n = 51)	1 (*2·0*)	50 (*98·0*)	0	97·8
Schedule B (n = 50)	3 (*6·0*)	47 (*94·0*)	0	93·2
Schedule C (n = 58)	5 (*8·6*)	53 (*91·4*)	0	90·2
S₁ btotal (n = 159)	9 (*5·7*)	150 (*94·3*)	0	93·6
95% confid interval(%)	2·1–9·3	90·7–97·9		
No prophylaxis (n = 84)	74 (*88·1*)	6 (*7·1*)	4·8	
95% confid interval(%)	81·2–95·0	1·6–12·7	0·2–9·3	

*A vs. control: χ = 95.4, P < .005; B vs. control: χ = 86.4, P < .005; C vs. control: χ = 87.8, P < .005; A vs. B, P = .30 (Fisher's); A vs. C, P = .14 (Fisher's); B vs. C, P = .4 (Fisher's).

(Courtesy of Beasley, R.P., et al.: Lancet 2:1099–1102, Nov. 12, 1983.)

temporal combinations of hepatitis B immune globulin (HBIG) and hepatitis B vaccine in preventing the perinatally transmitted hepatitis B surface antigen (HBsAg) carrier state in Taipei. Infants of e-antigen-positive HBsAg carrier mothers received HBIG immediately after birth, followed by vaccination at age 3 months with a second dose of HBIG (group A); vaccination at age 4 to 7 days (group B); or vaccination at about age 1 month (group C).

The results are given in the table. No differences in efficacy were apparent among the different vaccination schedules. Their overall efficacy was 94%, compared with 71% for HBIG alone and 75% for vaccination alone. Persistent HBs antigenemia developed in 6% of 159 infants given prophylaxis and in 88% of control infants. Antibodies developed in all infants who did not become antigenemic. The only factor found to predict immunization failure was a moderate to high level of circulating HBsAg at the time of vaccination. No adverse reactions to vaccination were observed.

Prophylaxis with HBIG and hepatitis B vaccine is highly effective in preventing perinatal transmission of HBsAg infection in an area with a high natural carrier rate. The control of perinatal transmission of HBV presumably can dramatically reduce the occurrence of hepatocellular carcinoma. The transmission of infection at birth makes immunoprophylaxis initiated at birth of value. It is thought that protection will be sustained, although long-term follow-up data remain to be collected. It is suggested that vaccination be initiated during confinement to maximize compliance and minimize costs.

▶ ↓ Because of the importance of the problem discussed in the preceding article, for the following article we have reproduced in its entirety the Recommendations of the Immunization Practices Advisory Committee that appeared in *Morbidity and Mortality Weekly Report* (33:285, 1984).—F.A.O.

Postexposure Prophylaxis of Hepatitis B
Immunization Practices Advisory Committee
Morbidity Mortality Weekly Rep. 33:285–290, June 1, 1984   2–28

Prophylactic treatment to prevent hepatitis B (HB) infection after exposure to hepatitis B virus (HBV) should be considered in several situations: perinatal exposure of an infant born to a hepatitis B surface antigen (HBsAg)-positive mother, accidental percutaneous or permucosal exposure to HBsAg-positive blood, or sexual exposure to an HBsAg-positive person. In each of these settings, the risk of HB infection is known to be high and justifies preventive measures. Previous recommendations for postexposure prophylaxis have relied on passive immunization with specific hepatitis B immune globulin (HBIG). However, the recent demonstration of high efficacy of HB vaccine combined with HBIG in preventing chronic HB infection in infants of HBsAg-positive mothers requires the revision of recommendations for postexposure prophylaxis (Table 1).

Passive immunization with HBIG alone has been partially effective in preventing clinical HB in studies of medical personnel after needlestick accidents and sexual exposure to partners with acute HB. In addition, HBIG prophylaxis has been shown significantly to reduce the percentage of infants who become chronic HBV carriers after perinatal exposure to HBsAg-positive mothers. For perinatal and needlestick exposures, however, HBIG alone is only about 75% effective even when given very soon after exposure, may provide only temporary protection, and is costly (over $150 per adult dose).

TABLE 1.—Hepatitis B Virus Postexposure Recommendations

| | HBIG | | Vaccine | |
| | | Recommended | | Recommended |
Exposure	Dose	timing	Dose	timing
Perinatal	0.5 ml IM	Within 12 hrs of birth	0.5 ml (10 μg) IM	Within 7 days* repeat at 1 & 6 mos
Percutaneous	0.06 ml/kg IM or 5 ml for adults	Single dose within 24 hrs	1.0 ml (20 μg) IM[†]	Within 7 days* repeat at 1 & 6 mos
	or[§]			
	0.06 ml/kg IM or 5 ml for adults	Within 24 hours repeat at 1 mo	—	—
Sexual	0.06 ml/kg IM or 5 ml for adults	Within 14 days of sexual contact	¶	—

*The first dose can be given the same time as the HBIG dose but at a separate site.
†For persons younger than age 10, use 0.5 ml (10 μg).
§For those who choose not to receive HB vaccine.
¶Vaccine is recommended for homosexually active males and for regular sexual contacts of chronic HBV carriers.
(Courtesy of Immunization Practices Advisory Committee: Morbidity Mortality Weekly Rep. 33:285–290, June 1, 1984.)

With the development of HB vaccine, the possibility arose that HB vaccine, alone or in combination with HBIG, might be useful for postexposure prophylaxis. Studies have shown that response to HB vaccine is not impaired by concurrent administration of HBIG and that the combination of HB vaccine and one dose of HBIG produces immediate and sustained high levels of protective antibody to the hepatitis B surface antigen (anti-HBs). A recent study examining the efficacy of HB vaccine combined with a single dose of HBIG in preventing perinatal transmission from HBsAg carrier mothers who were also positive for hepatitis B "e" antigen (HBeAg) showed this combination to be highly effective in preventing the HBV carrier state in infants and significantly more effective than multiple doses of HBIG alone.

Perinatal Transmission

Transmission from mother to infant during birth is one of the most efficient modes of HBV transmission. If the mother is positive for both HBsAg and HBeAg, about 80%–90% of infants will become infected. Although infection is rarely symptomatic in the acute phase, approximately 90% of these infected infants will become chronic HBV carriers. It has been estimated that 25% of these chronic carriers may die of cirrhosis or primary hepatocellular carcinoma. In addition, such persons are infectious, and female carriers may subsequently perpetuate the cycle of perinatal transmission. If the HBsAg-positive carrier mother is HBeAg-negative or if anti-HBe is present, transmission occurs in less than 25% and 12% of cases, respectively. Such transmission rarely leads to chronic HBV carriage; however, severe acute disease, including fatal fulminant hepatitis in the neonate, has been reported. Even if perinatal infection does not occur, the infant may be at risk of subsequent infection from other family contacts. For these reasons, prophylaxis of infants from all HBsAg-positive mothers is recommended, regardless of the mother's HBeAg or anti-HBe status.

The primary goal of postexposure prophylaxis for exposed infants is prevention of HBV carrier state. In addition, there is a need to prevent the rare occurrence of severe clinical hepatitis in some of these infants. Administration of 0.5 ml HBIG to an infant of an HBsAg, HBeAg-positive mother soon after birth and repeated at 3 months and 6 months reduces the probability of chronic infection from about 90% to about 25% (efficacy about 75%). The concurrent use of HB vaccine and various combinations of HBIG increases the efficacy to close to 90%. Since approximately 5% of perinatal infection may occur in utero, it appears likely that no form of postnatal prophylaxis will be 100% effective in this circumstance.

Concurrent HBIG and vaccine administration does not appear to interfere with vaccine efficacy. HB vaccine has been shown to be equally immunogenic in neonates, whether given in 10-μg or 20-μg doses. The use of HB vaccine in combination with HBIG in the perinatal setting has the advantages of increasing efficacy, eliminating the need for the second and third doses of HBIG, and providing long-term immunity to those who are not infected during the perinatal period.

Maternal Screening

Since efficacy of this regimen depends on administering HBIG on the day of birth, it is vital that HBsAg-positive mothers be identified before delivery. Mothers belonging to groups known to be at high risk of HB infection (Table 2) should be tested routinely for HBsAg during a prenatal visit. If a mother belonging to a high-risk group has not been screened prenatally, HBsAg screening should be done at the time of delivery or as soon as possible thereafter.

Management of HBsAg-Positive Mothers and Their Newborns

The appropriate obstetric and pediatric staff should be notified directly of HBsAg-positive mothers, so the staff may take appropriate precautions to protect themselves and other patients from infectious material, blood, and secretions, and so the neonate may receive therapy without delay after birth.

Recent studies in Taiwan and the United States have confirmed the efficacy of the regimen shown in Table 3. Other schedules have also been effective. The major consideration for all these regimens is the need to give HBIG as soon as possible after the infant has physiologically stabilized after delivery.

HBIG (0.5 ml) should be administered intramuscularly (IM) after physiologic stabilization of the infant and preferably within 12 hours of birth. HBIG efficacy decreases markedly if treatment is delayed beyond 48 hours. HB vaccine should be administered IM in three doses of 0.5 ml of vaccine (10 μg) each. The first dose should be given within 7 days of birth and may be given concurrently with HBIG but at a separate site. The second and third doses should be given 1 month and 6 months, respectively, after the first (Table 1). HBsAg testing at 6 months may be done for counseling purposes, since HBsAg-positivity at 6 months indicates a therapeutic failure, and the third vaccine dose need not be given if HBsAg-positivity is found. If a mother's HBsAg-positive status is not discovered until after delivery, prophylaxis should still be administered if a venous (not cord)

TABLE 2.—WOMEN FOR WHOM PRENATAL HBsAg SCREENING
IS RECOMMENDED

1. Women of Asian, Pacific Island, or Alaskan Eskimo descent, whether immigrant or U.S.-born.
2. Women born in Haiti or Sub-Saharan Africa.

and

Women with histories of:

3. Acute or chronic liver disease.
4. Work or treatment in a hemodialysis unit.
5. Work or residence in an institution for the mentally retarded.
6. Rejection as a blood donor.
7. Blood transfusion on repeated occasions.
8. Frequent occupational exposure to blood in medico-dental settings.
9. Household contact with an HBV carrier or hemodialysis patient.
10. Multiple episodes of venereal disease.
11. Percutaneous use of illicit drugs.

(Courtesy of Immunization Practices Advisory Committee: Morbidity Mortality Weekly Rep. 33:285–290, June 1, 1984.)

blood sample from the infant is HBsAg-negative. Testing for HBsAg and anti-HBs is recommended at 12–15 months to monitor the final success or failure of therapy. If HBsAg is found, it is likely the child is a chronic carrier. If HBsAg is not detectible, and anti-HBs is present, the child has been protected. Since maternal antibody to the core antigen (anti-HBc) may persist for more than 1 year, testing for anti-HBc may be difficult to interpret during this period. HB vaccine is an inactivated product, and it is presumed that it will not interfere with other simultaneously administered childhood vaccines. HBIG administered at birth should not interfere with oral polio and diphtheria-tetanus-pertussis vaccines administered at about 2 months of age (Table 3).

Acute Exposure to Blood Containing HBsAg

There are no prospective studies directly testing the efficacy of a combination of HBIG and HB vaccine in preventing clinical HB following percutaneous or mucous-membrane exposure to HBV. However, since health-care workers at risk to such accidents are candidates for HB vaccine and since combined HBIG plus vaccine is more effective than HBIG alone in perinatal exposures, it is reasonable to recommend both HB vaccine and HBIG after such exposure. This combination will provide prolonged immunity to subsequent exposures and may also increase efficacy in preventing HB in such postexposure situations. In addition, because the second dose of HBIG is not considered necessary if the vaccine is used, the cost of combination treatment is usually less than that of two HBIG doses alone. If exposure to blood occurs in situations where the HBsAg status of the blood is unknown, refer to "Immune Globulins for Protection against Viral Hepatitis." If HBsAg testing reveals the source of the blood to be positive, the following treatment schedule should be instituted as soon as possible.

For percutaneous (needlestick), ocular, or mucous-membrane exposure

TABLE 3.—ROUTINE PEDIATRIC VACCINATION SCHEDULE AND HBV PROPHYLAXIS
FOR INFANTS OF HBsAG-POSITIVE MOTHERS

Age (months)	Hepatitis B prevention schedule		HBV marker screening	Routine pediatric schedule
Birth	HBIG*	HB vaccine[†]		
1		HB vaccine		
2				DPT[§], Polio
4				DPT, Polio
6		HB vaccine	HBsAg test[¶] **	DPT
12-15			HBsAg** & anti-HBs[††] test	
15				MMR[§§]
18				DPT, Polio

*Hepatitis B immune globulin, 0.5 ml IM within 12 hours of birth.
†HB vaccine, 0.5 ml IM within 7 days of birth.
§Diphtheria-tetanus-pertussis.
¶Optional. If positive, indicates infection, and a third HB vaccine does not need to be given.
**HBsAg-positive indicates therapeutic failure.
††Anti-HBs-positive indicates therapeutic success.
§§Measles-mumps-rubella.
(Courtesy of Immunization Practices Advisory Committee: Morbidity Mortality Weekly Rep. 33:285–290, June 1, 1984.)

to blood known to contain HBsAg and for human bites from HBsAg carriers that penetrate the skin, a single dose of HBIG (0.06 ml/kg or 5.0 ml for adults) should be given as soon as possible after exposure and within 24 hours if possible. HB vaccine 1 ml (20 μg) should be given IM at a separate site as soon as possible, but within 7 days of exposure, with the second and third doses given 1 month and 6 months, respectively, after the first (Table 1). If HBIG is unavailable, immunoglobulin (IG [formerly ISG or "gamma globulin"]) may be given in an equivalent dosage (0.06 ml/kg or 5.0 ml for adults). If an individual has received at least two doses of HB vaccine before an accidental exposure, no treatment is necessary if serologic tests show adequate levels (>10 S/N by RIA) of anti-HBs. For persons who choose not to receive HB vaccine, the previously recommended two-dose HBIG regimen may be used.

HBIG for Sexual Contacts of Persons With Acute HBV Infection

Sexual contacts of persons with acute HB infection are at increased risk of acquiring HB infection. Two published studies have assessed the value of postexposure prophylaxis for regular sexual contacts of persons with acute HB infection. One showed that HBIG was significantly more effective than IG that contained no measureable anti-HBs in preventing both HB infection and clinical illness. The second study, however, showed comparable disease rates in persons receiving HBIG and IG containing the increased levels of anti-HBs found in currently available lots. Because data are limited, the period after sexual exposure during which HBIG is effective is unknown, but extrapolation from other settings makes it unlikely that this period would exceed 14 days. The value of HB vaccine alone in this setting is unknown. However, since about 90% of persons with acute HB infections become HBsAg-negative within 15 weeks of diagnosis, the potential for repeated exposure is usually self-limited. HB vaccine is not routinely recommended for such exposures.

Prescreening sexual partners for susceptibility before HBIG treatment is recommended if it does not delay HBIG administration beyond 14 days after last exposure. In one study, 27% of regular sexual partners (heterosexual) were positive for HBsAg or anti-HBs at the time they presented for evaluation. Among homosexually active males, over 50% have markers indicating prior infection, and 5%–6% are HBsAg positive. Testing for anti-HBc is the most efficient prescreening test to use in this population group.

A single dose of HBIG (0.06 ml/kg or 5 ml for adults) is recommended for susceptible individuals who have had sexual contact with an HBsAg-positive persons if HBIG can be given within 14 days of the last sexual contact, and for persons who will continue to have sexual contact with an individual with acute HB before loss of HBsAg in that individual (Table 1). In exposures between heterosexuals, a second HBIG dose should be given if the index patient remains HBsAg-positive 3 months after detection. If the index patient is a known HBV carrier or remains HBsAg-positive for 6 months, HB vaccine should be offered to regular sexual contacts. For exposures among homosexual men, the HB vaccine series should be initiated at the time HBIG is given following a sexual exposure, since HB vaccine is recommended for all susceptible homosexual men. Additional doses of HBIG are unnecessary if vaccine is given. Because current lots of IG contain anti-HBs, it remains an important alternative to HBIG when HBIG is unavailable.

DTP-Associated Reactions: Analysis by Injection Site, Manufacturer, Prior Reactions, and Dose
Larry J. Baraff, Christopher L. Cody, and James D. Cherry (Univ. of California, Los Angeles)
Pediatrics 73:31–36, January 1984   2–29

The effects of injection site, previous reactions, and dose reduction on reactions to diphtheria-tetanus-pertussis (DTP) immunization were examined in children, aged 6 years and younger, scheduled for routine immunization in 1978 and 1979. A total of 15,752 immunizations were carried out in this 2-year period. Commercially available DTP vaccines were used. A subset of 772 children received two or more doses of DTP vaccine during the study. Some children with a history of previous reaction were given a half-dose immunization.

The relation between immunization site and reactions is given in Table 1. No clear patterns of reaction were apparent in relation to different vaccine manufacturers, and there were no significant differences in rates of more serious reactions. Children with a previous reaction more often had fever, local redness, and persistent crying after subsequent DTP immunizations (Table 2). The effect of dose reduction on reaction rates is shown in Table 3. All local reactions were significantly less frequent after reduced-dose immunization.

Children who have reacted adversely to DTP immunization are at an

---

TABLE 1.—EFFECT OF IMMUNIZATION SITE ON REACTION RATE AFTER 12,327 PRIMARY DTP IMMUNIZATIONS

Reaction	Reaction Rates (%) by Immunization Site			P Value
	Midanterior Thigh (N = 5,889)	Upper Lateral Thigh (N = 1,896)	Buttock (N = 4,542)	
Local reaction				
Redness	36.7	25.7	38.9	<.0001
Swelling	42.2	37.5	33.7	<.0001
Pain	53.6	45.1	35.9	<.0001
Systemic reaction				
Temperature ≥38°C	47.3	52.6	40.4	<.0001
Drowsiness	30.2	39.8	36.4	<.0001
Fretfulness	53.7	66.0	54.1	<.0001
Vomiting	6.6	7.7	6.4	>.0500
Anorexia	19.2	26.2	19.5	<.0001
Persistent crying	6.5	8.1	10.9	<.0001

(Courtesy of Baraff, L.J., et al.: Pediatrics 73:31–36, January 1984. Copyright American Academy of Pediatrics 1984.)

TABLE 2.—Reaction Rates to Subsequent DTP Immunizations as Function of Prior Similar Reactions in 772 Children

Reaction	Reaction Rate (%), Subsequent DTP		P Value
	No Prior Reaction	Prior Reaction	
Temperature ≥39°C	7.5 (25/332)*	20.0 (3/15)†	<.0800
Local redness >2.5 cm	8.7 (57/657)	21.7 (25/115)	<.0001
Persistent crying	2.6 (19/732)	5.0 (2/40)	<.8000

*No. patients with reaction on subsequent DTP/no. without prior similar reaction.
†No. patients with reaction on subsequent DTP/no. with prior similar reaction.
(Courtesy of Baraff, L.J., et al.: Pediatrics 73:31–36, January 1984. Copyright American Academy of Pediatrics 1984.)

TABLE 3.—Effect of Reduced Dose on Reaction Rates (%) After DTP Immunization

Reaction	Full Dose (N = 15,426)*	Half Dose (N = 100)	P Value
Local reactions			
Redness	37.8	26.0	<.0200
Swelling	41.1	30.0	<.0250
Pain	51.1	30.0	<.0005
Systemic reactions			
Temperature ≥38°C	46.3	38.0	<.1000
Drowsiness	31.6	23.0	<.1000
Fretfulness	53.5	53.0	>.5000
Vomiting	6.2	6.0	>.5000
Anorexia	20.7	22.0	>.5000
Persistent crying	3.1	0.0	<.1000

*Fever was evaluated after 7,592 full-dose and 49 half-dose DTP immunizations. Only children whose temperature was recorded at 3 and 6 hours after immunization are included.
(Courtesy of Baraff, L.J., et al.: Pediatrics 73:31–36, January 1984. Copyright American Academy of Pediatrics 1984.)

increased risk of reacting similarly to subsequent immunization. Less serious local reactions can be expected in such children when a half-dose of DTP vaccine is administered. The effect of such a practice on protection, if any, is unknown. Analysis of the potential risk-benefit ratio for pertussis vaccination clearly favors routine immunization.

▶ The possible role of pertussis immunization in the etiology of infantile spasms was investigated by analysis of 269 cases reported to the National Childhood Encephalopathy Study in the United Kingdom. In 34% of the cases an antecedent factor that may have caused infantile spasms was identified. The most common identified causes were perinatal hypoxia and tuberous sclerosis. Case-control studies showed no significant association between infantile spasms and pertussis immunization in the 28 days before onset. The authors suggest, from the patterns observed, that the vaccine does not cause infantile spasms but may trigger their onset in children in whom the disorder is destined to develop (Bellman, M. H., et al.: *Lancet* 1:1031, 1983).

Help is on the way for those that are not reassured by such findings. A new vaccine, developed by the Japanese, against *Bordetella* pertussis cell wall antigens has been shown to be as effective and produces less side effects than does the current whole-cell vaccine. This new vaccine presently is being used for mass immunization in Japan (Sato, Y., et al.: ibid. 1:122, 1984).

In the meantime, it would be prudent to follow the suggestions of the Immunization Practices Advisory Committee regarding contraindications for the use of pertussis vaccine, which follow.—F.A.O.

Supplementary Statement of Contraindications to Receipt of Pertussis Vaccine
Immunization Practices Advisory Committee
Morbidity Mortality Weekly Rep. 33:169–171, Apr. 6, 1984   2–30

The following statement updates some of the previous recommendations regarding pertussis vaccine. The Immunization Practices Advisory Committee (ACIP) reviewed the available data concerning the risks of pertussis disease and pertussis vaccine to infants and children with personal or family histories of convulsions. Based on available evidence, the ACIP does not consider a family history of convulsion to be a contraindication to receipt of pertussis vaccine. However, a personal history of a prior convulsion should be evaluated before initiating or continuing immunization with vaccines containing a pertussis component (i.e., diphtheria and tetanus toxoids with pertussis vaccine [DTP] (table).

Deferral of DTP for Infants and Children With Personal Histories of Convulsion(s)

Although there are uncertainties in the reported studies, recent data suggest that infants and young children who have previously had convulsions (whether febrile or nonfebrile) are more likely to have seizures following pertussis vaccination than those without such histories. Available data do not indicate that seizures temporally associated with vaccine administration predispose to permanent brain damage or exacerbate existing conditions. The incidence of pertussis in most areas of the United States is presently quite low. Consequently, for infants and young children who have histories of seizures before initiation of DTP immunization or who develop seizures before the four-dose primary series is completed, initiating or continuing pertussis immunization should be deferred until it can be determined that there is not an evolving neurologic disorder present. If such disorders are found, the infants or children should be given diphtheria and tetanus toxoids (DT) instead of DTP. If DT is used, three doses at least 4 weeks apart, followed by a fourth dose 6–12 months later, are recommended for infants. For children 1 year of age or older, two doses of DT at least 4 weeks apart, followed by a third dose 6–12 months later, are recommended.

Recommendations for Beginning or Continuing DTP After Deferral

For infants and children whose DTP immunizations are deferred because of histories of convulsion(s), the decision whether to proceed with DTP

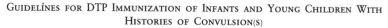

GUIDELINES FOR DTP IMMUNIZATION OF INFANTS AND YOUNG CHILDREN WITH HISTORIES OF CONVULSION(S)

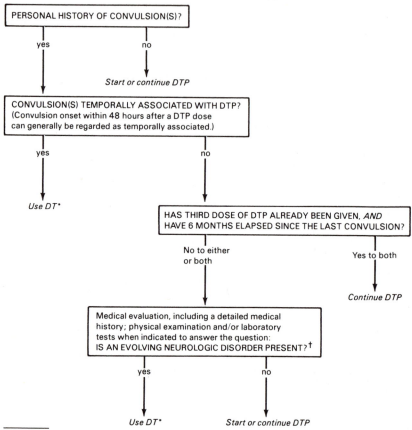

Note: These guidelines cannot cover every situation. Individualized medical judgment in specific cases may indicate a different course of action.

*For infants and children who received diphtheria-tetanua (DT), but who, on further evaluation, can be given pertussis vaccine, a separate pertussis vaccine is available. It is distributed by the Michigan State Department of Public Health.

†If the presence or absence of an evolving neurologic disorder cannot be established within 6 months after deferral of DTP, DT should be given rather than further delaying immunization.

(Courtesy of Immunization Practices Advisory Committee: Morbidity Mortality Weekly Rep. 33:169–171, Apr. 6, 1984.)

immunization can usually be made within the next few months. For infants who have received fewer than three doses of DTP, such a decision in most instances should be made no later than at 1 year of age. Following individual assessment, it may be decided to proceed with DTP, because infants and young children with convulsive disorders also appear to be at higher risk of adverse outcomes if they contract pertussis disease. Further, if unimmunized infants attend day-care centers, special clinics, and residential-care settings where other children may be unimmunized or if they travel to or reside in areas where the disease is endemic, they may be at increased risk of exposure to pertussis.

For infants and children with stable neurologic conditions, including well-controlled seizures, the benefits of pertussis immunization outweigh the risks, and such children may be vaccinated. The occurrence of single seizures (temporally unassociated with DTP) in infants and young children, while necessitating evaluation, need not contraindicate DTP immunization, particularly if the seizures can be satisfactorily explained. An example might be a febrile seizure in the course of exanthem subitum in a 14-month-old child. As with all infants or children with one or more febrile seizures, consideration of continuous anticonvulsant prophylaxis may be warranted.

Parents should be fully informed of the benefits and risks of immunization with DTP. Parents of infants and children with histories of convulsions should particularly be made aware of the slightly increased chance of post-immunization seizures. A minimum of three doses of DTP given at intervals of at least 4 weeks is necessary to provide adequate protection against pertussis. A fourth dose 6–12 months later is also recommended.

Contraindications to Pertussis Vaccine

Hypersensitivity to vaccine components, presence of an evolving neurologic disorder, or a history of a severe reaction (usually within 48 hours) following a previous dose all remain definitive contraindications to the receipt of pertussis vaccine. Severe reactions include collapse or shock, persistent screaming episode, temperature 40.5 C (105 F) or greater, convulsion(s) with or without accompanying fever, severe alterations of consciousness, generalized and/or local neurologic signs, or systemic allergic reactions. Although hemolytic anemia and thrombocytopenic purpura have previously been considered contraindications by the ACIP, the evidence of a causal link between these conditions and pertussis vaccination is not sufficient to retain them as contraindications.

Other Immunizations for Infants and Children for Whom Pertussis Vaccine Is Contraindicated

Immunization with DT and/or oral polio vaccine is not known to be associated with an increased risk of convulsions. Therefore, a history of prior convulsions is not a contraindication to receipt of these toxoids and vaccine. In addition, a history of prior convulsion(s) is not a contraindication for measles-mumps-rubella (MMR) vaccine. Further details concerning DTP vaccine or DT toxoids can be found in the 1981 ACIP statement.

Age-Related Changes in T and B Lymphocyte Subpopulations in the Peripheral Blood

Mary Jane Hicks, James F. Jones, Linda L. Minnich, Kristen A. Weigle, A. Cole Thies, and Jack M. Layton (Univ. of Arizona)
Arch. Pathol. Lab. Med. 107:518–523, October 1983

TABLE 1.—LYMPHOCYTE TYPING RESULTS FOR EACH AGE GROUP*

Age Group (N)	% Cells				Cell Counts ×10³/cu mm				
	T	B*	IgM	IgG	Total Lymphocytes	T	B	IgM B	IgG B
Newborns (12)	75 ± 7	13 ± 6	11 ± 6	1.2 ± 1	4.2 ± 2.0	3.1 ± 1.5	0.62 ± 0.6	0.49 ± 0.4	0.05 ± 0.06
<6 mo (10)	77 ± 6	17 ± 5	14 ± 4	0.82 ± 1	6.8 ± 1.7	5.2 ± 1.3	1.2 ± 0.5	0.94 ± 0.4	0.06 ± 0.07
6 mo-2 yr (17-18)	75 ± 6	16 ± 5	12 ± 5	0.88 ± 0.9	6.0 ± 1.5	4.5 ± 1.1	0.96 ± 0.4	0.71 ± 0.3	0.04 ± 0.04
2-4 yr (14-16)	76 ± 8	13 ± 4	9 ± 4	1.1 ± 0.8	4.7 ± 1.2	3.6 ± 0.9	0.58 ± 0.2	0.41 ± 0.2	0.05 ± 0.04
4-11 yr (15-19)	77 ± 6	11 ± 5	8 ± 6	1.5 ± 2	3.3 ± 1.0	2.6 ± 0.8	0.37 ± 0.2	0.27 ± 0.2	0.04 ± 0.06
13-21 yr (10-14)	79 ± 6	10 ± 7	8 ± 7	1.4 ± 1.6	2.3 ± 0.7	1.9 ± 0.6	0.30 ± 0.3	0.25 ± 0.2	0.04 ± 0.06
>21 yr (52-67)	79 ± 8	7 ± 4	5 ± 3	1.1 ± .1	1.9 ± 0.5	1.5 ± 0.4	0.14 ± 0.1	0.10 ± 0.07	0.02 ± 0.03

*Values are expressed as mean ± 1 SD.

†Surface immunoglobulin-bearing cells detected with polyvalent antiserum.

(Courtesy of Hicks, M.J., et al.: Arch. Pathol. Lab. Med. 107:518–523, October 1983; copyright 1983, American Medical Association.)

Quantitation of T and B lymphocytes in infants and children is important for the diagnosis of suspected immunodeficiency. Previous studies have indicated that the absolute and relative numbers of these cells vary with age, but the data regarding children are incomplete and often contradictory. In this investigation, the relationship between age and lymphocyte subpopulations was studied in 156 healthy subjects ranging in age from birth to 75 years. Common methods, including recent methodologic improvements, were used.

TABLE 2.—AGE GROUPS COMPARED WITH ADULT POPULATION*

Lymphocyte Value	Group					
	Newborns	<6 mo	6 mo-2 yr	2-4 yr	4-11 yr	13-21 yr
WBCs / cu mm	+	+	+	+	+†	−
% Lymphocytes	−	+	+	+	+	−
Lymphocytes / cu mm	+	+	+	+	+	−
% T cells	−	−	−	−	−	−
T cells / cu mm	+	+	+	+	+	−
% B cells (polyvalent)	+	+	+	+	+†	−
B cells / cu mm	+	+	+	+	+†	−
% IgM B cells	+	+	+	+†	+‡	−
IgM B cells / cu mm	+	+	+	+	+‡	−
% IgG B cells	−	−	−	−	−	−
IgG B cells / cu mm	−	−	−	−	−	−

*Symbols: + indicates significant difference ($P < .001$, unless otherwise specified); −, no significant difference.
†.001 < P ≤ .01.
‡.01 < P ≤ .05.
(Courtesy of Hicks, M.J., et al.: Arch. Pathol. Lab. Med. 107:518–523, October 1983; copyright 1983, American Medical Association.)

TABLE 3.—CORRELATION BETWEEN AGE
AND LYMPHOCYTE VALUES*

Lymphocyte Value	Spearman's ρ	P
WBCs / cu mm	−0.47	.001
% Lymphocytes	−0.69	.001
Lymphocytes / cu mm	−0.77	.001
% T cells	0.17	.07
T cells / cu mm	−0.75	.001
% B cells (polyvalent)	−0.46	.001
B cells / cu mm	−0.73	.001
% IgM B cells	−0.43	.001
IgM B cells / cu mm	−0.71	.001
% IgG B cells	0.15	.10
IgG B cells / cu mm	−0.07	.28

*In subjects aged 21 years and older, there was no correlation with age; newborns were excluded from correlation analysis.
(Courtesy of Hicks, M.J., et al.: Arch. Pathol. Lab. Med. 107:518–523, October 1983; copyright 1983, American Medical Association.)

TABLE 4.—SELECTED REVIEW OF PREVIOUS STUDIES

	Mean %*		Results	Comments
	B Cells	**T Cells**		
Clot et al	DFA-SIg	E rosette	No difference in % T and % B cells in newborns v infants; % B cells higher; % T cells lower in infants and children v adults	No 37 °C incubation of cells prior to SIg staining; only neonates and 3-mo-old infants studied
3-21 days (N = 26)	14	55		
3 mo (N = 12)	13	53		
Adults (N = 40)	11	70		
Campbell et al	DFA-SIg	E rosette	% B cells higher; % T cells lower in newborns v adults	No 37 °C incubation of cells; only compared cord blood results with adult values
Cord blood (N = 24)	32	53		
Adults (N = 29)	22	65		
Fleisher et al	EAC rosette	E rosette	% B cells higher; % T cells lower in infants (≤18 mo) v older children and adults	EAC method not specific for B cells, did not separate younger from older children
1 wk-18 mo (N = 9-18)	26	50		
18 mo-10 yr (N = 20-23)	23	57		
Adults (N = 30-42)	27	64		
Diaz-Jouanen et al	DFA-SIg	IFA-E rosette	Variable % T-cell result depending on method; no difference in % B cells in newborns v adults	No 37 °C incubation of cells; only compared cord blood results with adult values; IFA results higher than E rosette results
Cord blood (N = 30)	≅25	≅68/≅40		
Adults (N = 50)	≅22	≅80/≅65		
Asma et al	DFA-SIg	E rosette	No difference in % T and % B cells in newborns and children v adults; % T cells lowest and % B cells highest in newborns	No 37 °C incubation of cells
Cord blood (N = 4)	20	67		
0-1/1-3 mo (N = 8)	21/17	≅74		
3-6/6-12 mo (N = 8)	13/16	≅76		
1-14 yr (N = 45)	≅17	≅73		
Adults (N = 21)	14	76		

	DFA-SIg	E rosette		
Ben-Zwi et al			% B cells higher and % T cells lower in newborns *v* adults; % B cells and % T cells similar to adults by 1 and 3 yr, respectively	No 37 °C incubation of cells; did not study infants 1-11 mo old
Cord blood (N = 16)	40	50		
1-11 yr (N = 17)	30	54		
Adults (N = 18)	28	59		
Handzel et al			No difference in % B and % T cells in newborns *v* children and adults	No 37 °C incubation of cells; did not study children (1-12 yr) and adults separately
Cord blood (N = 10-11)	16	55		
Children and adults (N = 10-14)	14	60		
Falcaõ			% B cells higher in newborns than adults with further increase until 1 yr, then decline to adult levels by 3 yr; % T cells lower in newborns and children, increasing to adult levels by 7 yr	E rosette preparations smeared and covered, possibly causing mechanical disruption
Cord blood (N = 7)	14	60		
1 mo-2 yr (N = 57)	14-18	59-60		
3 yr-8 yr (N = 36)	12-13	63-67		
Adults (N = 51)	12	67		
Present study			% B cells higher in newborns than adults with further increase for 6 mo, then decline to adult levels by ≅13 yr; % T cells lower in newborns and children, increasing to adult levels by ≅13 yr	See Table 1
Cord blood (N = 12)	13	75		
<6 mo-2 yr (N = 27-28)	17-16	77-75		
2 yr-11 yr (N = 31-35)	13-11	76-77		
12 yr-21 yr (N = 10-14)	10	79		
Adults (N = 52-67)	7	79		

*In studies using more than one method, results given are those obtained using only the method indicated: DFA-SIg indicates direct fluorescent antibody technique for surface immunoglobulin using whole antibody reagents; E rosette, spontaneous sheep red blood cell rosette; EAC rosette, erythrocyte-antibody-complement rosette for detecting complement receptors; IFA, indirect fluorescent antibody staining with anti-human thymocyte serum.
(Courtesy of Hicks, M.J., et al.: Arch. Pathol. Lab. Med. 107:518–523, October 1983; copyright 1983, American Medical Association.)

Absolute numbers of T and B cells followed the same trend as the total lymphocyte count, which was elevated at birth, increased in the first 6 months, and then gradually decreased to adult levels at approximately age 13 years (Table 1). Compared with adult values, the percentage of B cells also was higher at birth and continued to increase for 6 months, followed by a gradual decrease to adult levels by late childhood or early adolescence. The percentage of T cells gradually increased from infancy to early adulthood. All values studied in subjects younger than 13 years, with the exception of the percentage of T cells and the percentage and absolute numbers of IgG-bearing B cells, varied significantly from those in persons older than age 21 years (Table 2). There were age-related trends for most lymphocyte values in subjects younger than age 21 years, excluding newborns (Table 3).

Previous studies (Table 4) provided conflicting and often incomplete data on relationships between age and relative proportions of lymphocyte subpopulations because of various experimental design problems, incomplete understanding of lymphocyte subpopulations, and use of older methods.

Common Variable Hypogammaglobulinemia in Children: Clinical and Immunologic Observations in 30 Patients
Christian Hausser (Ste-Justine Hosp., Montreal), Jean-Louis Virelizier, Diego Buriot, and Claude Griscelli (Hôp. des Enfants Malades, Paris)
Am. J. Dis. Child. 137:833–837, September 1983 2–32

Clinical and immunologic studies were made of 17 male and 13 female hypogammaglobulinemic patients for 1 to 16 years. Mean age at diagnosis was 10.5 years, 5 years after clinical onset.

Infectious manifestations in these patients are listed in Table 1. Upper and lower respiratory tract infections were observed most frequently, with chronic diarrhea of infectious origin the second most frequent manifestation. Lower respiratory tract damage with recurrent pneumonia was the most severe complication. *Candida albicans* was isolated repeatedly from bronchial secretions or stools of one third of the patients and reappeared every time antifungal therapy was discontinued. Noninfectious manifestations associated with common variable hypogammaglobinemia (CVHG) were numerous and diverse and included involvement of the digestive tract, hematologic disorders, lymphoid tissue hypertrophy, atopy-allergy, joint involvement, and short stature secondary to chronic illness (Table 2).

Immunologic findings included lymphoid hyperplasia with splenomegaly in 6 patients, seen in association with autoimmune hemolytic anemia in 1 and hyperplenism in another. Levels of serum immunoglobulin at the time of diagnosis are shown in Figure 2–14. The number of patients with a normal B lymphocyte count, compared with control children assayed on the same day, is shown in Table 3.

Total lymphocyte counts were normal in all but 3 patients, who had

TABLE 1.—INFECTIOUS MANIFESTATIONS
IN PATIENTS WITH CVHG

Infection	No. (%) of Patients
Pneumonia	26 (87)
Sinusitis	18 (60)
Diarrhea	17 (57)
Bronchiectasis	16 (53)
Otitis media	14 (47)
Pharyngitis-tonsillitis	13 (43)
Eye infections	8 (27)
Rhinitis	8 (27)
Cutaneous infections	4 (13)
Meningitis	4 (13)
Septicemia	4 (13)
Adenitis	2 (7)
Vaginitis	1 (3)
Pyelonephritis	1 (3)
Parotitis	1 (3)
Encephalomyelitis	1 (3)
Periodontitis	1 (3)

(Courtesy of Hausser, C., et al.: Am. J. Dis. Child. 137:833–837, September 1983; copyright, 1983, American Medical Association.)

repeated episodes of lymphopenia. Proliferative responses to mitogens and antigens and delayed cutaneous hypersensitivity (Table 4) showed normal response to mitogen stimulation, contrasting with lowered response to antigens in patients successfully vaccinated with BCG or infected with *Candida* organisms.

Three patients died, 1 of chronic respiratory insufficiency, 1 of chronic persisting hepatitis, and 1 of osteogenic sarcoma.

This study indicates that CVHG can occur in very young patients. Besides the two major complications (chronic bronchitis and chronic diarrhea), other complications observed were arthropathy, autoimmune hemolytic anemia, chronic hepatitis, and malignant neoplasms. Only symptoms can be treated, as the cause of CVHG is unknown; γ-globulin therapy, plasma infusion, antibiotic therapy, and respiratory kinesitherapy are the most useful treatments. Search for subtle defects of immunoregulation and study of familial cases (8 families had a history of immunodeficiency) may help explain the pathogenesis of this heterogeneous group of hypogammaglobulinemias.

▶ Doctor Micheal Miller, Professor and Chairman, Department of Pediatrics, University of California at Davis, helped us with this one. Doctor Spike writes:

TABLE 2.—Noninfectious
Manifestations Associated With CVHG

Manifestation	No. of Patients
Digestive involvement	
Sprue	3
Gastritis	3
Colitis	4
Hepatomegaly	3
Cholelithiasis	2
Stomatitis	2
Parotitis	1
Hematologic disorders	
Autoimmune hemolytic anemia	2
Idiopathic thrombocytopenia purpura	1
Pancytopenia	1
Lymphoid tissue hypertrophy	
Splenomegaly	6
Adenomegaly	4
Nodular lymphoid hyperplasia	7
Atopy-allergy	8
Joint involvement	7
Other diseases	
Alopecia	2
Psoriasis	2
Addison's disease	1
Keratoconjunctivitis	2
Malignant neoplasm	1
Short stature (secondary to chronic illness)	7

(Courtesy of Hausser, C., et al.: Am. J. Dis. Child. 137:833–837, September 1983; copyright 1983, American Medical Association.)

"Although there is not a great deal of new information in this report, the data provide the pediatrician with a very comprehensive and well-documented compendium of the likely types of clinical problems to be seen in patients with primary or secondary B cell deficiency. The degree of heterogeneity of the diagnostic category known as "common variable hypogammaglobulinemia" (CVHG) is of continuing importance to the clinical and basic immunologist. From a clinical point of view, however, it is interesting to note the similarity of clinical findings independent of mechanisms. In other words, regardless of whether the particular patient defect may lie in a suppressor T cell abnormality,

TABLE 3.—NUMBER (%) OF PATIENTS WITH VARIOUS B LYMPHOCYTE COUNTS

Detection Method	% of Cells With B-Lymphocyte Markers in Controls*	Total	B-Lymphocyte Count		
			Low	Normal	Elevated
C3 receptor	6-30	30	9 (30)	17 (57)	4 (13)
Fc receptor	10-22	25	6 (24)	17 (68)	2 (8)
Surface immunoglobulin					
μ	8-15	26	9 (34)	15 (58)	2 (8)
δ	5-15	11	4 (36)	6 (55)	1 (9)
γ	1-3	24	6 (25)	16 (66)	2 (9)
α	0.5-2	26	8 (31)	16 (62)	2 (7)

*Normal values in authors' laboratory.
(Courtesy of Hausser, C., et al.: Am. J. Dis. Child. 137:833–837, September 1983; copyright 1983, American Medical Association.)

TABLE 4.—PROLIFERATIVE RESPONSE AND DELAYED CUTANEOUS HYPERSENSITIVITY TO MITOGENS AND ANTIGENS IN PATIENTS WITH CVHG

Mitogen/Antigen	No. of Patients	
	Positive Proliferative Response	Positive Delayed Cutaneous Hypersensitivity
PHA	29/30	18/20
PWM	26/28	. . .
Concanavalin A	25/26	. . .
Allogeneic leukocytes	23/23	. . .
Tuberculin	5/12	12/21
Candida albicans	6/11	. . .
DNCB	. . .	7/8
Candidin	. . .	17/21
SKSD	. . .	5/10

PHA, phytohemagglutin, PWM, pokeweed mitogen; DNCB, dinitrochlorobenzene, and SKSD, streptokinase-streptodornase. Proliferative response was considered positive when it was more than 50% of that in normal controls.
(Courtesy of Hausser, C., et al.: Am. J. Dis. Child. 137:833–837, September 1983; copyright 1983, American Medical Association.)

a primary B cell abnormality, or a secondary phenomenon such as protein loss, the patient's symptoms appear quite similar. Thus, the "phenotype" is very predictable and the clinician should feel comfortable in making a tentative diagnosis of hypogammaglobulinemia regardless of the cause. The important clinical question that remains is how to develop more specific therapeutic approaches for individual patients with CVHG. The advent of intravenous γ-globulin along with the more traditional intramuscular and/or plasma preparations has increased the types of γ-globulin replacement available, but it may well be that some of these patients are better treated by a therapy dealing more directly with the underlying mechanism. With a more basic understanding of the

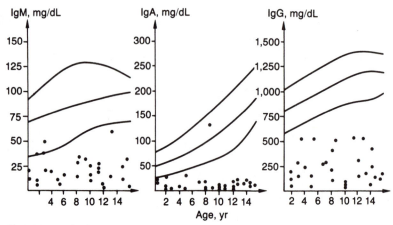

Fig 2–14.—Levels of IgM, IgA, and IgG at time of diagnosis in 30 patients with common variable hypogammaglobulinemia, compared with normal range curves (mean ± 2 SDs). (Courtesy of Hausser, C., et al.: Am. J. Dis. Child. 137:833–837, September 1983; copyright 1983, American Medical Association.)

individual mechanisms involved within this group, we can anticipate improved treatment for selected patients in the near future."

Hyperimmunoglobulin E Recurrent Infection (Job's) Syndrome: Review of NIH Experience and the Literature

Haig Donabedian and John I. Gallin (Natl. Inst. of Health)
Medicine (Baltimore) 62:195–208, July 1983   2–33

Findings were reviewed in 13 patients seen in the past 13 years with hyperimmunoglobulin E recurrent infection (HIE) syndrome, which is also termed "Job's syndrome" because of the presence of widespread "sore boils."

The patients had had recurrent bacterial sinopulmonary and skin infections from birth or early childhood and had serum IgE levels at least 10 times greater than the upper limit of normal (above 2,000 IU/ml). The findings in the 13 study patients and 3 others classified as having variants of HIE are summarized in Table 1. The cold abscesses can occur in any part of the body. Recurrent bronchitis and pneumonia are frequent (Table 2). Deep-seated infections other than pneumonias are unusual. The laboratory findings are given in Table 3. Preliminary HLA-typing studies have indicated no remarkable incidence of any one haplotype.

No treatment has been found more effective than antibiotics, local care, and surgical incision and drainage. Antibiotics effective against staphylococci or *Hemophilus,* or both, are given intravenously. Chronic hidradenitis suppurativa is a major problem in a few cases. Chronic onychomycosis has responded well to ketoconazole therapy. A trial of levamisole in 8 cases was stopped prior to projected termination when an increase in

TABLE 1.—CLINICAL PRESENTATION OF PATIENTS WITH HIE AND HIE VARIANTS

Patient	Sex	Race	Year of birth	Age at onset of 1st infection	Coarse facies?	History of cold abscesses?	History of pneumonias?	History of mucocutaneous candidiasis	Other infections
#1 JB	F	W	1967	1 month	Yes	Yes	Yes	Yes	Otitis externa
#2 AB	F	W	1971	4 months	Yes	Yes	Yes	Yes	Otitis externa and media, mastoiditis
#3 CC	F	W	1959	1 month	Yes	Yes	Yes	Yes	Otitis externa and media, lymphadenitis, osteomyelitis of ischium and maxilla
#4 KC	F	W	1967	1 month	Yes	Yes	Yes	Yes	Lymphadenitis
#5 WC	M	W	1959	Early childhood	No	Yes	No	No	Cellulitis of leg
#6 MD	M	W	1956	3 months	Yes	No	Yes	No	Cellulitis of arm
#7 MBD	F	W	1956	Early childhood	No	Yes	Yes	No	Otitis externa and media
#8 DL	M	W	1949	Early childhood	Yes	Yes	Yes	Yes	Otitis externa, bronchopleural fistula
#9 CP	F	W	1968	1 month	Yes	Yes	Yes	No	Bronchopleural fistula, prostatitis
#10 CS	F	B	1962	3 months	No	Yes	Yes	No	Otitis externa, parotitis, lymphadenitis
#11 JS	F	W	1973	3 months	No	Yes	Yes	Yes	Chalazia, otitis media
#12 SW	F	W	1953	2 years	Yes	Yes	Yes	No	Otitis externa, facial cellulitis
#13 KZ	F	W	1939	1 year	Yes	Yes	Yes	Yes	Osteomyelitis of finger
#14 CB	F	W	1978	1 month	No	No	No	No	Impetigo
#15 TC	F	B	1959	3 years	Yes	Yes	Yes	No	Osteomyelitis of finger
#16 TL	M	O	1961	17 years	No	No	Yes	No	Renal and hepatic abscesses

(Courtesy of Donabedian, H., and Gallin, J.I.: Medicine (Baltimore) 62:195–208, July 1983.)

TABLE 2.—Incidence of Major and Minor
Infections in Patients With HIE*

Patient #	Period of observation (mos.)	Major and minor infections	# Major infections
1	24	Pneumonia-1	0
		Soft tissue abscess-1	
		Furunculosis-5	
2	17	Sinusitis-1	1
		Bronchitis-1	
		UTI†-1	
3	20	Abscessed tooth and maxillary osteomyelitis-1	2
		Otitis media-1	
		Bronchitis-2	
7	24	Soft tissue abscess-1	1
		Otitis externa-1	
		Bronchitis-5	
10	11	Soft tissue abscess-3	3
		Pneumonia-1	
11	18	Pneumonia-1	3
		Bronchitis-2	
		Impetigo-1	
		UTI-3	
12	19	Soft tissue abscess-4	1
		Furunculosis-2	
		Cellulitis-1	
		Sinusitis-1	
		Paronychia-1	

*Major infection = infection that required intravenous antibiotics or inpatient surgical procedure, or both. Minor infection = infection that required only oral antibiotics or outpatient surgical procedure, or both.

†UTI = urinary tract infection.

(Courtesy of Donabedian, H., and Gallin, J.I.: Medicine (Baltimore) 62:195–208, July 1983.)

major infections was recognized. The threshold for surgical drainage of abscesses in patients with HIE should be lower than that for other patients.

The HIE syndrome is characterized by recurrent bacterial infections of the skin and sinopulmonary tract. A variable chemotactic defect is observed; the mononuclear cells variably produce an inhibitor of neutrophil chemotaxis. The reason for recurrence of infections, however, remains uncertain. Early surgery is used to treat the infections, and prolonged intravenous antibiotic therapy is given.

► I wrote to Dr. Ralph Wedgewood, Professor of Pediatrics, University of Washington, for a comment. Who better? Doctor Wedgewood was there when the entity was named. Doctor Wedgewood writes:

"I prefer the term 'Job's syndrome,' as 'hyper-IgE' gives inappropriate emphasis and hints at a causal relationship that may interfere conceptually with our understanding of the problem; the elevated IgE, may be, in fact, no more

TABLE 3.—EOSINOPHILIA, SERUM IgE LEVELS AND
INCIDENCE OF ABNORMAL NEUTROPHIL
CHEMOTAXIS IN PATIENTS WITH HIE
AND HIE VARIANTS

Patient number	Average* percentage of eosinophils	Average number of eosinophils/ mm³	Average IgE level (IU/ml)	Incidence of abnormal neutrophil chemotaxis†
1	9.0	814	25,500	4/7
2	7.9	776	26,165	5/12
3	6.6	547	11,287	11/16
4	12.5	1720	4,833	1/1
5	21.0	1554	35,000	0/2
6	3.3	57	19,000	2/2
7	11.6	1436	37,962	17/22
8	10.7	1193	7,292	3/3
9	8.4	667	30,041	6/13
10	9.5	666	50,946	17/17
11	2.8	294	9,260	5/5
12	6.1	442	26,325	4/8
13	9.4	181	3,200	2/5
Total (1–13)	9.1±1.3‡	796±147	22,067±4023	77/133§
14	16.8	1412	2,598	7/7
15	5.5	376	306	10/14
16	17.0	1614	32,500	3/5
Total (14–16)	13.1±3.8	1134±383	11801±10370	20/26

*Average of each patient's value determined by averaging first value
for each test obtained on each admission to National Institutes of Health.
†Number of abnormal studies divided by total number of studies.
‡Mean ± SEM.
§Total.
(Courtesy of Donabedian, H., and Gallin, J.I.: Medicine (Baltimore)
62:195–208, July 1983.)

than an epiphenomenon related to the type of chronic antigenic stimulation. Job is more deserving of a place in the sun—and he came first. The appearance of boils, not hyper-IgE, is the hallmark of the problem, although I suppose that this emphasis may also not be entirely accurate. The devastating pulmonary problems, as is true in so many immunodeficiency syndromes, are the major cause of morbidity and mortality. Most of our cases in the long term have had pulmonary abscesses and pneumatoceles; one of our original patients died a few years ago from chronic lung disease.

"Long-term follow-up of the other original patient also has been informative. Her firstborn son died at age 3 days with respiratory distress and pulmonary infiltrates. Her second son, now aged 6 years, developed respiratory diseases with wheezing by age 1 week; at age 2 weeks he had severe, secondarily infected (Staphylococcus) generalized eczema. Throughout infancy he had recurrent pulmonary problems, eczema, and staphylococcal skin infections. His IgE level was 10 IU/ml at age 2½ weeks, 18 IU/ml at age 8 weeks, 200 IU/ml at age 20 weeks, 2,560 IU/ml at age 1 year, 104,000 IU/ml at age 2 years, and 21,200 IU/ml at age 3 years. From birth, his chemotaxis was abnormal. A third son, by a different father, is normal (Clin. Res. 29:123A, 1980). The extraordinary rise in IgE concentration followed rather than preceded clinical symptoms. In this instance, the syndrome was hereditary (as in others) and the hyper-IgE was presumably a secondary phenomenon. Perhaps we might learn more about the syndrome if we quit perseverating on hyper-IgE as a prerequisite for diagnosis and paid more attention (as Gallin, Hill, Quie, and others have) to the sometimes evanescent, enigmatic aberrations in chemotaxis. Use of the term 'Job's syndrome' makes this easier."

Acquired Immunodeficiency Syndrome in Infants

Gwendolyn B. Scott, Billy E. Buck, Joni G. Leterman, Frederick L. Bloom, and Wade P. Parks (Univ. of Miami)
N. Engl. J. Med. 310:76–81, Jan. 12, 1984   2–34

A cellular immune deficiency state similar to that of adults with acquired immunodeficiency syndrome (AIDS) recently has been described in children in the United States and Canada. The authors report data on 14 infants with profound cellular immune deficiency who were seen at Jackson Memorial Hospital in a 32-month period in 1980 to 1983. Most had been born to Haitian parents in Miami. In the absence of usual causes of immunosuppression, AIDS was defined as the occurrence of an opportunistic infection or Kaposi's sarcoma, or both.

Clinical data are given in Table 1. Nine infants met strict criteria of the Centers for Disease Control for AIDS; the others did not have demonstrable opportunistic infection. Severe failure to thrive was the most consistent clinical feature. All but 2 patients had persistent *Candida albicans* infection of the oral mucosa. The most common types of opportunistic infection were *Pneumocystis carinii* pneumonitis and cytomegalovirus pneumonia. Ten of 13 infants had elevated immunoglobulin levels, and 6 had elevated levels of circulating immune complexes. Several patients exhibited autoimmune phenomena. In contrast to adults with AIDS, most patients had normal absolute lymphocyte counts. Two had normal T4/T8 ratios when *P. carinii* pneumonitis was diagnosed. An earlier T cell study in 1 patient showed a T4/T8 ratio of 1.0, and a repeat T cell study in another showed a T4/T8 ratio of 1.4. Five patients had a positive antinuclear antibody test, 3 had positive Coombs' tests, and 1 had antiplatelet antibodies during thrombocytopenia. The spectrum of infections is shown in Table 2. Bacterial infections were quite frequent. With 1 exception, blood transfusions were given when clinical disease was already evident.

Gram-negative sepsis was the major cause of the 7 deaths. Two infants had autopsy evidence of disseminated lymphadenopathic Kaposi's sarcoma.

These cases suggest the likelihood of transplacental, perinatal, or postnatal transmission of an unidentified infectious agent that causes acquired immunodeficiency syndrome in infants. One mother has clinical AIDS. The involvement of an unusual agent such as human T cell leukemia retrovirus in AIDS has been proposed.

▶ The fact that AIDS occurs in infants and children was first brought to our attention by James Oleske and co-workers (*JAMA* 249:2345, 1983) and Arye Rubinstein and associates (ibid., p. 2350) and was discussed in the 1984 YEAR

TABLE 1.—CHARACTERISTICS OF INFANTS WITH AIDS*

PATIENT NO.	NONBACTERIAL INFECTION *	SOURCE	BACTERIAL INFECTION *	SOURCE †
1	*Pneumocystis carinii* (p)	Tracheal aspirate	*Escherichia coli*	Blood
2	Cytomegalovirus (p) Herpes simplex (c) Hepatitis B (s)	Lung, liver Oral mucosa	*E. coli* *Pseudomonas aeruginosa*	Middle ear Blood (T)
3	*P. carinii* (p)	Lung biopsy	None	
4	Cytomegalovirus *P. carinii* (p)	Urine, lung Lung biopsy	None	
5	Cytomegalovirus (p)	Lung, liver GI tract	*E. coli* and *Bacillus fragilis*	Blood (T)
6	Cytomegalovirus Epstein–Barr virus (s)	Urine, lung	*Streptococcus pneumoniae*	Blood
7	None		None	
8	*P. carinii* (p)	Lung biopsy	None	
9	Herpes simplex	Lung	*P. aeruginosa*	Blood (T)
10	None		*E. coli* *Mycobacterium tuberculosis* (p)	Urine CNS, lung
11	Herpes simplex ‡ Cytomegalovirus (s) ‡ Epstein–Barr virus (s)	Oral mucosa	*Hemophilus influenzae* *Staphylococcus aureus*	Blood Blood
12	Varicella zoster (c)	L-5 dermatome	*Str. pneumoniae* *Staph. epidermidis* *H. influenzae*	Blood Blood Blood
13	None		*E. coli*	Blood
14	Cytomegalovirus (s) ‡ Herpes simplex ‡ Epstein–Barr virus (s)	Oral mucosa	*Str. pneumoniae* *Str. pneumoniae* *P. aeruginosa*	CSF Blood External-ear-canal abscess

*H = Haitian, PCP = *Pneumocystis carinii* pneumonia, FTT = failure to thrive, CA = persistent infection of oral mucosa with *Candida albicans*, PPI = persistent pulmonary infiltrates, Hep = hepatosplenomegaly, PD = protracted diarrhea, CMV = cytomegalovirus, CE = *Candida* esophagitis, Lym = lymphadenopathy, RD = recurrent diarrhea, B = American black, Clb = clubbing, W = white, KS = Kaposi's sarcoma, and HSV = herpes simplex virus.

(Courtesy of Scott, G.B., et al.: N. Engl. J. Med. 310:76–81, Jan. 12, 1984. Reprinted by permission of the New England Journal of Medicine.)

BOOK (pp. 22–24). The group of patients described by Scott and others puts this problem in sharp clinical focus.

The story is rapidly unfolding, so that what is written in 1984 may be hopelessly out of date as you read these words in 1985. The syndrome was first identified in 1981, and an intense search for its cause was begun. The May 4, 1984, issue of *Science* contained four reports that appear to have identified the virus responsible for the syndrome. It appears that a recently discovered subgroup of the human T cell leukemia virus family, termed "HTLV-III," is linked to the disease. The virus was isolated from lymphocytes of 36% of

TABLE 2.—INFECTIONS OCCURRING IN INFANTS WITH AIDS

PATIENT NO.	SEX	ETHNIC GROUP (MOTHER/FATHER)	AGE AT FIRST ADMISSION (Mo)	OPPORTUNISTIC INFECTION AND/OR KAPOSI'S SARCOMA	CLINICAL FEATURES	OUTCOME
AIDS with opportunistic infection and/or Kaposi's sarcoma						
1	F	H/H	1	PCP	FTT, CA, PPI, Hep, PD	Living
2	F	H/H	1	CMV, CE	FTT, CA, PPI, Hep	Death (at 6 mo)
3	F	H/H	1	PCP, CMV	FTT, PPI, Hep, Lym, RD	Living
4	F	H/H	Birth	PCP, CE, CMV	FTT, CA, PPI, Hep, Lym, PD	Living
5	F	H/H	2	CMV	FTT, CA, Hep	Death (at 4 mo)
6	F	B/B	4	CMV	FTT, PPI, Clb	Living
7	F	W/B	6	CE	FTT, CA, PPI, Hep, Lym	Death (at 16 mo)
8	M	H/H	6	PCP, KS	FTT, CA, Hep	Death (at 9 mo)
9	M	H/H	1	HSV, KS	FTT, CA, PPI, Hep, RD	Death (at 8 mo)
AIDS-like illness (without opportunistic infection or Kaposi's sarcoma)						
10	M	B/H	4	None	FTT, CA, PPI, Clb, Hep, Lym, PD	Living
11	M	H/H	1	None	FTT, CA, PPI, Hep, RD	Living
12	F	H/H	6	None	FTT, CA, PPI, Clb, Hep, PD	Death (at 18 mo)
13	M	H/H	2	None	FTT, CA, Hep, PD	Death (at 3 mo)
14	M	H/H	7	None	FTT, CA, PPI, Hep, Lym, PD	Living

*Organism identified by culture unless indicated as follows: p = pathologic findings consistent with diagnosis; s = serologic diagnosis (more than fourfold titer rise); and c = clinical diagnosis.

†T = terminal event—positive culture associated with fulminant sepsis and subsequent death. CNS = central nervous system, CSF = cerebrospinal fluid.

‡Self-limited, localized, or subclinical infection that did not qualify as opportunistic.

(Courtesy of Scott, G.B., et al.: N. Engl. J. Med. 310:76–81, Jan. 12, 1984. Reprinted by permission of the New England Journal of Medicine.)

patients with AIDS and from 86% of patients with closely related disorders (Gallo, R. C., et al.: *Science* 224:500, 1984). Antibody to HTLV-III occurs with very high prevalence among groups with a high prevalence of AIDS (Kalyanaraman, V. S., et al.: ibid. 225:321, 1984). Transmission is still believed to occur only as a result of intimate contact, sharing of contaminated needles, or, less frequently, through transfusions of blood or blood products.—F.A.O.

3 Allergy and Dermatology

Prophylaxis of Atopic Disease by Six Months' Total Solid Food Elimination: Evaluation of 135 Exclusively Breast-Fed Infants of Atopic Families
Merja Kajosaari and Ulla M. Saarinen (Helsinki)
Acta Paediatr. Scand. 72:411–414, May 1983   3–1

Evaluation was made of 135 infants of atopic parents who were exclusively breast-fed for 6 months without receiving any cow's milk-based supplements. Seventy infants received no nourishment except for breast milk during the 6 months, and 65 were first given solid foods at age 3 months. The diet for all infants was similar during ages 6–12 months.

Atopic eczema occurred in 33 (24%) of the 135 infants. Eczema was more common in the solid food group (35%) than in the exclusively breast milk group (14%) ($P < .01$) (Fig 3–1). Food allergy was less common (7%) in the exclusively breast milk group than in the solid food group (37%). Egg allergy was the most frequent finding (table). Symptoms usually included urticaria in children with egg and fish allergy, and skin rash in those with other allergies. All children with positive histories of fish, egg, and citrus fruit allergy were controlled by challenge and rechallenge. The difference between the exclusively breast milk group and the solid food group was evident with regard to positive history ($P < .01$).

These results suggest that late introduction of solid foods is prophylactic

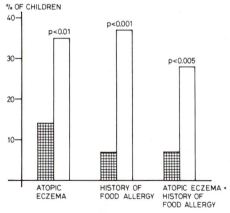

Fig 3–1.—Atopic eczema and history of food allergy at age 1 year, evaluated separately and together in 135 children. Shaded areas designate the exclusive breast milk group; white areas designate the solid food group. (Courtesy of Kajosaari, M., and Saarinen, U.M.: Acta Paediatr. Scand. 72:411–414, May 1983.)

History of Allergy to Different Foods at Age
1 Year

Food antigen	Exclusive breast milk group (n=70)	Solid food group (n=65)
Egg	2	10
Citrus fruit	2	3
Fish	1	4
Tomato	1	5
Strawberry	1	5
Cow's milk	1	5
Peas	–	4
Chocolate	1	3
Raspberry	–	2
Cereals	–	1

(Courtesy of Kajosaari, M., and Saarinen, U.M.: Acta Paediatr. Scand. 72:411–414, May 1983.)

---

for food allergy and atopic eczema in breast-fed infants at hereditary risk. The occurrences of food allergy and atopic eczema were significantly lower in the exclusively breast milk group than in the solid food group. The influence of early or late introduction of solid food seemed to be nonspecific, because the food items given were in general not responsible for the atopic symptoms. The prophylactic effect of postponing the introduction of solid foods seemed to last for up to age 1 year with regard to development of atopic eczema.

▶ As early as 1936, it was proposed that prolonged breast-feeding would reduce the incidence of atopic eczema (Grulee, C. G., et al.: *J. Pediatr.* 9:223, 1936). The Finnish group, the authors of the above article, have pursued this problem continuously (see 1981 Year Book, pp. 131–134) and have arrived at helpful conclusions. Failure of prevention may be a consequence of fetal exposure to excessive antigens from the maternal diet (see 1984 Year Book, p. 125) or exposure to antigens that are transferred in maternal milk. Not everyone agrees that prolonged and exclusive breast-feeding will prevent atopic disease (Fergusson, D. M., et al.: *Clin. Allergy* 11:325, 1981; and Hide, D. W., et al.: *Arch. Dis. Child.* 56:172, 1981).

Helenor Pratt has followed 198 infants from birth until age 4½ to 5 years to observe the development of eczema and asthma and its relationship to infant feeding. She found that the incidence of eczema decreased in infants with an immediate family history of atopy when *exclusive* breast-feeding was continued beyond age 12 weeks, whereas the incidence of eczema rose in all breast-fed infants, regardless of their atopic family history, when breast-feeding combined with other foods was continued beyond age 12 weeks (Pratt, H. F.: *Early Hum. Dev.* 9:283, 1984).

Sequential studies of infants with a family history of atopy have demonstrated that in infants in whom atopic eczema subsequently developed, the number of T-suppressor lymphocytes was reduced and that this defect in T cell regulation preceded overt clinical disease (Chandra, R. K., et al.: *Lancet* 2:1393, 1983).

What can we do with all this information? In families with a history of atopic disease, should we have mother's exclusively breast-feed their infants for as long as possible and for at least 6 months? In contrast, in families with no history of atopy, should we have mothers exclusively breast-feed their infants for as long as possible?—F.A.O.

Predictive Value of Cord Blood IgE Levels in "At-Risk" Newborn Babies and Influence of Type of Feeding
L. Businco, F. Marchetti, G. Pellegrini, and R. Perlini
Clin. Allergy 13:503–508, November 1983   3–2

Asthma develops more frequently in children with wheezy bronchitis and high levels of IgE than in children with normal IgE levels. Results of prospective studies suggest that dietary control in the first months of life may protect against the development of atopy. The authors determined cord serum levels of IgE in 101 neonates born of atopic parents; the infants were examined every 3 months thereafter until age 2 years to assess any relationship between IgE levels and signs and symptoms of allergic rhinitis, bronchial asthma, atopic dermatitis, urticaria, and food allergy.

Mean cord blood IgE concentrations were 1.06 ± 1.02 units per ml in infants with atopic disease and 0.34 ± 0.79 unit per ml in nonatopic infants ($P < .001$); 57% of the newborns had no detectable level of IgE. Among breast-fed infants, 37.5% of those with cord blood IgE levels of more than 0.8 unit per ml and 11.5% of those with an IgE level below 0.8 unit per ml had atopic disease. The corresponding percentages for soy-fed infants were 33.3% and 15.8%. Of the infants fed cow's milk, 90% with a cord blood IgE level of more than 0.8 unit per ml and 16% with an IgE level of less than 0.8 unit per ml became atopic. There was no correlation between IgE levels in maternal blood and those in the respective infant's cord blood.

The measurement of IgE antibody in cord blood is helpful in the early diagnosis of atopy. The total IgE level should be determined in all neonates at risk for atopy.

▶ This is an exciting observation and may be the predictor we have been looking for. It would appear that the development of atopy in babies with large amounts of IgE in their cord blood can be influenced by the type of feeding during early infancy. Please note that 90% of infants with a cord blood IgE level of more than 0.8 units per ml who were fed cow's milk developed atopy.

Only 1 newborn had cow's milk-specific IgE antibodies and none was present in the mother, thus suggesting intrauterine sensitization. When fed a cow's milk formula at age 20 days, this infant displayed wheezing, diarrhea, and vomiting. It appears that IgE antibodies, synthesized by the fetus, are responsible for atopic disease in early infancy.

Total IgE measurements may be a very useful determination to perform on cord blood, particularly in those babies at risk for atopy.—F.A.O.

Nitrofurantoin-Induced Cholestatic Hepatitis From Cow's Milk in a Teen-aged Boy

William R. Berry, George H. Warren, and Juerg Reichen (Univ. of Colorado)
West. J. Med. 140:278–280, February 1984   3–3

Acute hepatotoxic reactions to nitrofurantoin are rare. A case is reported of nitrofurantoin-induced cholestatic hepatitis in which the drug unknowingly was ingested in cow's milk.

Boy, 16, had had cramping epigastric and right upper quadrant pain for 3 days, associated with nausea and vomiting, and an erythematous rash of the palms and soles. Jaundice and chills occurred on the day of admission. Temperature was 38.3 C. Icterus and a maculopapular eruption were observed. The white blood cell count was 15,900/μl, with 68% segmented neutrophils. The serum alkaline phosphatase activity was 33 IU/L. The bilirubin concentration was 15.4 mg/dl, with a direct-reacting fraction of 8.2 mg/dl. The patient remained intermittently febrile. Liver biopsy after 1 week showed findings of toxic hepatitis, with moderate centrilobular cholestasis. Most portal tracts were edematous and infiltrated by neutrophils and eosinophils. It was learned that the patient had taken milk from cows treated parenterally with nitrofurantoin in the week before he became ill. He became afebrile in the next few days and has remained asymptomatic for over a year.

The histologic findings in this case were consistent with nitrofurantoin-induced cholestatic injury. The drug was present in milk from treated cows that the patient consumed. Transmission of drug toxicity via milk is a well-recognized phenomenon. An immune, possibly genetically mediated injury has been proposed in nitrofurantoin-induced liver cell damage, but the evidence is inconclusive. Furane derivatives are hepatotoxic in mice.

▶ *Cherchez la vache* when things go wrong. There was no chance that this article would pass by unselected.—F.A.O.

Allergic Form of Meadow's Syndrome (Munchausen by Proxy)

J. O. Warner and M. J. Hathaway (London)
Arch. Dis. Child. 59:151–156, February 1984   3–4

"Munchausen's syndrome by proxy" is a label attached to children presented by their mothers with a variety of fabricated disorders, leading to extensive unnecessary investigations. It now is known as "Meadow's syndrome." Seventeen children from 11 families who had the allergic form of Meadow's syndrome were evaluated (table). All the mothers believed that severe allergic disease was present. Foods were implicated in 16 cases and house dust mites in 1. Maternal obsession with avoiding allergens had led to bizarre diets and life-styles. Ten children had mild atopic disorders, but none had objective evidence of food intolerance or allergy. Double-blind food challenges yielded no reaction in all 6 children tested. Single-blind challenges were made in 2 other cases.

Most of the mothers were articulate, middle-class women. Marital problems were frequent; 3 mothers were single parents. A limpet-like attachment to the child was characteristic. The mothers insisted on many medical consultations. In only 3 cases was the outcome totally satisfactory. Three children improved while away from their mothers. In 5 cases in which double-blind challenge studies had been done the mothers were angered by the results and rejected every attempt to redirect treatment. They subsequently failed to attend for outpatient visits. No case of physical abuse or cot death has occurred to date.

In most of these cases of allergic Meadow's syndrome the obsession with allergy had originated with physicians. Management was extremely difficult. Many children remained on a diet and did not return for follow-up despite the careful exclusion of allergic disorder. Prevention seems to be the best approach. Appropriate initial management may prevent mothers from developing entrenched beliefs regarding the cause of their children's symptoms.

▶ The term "Meadow's syndrome" has not yet caught on in the United States, but certainly the problem that is described by this term is well recognized and, in fact, may be epidemic.

S. R. Meadow, of the Department of Pediatrics and Child Health, St. James University Hospital, Leeds, England, wrote these comments after the manuscript of Warner and Hathaway:

"Clinicians are familiar with parents who exaggerate their child's illness, are exceedingly anxious about minor symptoms, or who report symptoms and signs that are not apparent to others in the family and to other trained observers. The mothers have to be treated with understanding and skill in order to avoid overinvestigating the child; such families are a regular part of every pediatrician's work. The mother's behavior becomes pathological and dangerous, however, when she resorts to extreme falsification or the fabrication of signs and when the child's growth and development are hampered by excessive hospitalization, investigations, or by restriction of activity and schooling by the mother.

"Warner selected 17 children from among several hundred allegedly allergic children who were found not to be allergic. The particular problem for these children, as study of the detail of the results and discussion sections of his paper shows, was the way in which extraordinary and unpleasant regimens were inflicted on the children because of the mothers' obsessions—for instance, the schoolchild who had to sleep on an upturned wardrobe wrapped in toilet paper and silver foil. Most of us would agree that that child was being abused fearfully.

"The mothers probably did not fabricate signs, and most readers are likely to conclude that the mothers did not *deliberately* falsify the illness story or the symptoms. Unfortunately there is no sharp dividing line between deliberate falsification (malingering for conscious gain) and abnormal illness behavior in which there is unconscious gain (hysterical behavior). The end result for the child is the same, and can be both cruel and dangerous, regardless of the origin of the mother's behavior.

"It is interesting that in the 11 families neither the children nor their siblings

DETAILS OF 13 CHILDREN WITH THE ALLERGIC FORM OF MEADOW'S SYNDROME*

Case No.	Age (years)	Sex	Presenting problems	Treatment at presentation	Reputed allergies	Previous consultations	Origin of allergic knowledge	Skin tests		Total IgE IU/ml	Radioallergo sorbent tests		Food challenge	Final diagnosis and outcome	Diet related
								Inhalant	Foods		Inhalant	Foods			
1	8	M	Asthma, 'hyperactive'	Intal diet	5 foods	11	Allergist Hyperactive Society	+ve	–ve	ND	ND	ND	refused	Mild asthma easily controlled, failed clinic attendances.	No
2	10	M	'Hyperactive', disturbed	Diet sublingual hypos.	10 foods	5	Clinical ecologist	+ve	–ve	340	ND	2 –ve	DB –ve	Mild asthma, refused psychiatric help and follow up	No
3	8	F	Nausea, abdominal pains	Diet	5 foods	4	Allergy Advisory Service	–ve	–ve	34	–ve	2 –ve	DB –ve	Mother angry, refused follow up	No
4	15	M	Hyperactive dyslexia	Diet	12 foods	3	Hyperactive Society	+ve	–ve	ND	ND	ND	ND	Mild hayfever, dyslexia; failed follow up	No
5	14	F	Migraine, hyperactive	Diet, hyposen.	Many foods, inconsistent	4	Allergist	–ve	–ve	18	ND	2 –ve	DB –ve	Anorexia, gradual relaxation of diet	Yes
6	10	F	Hyperactive, nocturnal enuresis	Diet Homoeopathy	6 foods	3	Homoeopath	+ve	–ve	90	+ve HDM	3 –ve	DB –ve	Mild perennial rhinitis; refused psychiatric help and follow up	No ⎫ siblings
7	8	M	Hyperactive, nocturnal enuresis	Diet Homoeopathy	5 foods	3	Homoeopath	–ve	–ve	40	–ve	3 –ve	DB –ve	Normal child; refused psychiatric help and follow up	No ⎭

8	7	M	ESN, recurrent urinary tract infections	Diet sublingual hypos.	4 foods	3	Clinical ecologist	–ve	–ve	ND	ND	ND	Open –ve	Relaxed diet as out-patient and stopped prescriptions; no change Megalencephaly and ESN	Yes
9	6	M	Hyperactive, petit mal	Diet, Homeopathy, Anticonvulsants	5 foods	1	Hyperactive Society	+ve	–ve	ND	ND	ND	DB –ve	Petit mal, disturbed, mild asthma; refused completion of tests and follow up	No
10	10	M	Hyperactive, asthma	Diet, 'aero-allergen'	6 foods HDM and feathers	6	USA allergist	+ve	–ve	319	+ve HDM	5 –ve	SB –ve	Mother very disturbed. Very mild asthma; frequent school absences; children taken into care	? } siblings
11	7	F	Hyperactive, asthma	Diet, 'aero-allergen'	6 foods HDM and feathers	6	USA allergist	+ve	–ve	ND	ND	ND	SB –ve		?
12	13	F	Rhinitis, 'very sickly'	'Aero-allergen'	HDM	2	St Mary's allergy clinic	+ve	–ve	ND	ND	NA	Mother hospital admission with 'nervous breakdown'. Mild allergic rhinitis	—
13	35	F	Meniere's disease	Diet	8 foods	3	Clinical ecology book	–ve	–ve	ND	ND	ND	ND	5 of 6 children on diet for diarrhoea etc; all relaxed diet without relapse	Children—Yes Mother—No

*ND, not done; DB, double blind; SB, single blind; NA, not applicable; HDM, house dust mite; Hypos, hyposensitization.
(Courtesy of Warner, J.O., and Hathaway, M.J.: Arch. Dis. Child. 59:151–156, February 1984.)

seem to have suffered from other forms of child abuse, for there is an important link between parentally induced factitious illness and nonaccidental poisoning, physical abuse, and sudden death.

'' 'Allergy' has been reported as an associated feature of many of the gross cases of Munchausen's syndrome by proxy reported from several different countries in recent years. Of 71 British cases for which I have details, 'allergy,' though rarely the most worrying presentation, was an additional main presentation in 22. After a false story of seizures and after factitious bleeding, it was the third most common presentation. The alleged allergies have been to a variety of substances—foods causing diarrhea, chemicals causing behavior problems, and chemicals, plasters, and procedures causing rashes. Allergy is one of several warning signals that may help the clinician to remember the possibility of factitious illness when dealing with a child who has prolonged, unexplained, and complex illness which has been solved by neither extensive investigation nor treatment.''

Is Migraine Food Allergy? Double-Blind Controlled Trial of Oligoantigenic Diet Treatment

J. Egger, C. M. Carter, J. Wilson, M. W. Turner, and J. F. Soothill
Lancet 2:865–868, Oct. 15, 1983   3–5

Cheese, chocolate, and red wine sometimes provoke migraine. The authors conducted a study in 88 children with severe migraine, giving them an oligoantigenic diet. In those who improved, the causative foods were identified by open reintroduction. Responses were confirmed by a double-blind controlled trial of reintroduction of causative foods. The oligoantigenic diet consisted typically of one meat (lamb or chicken), one carbohydrate (rice or potato), one fruit (banana or apple), one vegetable (brassica), water, and vitamin supplements for 3–4 weeks, depending on the frequency of headaches. Normal daily helpings of excluded foods were reintroduced singly, one a week. Each patient who responded to foods for which test reagents were available was asked to enter a double-blind, placebo-controlled, crossover trial that tested the response to 1 of the foods that provoked symptoms.

Of the 88 participating children, 6 did not improve at all, 78 recovered completely on the first or second oligoantigenic diet, and 4 improved greatly. Of the 82 who improved, all but 8 relapsed on reintroduction of one or more foods; these 8 have remained well. The 74 who relapsed were considered for the controlled trial, but 28 were excluded. The trial was closed when 40 patients had completed it. The 88 patients (40 boys and 48 girls) were aged 3–16 years (mean, 9.83 years) and had had migraine for 6 months to 11 years. Of these, 39 had migraine with typical prodromal symptoms, and 49 had common migraine. Associated symptoms are shown in Table 1. There was no significant order effect in the occurrence of headaches or any migraine-associated symptom, but there were highly significant relations between the active material and symptoms (Table 2).

TABLE 1.—Associated Symptoms and Signs

| | Patients completing oligoantigenic diet (88) | | Patients completing trial (40) | |
	Before diet	On diet	Group AP	Group PA
Abdominal pain, diarrhoea, flatulence	61	8	14	19
Behaviour disorder	41	5	12	16
Aches in limbs	41	7	12	17
Fits	14†	2	5	5
Permanent neurological signs	6	6	1	4
Rhinitis	34	15	5	9
Recurrent mouth ulcers	15	2	4	6
Vaginal discharge	11	1	3	5
Asthma	7	3	1	1
Eczema	6	3	3	4

*Group AP received food first, then placebo after "washout" period; group PA received placebo first.

†Sometimes coinciding with headaches in all 14; 9 had generalized or partial seizures, coinciding with headaches in all but 1.

(Courtesy of Egger, J., et al.: Lancet 2:865–868, Oct. 15, 1983.)

TABLE 2.—Occurrence of Headache or Migraine-Related Symptoms and Preference for Active or Placebo Foods*

| | Headaches | | | Migraine-associated symptoms | | | Preference | | |
	AP	PA	Total	AP	PA	Total	AP	PA	Total
Neither food	2	6	8	1	2	3	1	2	3
Active food	14	12	26†	12	15	27†	0	2	2†
Placebo	0	2	2†	0	2	2†	16	19	35†
Both foods	1	3	4	4	4	8	..	..	..
Total	17	23	40	17	23	40	17	23	40

*AP indicates group AP, who received food first and then received placebo after "washout" period; PA indicates group PA, who received placebo first.

†Difference between active and placebo foods is significant ($P < .001$).

(Courtesy of Egger, J., et al.: Lancet: 2:865–868, Oct. 15, 1983.)

Fifty-five foods provoked symptoms on reintroduction (Table 3). Thirty-eight of the patients successfully treated by diet reported nondietary provocation before treatment (Table 4). During the trial, smoke and perfume still provoked migraine. Forty-five (52%) patients had positive skin-prick tests to one or more of the five antigens used to identify atopic subjects. Of the 64 patients tested, 28% had high serum IgE levels; however, IgE antibodies were not helpful in identifying causative foods (Table 5).

This trial showed that most children with severe frequent migraine recover on an appropriate diet and that so many foods can provoke attacks that any food or combination of foods may be the cause. Intolerance to such a wide range of foods suggests allergic disease rather than metabolic idiosyncrasy.

TABLE 3.—Number of Children in Whom Foods
Caused Symptoms*

Food	n	Food	n	Food	n	Food	n
Cows' milk	27	Soya	7	White wheat flour	3	Vegetable oils	2
Egg	24	Tea	7	Artificial milk		Lentils	2
Chocolate	22	Oats	6	substitute	3	Peas	2
Orange	21	Goats' milk	6	Banana	3	Ice cream	2
Wheat	21	Coffee	6	Strawberries	3	Rabbit	1
Benzoic acid	14	Peanuts	5	Melon	3	Dates	1
Cheese	13	Bacon	4	Carrots	3	Avocado	1
Tomato	13	Potato	4	Lamb	2	Rhubarb	1
Tartrazine	12	Yeast	4	Rice	2	Leek	1
Rye	12	Mixed nuts	4	Malt	2	Lettuce	1
Fish	9	Apple	4	Sugar	2	Cucumber	1
Pork	9	Peaches	4	Ginger	2	Cauliflower	1
Beef	8	Grapes	4	Honey	2	Mushrooms	1
Maize	8	Chicken	3	Pineapple	2	Runner beans	1

*(Courtesy of Egger, J., et al.: Lancet: 2:865–868, Oct. 15, 1983.)

TABLE 4.—Nonspecific Provokers of Migraine in
38 Patients*

	Before diet	On diet
Exercise	13	1
Trauma	11	1
Emotional	10	0
Perfumes and/or cigarette smoke	10	9
Travel	9	0
Bright light	5	0
Heat	2	1
Noise	2	0

*(Courtesy of Egger, J., et al.: Lancet 2:865–868, Oct. 15, 1983.)

TABLE 5.—Association of Positive Skin-Prick Tests
and IgE Antibodies to Foods With Provocation
of Childhood Migraine

	Skin-prick* test	IgE antibodies†
Number of tests positive for a provoking food	57	8
Number of tests negative for a provoking food	141	152
Number of tests positive for a non-provoking food	80	24
Patients who would be cured by avoidance of indicated foods	3	0

*Twenty-one food antigens tested in 87 patients. Wheal diameter greater than 3 mm was taken as positive.
†Fifteen food antigens tested in 76 patients. Binding greater than twice cord serum value was taken as positive.
(Courtesy of Egger, J., et al.: Lancet 2:865–868, Oct. 15, 1983.)

▶ To avoid even more cases of Meadow's syndrome, we need rigorous studies of this type. It is unfortunate that no tests are presently available for identifying the causative food, or foods, because the diet, by the authors' own admission, is quite demanding. Dietary responses were observed not only for symptoms such as headache, but also for epilepsy and limb pains, disease manifestations not usually associated with food allergy.

Other investigators also have failed to find any relationship between IgE and IgG4 antibodies and their relationship to dietary or nondietary migraine, suggesting that this food-associated problem is probably not mediated by classic allergic mechanisms (Merrett, J., et al.: *J. Neurol. Neurosurg. Psychiatry* 46:738, 1983).

For more on childhood migraine, see Chapter 15, Neurology and Psychiatry.—F.A.O.

Routine Elective Penicillin Allergy Skin Testing in Children and Adolescents: Study of Sensitization

Louis M. Mendelson, Charlotte Ressler, James P. Rosen, and Jay E. Selcow (Univ. of Connecticut, Farmington)
J. Allergy Clin. Immunol. 73:76–81, January 1984   3–6

The authors investigated whether resensitization to penicillin can occur in children and adolescents subjected to skin testing and challenge. A total of 240 healthy pediatric patients with a history of reaction to penicillin or an analogue were skin-tested with penicillin G (PEN G), commercial benzylpenicilloyl polylysine (PPL), and a minor determinant mixture (MDM) of sodium benzylpenicilloate and sodium benzylpenilloate. Testing was carried out during routine office visits when there was no immediate need for penicillin.

No systemic reactions to skin testing occurred, but 8.75% of patients had positive intradermal tests. Three reacted only to the MDM, and 1

CORRELATION WITH DRUG ALLERGY HISTORY OF REACTIVITY TO VARIOUS SKIN TEST COMPONENTS IN 23 SKIN TEST-POSITIVE PATIENTS

	No. of patients					
	Drug allergy history					
	PEN G		Ampicillin/amoxicillin		Cephalosporin	
Skin test components	Initial	Retest	Initial	Retest	Initial	Retest
PPL only	5	1	4	0	1	0
PEN G only	0	0	0	0	0	0
MDM only	3	0	0	0	0	0
All (PPL/PEN G/MDM)	0	1	2	0	0	0
PPL/PEN G	1	0	1	0	0	0
PPL/MDM	3	0	1	0	0	0
	12	2	8	0	1	0

(Courtesy of Mendelson, L.M., et al.: J. Allergy Clin. Immunol. 73:76–81, January 1984.)

reacted only to the benzylpenilloate component. A 10-day oral course of penicillin was given to 219 subjects with negative skin tests. Three (1.4%) had a mild exanthem after 7 to 10 days. All the skin test-negative patients were retested a month or longer after the oral challenge. Only 2, both of whom tolerated the oral challenge, had positive repeat skin tests. No patient with a history of reaction to a penicillin analogue had a positive skin test after the oral challenge. Responses of the reactors to various components of the skin test reagents are given in the table.

Children and adolescents with a history of reaction to penicillin or an analogue should not be labeled as penicillin allergic for the rest of their lives without being skin tested. It is usually impractical to perform skin tests at times that penicillin is needed. Testing can be carried out reliably at routine office visits. The chance of resensitization occurring appears to be low and no greater than that in the general population lacking knowledge of personal penicillin sensitivity.

Frequency and Severity of Cat vs. Dog Allergy in Atopic Children
Andrew B. Murray, Alexander C. Ferguson, and Brenda J. Morrison (Univ. of British Columbia)
J. Allergy Clin. Immunol. 72:145–149, August 1983   3–7

A study was done of 1,238 children, whose mean age was about 6½ years and who had respiratory tract symptoms, to establish whether allergic symptoms after exposure to cats are more common or severe than those after exposure to dogs and whether animal sensitivities change with age. Detailed histories were taken, and skin-prick tests were performed with extracts of inhalant allergens commonly responsible for allergic respiratory tract disease. One-second forced expiratory volume and maximal mid-expiratory flow rate were determined in children, aged 7 years and older, with histories of asthma.

Considerably more children had allergic symptoms caused by cats than by dogs (Table 1). The difference was most marked in those who were probably atopic, i.e., children who had at least one positive prick test to an inhalant allergen; 15.4% had allergic symptoms when exposed to cats, 4.6% when exposed to dogs, and 16.9% when exposed to either cats or dogs. Of 1,161 children on whom skin-prick tests were performed, 166 (14.4%) had reactions to cats, only 9 (0.8%) to dogs, and 42 (3.6%) to both cats and dogs.

The proportion of symptoms caused by cats and dogs was the same (12%) in children younger than age 4. Of those aged 11 years or older, 30.7% had symptoms from cats and 18.8% from dogs; 24.6% had positive cat allergen tests and 6% had positive dog allergen tests. This increased prevalence of cat allergy does not seem to be due to greater exposure of children to cats, for a significant majority of subjects who owned pets owned dogs (Table 2). Increased intimacy of exposure to cats could be a factor, because cats are more likely to be in the house than dogs, and cats

TABLE 1.—PREVALENCE OF ALLERGIC SYMPTOMS
CAUSED BY CATS VS. DOGS IN PROBABLY ATOPIC
AND POSSIBLY ATOPIC SUBGROUPS OF TOTAL
POPULATION OF 1,238 CHILDREN*

Children reporting symptoms

	Probably atopic		Possibly atopic	
Allergen	**No.**	**%**	**No.**	**%**
Cat only	100	15.4(a)	36	6.1(c)
Cat and dog	110	16.9	33	5.6
Dog only	30	4.6(b)	14	2.4(d)
Neither	410	63.1	505	85.9
	650	100.0	588	100.0

*Probably atopic: at least 1 positive prick test to inhalant allergen; possibly atopic: no positive tests. Possibly atopic subgroup included 77 subjects on whom skin testing was not performed. Significance of difference of proportions between symptoms from cats alone vs. dogs alone: (1) probably atopic (difference between a and b), $Z = 6.466$, $P = .000$; (2) whole study group (difference between a + c and b + d), $Z = 7.129$, $P = .000$.

(Courtesy of Murray, A.B., et al.: J. Allergy Clin. Immunol. 72:145–149, August 1983.)

TABLE 2.—PROPORTIONS OF CHILDREN OWNING
CATS VS. DOGS, BOTH IN TOTAL OF 1,234
SUBJECTS AND IN SUBGROUP OF 392 IN WHOM
ATOPY DID NOT AFFECT CHOICE
OF PET ANIMAL*

**Symptoms from cats or dogs
and/or the presence of atopy in
the immediate family**

	Yes		No	
Ownership	**No.**	**%**	**No.**	**%**
Cat only	115	13.7(a)	67	17.1(c)
Cat and dog	108	12.8	55	14.0
Dog only	193	22.9(b)	87	22.2(d)
Neither	426	50.6	183	46.7
	842	100.0	392	100.0
		Total: 1234†		

*Significance of difference between proportions of ownership of cat alone vs. dog alone: (1) total study group (difference between a + c and b + d), $Z = 5.056$, $P = .000$; (2) no symptoms from cats or dogs and no atopy in family (difference between c and d), $Z = 1.797$, $P = .036$.

†Data missing on 4 subjects.

(Courtesy of Murray, A.B., et al.: J. Allergy Clin. Immunol. 72:145–149, August 1983.)

are significantly $(P = .032)$ more likely to be in the bedroom (46%) than dogs (32%).

Two subgroups were examined to determine whether those with cat sensitivity who owned cats had more severe symptoms than those with dog sensitivity who owned dogs. Those in the cat subgroup more frequently had persistent allergic nasal symptoms (prolonged nasal obstruction, rhinorrhea, itching, and sneezing) and abnormally low spirometric measurements than did those in the dog subgroup.

The findings seem to indicate that it may be preferable for an atopic child to own a dog rather than a cat.

▶ Richard K. Sheehan, Associate Clinical Professor of Pediatrics, State University of New York Upstate Medical Center, and a very busy and successful allergist, provides the following comment:

"After 25 years in the practice of clinical allergy, I feel it can be said with some degree of certainty that cat dander allergen (all other factors being equal) does seem to cause more allergic problems in atopic children than does dog dander.

"The authors of this article would seem to be quite correct in assigning as the main reason for this the factor of increased potency of cat dander plus the increased intimacy and increased time of exposure to cat dander.

"Extensive patient surveys would suggest that cats have a tendency both to stay indoors more than dogs and particularly to sleep more in children's bedrooms at night. When one considers just the pure numbers involved—the average small child would probably breathe 16 times per minute at night and sleep approximately 10 hours. This comes to 9,600 breaths taken at night in a room where every cubic foot of air would contain at least some degree of cat allergen (coming from either dander or saliva). This serves as a tremendous "priming effect" for the child to have symptoms either at night or shortly after arising in the morning, particularly if additional inhalant exposures are encountered in other categories.

"In summary, I feel the authors have stated the case very well, but I tend to disagree with the conclusion—that if a child is sensitive to cats, then a dog would be an acceptable substitute. My personal feeling is that when an atopic child has acquired sensitivity to one animal dander (cat), then sensitivity to other animal danders (dogs, guinea pigs, gerbils, parakeets, etc.) is really not far behind. I think a more logical conclusion should be that when a child has encountered some sensitivity to cat dander, then no animal with fur or feathers should be allowed in the internal home environment. . . . When you really think about it, snakes as house pets are really not all that bad."

Chronic Urticaria in Childhood: Natural Course and Etiology
Alan Harris, Frank J. Twarog, and Raif S. Geha (Harvard Med. School)
Ann. Allerg. 51:161–165, August 1983   3–8

A retrospective study was done of 94 children younger than age 16 with urticaria of more than 6 weeks' duration. Median age of onset of urticarial symptoms was 6.8 years. Urticaria alone was present in 79 (85%) of patients, 9 (9%) had angioedema alone, and 6 (6%) had both urticaria and angioedema; 6 patients (6%) had concurrent arthralgia.

Results of laboratory investigations are given in Table 1. Of 81 patients, 17 had an erythrocyte sedimentation rate (ESR) greater than 20 mm; of these, 2 had a diagnosis of collagen vascular disease, and 1 had immune complexes which resolved together with the high ESR with clearing of the urticaria. None of the abnormal laboratory values had predictive correlation with outcome of the urticaria.

A presumptive cause for urticaria was identified or suspected in 15 patients (Table 2). These included 8 patients with cold urticaria confirmed by an ice cube challenge test; none had cryofibrinogens or cryoglobulins in the serum. Two patients each had infections (hepatitis, sinusitis) and food allergies. Three patients had immunologically related disease: 1, juvenile rheumatoid arthritis; 1, elevated ESR, positive antinuclear antibody titer and arthralgia; and 1, low levels of total hemolytic complement but normal serum C3 and C4 levels and negative assays for immune complexes.

Fifty-two patients were followed for 12 months or longer. Median duration of urticarial symptoms was 16 months. Nineteen patients (37%) followed for more than 12 months had no urticarial symptoms after not receiving therapy for 12 months, 11 (21%) had no symptoms after not receiving therapy for 6 months and were considered to have inactive disease, whereas 22 (42%) continued to have symptoms within 6 months and were considered to have active disease.

Girls had a higher rate of resolution than boys (41% vs. 33%) and children younger than age 8 had a higher resolution rate than children

TABLE 1.—RESULTS OF LABORATORY INVESTIGATIONS IN PATIENTS
WITH CHRONIC URTICARIA

	Number studied	Percent with abnormal results
WBC	87	8% leukopenia
Eosinophil count	87	10% elevated
ESR	81	21% elevated
IgG	68	8% low
IgA	68	4% low
C3, C4	68	0
Antitrypsin	68	0
ANA	20	0
C1 inhibitor	14	0
Throat culture	13	0
Ice cube test	10	80% positive (8/10)
Thyroid function studies	5	0
Raji cell assay	5	0
$C1_q$ binding assay	4	25%
Chest X-ray	13	0
Stool for ova + parasite	2	0
IgE	48	13% elevated

(Courtesy of Harris, A., et al.: Ann. Allerg. 51:161–165, August 1983.)

TABLE 2.—Possible Underlying Diagnosis in 94 Children
With Chronic Urticaria

Etiology	Number of Patients
Physical	
Cold	8
Infectious	
Sinusitis	1
Hepatitis	1
Immunologic	
Juvenile rheumotoid arthritis	1
Arthralgia with positive ANA	1
Complement defect (low CH_{50})	1
Allergic	
Food	2
Unknown	79

(Courtesy of Harris, A., et al.: Ann. Allerg. 51:161–165, August 1983.)

older than 8 years (50% vs. 22%). There was little objective evidence for the impression reported by many patients (21%) that their urticaria was precipitated by foods.

Urticaria is a manifestation of mediator release from cutaneous mast cells that can be activated by several mechanisms, i.e., interaction of antigen with IgE on the mast cell surface, complement activation with formation of the anaphylatoxins C3a and C5a, and physical factors, substances, and drugs.

It appears that chronic urticaria in children is a benign condition often of unknown etiology. Extensive workup usually is indicated only when systemic symptoms such as infection or collagen vascular disease are present.

▶ It may be comforting to the frustrated physician to learn that 85% of children with chronic urticaria go undiagnosed and most get better, but this news will not comfort the patient or their families. It would appear that the primary diagnostic tool in the evaluation of a patient with chronic urticaria remains a detailed history with emphasis on precipitating events. Do physical events precipitate an attack, i.e., exercise, exposure to cold, exposure to sunlight? Any link with meals? Incidentally, the authors did not explore the possible role of salicylates, food colorings, or food preservatives in the genesis of the problem (Michaelson, G., et al.: Br. J. Dermatol. 88:525, 1973). Laboratory studies need not be extensive because they are rarely useful—start out with a determination of the sedimentation rate and a complete blood count. In other parts of the world, a search for parasites may be justified.

Continuous administration of agents such as hydroxyzine and azatadine may be helpful. Systemic administration of corticosteroids should only be used for acute and severe exacerbations.

In this—like all else—no matter which way you ride, it's uphill and against the wind.—F.A.O.

Ketoconazole Treatment of Nail Infection in Chronic Mucocutaneous Candidiasis

D. M. Roberton and C. S. Hosking (Royal Children's Hosp., Parkville, Australia)
Aust. Paediatr. J. 19:178–181, September 1983   3–9

Chronic mucocutaneous candidiasis (CMC) is an immunodeficiency disorder that has significant morbidity due to mucous membrane, skin, and nail infection. Studies of the immunologic abnormalities involved have had only limited success. The authors tested the newly available imidazole antifungal agent, ketoconazole, in 4 children with CMC who had severe nail infection. Ketoconazole was given prior to the evening meal in a single daily dose of 100 mg for children weighing between 15 to 30 kg and 200 mg for those weighing more than 30 kg. Two of the 4 cases are described below.

CASE 1.—Girl, 12, developed chronic *Candida albicans* infection of the oral mucous membranes at age 1 year; at age 4 the nails of both index fingers became infected; eventually she had infection and deformity of the nails of four fingers and seven toes. Mucous membrane and nail infections failed to respond to topical antifungal agents or administration of iron. Reinfection was not prevented by application of 40% urea paste to affected nails, followed by curettage. After biochemical and histologic resolution of chronic active hepatitis, she was given ketoconazole, 200 mg daily. Oral infection cleared within days; first evidence of nail

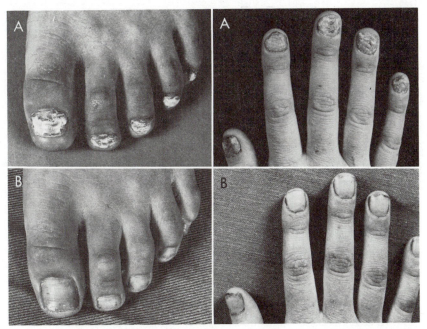

Fig 3–2 (left).—Toenails of girl aged 12 years before treatment (**A**) and after 8 months of treatment (**B**).
Fig 3–3 (right).—Fingernails of boy aged 13 years before treatment (**A**) and after 4 months of treatment (**B**).

(Courtesy of Roberton, D.M., and Hosking, C.S.: Aust. Pediatr. J. 19:178–181, September 1983.)

improvement was seen at 6 weeks. After 8 months of therapy there was complete resolution of involvement of all infected nails (Fig 3–2).

CASE 3.—Boy, 13, developed oral and diaper-area infections due to *C. albicans* from age 6 weeks. When he was nearly age 7 years he had adrenal failure and began replacement therapy; at age 7 he developed *Trichophyton mentagrophytes* infection of the skin of the left forearm and left knee. These lesions cleared when treated with grisefulvin, but later recurred. In the next 4 years he developed persistent *Candida* infection of all nails of both hands and persistent oral candidiasis. Transfer factor was not effective. After he received ketoconazole, 200 mg daily, the oral candidiasis and *Trichophyton* skin lesions cleared rapidly. Nail lesions improved within 3 weeks and had resolved completely within 4 months (Fig 3–3).

Laboratory tests showed 3 of the children had negative skin test responses to *Candida* antigen; 1 was weakly positive. There were no changes suggestive of drug toxicity with respect to hematologic, hepatic, or renal function during treatment.

It is concluded that ketoconazole represents a significant advance in treatment of fungal infection of mucous membranes, skin, and nails in CMC. Prolonged therapy may be required for complete resolution of nail lesions. Careful consideration of alternative agents may prevent the development of drug resistance and preserve the efficacy of ketoconazole in CMC as well as in life-threatening or chronic mycotic infections.

▶ This is one new drug that really does make a difference for patients with chronic mucocutaneous candidiasis. The drug is water-soluble, is well absorbed after oral administration, and only needs to be given once a day. Side effects are minimal, although 10% of patients may display transient liver function abnormalities (Heel, R. C., et al.: *Drugs* 23:1, 1982). We always advise that everyone use a drug while it is new. When new, it is still 100% effective and free of all side effects. If you wait, the drug no longer works as well as you originally had believed and starts causing all kinds of problems. Ketoconazole may be an exception.—F.A.O.

Herpetic Whitlow
Henry M. Feder, Jr. (Univ. of Connecticut), and Sarah S. Long (Temple Univ., Philadelphia)
Am. J. Dis. Child. 137:861–863, September 1983   3–10

Herpetic whitlow is a herpes simplex virus infection of the distal phalanx that occurs primarily in medical personnel and in patients with herpetic gingivostomatitis or genital herpes. It follows direct inoculation or reactivation of latent virus and is characterized by pain, swelling, erythema, and formation of nonpurulent vesicles. The authors report data on 7 cases to increase awareness of herpetic whitlow as a pediatric disease, to emphasize characteristic clinical findings and laboratory tests, and to suggest appropriate treatment. One case is described below.

Infant, aged 6 months, had tenderness and erythema of the distal part of the third finger for 24 hours. Temperature was 39.4 C. The pulp area of the distal phalanx was swollen, erythematous, and tender, and a 2-cm epitrochlear node was present; the mouth was normal. Cellulitis was presumed and treatment with dicloxacillin sodium was begun. The patient became afebrile in the next 7 days; a vesicle developed over the fingertip. There was no history of herpes simplex exposure. The finger remained swollen and erythematous and had vesicles on the distal phalanx; a brown crust covered the dorsal aspect of the terminal phalanx (Fig 3–4). No tenderness or lymphadenopathy was present. A Tzanck test of a vesicular base revealed many multinucleate giant cells (Fig 3–5). Gram's stain and bacterial culture of vesicular fluid were negative. Antibiotic therapy was discontinued and swelling and erythema resolved shortly. The finger was normal 2 weeks later, but the patient had a recurrence after 2 months, which was less severe.

This case and another show that herpetic whitlow can occur without predisposing factors and that clinical recognition is important to avoid potentially harmful surgery. Also described are 2 cases of herpetic whitlow associated with oral herpes and 1 associated with genital herpes. Two cases in medical personnel were secondary to contact with patients who had herpes simplex infections. In all instances, the patients had uneventful recoveries although there were some milder recurrences.

Patients with herpetic whitlow initially have pain and tingling or burning of a distal phalanx, followed by digital swelling and erythema. There may be fever, lymphadenopathy, lymphangitis, and constitutional symptoms.

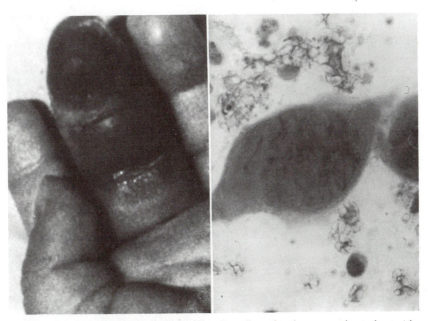

Fig 3–4 (left).—Resolving herpetic whitlow. Finger is swollen and erythematous and secondary vesicles are seen. Distal phalanx that was site of primary vesicular eruption is crusted.

Fig 3–5 (right).—Tzanck test from base of vesicular lesion shows characteristic multinucleate giant cell. Modified hematoxylin-eosin; original magnification ×1000.

(Courtesy of Feder, H.M., Jr., and Long, S.S.: Am. J. Dis. Child. 137:861–863, September 1983; copyright 1983, American Medical Association.)

Vesicles appear to contain pus but usually have clear, opalescent, or serosanguineous fluid that helps to distinguish herpetic whitlow from bacterial felon or paronychia. Vesicles remain about 10 days and are followed by crusting and peeling that reveals normal skin. About 20% of patients have recurrences that are usually less severe.

In infants and children, herpetic whitlow is usually a secondary, autogenous infection associated with primary herpes gingivostomatitis. A severely traumatized digit may become infected with herpes simplex derived from exogenous or autogenous sites.

The Tzanck test is simple and inexpensive, and results are available immediately; it identifies about 70% of infections confirmed by cultures. Treatment is symptomatic; dry dressings are suggested and analgesics may be needed. Deep incisions or débridement of lesions should be avoided because the infection is self-limited and surgical intervention may predispose patients to secondary bacterial infections.

Immunogenetics of Neonatal Lupus Syndrome

Lela A. Lee, Wilma B. Bias, Frank C. Arnett, Jr., J. Clark Huff, David A. Norris, Catherine Harmon, Thomas T. Provost, and William L. Weston
Ann. Intern. Med. 99:592–596, November 1983   3–11

Infants with neonatal lupus erythematosus have congenital heart block, transient cutaneous lesions, or both. Mothers of these infants have SSA/Ro autoantibodies that are passed across the placenta to the fetus and that have been temporarily associated with the syndrome. Seven children from six families with neonatal lupus were studied by human leukocyte antigen (HLA) typing. Cutaneous lupus lesions were defined as annular, erythematous, scaly plaques with raised borders occurring predominantly on sun-exposed skin (Fig 3–6). All of the mothers were examined clinically, serologically, and by HLA typing.

The results are listed in the table. All 7 infants were female and had cutaneous eruptions consistent with lupus; 5 had sun-induced lesions by history. Two had congenital heart block, but neither required a pacemaker. One had hepatic or hematologic abnormalities. Five mothers were asymptomatic, and 1 had Sjögren's syndrome. All infants except for 1 had antibodies to SSA/Ro. None of the 71 control infants had antibodies to SSA-Ro or SSB/La. All mothers had antibodies to SSA/Ro. Four infants were followed serologically at least for 2 years; by age 6 months, all were seronegative. Five fathers and 2 unaffected siblings were also studied; there were no apparent HLA associations in the affected infants, fathers, or unaffected siblings.

Examining the families of infants with neonatal lupus provides an opportunity to study the components of immunologic injury, because antibody production occurs in the mother but tissue damage is expressed in the infant. Apparently, specific HLA antigens occur with increased frequency in the mothers but not in the infants, suggesting that HLA antigens DR3, B8, MB2, and MT2 may be associated with autoantibody production

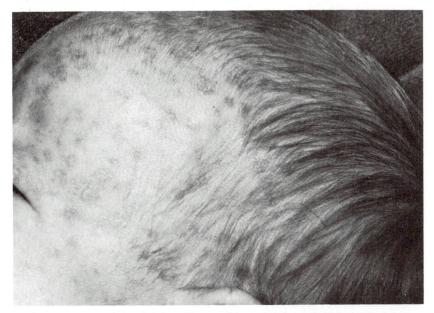

Fig 3–6.—Cutaneous lesions in infant with neonatal lupus. Annular, erythematous, scaly plaques are seen on the scalp and forehead. (Courtesy of Lee, L.A., et al.: Ann. Intern. Med. 99:592–595, November 1983.)

but are not otherwise significantly associated with the expression of tissue injury.

▶ Paul J. Honig, Associate Professor of Pediatrics, University of Pennsylvania, and Director, Pediatric Dermatology, Children's Hospital of Philadelphia, comments:

"The authors have focused on an intriguing aspect of neonatal lupus erythematosus (NLE), that is, the manner by which genetic factors modulate susceptibility to the disorder. It is clear that a female predominance exists in both infants and adults affected by lupus erythematosus. This is true in infants despite the fact that current studies indicate that the disease is transmitted from mother to fetus via passively transferred antibodies, such as SSA/Ro or SSB/La (Franco, H. L., et al.: *J. Am. Acad. Dermatol.* 4:67, 1981). A question that must be answered, therefore, is why infants of both sexes are not affected equally. Why is the female to male ratio 14:1 in those infants with manifestations of NLE limited to the skin, whereas the ratio drops to 2:1 when congenital heart block is present (Karkij, W., and Soltani, K.: *Pediatr. Dermatol.* 1:189, 1984)?

"In seeking answers to these questions, a report by Sontheimer et al. (*Ann Intern. Med.* 97:664, 1982) seemed promising. They found an increased incidence of HLA antigens DR3 and B8 in a subset of systemic lupus erythematosus (SLE) characterized by photosensitivity, negative antinuclear antibody, and antibodies to SSA/Ro and SSB/La. Since gene products of the HLA-DR

CLINICAL AND LABORATORY CHARACTERISTICS OF INFANTS WITH THE NEONATAL LUPUS SYNDROME AND THEIR MOTHERS*

| | Race | Clinical Findings | Autoantibodies | HLA | | | | | |
				A	B	C	DR	MB	MT
Infants									
1	Black	Congenital heart block, cutaneous lesions	SS-A	26,28	8,42	7	3	1,2	2
2	Mexican-American	Cutaneous lesions	SS-B	28,32	35,38	4	4,8	3,1	2
3	White	Cutaneous lesions	SS-A	23,33	53,14	6,4	9,7	2	2
4	White	Cutaneous lesions	SS-A	1,2	7,63	7	2,6	1	x
5	White	Congestive heart block, cutaneous lesions	SS-A,SS-B	2,33	14,62	3,8	1,4	1,3	
6	White	Cutaneous lesions	SS-A	26,29	27,60	1,3	5,6	3,1	2
7	White	Cutaneous lesions	SS-A	28,1	44,8	7	5,3	3,2	2
Mothers									
1	Black	···	SS-A	19,28	8,45	6,7	3,9	2	2
2	Mexican-American	···	SS-A,SS-B	32,1	8,38	···	6,8	1,3	2
3	White	···	SS-A	33,1	8,14	7,8	3,7	2	2
4	White	Sjögren's syndrome	SS-A	1,2	8,7	7	3,2	2,1	2
5	White	···	SS-A,SS-B	1,2	8,62	3,7	3,4	2,3	2,x
6	White	···	SS-A	29,1	8,60	3,7	3,6	2,1	2

*Infants 6 and 7 are siblings; x = antigen not characterized.
(Courtesy of Lee, L.A., et al.: Ann. Intern. Med. 99:592–596, November 1983.)

locus have been associated with autoimmune disorders, this seemed to be an encouraging direction to pursue (especially because newborns with NLE also had antibodies to SSA and SSB antigens). Unfortunately, the infants with NLE studied by Doctor Lee did not show a consistent HLA pattern. Other approaches must be taken to further delineate genetic influences on this disorder if we are to uncover an etiology.

"Now that NLE has been clearly described in the literature, many more cases will be identified. It is important for the clinician to realize that mothers with syndromes other than SLE (e.g., Sjögren's syndrome, rheumatoid arthritis, mixed connective tissue disease, and other undifferentiated connective tissue diseases) may give birth to infants with NLE. Practitioners should not forget, however, that 20%–30% of mothers who deliver infants with NLE are completely asymptomatic.

"One of the more serious manifestations of infants with NLE is congenital heart block. This association has led to the screening of infants with unexplained congenital heart block for NLE. Reed et al. (*J Pediatr.* 103:889, 1983) concluded, in one such study, that a large percentage of infants born with 'idiopathic' congenital heart block have NLE as an underlying process.

"Two other factors are important to keep in mind. Neonatal lupus erythematosus may occur in successive pregnancies; additionally, infants with NLE may go on to develop SLE later in life. Two infants with NLE were well until ages 13 and 19 years, respectively, when they developed SLE (Fox, J. R., et al.: *Arch. Dermatol.* 115:340, 1979; and Jackson, R., et al.: *Br. J. Dermatol.* 101:81, 1979).

"The following conclusions can be drawn:

"1. Neonatal lupus erythematosus must be considered in young patients with annular erythemas, vasculitic lesions, etc., especially when these changes occur on the face and head.

"2. Consider NLE in young infants who manifest photosensitivity-type facial rashes.

"3. All infants born with heart block should be checked for NLE (and their mothers for collagen vascular disease).

"4. Do not forget to consider NLE even if the infant's mother is asymptomatic and her antinuclear antigen titer is negative.

"5. Anti-SSA and anti-SSB titers should be obtained in newborns, or young infants, considered to have NLE (as well as their mothers)."

Topical Erythromycin vs. Clindamycin Therapy for Acne: Multicenter, Double-Blind Comparison
Alan R. Shalita, Edgar B. Smith, and Eugene Bauer
Arch. Dermatol. 120:351–355, March 1984   3–12

A double-blind study was done to compare topical 1.5% erythromycin solution to 1% clindamycin phosphate solution in 126 female and 52 male patients aged 12–45 years with moderate facial acne seen at three university hospital outpatient clinics and a private dermatology test facility. The patients had at least 10 papules or pustules and at least 5 open or closed comedones. Eighty-eight patients were randomized to erythromycin treatment and 90 to clindamycin therapy. The groups were demographically and clinically comparable, and similar numbers of patients had received systemic antibiotics. Medication was applied on arising in the morning and at bedtime for 12 weeks.

Changes in inflammatory lesion counts are compared in Table 1. Counts fell by about 60% by the end of treatment in both groups. Significant reductions (about 40%) in the number of noninflammatory lesions also occurred in both treatment groups (Table 2). There were generally fewer

TABLE 1.—Mean* ± SE Inflammatory Lesion Count

Treatment	Weeks of Treatment					P (Effects Over Time)
	Initial	2	4	8	12	
1.5% erythromycin solution	22.1^A ± 1.1 (n = 80)†	18.4^B ± 1.2 (n = 80)	14.3^C ± 1.2 (n = 77)	11.1^D ± 1.3 (n = 74)	8.4^E ± 1.2 (n = 74)	.001
1.0% clindamycin phosphate solution	20.3^A ± 1.0 (n = 86)	14.8^B ± 1.0 (n = 86)	12.2^C ± 0.9 (n = 86)	10.4^D ± 1.0 (n = 83)	8.4^E ± 0.9 (n = 80)	.001
P (difference between treatments)	.26	.02	.20	.64	.95	...

*For each drug, means with one or more common superscripts (A, B, C, etc.) are not significantly different by Duncan's procedure ($P \leq .05$).
†Numbers in parentheses indicate number of observations.
(Courtesy of Shalita, A.R., et al.: Arch. Dermatol. 120:351–355, March 1984; copyright 1984, American Medical Association.)

TABLE 2.—Mean* ± SE Noninflammatory Lesion Count

Treatment	Weeks of Treatment					P (Effects Over Time)
	Initial	2	4	8	12	
1.5% erythromycin solution	53.4^A ± 7.0 (n = 80)†	42.4^B ± 4.6 (n = 80)	39.2^{BC} ± 3.9 (n = 77)	36.5^{BC} ± 4.2 (n = 74)	30.3^C ± 2.8 (n = 74)	.001
1.0% clindamycin phosphate solution	55.8^A ± 7.0 (n = 86)	43.7^B ± 5.4 (n = 86)	35.1^{BC} ± 3.5 (n = 86)	35.3^{BC} + 4.0 (n = 83)	34.2^C ± 3.9 (n = 80)	.001
P (difference between treatments)	.92	.93	.32	.79	.57	...

*For each drug, means with one or more common superscripts (A, B, C, etc.) are not significantly different by Duncan's procedure, $P \leq .05$.
†Numbers in parentheses indicate number of observations.
(Courtesy of Shalita, A.R., et al.: Arch. Dermatol. 120:351–355, March 1984; copyright 1984, American Medical Association.)

good and excellent clinical responses to clindamycin, but the differences were not significant. Side effects occurred in 23% of the erythromycin group and in 13% of the clindamycin group. Dryness was the most common side effect in both treatment groups. A reduction in the frequency of treatment because of side effects did not compromise the overall clinical outcome.

Treatment of moderate acne with 1.5% erythromycin solution is as effective as the use of 1% clindamycin solution is. Side effects were somewhat more frequent with erythromycin, but serious local side effects did not occur.

▶ Systemic antibiotics, erythromycin or tetracycline, were the mainstays in the treatment of acne prior to the introduction of benzoyl peroxide. Now systemic antibiotics are reserved, in general, for those persons sensitive to benzoyl peroxide or resistant to topical therapy. In inflammatory acne, both antibiotics appear to be equally effective.

Recently, topical antibiotic therapy has become widely used. The use of topical antibiotic therapy produces a fall in surface free fatty acid concentrations but not necessarily any change in the *Cornyebacterium acnes* colonization. The means by which topically applied antibiotics exert a beneficial effect in the treatment of acne is uncertain.

Most dermatologists prefer topical clindamycin therapy to topical erythromycin therapy. This controlled study demonstrates that the two topically applied antibiotics are equally effective in reducing the clinical manifestations of the acne in patients with moderate disease. This is another example of six being as good as a half-dozen.

Lois Matsuoka, in a recent review of acne (*J. Pediatr.* 103:849, 1983), refers to the fact that although only about 10% of topically applied clindamycin is absorbed systemically, there have been case reports of associated pseudomembranous colitis.—F.A.O.

Topical Cholesterol Treatment of Recessive X-linked Ichthyosis
Gert Lykkesfeldt and Henrik Høyer (Univ. of Copenhagen)
Lancet 2:1337–1338, Dec. 10, 1983   3–13

In an open prospective half-side trial, creams containing 10% cholesterol or 10% urea were applied to lesions in 20 steroid-sulfatase-deficient male patients with recessive X-linked ichthyosis (RXLI). Thirteen of the 20 were children aged 1 to 13 years; the other 7 were aged 17 to 39. Diagnosis of RXLI was based on the virtual absence of steroid sulfatase. Blinding was impossible because of the obvious difference in appearance of the two creams. Patients were instructed to apply the cholesterol-containing cream twice daily to the skin of the arm and leg of one side and the urea-containing cream to the other side. Patients were examined every 2 weeks.

Treatment with cholesterol cream produced significantly better results than treatment with urea cream (table). Among the 13 patients who responded more favorably to cholesterol than to urea, lesions were cleared

Clinical Half-Side Trial of 10% Cholesterol
Cream Versus 10% Urea Cream in Patients With
Recessive X-linked Ichthyosis and Steroid
Sulfatase Deficiency

Patients	Cholesterol superior to urea	Urea superior to cholesterol	No difference
Children (13)	8	0	5
Adults (7)	5	0	2
Total (20)	13	0	7

(Courtesy of Lykkesfeldt, G., and Høyer, H.: Lancet 2:1337–1338, Dec. 10, 1983.)

completely in 7 children and 1 adult; in 1 child and 4 adults the lesions were significantly improved. This difference was seen after an average treatment period of 3 weeks in children and 5 weeks in adults. Among the 7 patients in whom no difference occurred between the two sides at the end of 6 weeks, lesions on both sides were almost cleared in 2 children and uniformly improved in 2 children and 1 adult. There was no clinical improvement in 1 child and 1 adult. Eighteen of the 20 patients responded well to the cholesterol treatment. No untoward effects were noted with either cream.

In this study, topical application of cholesterol had a beneficial effect on the skin of patients with RXLI and gave superior results when compared to treatment with urea. Once a clearing of the scaly lesions has been achieved, the application of cholesterol cream twice weekly may be sufficient to maintain benefit. However, the outcome of extended clinical trials and experimental investigations must be awaited before the value of cholesterol in treatment of this disorder can be established.

Foot Dermatitis in Children
Janet A. Weston, Kathleen Hawkins, and William L. Weston (Univ. of Colorado)
Pediatrics 72:824–827, December 1983   3–14

Redness and scaling of the feet in prepubertal children probably represents a disease other than tinea pedis. When the dorsum of the foot is involved, allergic contact dermatitis is a likely cause. The incidence of allergic contact dermatitis was assessed in 34 children (aged 0 to 14 years) treated for dermatitis involving the feet. The dermatitis was present for more than 2 weeks and was characterized by erythema with vesiculation, lichenification, scaling, or fissures.

In 19 children the dermatitis was limited to the dorsum of the feet (group A); in 15, dermatitis developed on the plantar surface of the feet (juvenile plantar dermatitis; group B). Average ages were 5.8 years in group A (range, 9 months to 14 years) and 8 years in group B (range, 11 months to 14 years). Approximately 50% of the children in each group were younger than age 5 years. Nine of the 19 children in group A, but none of the 15 in group B, had a positive result on patch testing ($P < .001$). None of the 9 children with a positive patch test result had the "angry back syndrome." One child had a 2+ positive patch test result to nickel, manifested by the appearance of papulovesicles, but there was no correlation with metal components of shoes; 6 had reactions to rubber antioxidants, and 2 were allergic to a leather tanning agent (potassium dichromate). The latter 8 children were given specific instructions and education on allergen avoidance. Follow-up examination of these 8 children 2 years later showed that 1 still had foot dermatitis because of failure to comply with allergen avoidance; 6 had complied and were free of dermatitis. The eighth child was not available for examination. Of the 10 children in group A with negative patch test results, 3 had recurrent foot dermatitis and the disease in 7 cleared. Six group B children had flexural eczema consistent with atopic dermatitis and 2 had generalized dermatitis; disease in 6 of the 15 group B children cleared, but in 3 it persisted.

Children with dermatitis involving the dorsum of the feet probably have allergic contact dermatitis; those with involvement of the weight-bearing areas of the feet are likely to have juvenile plantar dermatitis. Allergy patch testing may lead to a successful outcome by indicating the specific allergens to avoid.

▶ This is a simple message. Dorsum of the foot—thick contact dermatitis. Involvement of the sole of the foot probably indicates the presence of juvenile plantar dermatosis, a term invented by dermatologists for dermatologists that signifies no precise etiology. We are encouraging our young to become athletes. Fortunately, they rarely get athlete's foot (Johnson, M.-L. T., et al.: *Vital Health Stat.* 212:1, 1978).—F.A.O.

▶ ↓ Starting with the 1983 YEAR BOOK, Dr. Walter W. Tunnessen, Jr., began preparing a summary of the highlights of the annual meeting of the Society for Pediatric Dermatology. This report has proved to be immensely popular and now, after only 3 years, a tradition is in place. Doctor Tunnessen, Professor and Vice-Chairman, Department of Pediatrics, State University of New York Upstate Medical Center, wrote the following summary.—F.A.O.

What's New in Pediatric Dermatology?

WALTER W. TUNNESSEN, JR.
Professor and Vice-Chairman, Department of Pediatrics, State University of New York Upstate Medical Center

The ninth annual meeting of the Society for Pediatric Dermatology was held June 28–30, 1984. Some highlights of the meeting are abstracted below for your interest.

Newer Neonatal Dermatoses

Ron Hansen, of Tucson, Arizona, reviewed some of the newer as well as some of the older neonatal dermatoses. Although most newborns peel, they do so after age 1 day. Peeling is not normal at the time of birth and should alert the physician to three possibilities: (1) intrauterine stress, (2) postmaturity, and (3) disorders of keratinization.

Pustules present in the first few days of life often cause much consternation. Erythema toxicum usually can be distinguished by the large area of macular erythema surrounding the papulopustular lesion. If the diagnosis is in doubt, the pustule can be opened and stained. Erythema toxicum is filled with eosinophils. Transient neonatal pustular melanosis may alarm the unwary that they are dealing with a staphylococcal skin infection. The pustules are filled with polymorphonuclear leukocytes, but the Gram stain is negative. This fairly common disorder is more common in blacks and may present as freckle-like macules rather than pustules. Congenital candidiasis is another diffuse pustular disorder that appears much more virulent than it really is. The lesions may be present at birth and represent contact of the skin with infected amniotic fluid. A simple potassium hydroxide preparation will readily yield the diagnosis. Miliaria pustulosa is seen in premature infants who have been coated with paraffin or other occlusives in an attempt to cut down on fluid loss from the skin. Not all pustules, then, are staphylococcal.

The Biologic Basis for Pigmentary Disorders

James Norlund, of Cincinnati, presented a fascinating review of pigment formation, replete with clinical examples of the system gone awry. Because pigment cells have their origins in the neural crest and then migrate to the leptomeninges, eye, cochlea of the ear, and the skin, defects in these cells in one area should signal our attention to look for problems in the other areas. Examples include Waardenburg's syndrome, which may include a white forelock, heterochromia, and deafness; the association of Piebaldism with Hirschsprung's disease or cerebellar ataxia; and Ito syndrome, in which swirls of depigmented skin may be associated with neurologic problems.

More on Neonatal Lupus

Neonatal lupus erythematosus (NLE) has become a popular topic in both the pediatric and the dermatologic literature. Doctor Nancy Barnett of Johns Hopkins University presented some of the data from studies carried out in Baltimore and other centers. It has become clear that Ro (SSA) and/or La (SSB) nuclear antibodies are the marker for NLE. About half of mothers of infants with NLE have positive titers of antinuclear antibody, but all have SSA. Almost half of the mothers whose offspring have NLE are asymptomatic. Therefore, if an infant presents with a macular or slightly elevated faintly erythematous eruption, particularly on the scalp, face, and upper part of the chest, consider this diagnosis.

It also has become increasingly clear that congenital heart block (CHB) is a marker for maternal SLE or other connective tissue disease. In one study 83% of mothers of infants with CHB had Ro antibody. In a series of 45 infants with structural heart disease none of the mothers had the presence of this antibody. The risk for siblings of NLE patients is variable. Although CHB is permanent and associated with a 22% to 30% mortality, the skin lesions of NLE are gone in 100% of the infants by age 1 year.

Allergic Contact Dermatitis

Bill Weston of Denver suggested that allergic contact dermatitis in children is much more common than many suspect. In one study, 20% of children aged 0 to 14 years who presented with dermatitis had contact allergy as the cause. Forty percent were younger than age 5 years! For potent allergens, sensitization takes place in 5 to 7 days; for weak allergens, however, it may take weeks or months to sensitize. Once the T lymphocytes have processed the antigens and have taken up residence in the dermis, a second exposure to the antigen results in the release of inflammatory mediators in a matter of hours.

The distribution of the dermatitis should suggest the possible culprit. Examples include: dorsum of the feet—shoes (rubber chemicals); earlobes, wrists, fingers—metal (nickel); face and eyelids—cosmetics; axillae—deodorants; perioral area—toothpaste, bubble gum, mouthwash; and clothing areas—formaldehyde.

A rule of thumb for treatment, in addition to allergen avoidance, is that if less than 10% of the body surface is involved, topical steroids can be used. If the disease is more extensive, systemic steroids may be necessary. Prednisone, .5 to 1.0 mg/kg/day, decreased gradually over 10 to 14 days, is usually effective.

Is There a Cure for TV?

Although most people agree that TV is in dire need of rehabilitation, "TV" here does not mean "television," but an old annoyance, tinea versicolor. Paul Jacobs of Stanford University presented some impressive data on the use of a single 400-mg dose of ketoconazole for TV. The infection cleared in most patients treated with a single tablet, although reinfections appear to be common months down the line. I hope others find this simple treatment just as effective. It sure beats slopping on the topical agents!

The Sexually Transmitted Disease Explosion—The Dust Settles

Sexual abuse in children has become a distressingly common problem, particularly since it has come out of the closet, so to speak. Sexually transmitted diseases, of course, follow suit. Ron Hansen highlighted some features of these problems. Statistics such as that (1) 20% to 30% of college females and 10% to 15% of males had been sexually abused as children and (2) 10% of males are gay or bisexual clearly indicate the extent of this social ill.

It has become increasingly clear that prepubertal children with gonococci do not acquire the bacteria by being innocent bystanders. The old toilet seat and wet towel explanations of transmission are passé. Hansen believes that acquired gonococcal infection in this age group is 99.9% sexual abuse.

It is also worth noting that 20% to 30% of patients with gonorrhea have nonspecific urethritis as well, generally caused by *Chlamydia*. Treatment of gonococcal urethritis, then, should be followed by a week of tetracycline.

Tinea in Tiny Tots

Alvin Jacobs, Dean of Pediatric Dermatology at Stanford University, reminded us of some of the vagaries of dermatophyte infections in young children. Often these infections cannot be diagnosed by inspection alone. A potassium hydroxide preparation and fungal culture should be done if the lesions look remotely suspicious. Gradually spreading circinate lesions in the diaper area are often mistaken for routine diaper dermatitis. Tinea pedis in the prepubertal child is not RARE, but it is unusual. The Wood's lamp is useless in diagnosing tinea in glabrous skin. But keep in mind that the dermatophytes have changed. *Trichophyton tonsurans* is responsible for most infections in the United States today and *T. tonsurans* does not fluoresce!

Lifelong Implications of Childhood Psoriasis

Eugene Farber of Stanford University discussed the heartbreak of psoriasis in childhood. Thirty-five percent of psoriasis begins before age 20 years and 2% of psoriatic patients report an onset before age 2. The etiology of psoriasis appears to be multifactorial, with exogenous causes such as trauma and phototoxic reactions and endogenous causes that include group A β-hemolytic streptococcal infections.

Approximately one third of patients with psoriasis go into spontaneous remission. Those who have a strong family history are more likely to have ongoing problems. Thirty-five percent of 5,000 patients with psoriasis had first-, second-, or third-degree relatives with the disease, but 59% of those with onset before age 2 years had a positive family history. Farber does not think that the early onset of the disease correlates with an increased severity, however.

Triggering factors of psoriasis include: (1) stress; (2) direct skin injury—bruises, cuts, burns, and phototoxicity; (3) drugs—antimalarials; (4) bacterial and viral infections; and (5) prolonged low humidity. Indoor living in the winter with prolonged periods of drying of the skin should be meticulously avoided. Farber makes a strong point for the use of humidifiers in the winter and the use of emollients. At Stanford University, parental education on the care of psoriatic skin has lessened morbidity. Oral psoralens and ultraviolet light (PUVA) should not be used in children.

The Therapeutic Hotline

This final session of the meeting is one of the favorites of most attendees. A wide variety of tips from the experts always proves helpful and enlightening.

SEBORRHEA

Severe, recalcitrant seborrheic dermatitis should suggest the possibility of biotin-responsive decarboxylase deficiency, especially if the infant has vomiting as well. Some cases of severe seborrheic dermatitis may be biotin sensitive without an apparent decarboxylase deficiency. Alvin Jacobs has had success with 600–900 μg of biotin daily.

ACNE AND ACCUTANE

Recent reports have made it strikingly clear that Accutane, the "wonder" drug for cystic acne, is a teratogen. All women who are started on this drug should have a pregnancy test beforehand, and most panelists require that they sign a written consent verifying that they have been informed of the dangers to the fetus should pregnancy occur. Contraceptives should be used and many physicians obtain routine pregnancy tests during the treatment course.

CONGENITAL NEVI AND MELANOMA

Controversy still persists regarding the removal of all congenital nevi. The risk of development of melanoma in the future is still not known for small nevi, although for large lesions it may be as high as 1 in 10. A few panelists remove all congenital nevi under local anesthesia when it can be done easily.

FREEZING WARTS

If one decides to subject warts to liquid nitrogen, the best results are obtained when the cotton swab is applied without pressure to the wart until a halo of white, 1–2 mm in width, and lasting 15 to 30 seconds, occurs after swab removal.

OUT, OUT DAMNED ITCH

The final word on itching or stinging lesions from bug bites, varicella, or herpes may be the following neat concoction: 20% isopropyl alcohol, 0.5% to 1% phenol, 0.5 to 1% menthol, and calamine lotion to make 4 oz. Try it, you and your patients may like it!

4 Dentistry and Otolaryngology

Oral Tissue Alterations Associated With the Use of Smokeless Tobacco by Teenagers: Part I. Clinical Findings
Robert O. Greer, Jr., and Todd C. Poulson (Univ. of Colorado)
Oral Surg. 56:275–284, September 1983   4–1

One hundred seventeen (10.45%) users of smokeless tobacco were identified among 1,119 students in grades 9 through 12. Students completed a questionnaire that provided information on number of years with the habit, daily exposure, brand of tobacco, site of application, smoking and drinking habits, subjective symptoms, and frequency of dental care. Examination of oral hard and soft tissues was performed without reference to the questionnaire.

Age and sex distribution of smokeless tobacco users is shown in the table. Fifty-seven (48.7%) had lesions of mucosa, periodontium, or teeth. Lesions were classified in 50 patients with mucosal alterations only as follows: degree 1, 25 with superficial lesion of color similar to surrounding mucosa and slight wrinkling; degree 2, 18 with superficial whitish or reddish lesions with moderate wrinkling; and degree 3, 7 with red or white lesions with obvious wrinkling and thickening. All lesions arose directly in the area of quid placement, with most in the anterior mandibular mucobuccal fold, extending from cuspid to cuspid.

Average intensity and length (only 2.72 years) of use of smokeless tobacco in this youthful study population were less than that found in adult populations; this accounts for the comparatively minor lesions that documented no gingival recession, periodontal destruction, or abrasion of teeth. Such severe changes in hard and soft tissues result from long-term use of the tobacco product in an adult population.

The study identified four distinct lesions associated with smokeless tobacco use: hyperkeratotic or erythroplakic lesions of oral mucosa; gingival or periodontal inflammation; a combination of oral mucosal lesions and periodontal inflammation; and cervical erosion of teeth.

No evidence of tobacco-associated dental caries was found. This may be due to the physical cleansing action of the accelerated salivary flow stimulated by tobacco use. Many smokeless tobacco products contain fluoride levels ranging from 0.91 ppm to 2.01 ppm, which may also contribute to suppression of dental caries. Most of this patient population (69.3%) had access to dental care; it is unclear whether the difficulty in recognizing early tobacco-related lesions (degree) prevented their recognition during dental examinations.

The suggestions that nitrosonornicotine, the first organic carcinogen

SEX AND AGE DISTRIBUTION AMONG 117 TEENAGE USERS
OF SMOKELESS TOBACCO

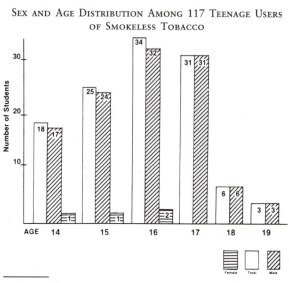

(Courtesy of Greer, R.O., Jr., and Poulson, T.C.: Oral Surg. 56:275–284, September 1983.)

isolated from unburned tobacco, may be responsible for verrucous carcinoma in users of smokeless tobacco and that oral epithelial changes may be predicted on the basis of histologic findings deserve further study.

▶ The authors write, "Tobacco has been smoked, chewed, and inhaled in various forms for more than 500 years." The historical development and folklore concerning the use of smokeless tobacco date back to the time of Columbus's first voyage to the New World. Smokeless tobacco has been, and still is, used worldwide. In the United States, its use has been well documented since the Revolutionary War period, and during the 1800s, three forms became quite popular: moist snuff, loose-leaf chewing tobacco, and plug or block chewing tobacco. In the 1800s the use of smokeless tobacco fell into disfavor, largely because Koch, Pasteur, Lister, Ehrlich and others popularized the "germ theory of infection" and characterized chewing tobacco as unsanitary. Most of the rest of the world does not view the United States as being particularly sanitary with regard to tobacco habits, and unfortunately this was substantiated by a resurgence in the use of all forms of smokeless tobacco during the 1970s. To be precise, sales of smokeless tobacco have increased about 11% annually since 1974, and there are now an estimated 22 million users in the United States. The revival of the use of smokeless tabacco among adolescents has aroused renewed interest in the health controversy concerning its use. Teenagers use smokeless tobacco either as dipping tobacco (snuff) or as rough-cut chewing tobacco. Snuff dipping consists of putting a pinch of powdered tobacco into the buccal sulcus, whereas the use of chewing tobacco consists of placing a leaf tobacco or a plug of tobacco near the inner cheek. A "chaw" is a golf-ball-sized quid of leaf or plug tobacco on which the chewer sucks. To me, the whole concept does the same thing. The only apparent benefit to chewing tobacco is the fact that it may help prevent dental caries, because there is some fluoride contaminating most tobacco leaves.

Despite the carcinogenic dangers of placing chewing tobacco or snuff in the oral cavity and leaving it in place for extended periods, the use of these crummy agents has found its way into middle schools, high schools, and college campuses as a socially acceptable and popular habit. It is even more unfortunate that most of this came about as a reaction to the dangers inherent in the actual smoking of tobacco. Perhaps the only way to handle this problem, because we seem to be so weak hearted about directly attacking the tobacco industry, is to ban all access to spittoons.—J.A.S., III

Iatrogenic Erosion of Teeth
Robert E. Sullivan and William S. Kramer (College of Dentistry, Univ. of Nebraska, Lincoln)
ASDC J. Dent. Child. 50:192–196, May–June 1983   4–2

A rheumatologist noted that many of his patients with juvenile rheumatoid arthritis (JRA) had teeth that looked yellower and darker than normal and had a "peculiar" size and shape; however, the literature contains no reports that JRA can cause dental abnormalities. Therefore, the authors examined the teeth of 27 female and 15 male patients, aged 3 to 20 years, who had JRA. All were receiving massive aspirin therapy, with some children swallowing aspirin tablets and some receiving chewable aspirin.

Some dentitions appeared normal and others showed varying degrees of erosion, i.e., loss of enamel and dentin structures as a result of dissolution of tooth substances by a nonbacterial chemical process. Where erosion was minimal and apparently early, the exposed dentin was yellowish. Where erosion had progressed, the dentin was yellowish-brown, brown, or black and appeared to have been extrinsically stained. In all cases, the dentin was hard, smooth, and had an eburnated appearance. In some teeth, the entire occlusal surface and morphological features had been lost, with as much as one third to one half of the occlusal part of the crown missing. In other teeth, the loss was confined to the area of the major occlusal pit, especially in first and second primary molars (Fig 4–1). The defects appeared on roentgenograms to resemble large caries lesions but clinically were found to be erosions lined by hard, smooth, stained dentin similar to flattened erosions (Fig 4–2). In neither case did the lesions appear to be carious. The clinical impression of erosion was quite definite.

Matching of the dental findings with the medical histories quickly showed that dental erosions occurred only in children who chewed aspirin tablets; those who swallowed tablets had unaffected teeth. The oral hygiene, excellent in 28 children and satisfactory in 14, appeared to be far superior to that seen in routine patients treated in the pedodontic clinic.

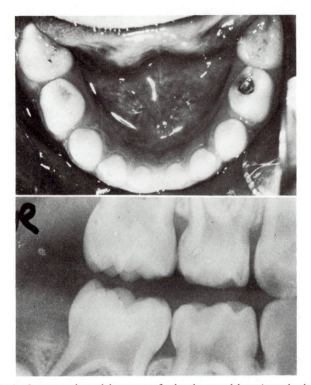

Fig 4–1 (top).—In some teeth, tooth loss was confined to the area of the major occlusal pit, especially in first and second primary molars.

Fig 4–2 (bottom).—The defects resembled large caries lesions on roentgenograms; clinically, however, they were found to be erosions lined by hard, smooth, stained dentin.

(Courtesy of Sullivan, R.E., and Kramer, W.S.: ASDC J. Dent. Child. 50:192–196, May–June 1983.)

Because of this topical effect of aspirin on teeth, children with JRA should be encouraged to swallow rather than chew aspirin tablets.

▶ It is important for physicians and dentists to understand the untoward affects of aspirin therapy for patients with juvenile rheumatoid arthritis. In most cases, substitute forms of therapy are not possible, so every effort should be made to teach the child to swallow rather than chew the tablets.

Tooth enamel will decalcify in acidic solutions when the pH is below 6.0. At pH values between 5.0 and 6.0, it takes several hours of accumulative exposure for clinically evident decalcification to occur, but it does occur. The past few years have taught us about a number of circumstances in which this phenomenon becomes important. As we note above, aspirin chewing will do this. The same thing has been observed among industrial workers exposed to acid fumes (*Morbid. Mortal. Weekly Rep.* 32:362, 1983), as well as among people consuming excessive quantities of acidic fruits, beverages, and other medications. In 1980 and in 1982, outbreaks of erosion of dental enamel were reported in swimmers who had been in prolonged contact with pool water that had been gas chlorinated. Gas chlorination of pools (unless adequately buffered with soda ash) produces a very acidic water. The American Public Health Association has set forth guidelines regarding proper maintenance of this sort of pool (ibid., p. 361).

One additional cause of erosion of the dental enamel is repetitive exposure to gastric acids. This is now being increasingly recognized in infants with gastroesophageal reflux who are old enough to have teeth and in teenagers with bulimia. These conditions are now sufficiently common that when you diagnose a child or teenager with these problems, you should pay careful attention to the dental complications. This is especially true since the teeth can be protected from stomach acid with an acrylic sealant (Rosenthal et al.: *Clin. Pediatr.* 22:818, 1983). The precise product used is a synthetic acrylic material called Prisma-Shield made by the L. D. Caulk Company in Delaware. Imagine having your teeth caulked? Even though it works, it is somewhat akin to having your car Ziebarted or treated by Rusty Jones.—J.A.S., III

Use of Pneumococcal Polysaccharide Vaccine in Preventing Otitis Media in Infants: Different Results Between Racial Groups
V. M. Howie, John Ploussard, John L. Sloyer, and James C. Hill
Pediatrics 73:79–81, January 1984   4–3

The data were reviewed on 133 children aged 6–11 months with at least one episode of otitis media who received one of two pneumococcal vaccines. One vaccine contained 25 μm of types 1, 3, 6, 7, 14, 18, 19, and 23, and the other, the control vaccine, contained 25 μm of types 2, 4, 5, 8, 9, 12, and 25. Sixty-five black and 68 white infants from Huntsville, Alabama, participated in the study. The subjects were distributed fairly evenly by race and socioeconomic class in the different vaccine groups.

Follow-up of the black infants showed significantly more visits for otitis media in those given the control vaccine, but no such difference was apparent for the white infants. Most episodes of otitis occurred in the first year after vaccination in both vaccinated and control infants. This is the first report of racial differences in clinical responsiveness to a vaccine. Confirmation of the findings would support the cost-effectiveness of pneumococcal vaccine in preventing otitis media in black children, but not in white children. It is possible that the difference in responsiveness is associated with a particular genotype in black children.

▶ The results of a pneumococcal polysaccharide vaccine trial for the prevention of otitis media in infants in Huntsville, Alabama, were reported previously (*Rev. Infect. Dis.* 3:S119, 1981). What this report does is to follow these results further in time. Although the conclusions are somewhat puzzlesome, they do show a statistically significant reduction in the recurrence rate of otitis media in black infants who have received the pneumococcal vaccine. All these infants had had one or more episodes of otitis media and then received the pneumococcal vaccine between ages 6 and 11 months. The recurrence rate of otitis media was reduced by about 50%. No such improvement was seen in a white control population who received the vaccine after one or more episodes of otitis media. The differences in the racial differences here are totally unexplained. Also peculiar is the fact that we have become accustomed to thinking that polysaccharide vaccines do not produce much of an immunogenic response in such young infants. Clearly, it must do something, because there was protection for a fair proportion of these children. Frankly, this report comes none too soon, because the prevalence of pneumococci relatively resistant to penicillin seems to be on the increase. M. A. Jackson et al. (*Pediatr. Infect. Dis.* 3:129, 1984) suggest that the prevalence of pneumococci relatively resistant to penicillins (at least in Dallas) is now running at about 8%. These numbers are sufficiently large that if you have any serious illness caused by pneumococci that can be documented by culture, the sensitivities to penicillin should be clearly documented.

The use of the pneumococcal vaccine for preventing otitis media obviously is not likely to produce dramatic results in the overall population. As noted, its effects in white infants are relatively poor at this age. Obviously, this approach does nothing to deal with the more significant problem of *Hemophilus influenzae* infection of the middle ear. Vaccines for this do not produce any dramatic effects either. Some infections are with nontypable strains, and the *H. influenzae* type B polysaccharide vaccine is definitely not very immunogenic in its current form in children younger than age 18 months. Over two thirds of cases of otitis media occur in this younger age group. As mentioned in previous YEAR BOOKS, one approach to this latter difficulty is to immunize a pregnant woman at 36 weeks with polysaccharide vaccines so that the infant is "passively immunized" by IgG antibody from the mother. This sort of passive immunization does produce significant antibody titers that can last up to a year or more. Clinical trials demonstrating the real efficacy of this, of course, are still pending. An absolutely superb review of neonatal passive immunization by maternal vaccination for all sorts of things may be found in an article by Amstey et al. (*Obstet. Gynecol.* 63:105, 1984). The major criticism of approaching a woman in this regard has been the fact that some of the polysaccharide vaccines were contaminated heavily with ABO antigens and could have provided isohemagglutinin stimulation and perhaps even clinical disease in the neonate. This no longer is a problem.

It is imperative that something be done about this problem with *H. influenzae* infection in the first 18 months of life because there has been a slow emergence of *H. influenzae* organisms that are now resistant to both ampicillin and chloramphenicol (*Morbidity Mortality Weekly Rep.* 33:66, 1984). The prevalence of this type of resistant organisms is still sufficiently low that we should not be changing our approach to disease caused by *H. influenzae,* but you should keep an eye out for worsening of this problem.

I believe it would be ideal if the sort of study that was done in black and white infants using the pneumococcal polysaccharide vaccine had been performed also in other racial groups, particularly among native American Indians. In the latter group of children, the problem of otitis media is of monumental proportions for reasons that are not entirely well understood. Presumably this is a true genetic difference in susceptibility and not a contamination by the white man or a change in life-style brought about by displacement of Indians from their own native locales. I believe the role of preventative vaccine could be tremendously important in this population. This also reminds me of the story of the tourist who asked a native American Indian in the Southwest what America was called by the Indians before the white man arrived. The reply was, "Ours."—J.A.S., III

Ventilation Tubes in Secretory Otitis Media: Randomized, Controlled Study of the Course, Complications, and Sequelae of Ventilation Tubes
Torben Lildholdt (Vejle, Denmark)
Acta Otolaryngol. [Suppl. 398] (Stockh.), 1–28, 1983   4–4

An evaluation was made of the use of ventilation tubes in the management of primary secretory otitis media in bilaterally affected patients who had a tube placed in one ear while the other was left intact. The 85 boys and 65 girls in the study had a mean age of 3.9 years. Tympanography was carried out the day before tube placement. Seven children with tympanosclerosis or atrophy were excluded from analysis. Tonsillectomy has been done or was done subsequently in 43% of patients and adenoidectomy in 25%. Mean follow-up was 3.2 years.

The tympanometric and audiometric findings were generally comparable in the intubated and control ears. Hearing losses are compared in Figure 4–3. Repeat operation was performed in 17% of patients, and follow-up otomicroscopic examination showed a higher rate of atrophy in these patients. Suppuration was observed in one fourth of intubated ears 2 months or more after operation. The later incidence of tympanosclerosis

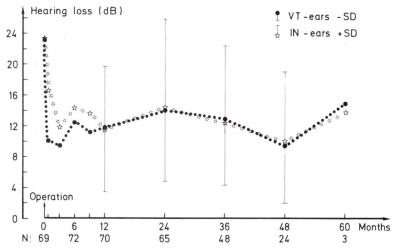

Fig 4–3.—Hearing level of two types of ear during observation. Hearing loss represents pure-tone average. *IN*, intact; *VT*, ventilation tube. (Courtesy of Lildholdt, T.: Acta Otolaryngol. [Suppl. 398] (Stockh.), 1–28, 1983.)

was increased. The overall findings at follow-up were considered to be normal in 83% of intact ears but in only 23% of treated ears. Nearly one third of the children had one ear considered to be diseased, and both ears were considered to be abnormal in 9% of the children. The children who had tonsillectomy initially had a poorer outcome. No permanent perforations were observed after spontaneous extrusion of the ventilation tubes.

Ventilation tube insertion probably has no overall therapeutic effect on serous otitis media, as judged from follow-up tympanography. Some patients, however, exhibit recurrent disease after extrusion of the ventilation tube, and intubation probably should be maintained for some time in these patients. Further work is needed to find ways of identifying these patients in the early phase of involvement. The high rate of adverse sequelae of ventilation tube use is an important consideration in most children with primary serous otitis media.

▶ If you haven't noticed that the pendulum is swinging away from being in favor of tympanostomy tubes, you haven't been following the debates sufficiently closely. It is not that tympanostomy tubes are out of favor at this point, but they may have reached their peak and are on the way down a bit. Since myringotomy became popular as a result of the work of Astley Cooper in the early 19th century, efforts have been made to remove secretions from the middle ear by making a semipermanent opening in the tympanic membrane. Attempts at this were made during the 19th century by using various foreign bodies, such as catgut strings (one of the 2,009 ways of utilizing dead cats), wires, and tubes. It was Politzer who described an islet made of hard rubber, which had grooves to fit into the tympanic membrane and a silk thread sewn on to it to prevent entry into the middle ear. None of this seemed to work very well until around 1954, when Armstrong began to insert small pieces of plastic tubes into myringotomy incisions. He described this as a new treatment for chronic otitis media, but warned that it was not a panacea and should be used only in chronic cases that had resisted all other forms of treatment (*Arch. Otolaryngol.* 59:653, 1954). I thought you might enjoy hearing this brief historical vignette on polyethylene tubes because the cautions of Armstrong have largely been either ignored or not believed. This is evidenced by the fact that here in the United States about 1 million children a year are treated for glue ears by this surgical approach. The study reported by Lildholdt and presented here seems to tell us that polyethylene tubes may not work as well as we might suspect they do. It is not easy to do the sort of study reported here, putting a tube in one ear and leaving the other ear unoperated on as a control. The data, however, do suggest that ventilation tube insertion probably has no overall therapeutic effect on serous otitis media. This is a pretty strong conclusion, but has been seconded by others. Nick Black reported from Oxford, England, that surgery for glue ear there was a modern epidemic (*Lancet* 1:835, 1984). Later in this same journal, surgery for glue ear was called a surgical approach for a nondisease (ibid., p. 1027). The number of letters to the editor regarding these sorts of comments was staggering last year. Comments such as the following appeared: "In 1984, no middle ear exudate, sticky or fluid, needs to be evacuated. When the infection has been defeated, the middle ear is biologically equipped to deal with resorption via enzymes, scavenger cells, and vascular permeability changes. Resorption is made easier by Politzer air inflation, which disperses exudate. Antibiotics must be continued until the hearing is normal" (ibid., p. 1235). These are pretty strong words for the British literature. In part, this is a response to the risk of cholesteatoma related to polyethylene tubes. In the United States, it has been roughly estimated that 1,000 to 10,000 cases of cholesteatoma resulting from violation of the tympanic membrane require secondary surgical procedures. What the antagonists of polyethylene tubes are trying to say is that with proper medical management, the outcome with respect to reinfection and resolution of fluid is not very different with or without the tubes.

What many of these negative reports fail to recognize, of course, is that one of the main rationales for surgery is to improve the child's hearing during a critical period for acquisition of speech and language. If we were to ask ourselves, "Are all myringotomies and grommet insertions really necessary?" The answer would have to be: "No." But there must be selected cases in which real benefits would accrue in terms of immediate improvement in hearing. Lildholdt was not able to show much difference in hearing, but I think it is the personal observation of many persons that this is so.

We pediatricians obviously are not in the driver's seat all the time when it comes to the final decision to put in polyethylene tubes, but it is our responsibility to direct the flow of traffic to the ear, nose, and throat specialist's office. What I really think we need are more options. It you want to see some of these options, read the excellent commentary by Charles Bluestone on how he medically manages the chronic draining ear (*Laryngoscope* 93:661, 1983). Here is a surgeon presenting an excellent medical approach to this problem. As another alternative to tubulation, you might try treatment with sulfur hexafluoride. This is a nontoxic inert gas that can be infused into the middle ear with a tuberculin syringe and acts as a gas cushion behind an intact ear drum in somebody who has a middle ear effusion. This technique was recently reported from Sweden (*Arch. Otolaryngol.* 109:358, 1983). The idea here is to put a type of gas into the middle ear that diffuses out only very slowly and allows a positive pressure to be present for a long time, helping to restore eustachian tube function and drainage within the middle ear (you might call this the "Firestone approach" rather than the "Bluestone approach" because the middle ear rides along on a cushion of air). Despite this report, somehow I just don't think that middle ear insufflation will ever catch on or, if it does, it will be about as successful as a hatcheck concession in a nudist colony.

What I would really like to see done as a controlled study as part of the management of serous otitis media is the "Wrigley approach." That's where you take 100 children with serous otitis media and get them to chew chewing gum continuously for 2 weeks and compare them with a control group of patients who are deprived of this pleasure. I am absolutely convinced that this technique would restore eustachian tube function if you had a patient old enough to use it.—J.A.S., III

Two Versus Seven Days' Penicillin Treatment for Acute Otitis Media: A Placebo Controlled Trial in Children

K.-I. Meistrup-Larsen, H. Sørensen, N.-J. Johnsen, J. Thomsen, N. Mygind, and J. Sederberg-Olsen
Acta Otolaryngol. (Stockh.) 96:99–104, July–Aug. 1983   4–5

One hundred three children aged 1–10 years were studied in a double-blind placebo-controlled trial testing the effect of penicillin V, 55 mg/kg/day, for 2 days versus 7 days in acute otitis media.

Pretreatment symptoms and symptoms on the first treatment day (when both groups received penicillin) were more pronounced in the "penicillin 2 days" group, but differences were not statistically significant. After 2 days of penicillin treatment, the patients were almost without symptoms and there was no difference between the two groups. There were no differences between the two treatment groups for course of disease and healing, results of tympanometry at 2-week follow-up, or common cold symptoms. In the "penicillin 7 days" group, 76% had a satisfactory course of the disease and in the "penicillin 2 days" group, 71% had a satisfactory course. The difference was not statistically significant.

The relatively small number of patients notwithstanding, it appears that in acute otitis media the effect of penicillin for an additional 5 days after initial treatment for 2 days can, at most, be marginal. The advantages of shortened treatment are several. Penicillin consumption in children with acute otitis media can be reduced to about 15% of the previous level without increasing the risk of serious complications.

▶ This past year or so has been an absolute banner one with respect to a plethora of reports on antibiotics for the management of otitis media. They are so numerous that it would be impossible to encapsulate them in 10 volumes of a YEAR BOOK. Some highlights are as follows: Giebink et al. found no significant differences between cefaclor and amoxicillin in the management of acute otitis media (*Am. J. Dis. Child.* 138:287, 1984). Using the same two drugs, John and Valle-Jones (*Practitioner* 227:1809, 1983) found that cefaclor was at least as effective as amoxicillin and perhaps a little better in that symptoms resolve slightly more quickly. I would call that a draw. Then there was the report of Liston et al. (*Pediatrics* 71:524, 1983) suggesting that sulfisoxazole was not able to be documented to be a good prophylactic agent for otitis media. The response to this was immediate and swift on the part of Paradise, who, in his letter to the editor of *Pediatrics* (77:583, 1983), provided what to me was a convincing retort suggesting that evidence does exist regarding the efficacy of antimicrobial prophylaxis. I don't think the boxing match is over in this regard; we are merely in round three or four now. And, as usual, a year could not pass without another report of anaerobes being a significant bacteriologic feature of serous otitis media (*Am. J. Otolaryngol.* 4:389, 1983). The authors who wrote this last article are absolute magicians; they can turn anything into an anaerobe.

Finally, there appeared the article presented above that challenged the current concept of duration of therapy for the management of otitis media. Stanford Schulman, Chief of the Division of Infectious Disease, Department of Pediatrics, Children's Memorial Hospital in Chicago, nicely critiques this study for us as follows:

"Defining optimal therapy for otitis media continues to provide great frustration. Data have been presented in recent years to show that decongestants and antihistamines are of little or no benefit in the treatment of acute otitis media or serous otitis, when studied in a controlled manner. To make matters worse, studies from northern Europe, including this one from otolaryngologists in Copenhagen and Elsinore, Denmark ('To treat or not to treat?'), suggest that antibiotic therapy may be superfluous and may expose children unnecessarily to antibiotic agents. Comparing 2-day and 7-day courses of oral penicillin V, the authors conclude that no benefit attributable to the additional 5 days of antibiotic could be identified. Although more subjects in the 2-day treatment group developed contralateral otitis media or spontaneous perforation after enrollment, these complications were apparent within the first 2 days of therapy, before any variation in treatment had occurred.

"In addition, the authors introduce a form of clinical management that they term 'masterful inactivity' (honest!). They apparently have moved now to a scheme for children with acute otitis, but without severe otalgia, in which patients are given one to three doses of analgesics over 8–12 hours (their 'masterful inactivity'), and then only the 50% with persisting earache are treated with four doses of penicillin V over 2 days. If symptoms still persist, myringotomy is performed by an otologist, and amoxicillin is prescribed 'when necessary.' This approach may work in Scandinavia, but to me it appears foolhardy to restrict so severely antibiotic usage for a disease in which bacteria (presumably important in its pathogenesis) can be isolated from middle ear aspirates in approximately 75% of instances. We showed that mastoiditis and even intracranial infections can result from unresolved otitis in the modern era (Venezio et al: *J. Pediatr.* 101:509–513, 1982), and Peter Wright recently pointed out that in 1936, prior to the availability of antibiotics, more deaths in the United States were attributable to otitis media and mastoiditis than to meningitis (*Pediatr. Ann.* 13:377–379, 1984).

"It is crystal clear that, as clinicians, we regularly overuse antibiotics and that we should try to minimize this practice. However, both simple pharyngitis and uncomplicated upper respiratory tract infection, for example, afford much more legitimate situations at present than otitis media in which to control unwarranted exposure to expensive, potentially sensitizing, and occasionally toxic antimicrobial agents. Before we curtail the usage of antibiotics for otitis media, convincing data from well-designed studies incorporating a more appropriate antibiotic than penicillin will be necessary."

Effect of Menthol on Nasal Resistance to Airflow
R. Eccles and A. S. Jones (Cardiff, Wales)
J. Laryngol. Otol. 97:705–709, August 1983   4–6

Menthol vapor is traditionally believed to be of use in the symptomatic treatment of nasal congestion, and preparations containing menthol are popular as over-the-counter remedies for relief of nasal congestion associated with coryza. They studied the effect of menthol vapor on nasal resistance to airflow by using standard rhinometric techniques to measure total nasal resistance before and after using menthol. A questionnaire was used to obtain a case history and determine the subjective effects of menthol. Thirty-one subjects were included in the study.

Exposure to menthol vapor had no consistent effect on total nasal resistance to airflow in these subjects. Nine of the 31 showed a significant decrease in nasal resistance, 9 showed a significant increase in nasal resistance, and 13 showed no change. Responses to menthol could not be correlated with any of the information obtained by the questionnaire. Twenty-two of the 31 subjects reported a subjective improvement in nasal airflow; 24 reported increased sensation of nasal airflow, and all 31 believed that airflow felt cool after menthol. Of the 9 subjects in whom menthol caused a significant increase in nasal resistance, 8 reported a subjective improvement in airflow.

Menthol exposure has no consistent effect on nasal resistance to airflow and therefore no consistent nasal decongestant action. The results indicate that menthol stimulates cold receptors in the nasal mucosa to create an increased sensation of airflow.

Odor Perception in Children in Relation to Nasal Obstruction
S. Nasrin Ghorbanian, Jack L. Paradise, and Richard L. Doty
Pediatrics 72:510–516, October 1983   4–7

To determine whether nasal obstruction in children results in impaired nasal function, olfactory sensitivity was assessed in 65 children seen at the Children's Hospital of Pittsburgh for various degrees of nasal obstruction and in 13 children without such obstruction; there were 45 boys and 33 girls aged 5–15 years.

Initially, degree of nasal obstruction, if any, was determined in all 78 subjects, as well as its relationship, if any, to impairment of smell sensitivity. The procedure was repeated 2–28 months later on 28 subjects who had had adenoidectomy for enlarged adenoids in the interim and on 16 subjects who initially had nasal obstruction and received no operative intervention. Assessment included clinical observation of mouth breathing and hyponasality, measurement of olfactory sensitivity, and clinical impressions based on nasal mucous membrane appearance, amount and character of nasal secretions, results of allergy skin tests and nasal smears for eosinophils, white blood cell and differential count, and lateral radiograph of the nasopharynx.

Twenty of the 28 subjects who had adenoidectomy showed generally commensurate reductions in nasal obstruction ratings and olfactory detection thresholds, whereas in the 16 subjects retested after 5–13 months without having received in the interim adenoidectomy, both nasal obstruction ratings and olfactory detection thresholds remained essentially unchanged. These results indicate that, in children, nasal obstruction will be associated with impairment of the ability to smell and reduction in the degree of obstruction will result in commensurate recovery of such ability. This effect of obstruction was observed whether the obstruction was within the nasal cavity or in the nasopharynx.

Ability to detect and discern odors enables children to: orient to the environment, recognize noxious or dangerous airborne substances, detect fire, and appreciate the flavor of foods and pleasant aromas. Whether impairment of the appreciation of food adversely affects nutrition, growth, or developmental processes is not known.

▶ This article and the preceding one deal with one or another aspect of "plugged-up" noses. The concept that nasal obstruction may give rise to developmental abnormalities with respect to otoperception is unique and intriguing. The authors speculate that the inability to smell can cause disorientation to the environment and limit the child's ability to detect noxious or dangerous substances. They also allude to the potential for an adverse effect on nutrition and development. Obviously, all this requires further study.

I found the report on menthol vapors to be absolutely fascinating. Ask any lay person whether menthol vapors unplug your nose and the response would more likely than not be: "Yes." Yet, we see that this does not happen at all. What we merely sense is the false illusion of coolness in our nose and associate this incorrectly with the passage of air through the nasal cavities. This is a form of hypnotism, as it were, of the nose. I can recall as a child having a goopy product rubbed over my chest at bedtime when I had a head cold (You all know the name of the product). These products actually may indeed work, because I (and most current children) screamed and hollered so much with the application that the vigors of the crying actually cleared the nose. There seems to be no safe way to handle this problem. Nose drops produce hypernatremia. Sympathomimetic vasoconstrictors also can cause trouble. Even ones such as xylometazoline (example: Neo-Synephrine II Long Acting Nose Drops) and oxymetazoline (example: Afrin Pediatric Nose Drops), which are among the newer-generation agents, are not totally free of complications. Sodeiman et al. (*Lancet* 1:573, 1984) reported excitation, sedation, and even a case of epileptiform convulsive attacks as well as hallucinations with the use of these drugs. Sometimes it is better to leave well enough alone, I suppose.—J.A.S., III

Prevalence of Lymphadenopathy of the Head and Neck in Infants and Children

Lynn W. Herzog (Children's Hosp. Med. Center, Boston)
Clin. Pediatr. (Phila.) 22:485–488, July 1983   4–8

The prevalence and distribution of palpable lymph nodes was assessed in 223 patients aged 3 weeks to 6 years seen in a 6-month period at a hospital-based primary care clinic for routine health examination (47%) or for acute illness. No child had a clinical diagnosis of rubella, lymphadenopathy as a presenting complaint, or serious systemic disease.

Palpable nodes were detected in 55% of children (Table 1). The most

TABLE 1.—Prevalence of Adenopathy by Age

Palpable Nodes

Age	Number of Patients	Occipital		Postauricular		Submandibular		Cervical		No Palpable Nodes	
		No.	(%)	No.	(%)	No.	(%)	No.	(%)	No.	(%)
0–6 months	52	17	(32)	7	(13)	1	(2)	1	(2)	32	(62)
7–12 months	31	8	(26)	4	(13)	1	(3)	8	(26)	16	(52)
13–23 months	39	4	(10)	3	(7)	7	(18)	11	(28)	20	(52)
2 years	35	3	(8)	2	(6)	7	(20)	16	(45)	11	(32)
3 years	27	2	(7)	0	(0)	7	(26)	9	(33)	11	(41)
4 years	20	0	(0)	0	(0)	5	(25)	11	(55)	7	(35)
5 years	19	0	(0)	1	(5)	4	(21)	12	(63)	5	(26)
Total	223	34	(15)	17	(8)	32	(14)	68	(30)	102	(45)

(Courtesy of Herzog, L.W.: Clin. Pediatr. (Phila.) 22:485–488, July 1983.)

common enlarged nodes were cervical, found in 30% of all children, followed by occipital nodes (15%), submandibular nodes (14%), and postauricular nodes (8%). Occipital nodes were found most often in infants, and cervical nodes were found most often in older children. Postauricular adenopathy was associated with occipital adenopathy in 47% of cases and was associated with a rash in 23%. Size of the nodes varied from 0.5 cm in infants (with the largest in patients with a rash) to 1.5 cm in older children (with the largest in patients with strep throat). None of the nodes had signs suggestive of infectious adenitis.

Forty-four percent of 105 children seen for routine health examination had palpable nodes, compared with 64% of those being seen for sick visits (Table 2), a difference significant only in children older than age 2 years. Prevalence of adenopathy was highest in children with a rash (84%), compared with 53% in children with nonspecific febrile illness or febrile upper respiratory tract infection.

In this series, infants and younger children commonly had occipital and postauricular adenopathy, whereas the older children for the most part had cervical and submandibular nodes. Enlarged occipital nodes are suf-

TABLE 2.—Prevalence of Adenopathy by Diagnosis

Age	Well-child Visit	Sick Visit (including rash)	Rash*
0–6 months	10/33†	10/19†	6/7†
7–12 months	7/16	8/15	3/3
13–23 months	6/13	13/26	3/3
2 years	12/18	12/17	2/2
3 years	5/12	11/15 ⎫	1/2
4 years	3/8	10/12 ⎬ ‡	0/0
5 years	3/5	11/14 ⎭	1/2
Total	46/105 (44%)	75/118‡ (64%)	16/19‡ (84%)

*Types of rash: eczema-seborrhea, 9; febrile illness, 3; nonspecific, 3; varicella, 1; impetigo, 1; scarlatina, 1; alopecia, 1.

†Number with adenopathy and number seen.

‡P < .01 when compared to well-child visit.

(Courtesy of Herzog, L.W.: Clin. Pediatr. (Phila.) 22:485–488, July 1983.)

ficiently rare in children older than age 2 years to be a useful diagnostic clue. Enlarged supraclavicular nodes are likely to be pathologic at any age.

▶ Jerome O. Klein, Professor of Pediatrics, Boston University School of Medicine, comments:

"Results of studies of normative values do not make exciting reading. The data are most important, however, for defining the usual so that the examiner may be able to identify at a subsequent time the unusual and potentially pathologic. Examination of the well child should include palpation of areas of lymph glands, and the record should identify negative as well as positive findings.

"The article by Herzog brings to mind that there are few studies of the prevalence or "natural history" of lymphadenopathy in children. This report should stimulate two types of investigations of value: prevalence studies of the presence and quality of nodes in various age groups, including neonates; and longitudinal studies (optimally beginning at birth) that would identify the time of appearance, evolution, and resolution of nodes and correlate this information with the presence of local or systemic infection. These studies could be performed by physicians in practice, and if any reading this commentary are interested, I would be happy to assist in developing protocols."

Acute Mastoiditis in Children: A Review of 54 Cases
Donald B. Hawkins, Denise Dru, John W. House, and Richard W. Clark (Los Angeles County-Univ. of Southern California Med. Center)
Laryngoscope 93:568–572, May 1983   4–9

A review was made of the management of 54 children seen in 1972 through 1982 with acute mastoiditis, diagnosed from physical findings of acute or subacute otitis media and postauricular swelling and clouding of the ipsilateral mastoid air cells seen on films. Age range was 2 months to 13 years; median age was 2 years. Forty children had no history of previous otitis media. Fifteen were receiving antibiotics at or shortly before admission. Duration of symptoms ranged from 2 days to 4 weeks. None of the patients appeared to be severely ill. The mean white blood cell count was 15,700/cu mm.

Myringotomy is done as soon as possible if the ear is not already draining, and intravenous antibiotic therapy is instituted, usually with ampicillin, 150 mg/kg daily. The antibiotic is continued for 24–48 hours after all physical signs of mastoiditis have resolved, and oral treatment then is continued for 2 weeks.

Thirty-one patients recovered on conservative management; 23 others had operations for a clinical diagnosis of subperiosteal abscess. No patient had intracranial or meningeal spread of infection. Five patients had incision and drainage of subperiosteal abscesses, and 2 of them recovered without further surgery. Mastoidectomy was done in 21 cases. Only 1 patient had a radical procedure, for tuberculous mastoiditis. Ventilation tubes usually were placed after mastoidectomy, and antibiotic therapy was continued intravenously for 2–3 days and then orally for 10–14 days.

Most children in this series with acute mastoiditis responded to early myringotomy and intravenous antibiotic therapy. Surgery was done when subperiosteal abscess was diagnosed clinically. Although large abscesses will require mastoid surgery, small, apparently fluctuant areas within a postauricular swelling sometimes resolve on conservative management.

▶ Charles Bluestone, Director of Otolaryngology, Children's Hospital of Pittsburgh, and Professor of Otolaryngology, University of Pittsburgh School of Medicine, writes:

"Mastoiditis can be classified into: (1) acute mastoiditis, (2) acute mastoiditis with periosteitis, (3) acute mastoid osteitis (with or without subperiosteal abscess), and (4) chronic mastoiditis. *Acute mastoiditis* is a natural extension of acute otitis media in which there are no specific signs or symptoms of mastoid infection. The condition is present in most children who have acute otitis media, since roentgenograms in such children are usually read as 'cloudly mastoids.' The process is reversible, as the infection in the middle ear cleft resolves, either as a natural process or as a result of treatment of the clinically evident acute otitis media. No mastoid surgery is indicated. However, the infection may progress. *Acute mastoiditis with periosteitis* results when the infection spreads to the periosteum covering the mastoid process. Classically, the child will have postauricular swelling, erythema, tenderness to touch, and loss of the postauricular crease, but no evidence of a subperiosteal abscess or roentgenographic evidence of mastoid osteitis. Management consists of tympanocentesis-myringotomy for identification of the causative organism(s) and to provide drainage of the middle ear cleft. This procedure, combined with the appropriate antimicrobial agent, administered parenterally, should result in rapid resolution of this suppurative complication. However, if the child fails to improve, mastoidectomy is indicated. *Acute mastoid osteitis,* commonly called acute 'coalescent' mastoiditis, is the progression of the infection causing rarefying osteitis of the mastoid. The presence of a fluctuant, subperiosteal abscess requires surgical drainage of the abscess, which is best achieved by a complete simple ('cortical') mastoidectomy, in addition to the management advocated when a child presents with only periosteitis. *Chronic mastoiditis* is almost always associated with chronic suppurative otitis media, which requires medical treatment or surgery, or both."

For more details on this topic, please refer to the review by C. D. Bluestone and J. O. Klein, "Intratemporal Complications and Sequelae of Otitis Media," in *Pediatric Otolaryngology,* edited by C. D. Bluestone and S. E. Stool (W. B. Saunders Co., Philadelphia, 1983, pp. 513–564).—J.A.S., III)

Maxillary Sinus Radiographs in Children With Nonrespiratory Complaints
Anthony L. Kovatch, Ellen R. Wald, Jocyline Ledesma-Medina, Darleen M. Chiponis, and Bruce Bedingfield (Univ. of Pittsburgh)
Pediatrics 73:306–308, March 1984   4–10

Although the presence of both clinical and radiographic findings of acute sinusitis imply the presence of bacterial infection, the significance of only those changes seen radiographically is unclear. An attempt was made to determine the frequency of abnormal findings on maxillary sinus radiographs in 112 unselected children aged 5 days to 16 years having diagnostic skull radiography for indications unrelated to respiratory infection. The indications for skull radiography are listed in Table 1. An occipitomental, or Water's, view was obtained in each case. Abnormal findings included an air-fluid level, partial or complete opacification, and mucosal thickening of 4 mm or more.

Fifty-nine children had evidence of respiratory inflammation. Abnormal maxillary sinus findings were frequent in children younger than age 1 year regardless of respiratory tract status (Table 2). In older children, only 2 of 31 with neither symptoms nor signs of respiratory inflammation had abnormal findings on sinus radiographs, compared with 8 of 14 having both symptoms and signs (Table 3). Crying in the absence of respiratory

TABLE 1.—INDICATIONS FOR SKULL RADIOGRAPHS
IN STUDY POPULATION

	<1 yr of Age	1–16 yr of Age	Total
Trauma	18	32	50
Skull growth	15	4	19
Craniosynostosis	14	3	17
Mass lesion	0	11	11
Seizures	1	5	6
Short stature	0	3	3
Shunt position	0	3	3
Developmental delay	2	1	3
Total	50	62	112

(Courtesy of Kovatch, A.L., et al.: Pediatrics 73:306–308, March 1984. Copyright American Academy of Pediatrics 1984.)

TABLE 2.—RADIOGRAPHIC FINDINGS WITH RESPECT TO
RESPIRATORY SYMPTOMS AND SIGNS IN CHILDREN
YOUNGER THAN 1 AGE YEAR*

No. of Children	History	Physical Examination	Maxillary Sinus Radiographs		
			Normal	Abnormal	Minor Abnormalities
22	−	−	12	8	2
11	+	−	1	10	0
3	−	+	2	1	0
14	+	+	8	6	0
50			23	25	2

*Symbols used are as follows: minus (−), normal; plus (+), abnormal.
(Courtesy of Kovatch, A.L., et al.: Pediatrics 73:306–308, March 1984. Copyright American Academy of Pediatrics 1984.)

TABLE 3.—RADIOGRAPHIC FINDINGS WITH RESPECT
TO RESPIRATORY SYMPTOMS AND SIGNS IN
CHILDREN AGED 1–16 YEARS*

No. of Children	History	Physical Examination	Maxillary Sinus Radiographs		
			Normal	Abnormal	Minor Abnormalities
31	−	−	28†	2	1
11	+	−	6	3	2
6	−	+	5	0	1
14	+	+	4†	8	2
62			43	13	6

*Symbols used are as follows: minus (−), normal; plus (+), abnormal.
†P < .005.
(Courtesy of Kovatch, A.L., et al.: Pediatrics 73:306–308, March 1984.
Copyright American Academy of Pediatrics 1984.)

symptoms or signs was not associated with abnormal results of sinus radiography in children older than age 1 year.

Abnormal findings on maxillary sinus radiographs in children aged 1 year or older generally are related to upper respiratory tract inflammation. Crying alone is not a cause of abnormal radiographic findings at this age level. Sinus radiographs are of limited use in younger infants.

Treatment of Acute Maxillary Sinusitis in Childhood: Comparative Study of Amoxicillin and Cefaclor

Ellen R. Wald, James S. Reilly, Margaretha Casselbrant, Jocyline Ledesma-Medina, Gregory J. Milmoe, Charles D. Bluestone, and Darleen Chiponis (Univ. of Pittsburgh)
J. Pediatr. 104:297–302, February 1984

4–11

Amoxicillin and cefaclor therapy were compared in children with clinical evidence of sinusitis that had been present for less than 30 days and abnormal maxillary sinus roentgenograms. Seventy-nine maxillary sinuses were aspirated in 50 patients aged 1 to 16 years, and quantitative culture of the aspirate showed at least one sinus to be infected in 35 children. The patients were randomized to receive either amoxicillin or cefaclor orally for 10 days in a dosage of 40 mg/kg daily. All patients also received a combination of chlorpheniramine maleate and pseudoephedrine, and oxymetazoline nasal spray.

The 31 boys and 19 girls had a mean age of 5 years. The microbiologic findings are given in the table. One fifth of the *Hemophilus influenzae* strains isolated and 27% of the *Branhamella catarrhalis* strains were β-lactamase positive and amoxicillin resistant. The clinical cure rates were 81% with amoxicillin and 78% with cefaclor. Three of the 4 failures were in children from whom a β-lactamase-producing organism was recovered. The x-ray courses were similar in the two treatment groups. The only

BACTERIAL SPECIES CULTURED FROM 79 SINUS ASPIRATES
IN 50 CHILDREN*

	Single isolates	Multiple isolates	Total
Streptococcus pneumoniae	14	8	22
Branhamella catarrhalis	13	2	15
Haemophilus influenzae	10	5	15
Eikenella corrodens	1	0	1
Group A streptococcus	1	0	1
Group C streptococcus	0	1	1
α-Streptococcus	1	1	2
Peptostreptococcus	0	1	1
Moraxella spp	1	0	1

*Table includes only cultures with at least 10^4 colony-forming units per ml.
(Courtesy of Wald, E.R., et al.: J. Pediatr. 104:297–302, February 1984.)

significant drug toxicity was an urticarial rash, developing on the tenth day of amoxicillin administration.

The bacteriologic nature of acute sinusitis in children is similar to that of acute otitis media. Amoxicillin and cefaclor were comparably effective in this study. Clinical failure in the presence of antibiotic-resistant sinus isolates strongly suggests a beneficial effect of appropriate antimicrobial therapy. If amoxicillin or cefaclor treatment is ineffective, erythromycin-sulfisoxazole is appropriate. Such therapy may be useful in areas where amoxicillin-resistant *H. influenzae* and *B. catarrhalis* are common and in patients allergic to penicillin.

▶ This study and the preceding one, both from the Children's Hospital of Pittsburgh, go a very long way in filling in the many gaps that exist concerning our knowledge of infants and children with sinusitis. The study of sinus x-ray films was undertaken for the purpose of clarifying several issues. Little has been known about the sensitivity and specificity of radiographic findings in the paranasal sinuses of children. It has been suggested that maxillary sinus radiographs are frequently abnormal in normal children. Others have speculated that sinuses may be rendered opaque radiographically during or after an episode of crying when these patients may be filled with tears. What we now see from these reports is that sinus radiographs are actually fairly specific. If you examine children older than age 1 year who have no history of signs or symptoms of respiratory inflammation, maxillary sinus radiographs will be normal. Thus, an abnormal radiograph after age 1 year does suggest inflammation of the upper respiratory tract. It is also apparent that crying alone is not a cause of abnormal maxillary sinus x-ray films in children older than age 1 year. Unfortunately, for infants younger than age 1 year there is a high frequency of abnormalities attributed to physiologic cloudiness of the sinuses caused by a relatively redundant normal mucous membrane. The conclusion of all this is that certain radiographic findings (air-fluid levels, partial or complete opacification, mucous membrane thickening of at least 4 mm) in conjunction with symptoms referable to the upper respiratory tract can predict the isolation of bacteria from a maxillary sinus aspirate in approximately 75% of cases in children.

The second study from Pittsburgh tells us even more. In addition to the usual case of sinusitis associated with severe headache, fever, facial pain, or periorbital swelling, two other presentations were seen in children. One was that of a child with "severe" symptoms in excess of what one normally would see in the course of a routine "cold" (for example, significant fever and purulent nasal discharge). A second presentation was that of persistent respiratory symptoms for longer than 10 to 30 days without improvement (such as a nasal discharge or frequent cough). Another conclusion of this study was that a particularly common infectious cause of sinusitis is *Branhamella catarrhalis*. This is important to recognize because an increased frequency of β-lactamase-producing *B. catarrhalis* has been noted recently in several cities. In this study, amoxicillin and cefaclor appeared to be of comparable efficacy for management of acute sinusitis in children. Erythromycin-sulfisoxazole is appropriate therapy when amoxicillin or cefaclor treatment fails, and this antimicrobial combination may be useful in geographic areas where amoxicillin-resistant *Hemophilus influenzae* and *B. catarrhalis* are common or in patients with penicillin allergy.

Despite the fact the authors of these two studies used topical decongestants and an antihistamine-decongestant combination orally, the need for these modalities of therapy in the management of sinusitis still has never been totally clarified. Likewise, it must be emphasized that although maxillary sinus aspirations were performed in all patients, these aspirations were done for the purposes of this study. Current clinical indications for maxillary sinus aspiration include life-threatening intracranial or intraorbital suppurative complications, maxillary sinusitis in an immunocompromised host, relief of intense pain, and failure of the usual medical management. When one says something is being done, usually it is being done for one of two reasons, a very good reason or the real reason. The only reason aspirations were done in this study was to establish correlations between infective organisms and response to therapy. Now that we know the answers to many of the questions regarding sinusitis, we can just go ahead and manage it medically using the guidelines taught to us by the Pittsburgh group.—J.A.S., III

Efficacy of Tonsillectomy for Recurrent Throat Infection in Severely Affected Children: Results of Parallel Randomized and Nonrandomized Clinical Trials

Jack L. Paradise, Charles D. Bluestone, Ruth Z. Bachman, D. Kathleen Colborn, Beverly S. Bernard, Floyd H. Taylor, Kenneth D. Rogers, Robert H. Schwarzbach, Sylvan E. Stool, Gilbert A. Friday, Ida H. Smith, and Carol A. Saez (Univ. of Pittsburgh)
N. Engl. J. Med. 310:674–683, Mar. 15, 1984   4–12

Tonsillectomy long has been the most common major operation done on children in the United States, but the indications remain uncertain and controversial, and regional operative rates vary widely. The few controlled trials done, all involving adenoidectomy as well, indicated lower throat

ISOLATED CERVICAL LYMPHADENOPATHY, SORE THROAT DAYS, AND SORE THROAT-ASSOCIATED SCHOOL ABSENCE, ACCORDING TO FOLLOW-UP YEAR AND TREATMENT GROUP*

FOLLOW-UP YEAR	TREATMENT GROUP	CERVICAL LYMPHADENOPATHY FOUND AT NON-THROAT-INFECTION VISIT (% of visits)		SORE-THROAT DAYS† (no. of days per year)		SORE-THROAT-ASSOCIATED SCHOOL ABSENCE‡ (no. of days per year)	
		RANDOMIZED TRIAL	NONRANDOMIZED TRIAL	RANDOMIZED TRIAL	NONRANDOMIZED TRIAL	RANDOMIZED TRIAL	NONRANDOMIZED TRIAL
First	Surgical	3.0 (38)	4.6 (44)	16.3±14.3 (31)	28.0±23.9 (42)	3.5±4.2 (29)	6.3±6.7 (41)
	Nonsurgical	12.2 (35)	14.2 (34)	18.9±14.6 (33)	20.8±20.2 (34)	6.7±6.9 (30)	7.4±8.6 (31)
Second	Surgical	3.1 (31)	5.6 (34)	10.8±13.4 (29)	13.4±13.7 (37)	4.5±4.5 (28)	4.4±5.6 (25)
	Nonsurgical	14.6 (29)	13.6 (28)	15.1±12.5 (27)	14.5±11.7 (28)	5.9±4.2 (26)	4.3±3.9 (25)
Third	Surgical	0.7 (22)	1.3 (15)	10.7±11.1 (22)	8.8± 7.0 (16)	5.1±5.7 (21)	4.0±5.9 (10)
	Nonsurgical	12.5 (20)	4.6 (13)	19.0±20.2 (21)	16.1±11.5 (13)	5.9±6.2 (21)	7.2±7.8 (13)

*Values are means ± 1 SD. Numbers in parentheses denote numbers of patients. For bracketed pairs of values, $P < .05$ by a chi-square analysis of distributions of patients.

†Limited to patients with at least 270 days of reportage in a follow-up year. Includes sore throat days immediately after surgery. Number of days for each patient for each follow-up year was standardized on the basis of 365 days.

‡Limited to patients aged 5 years or older with at least 130 days of reported school attendance or absence in a follow-up year. School absence immediately after surgery was excluded. Number of days for each child for each follow-up year was standardized on the basis of a 180-day school year.

(Courtesy of Paradise, J.L., et al.: N. Engl. J. Med. 310:674–683, Mar. 15, 1984. Reprinted by permission of the New England Journal of Medicine.)

infection rates in surgically treated children in the ensuing 2 years, but rates of infection in control children were not impressively high. The authors examined the efficacy of tonsillectomy, alone or combined with adenoidectomy, in 187 children seen with severe recurrent throat infections between 1971 and 1982. Overall, 91 children were randomly assigned to surgical or medical management and 96 were assigned according to parental preference.

The effects of operation were similar in the randomized and nonrandomized trials. Throat infection in the first 2 years of follow-up was significantly less frequent in the surgical groups, and third-year differences, though usually not significant, consistently favored the surgical groups. Many children in the nonsurgical group, however, had fewer than three episodes of infection in each follow-up year, and most episodes were mild. The results are summarized in the table. Surgery-related complications occurred in 14% of the 95 children operated on. All were self-limited or easily managed. None of the 4 children who bled required transfusion.

These findings warrant elective tonsillectomy in selected children, but they also provide support for nonoperative management of those with recurrent throat infections. Management should be individualized. Decisions can take into consideration such factors as parent and child preferences, anxieties, school performance, and cost. It would appear that many children who currently undergo tonsillectomy have throat infection experiences that, at most, conform to the more permissive guidelines of a number of present quality-of-care standards.

▶ Winston Churchill once remarked, "I am easily satisfied with the very best." Had Winston been alive to read the results of this study on the efficacy of tonsillectomy, he would have been very satisfied. It indeed is the very best.

Among the currently sanctioned indications for tonsillectomy, recurrent throat infection is at once the most frequently invoked and the most problematic. Not only do opinions differ over the number of episodes, their character, and the period of time that constitute grounds for tonsillectomy, but one standard pediatric textbook (Nelson's 12th edition) rejects recurrent throat infection altogether as a valid indication. To some extent, these differences of opinion reflect differences in physicians' training, experience, and personal attitudes and values; but more fundamentally they reflect the fact that the degree of benefit conferred by tonsillectomy in reducing the recurrence of throat infection has not been established, at least not until now. It is incumbent on all of us to take the time to read the results of this clinical trial carefully. The conclusions of this report can only be understood in light of the exact construct of the study. For example, for a child to be eligible, his or her episodes of tonsillitis had to meet very defined standards in each of four categories: frequency of occurrence—seven or more episodes in the preceding year, five or more in each of the 2 preceding years, or three or more in each of the 3 preceding years; clinical features—each episode characterized by one or more of the following: oral temperatures of at least 38.3 C, cervical adenopathy (enlarged greater than 2 cm) or tender cervical nodes, tonsillar or pharyngeal exudates, or positive culture for group A β-hemolytic *Streptococcus;* treatment—antibiotics administered in conventional dosage for proved or suspected streptococcal episodes; and documentation—each episode and its qualifying features substantiated by concurrent notation in a clinical record. Now that was one long sentence! With all these caveats in place, it can be stated confidently that tonsillectomy does afford clinical benefits. It also can be stated confidently that many children also will get better on their own during a period of follow-up. The authors do not go overboard in their conclusions.

This study won't make everybody happy. That is not possible in an area such as this. But it makes some of us happy, and for that we are grateful.— J.A.S., III

Unique Pattern of Epstein-Barr Virus-Specific Antibodies in Recurrent Parotitis

Izumi Akaboshi, Jiro Jamamoto, Takato Katsuki, and Ichiro Matsuda (Univ. Medical School, Kumamoto, Japan)
Lancet 2:1049–1051, Nov. 5, 1983   4–13

Serums from 19 boys and 15 girls with recurrent parotitis were analyzed and antibody levels to several Epstein-Barr virus (EBV) antigens were measured by indirect immunofluorescence technique. The 34 patients were aged 2–12 years when seen in 1979–1982. All had had unilateral or bilateral recurrent swelling of the parotid gland more than four times.

Results showed 5 patients (15%) were seronegative for IgG class antibody to EBV-capsid antigen (VCA), suggesting that they had not had the experience of primary infection with EBV. There were no differences between the seropositive and seronegative patients in clinical features. Among 29 seropositive patients, 3 had IgM antibody to VCA and also IgG antibody to the D or R component, or both, of early antigen (EA). Nineteen were positive for EA (R + D) = IgG, and 18 had higher titer to R than D. A total of 20 had IgA class antibody to VCA. High titers of VCA-IgG and EBV-associated nuclear antigen antibody were found in 18 (53%) and 14 (41%) RP patients, respectively. None of the 8 patients who were followed up had significant changes in antibody titer to EBV. Titers of antibody to mumps virus were negative or not raised in all patients.

The results clearly show that EBV infection may be important in the pathogenesis of recurrent parotitis. The abnormal antibody patterns seen in these patients to EBV-associated antigens persisted even in the symptomless period. The results suggest that suppressor T cell dysfunction, besides resulting in repeated active multiplication of EBV in parotid gland, may amplify the antibody response to EBV-associated antigen in patients with recurrent parotitis.

▶ The Epstein-Barr virus (EBV) has overtaken syphilis as holder of the record of the infectious agent that can produce the most signs and symptoms. Recurrent parotitis is hardly a common problem, but when it does present itself it is most perplexing. This is a disorder mostly of children younger than age 10 years. The frequency and severity of recurrence are variable and not of prognostic significance. The tendency is toward spontaneous remission at puberty. Various etiologies have been suspected to cause recurrent parotitis in children. These suggestions include congenital malformation of the parotic glands, primary or secondary infection, allergy, and localized manifestation of some systemic immunologic disorder. If you believe the results of this study, the vast majority of cases of recurrent parotitis are related to EBV infection. The episodes are due to bouts of multiplication of EBV in EBV carriers who for some unknown reason are immunosuppressed and have abnormal T suppressor cell function. No one will argue that EBV is a bad actor. More about this virus is discussed in Chapter 10, Oncology.—J.A.S., III

Management of Tracheobronchial and Esophageal Foreign Bodies in Childhood

James A. O'Neill, Jr., George W. Holcomb, Jr., and Wallace W. Neblett
J. Pediatr. Surg. 18:475–479, August 1983   4–14

The authors reviewed their experience in the management of esophageal and tracheobronchial foreign bodies in 140 infants and children seen at Vanderbilt University Medical Center from 1971 to 1981. Esophageal foreign bodies were present in 72 children, and 68 others had tracheobronchial foreign bodies. The 72 children with esophageal foreign bodies ranged in age from 6 months to 14 years (mean, 3.8 years). Of these, 60 had a history suggestive of ingestion of a foreign body; in the other 12, this possibility was suggested only by the presence of dysphagia. Foley balloon catheter extraction, attempted in 62 of 66 children with a previously normal esophagus, was successful in 52; in the other 10, the foreign body moved to the stomach and was later passed uneventfully. Esophagoscopy was successful in the remaining 4 children and in the 6 with previous esophageal pathology. There were no complications.

The 68 children with tracheobronchial foreign bodies ranged in age from 12 months to 7 years (mean, 2.5 years), and all but 2 had a relevant history. A chest roentgenogram was the most helpful diagnostic study, but in 29 children, all with a short history of symptoms, no diagnostic radiologic sign of a foreign body was noted. Bronchoscopy was indicated in 67 children because of a strong suspicion of the presence of a foreign body. Postural drainage was successful in only 1 of 30 children (table). Fogarty extraction was successful in 55 of 60 children, and forceps extraction was successful in 7 of 12. Of the 5 children in whom endoscopic removal was unsuccessful, 2 underwent lobectomy and 3 had bronchotomy. Of the 67 children who underwent bronchoscopy, 18 had sufficient croup or airway edema to require steroid treatment and mist-tent therapy; these complications resolved within 48 hours without additional therapy. Complications related to the foreign body itself occurred more often, with 12 children having evidence of pneumonia and 17 having varying degrees of atelectasis. In 1 of the 3 children who underwent bronchotomy a temporary bronchial stricture developed; there were no complications in the 2 who underwent lobectomy.

Because more than 90% of the children in this series had no evidence of intrinsic esophageal disease, and more than 90% of the esophageal foreign bodies had smooth surfaces, Foley balloon catheter extraction in the awake patient was the preferred approach in management. In patients with tracheobronchial foreign bodies, Fogarty balloon catheter extraction

TRACHEOBRONCHIAL FOREIGN BODIES	
Treatment and Results	Number of Patients
Postural drainage	30
Successful	1/30
Bronchoscopy	67
Fogarty extraction successful	55/60
Forceps extraction successful	7/12
Both methods successful	5
Thoracotomy	5
Lobectomy	2
Bronchotomy	3
Total	68

(Courtesy of O'Neill, J.A., Jr., et al.: J. Pediatr. Surg. 18:475–479, August 1983; reproduced by permission of Journal of Pediatric Surgery.)

in association with magnification bronchoscopy is not only useful for dislodging and removing foreign bodies, but is also effective in dilating a narrow bronchus and stripping away adherent granulations.

▶ It is amazing what balloons are being used for these days. We all thought it was terribly innovative when the Rashkind procedure was used to create an atrial septostomy with a balloon catheter. Now we see balloons used to dilate narrowed renal arteries and correct hypertension, to widen pulmonary valves, and for a variety of other angioplastic procedures. Such catheters, including the Foley-type catheter, have been used for awhile now to remove foreign bodies from the airway or the esophagus. The series presented here, however, is one of the largest that shows the simplicity of the technique. Obviously, the inflated Foley catheter is successful mostly with smooth objects. Needless to say, an open safety pin is liable to burst your bubble.

The more difficult situation is that of the child who acutely "chokes." C. S. Harris et al. (*JAMA* 251:2231, 1984) summarized the findings in the deaths of 703 infants and children, aged 0 to 9 years, who died of food asphyxiation between 1979 and 1981. The most commonly implicated foods, in order, were hot dogs, candy, nuts, grapes, cookies or biscuits, carrots, popcorn, and peanut butter and jelly sandwiches. Forty percent of the deaths could be accounted for by hot dogs, candy, nuts, and grapes. The number of deaths from choking on food was roughly comparable to deaths from poisoning in the age group examined. There seems to be no easy solution to this problem. It only highlights our need to make the public aware of appropriate procedures to help manage the choking subject. If you want to hear more about the pros and cons of first aid treatment of the choking child, see the very nice discussion of S. B. Torrey, who summarizes the statement of the American Academy of Pediatrics. Torrey additionally reviews the medical literature and the controversy over the Academy's approach versus the Heimlich maneuver. He concludes that there are no compelling data that contradict the recommendations of the American Academy of Pediatrics for the treatment of the choking child. All this may be found in *Clinical Pediatrics* (22:751, 1983).—J.A.S., III

Congenital Laryngeal Webs

Bruce Benjamin (Royal Alexandra Hosp. for Children, Sydney)
Ann. Otol. Rhinol. Laryngol. 92:317–326, July–Aug. 1983   4–15

Congenital laryngeal webs are less prevalent than previously thought, and thorough assessment is necessary before any form of surgical treatment is planned. The findings were reviewed in 29 cases of congenital laryngeal web seen in 1960 to 1982. Twenty-one patients presented at birth; 3 others presented in the first month of life. All patients but 1 were seen by age 8 months. There were 16 female and 13 male patients in the series. The chief features were an abnormal cry or voice, "respiratory distress," and stridor. Three patients with glottic webs and subglottic stenosis had recurrent or atypical "croup." Seventeen patients had other major congenital anomalies, chiefly of the upper respiratory tract. The endoscopic appearances in 6 patients are shown in Figure 4–4.

Of the 9 patients who required endotracheal intubation at birth, 7 had tracheotomy soon afterward; the other 2 died of other causes. All 5 patients with interarytenoid fixation eventually required tracheotomy. One patient had a tracheotomy at birth after intubation failed. In all, 10 patients had tracheotomies. Twelve webs were treated by simple means, usually division with a scissors. Four were treated with the carbon dioxide laser, and 1 was managed by laryngofissure with insertion of a silicone rubber keel. Three of these 17 patients had no apparent change, 3 had some improvement, and 11 had a good outcome subjectively. Patients with smaller

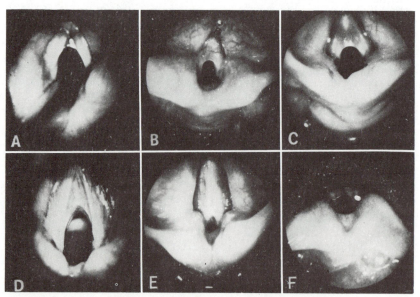

Fig 4–4.—Endoscopic view of congenital laryngeal webs. **A,** thin web in newborn; **B,** thicker web in newborn; **C,** medium web; **D,** thick web with subglottic stenosis; **E,** severe web with small glottic opening; **F,** congenital interarytenoid web. (Courtesy of Benjamin, B.: Ann. Otol. Rhinol. Laryngol. 92:317–326, July–Aug. 1983.)

anterior glottic webs generally had the best results. Six patients still have tracheotomies. There were no complications of treatment, and no patient was made worse by treatment.

The cause of congenital laryngeal web is unknown. Severely affected patients may require an artificial airway soon after birth. Tracheotomy has not been necessary for webs involving only the glottic region. Some webs do not have to be treated. Only 11 of 17 treated patients in the present study had a good outcome. The carbon dioxide laser no longer is considered useful in treating difficult cases of congenital laryngeal web. Endoscopic placement of a keel may be useful for thin webs, but simpler satisfactory methods are already available.

Epiglottitis: Duration of Intubation and Fever
Peter Rothstein and George Lister (Yale Univ.)
Anesth. Analg. (Cleve.) 62:785–787, September 1983   4–16

Nasotracheal intubation has reduced the period of airway support and hospitalization in children with epiglottitis, compared with tracheostomy, but the duration of intubation has varied. The course of 23 pediatric patients with epiglottitis was reviewed in an attempt to define criteria for the duration of intubation. Nasotracheal intubation was done in the operating room, and direct laryngoscopy was done with the use of thiopental anesthesia each morning. Extubation was allowed when the estimated thickness of the proximal part of the epiglottis was 3–4 mm or less. All the children received ampicillin or chloramphenicol; steroids were not used. The children breathed a warmed, humidified gas mixture with an inspired oxygen fraction of 0.3–0.4 while intubated. The mean age was 41 months.

All but 1 of the children were febrile when admitted. The mean time to defervescence was 42 hours. Blood cultures were positive for *Hemophilus influenzae* in 87% of cases. Airway swelling often showed little improvement in the first 12 hours. Extubation was carried out after an average of 36 hours; no child had to be reintubated. The duration of intubation did not correlate significantly with the time it took for fever to resolve.

These patients were similar to those in other series with respect to age and the incidence of isolation of *H. influenzae*. The children were extubated an average of 36 hours after nasotracheal intubation. Extubation after 12 hours is not recommended unless a marked reduction in size of the epiglottis is documented. Extubation in the late evening or at night does not offer a major advantage, because the child generally breathes comfortably with the tube in place without the need for sedation.

▶ Robert K. Kanter, Assistant Professor of Pediatrics and Director of the Pediatric Intensive Care Unit, State University Hospital, Syracuse, New York, comments on this report:

"While placement of an artificial airway has become standard therapy for epiglottitis, we still lack data on clinical end points to decide when to extubate these children. Rothstein and Lister have added convincing evidence for the safety of early extubation. They confirm the observations of several groups that a brief period of airway protection, averaging only 36 ± 14 (SD) hours, successfully prevents airway obstruction.

"The authors also have provided us with the most objective evaluation of specific criteria for extubation available thus far. Several presumptive indicators for extubation have been used by clinicians, including reduction in edema of the epiglottis, defervescence, and resolution of 'toxemia.' The criterion used in this study was reduction in thickness of the proximal epiglottis to 3–4 mm or less. This approach successfully limited duration of airway support to 67 hours or less, while avoiding any premature extubations; however, some questions remain.

"Will duplication of these results be difficult because of the subjective nature of anatomical observations? Tos (*Arch. Otolaryngol.* 97:373, 1973) reported that edema of the epiglottis persisted for an average of 6 days in his patients. Extubation according to subsiding edema of the epiglottis resulted in longer mean duration of intubation of 67 hours in another study (Battaglia and Lockhart: *Am. J. Dis. Child.* 129:334, 1975).

"Hannallah and Rosales (*Can. Anaesth. Soc. J.* 25:84, 1978) found no relation between the size of the epiglottis and the degree of respiratory difficulty. What criteria should we use for extubation of the child with airway obstruction due to supraglottitis who may have very little edema of the epiglottis?

"Is persistence of fever an indication that airway obstruction may recur? Because Rothstein and Lister did not utilize defervescence as a criterion for extubation, it is not surprising that they found no correlation between the duration of fever and the duration that endotracheal tubes remained in place. Would defervescence more adequately indicate safe timing for extubation if a temperature of 38.5 C rather than 38.0 C is used to define fever? While some authors advocate extubation at the time of defervescence and resolution of 'toxemia,' more thorough study is required to clarify this issue. It is worth noting that one unsuccessful extubation on day 3 occurred in a child with both persistent fever and swelling of the epiglottis (Breivik: *Br. J. Anaesth.* 50:505, 1978).

"What should we conclude from this study? Patients with epiglottitis should be extubated on the first morning that thickness of the epiglottis has diminished to 4 mm or less. Laryngoscopy can be performed without general anesthesia with the use of a flexible fiberoptic instrument (Nussbaum: *J. Pediatr.* 102:269, 1983). The potential danger when fever or lethargy persists has not been defined adequately, and these findings suggest delaying extubation. Too little experience is available to advocate extubation after fewer than 12 hours of antibiotic therapy."

C-Reactive Protein in Rapid Differentiation of Acute Epiglottitis From Spasmodic Croup and Acute Laryngotracheitis: Preliminary Report
Heikki Peltola (Children's Hosp., Helsinki)
J. Pediatr. 102:713–715, May 1983   4–17

Serum C-reactive protein (CRP) is capable of distinguishing an invasive bacterial disease from a viral infection. However, factors other than bacteria can produce elevated CRP values. This nonspecificity, as well as the impracticality of quantitating CRP in routine practice, has resulted in less use of the CRP test. However, new technical modifications that allow rapid measurement of CRP have eliminated this obstacle. Because quantitation of CRP may help in the rapid distinction between acute epiglottitis and spasmodic croup or acute laryngotracheitis, the author prospectively and retrospectively (50% of patients with epiglottitis) determined serum CRP levels in 10 children with acute epiglottitis, 9 with spasmodic croup, and 16 with acute laryngotracheitis. A rapid turbidimetric or nephelometric technique was used to measure CRP; values below 20 mg/L were considered normal.

The CRP level was invariably elevated in the 10 children with acute epiglottitis, ranging from 23 mg/L to 252 mg/L (Fig 4–5). Body temperatures varied from normal to slightly elevated to highly increased values. All 10 children received antimicrobial therapy. In the 9 children with spasmodic croup, CRP levels were invariably normal, all values being less than 10 mg/L. No child had fever, but leukocyte counts varied considerably. None received antimicrobial therapy. The CRP level was elevated in 3 of the 16 children with acute laryngotracheitis. One of the 3, whose CRP level was 22 mg/L, had *Mycoplasma pneumoniae* infection. No cause for the elevated CRP levels was found in the other 2 children. Symptoms in these 3 children subsided within 3 days without antimicrobial therapy. Five others with laryngotracheitis were admitted to the intensive care unit and 4 received antimicrobial therapy. Causes of laryngotracheitis, identified in 5 children, included respiratory syncytial virus, parainfluenza virus 2, measles virus, and *M. pneumoniae* infection. The CRP levels in children

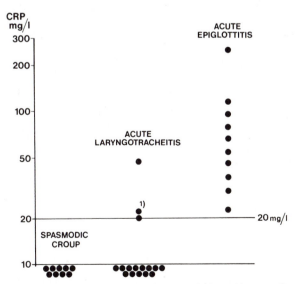

Fig 4–5.—Individual C-reactive protein (CRP) values in 9 children with spasmodic croup, 16 with acute laryngotracheitis, and 10 with acute epiglottitis. A CRP level of less than 20 mg/L is considered normal. 1 = child with *Mycoplasma pneumoniae* infection and a CRP value of 22 mg/L. (Courtesy of Peltola, H.: J. Pediatr. 102:713–715, May 1983.)

with acute epiglottitis were significantly higher than those in children with acute laryngotracheitis ($P < .001$); this difference was even more pronounced when CRP values in children with epiglottitis were compared with those in children with croup.

The possibility of epiglottitis should be considered carefully in patients having an elevated CRP value. Spasmodic croup probably can be excluded in the presence of elevated CRP levels. A normal CRP value is even more informative, as it probably indicates the absence of epiglottitis, regardless of the extent of breathing difficulties. If this finding is confirmed, CRP determinations would then be particularly useful in distinguishing epiglottitis from serious acute laryngotracheitis.

▶ It is difficult to be totally certain about what one should do with the information gained from this study. I have no hesitation in believing this information. It is just that I do not think that I would rely on the C-reactive protein (CRP) concentration to tell me what I should do or not do with a patient. Despite the data from this study, if a patient acts like he or she has epiglottitis, a normal CRP determination will not prevent me from having the right person examine the epiglottis under the right conditions. On the other hand, an elevated CRP value in a patient who acts like he or she has run-of-the-mill acute laryngotracheal bronchitis isn't going to make me want to treat that patient any differently. So, as interesting as all these data are, I don't know how to translate them into any useful information. One would have liked to have seen additional data in subjects with tracheitis. If these subjects had markedly elevated CRP levels such as the patients with epiglottitis, that truly would be helpful, because lateral neck films and a quick look at the upper airway do not help very much in making the latter diagnosis.

The CRP determination has been around for a long time. It has been purported to help diagnose neonatal sepsis and meningitis differentially from noninfectious situations (Philip et al.: *J. Pediatr.* 102:715, 1983). Here, too, not many would hang their hats on the CRP assay as the sole laboratory test to determine treatment. I have the suspicion that the CRP value ultimately will fall into the same class of interesting but not convincing tests as the old NBT (nitro-blue tetrazolium) dye test in the differential diagnosis of bacterial infection. If I were a betting person, I would say that the CRP determination has about as much chance of getting somewhere in the long run as a guy with a wooden leg in a forest fire.—J.A.S., III

5 The Respiratory Tract

Respiratory Response to Intraesophageal Acid Infusion in Asthmatic Children During Sleep
Ray S. Davis, Gary L. Larsen, and Michael M. Grunstein (Univ. of Colorado)
J. Allergy Clin. Immunol. 72:393–398, October 1983   5–1

Gastroesophageal reflux (GER) is frequent in asthmatic children, especially those with predominantly nocturnal wheezing. Acid-sensitive vagal nerve endings in the distal esophagus may reflexly cause bronchoconstriction in response to GER, but a causal relationship between GER and nocturnal bronchoconstriction has not been established. The authors infused 0.1N hydrochloric acid into the distal esophagus in 9 asthmatic children with documented GER during sleep and monitored respiration continuously by inductance plethysmography. The children, aged 8–14 years, all had a history of recurrent nocturnal cough or wheezing as well as documented GER. All were on maintenance bronchodilator therapy. Infusion studies were done only after the patients had been clinically stable for 48 hours. Both 30 ml of normal saline and 30 ml of 0.1N hydrochloric acid were infused at about midnight and again at 4–5 A.M.

The saline and midnight acid infusions did not affect patients with either a positive or a negative Bernstein test result, but all patients with a positive test result had significant respiratory changes indicating bronchoconstriction as well as overt wheezing when acid was infused at 4–5 A.M. Acid infusion at this time had no effect on respiration in patients with a negative Bernstein test result. The symptomatic patients responded well to discontinuance of the acid infusion and nebulized bronchodilator therapy.

These findings support the concept that GER may be an important mechanism precipitating nocturnal asthma in patients whose asthma is complicated by esophagitis. Theophylline therapy may facilitate reflux through its relaxing effect on the lower esophageal sphincter. Antacids, cimetidine, an altered feeding schedule, and elevation of the head of the bed may help patients with nighttime respiratory symptoms. If these measures fail, esophagoscopy should be considered.

▶ This excellent article helps us better understand the nature of nocturnal wheezing in some of the asthmatics that we care for. I think we all have tended to believe that this could be the result of mild gastroesophageal reflux, but this study seems to document it. A touch of acid in the distal esophagus does produce bronchial spasm in infants with this problem. It is a shame that this was not pursued with a clinical trial of antacids or cimetidine. If you try this in your practice, recall that cimetidine alters the pharmacology of a number of agents used to treat asthma, so you may have to adjust the dosage of bronchodilator being used.

While dealing with the topic of the esophagus, acids, and asthma, one might recall the recent letter to the editor of the *New England Journal of Medicine* (310:261, 1984). A fellow was described in whom a sustained-action theophylline tablet became stuck in the esophagus. When he awoke the next morning, he had typical signs of severe esophagitis that lasted for some weeks. Orally administered theophylline must be added to the long list of agents, including aspirin, potassium preparations, tetracycline, etc., that will irritate and ulcerate the esophagus. From what we know from this article by Davis et al., if somebody has this problem from taking theophylline preparations, they are in for a lot of trouble with their asthma. On the other hand, there is one acid that, in fact, may be helpful in the management of asthmatic patients. This is vitamin C. It has been reported that in adult volunteers bronchoconstriction caused by inhalation of histamine aerosols in textile dust was significantly reduced by the prior administration of 1 gm of ascorbic acid. A study in Nigeria suggested that ingestion of vitamin C by children with bronchial asthma in whom the attacks were precipitated by viral infections would decrease the frequency and severity of asthmatic episodes (Anah, C. O., et al.: *Trop. Georg. Med.* 32:132, 1980). Although this is highly controversial, one more study done in 16 white children also showed a similar effect (Anderson, R., et al.: *S. Afr. Med. J.* 63:649, 1983). If vitamin C works at all, it's obviously not clear whether it does this through its own mild bronchodilator effect or through some minor immune-mediated effect. There seems to be no harm in trying the 1 gm daily dose (unless it also gets caught in the esophagus).

Also known to stimulate wheezing in addition to acids is the inhalation of cold air. This has been commented on before in the YEAR BOOK. F. J. McLaughlin have capitalized on this phenomenon and, using a very rigidly controlled protocol, have demonstrated that the response to inhalation of cold air is a safe and simple test for diagnosing asthma in children. One simply does basic pulmonary function tests before and after the inhalation of cold air. Asthmatics show significant deterioration compared to controls, without actually having a frank asthmatic episode (*Pediatrics* 72:503, 1983). If you have to breathe cold air, the best kind of air to breathe is air that is heavily ionized. You know what I mean by this—the kind of air you smell after an electric storm. The ionic charge of the air has long been thought to affect various biologic systems, including the respiratory system. Haven't you noticed how much better you seem to breathe right after walking outside on a fresh night after a lightning storm? Well, that wasn't a false feeling, because Ben-Dov et al. have demonstrated clearly that negative ionization of inspired air remarkably improves pulmonary function in children who have exercise-induced asthma (*Thorax* 38:584, 1983).

Don't ask how ions in the air help relieve asthma. Nobody seems to know. You can bet, however, that there will be much future controversy in this regard or, as I would say, you will see a lot of "ions in the fire."—J.A.S., III

Bronchodilator Effects and Pharmacokinetics of Caffeine in Asthma
Allan B. Becker, Keith J. Simons, Catherine A. Gillespie, and F. Estelle R. Simons (Univ. of Manitoba)
N. Engl. J. Med. 310:743–746, Mar. 22, 1984   5–2

Because the effects, if any, of caffeine treatment in asthmatic children are unknown, a single-dose, double-blind study was undertaken to compare the bronchodilator effects and pharmacokinetics of orally administered caffeine and theophylline. There were 23 studies done in asthmatic children aged 8–18 years with reversible obstructive airway disease; all required continuous bronchodilator therapy. Thirteen studies were done with caffeine, 10 mg/kg, and 10 with theophylline, 5 mg/kg. Studies were done 48 hours after the discontinuance of methylxanthines and β_2-adrenergic agonists. The two groups were similar clinically and with regard to past treatment.

All measures of pulmonary function showed significant improvement after both caffeine and theophylline treatment. Peak improvement occurred at 2 hours, and lung function remained significantly better than at baseline 6 hours after drug ingestion. The bronchodilator effect of caffeine did not differ significantly from that of theophylline. The mean elimination half-time for caffeine was 3.9 hours and for theophylline, 5.8 hours. Adverse effects were comparable in the two groups, although increased shakiness and tremor were more evident after caffeine ingestion. All side effects were mild and transient. No nausea or vomiting occurred with either drug, and vital signs did not change significantly.

Caffeine is as effective a bronchodilator as theophylline is in young asthmatic patients. A patient weighing 50–60 kg would have to drink at least two cups of strong-brewed coffee in order to obtain a bronchodilator effect. Caffeine is not recommended for regular use as a bronchodilator, but it may have value for temporary use when prescribed antiasthma medications are not readily available.

▶ Well, it appears that two cups of coffee can keep the doctor away. It really isn't surprising that caffeine should nicely produce bronchodilations. Methylxanthines in general will do this. It's nice knowing that this phenomenon occurs, however. As the authors suggest, if a patient runs out of a bronchodilator, one can always suggest that a caffeinated product be used on an interim basis. If such products must be used, I think a cola product is more appropriate than coffee, for lots of reasons. First, standard colas have relatively reproducible amounts of caffeine, unlike coffee that may vary from coffeepot to coffeepot. Secondly, no one has described an association between colas and pancreatic cancer or birth defects, to which coffee has been related (*N. Engl. J. Med.* 310:783, 1984). Finally, children are much more likely to take cola than coffee.

One should recognize that caffeine may be a metabolic by-product in vivo of theophylline. Several reports have indicated that young infants receiving therapeutic doses of theophylline for apnea will accumulate caffeine as a metabolite in the blood. The hypothesis is that the metabolic pathway of theophylline to caffeine is intact in tiny infants but such infants may not have a sufficiently well-developed cytochrome P-450 system to metabolize caffeine out of the body (Nahata, M. C., et al.: *Ther. Drug Monitoring* 5:269, 1983). This may not have any really practical implications clinically, except for the fact that some feel caffeine may be a more potent central nervous system stimulator than theophylline is. Indeed, one recent study (Aranda, J. V., et al.: *J. Pediatr.*

103:975, 1983) showed that caffeine was as good as theophylline in acting as a central nervous system stimulant to control infantile apnea. If you go the caffeine route, recall that rapid changes in caffeine elimination occur in the first 6 months of life; the plasma half-life of caffeine in the newborn infant is about 100 hours and changes to about 3 hours by age 6 months. Thus, doses will require constant adjustment in the young infant with apnea.

In case the use of caffeine to treat asthma seems new to you, let me quote the following: "One of the commonest and best reputed remedies of asthma, one that is almost sure to have been tried in any case that may have come under our observation, and one that in many cases is more efficacious than any other, is strong coffee." The reference for this is an article by H. Salter, "On Some Points in the Treatment and Clinical History of Asthma" (*Edinburgh Med. J.* 4:1109, 1859). Yes, this was typed correctly; the year was *1859!*— J.A.S., III

Aerosol Treatment of Bronchoconstriction in Children, With or Without Tube Spacer
Søren Pedersen (Aalborg, Denmark)
N. Engl. J. Med. 308:1328–1330, June 2, 1983   5–3

The advantages of adding an extension tube to a conventional pressurized aerosol container for drug inhalation therapy was assessed in 20

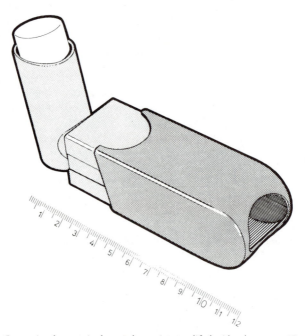

Fig 5–1.—Conventional pressurized aerosol container modified with tube spacer. (Courtesy of Pedersen, S.: N. Engl. J. Med. 308:1328–1330, June 2, 1983. Reprinted by permission of the New England Journal of Medicine.)

children with acute bronchoconstriction. The children were treated under double-blind conditions with either placebo or terbutaline (0.25 mg per activation) delivered by either a conventional aerosol container or one having a tube spacer attached (Fig 5–1).

Compared with placebo, both methods of terbutaline administration produced a significant increase in forced expiratory volume in 1 second (Fig 5–2). However, aerosol treatment with the tube spacer resulted in significantly greater improvement ($P < .01$) than did treatment by conventional means. Treatment with aminophylline was required by 5 children after administration of terbutaline from the conventional aerosol, whereas only 1 child needed such treatment after using the aerosol with the spacer. Breath-holding periods did not differ significantly among treatments. Rapid submaximal inspiration after activation occurred more often after conventional aerosol treatment than after use of the aerosol with the spacer ($P < .002$). In addition, the number of errors in inhalation technique was significantly reduced when the modified aerosol dispenser was used, especially the number of incidents in which the release of cold aerosol particles into the mouth caused the patient to stop inspiration and exhale ($P < .05$). There were no side effects. Nine children preferred treatment with the modified aerosol container and 3 preferred to use the conventional container; 8 had no preference.

Treatment in this series reflected the normal day-to-day situation in the life of the asthmatic child. Most of the children benefited from aerosol treatment during periods of exercise-induced asthma, but improvement

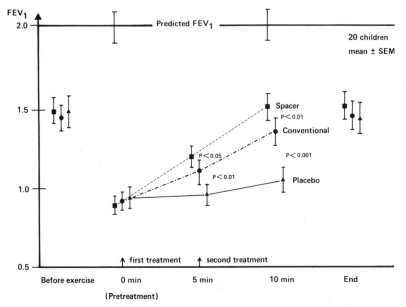

Fig 5–2.—Measurements of forced expiratory volume in 1 second (FEV₁) in 20 children with acute bronchoconstriction. (Courtesy of Pedersen, S.: N. Engl. J. Med. 308:1328–1330, June 2, 1982. Reprinted by permission of the New England Journal of Medicine.)

was significantly greater when an aerosol container having a tube spacer was used; the reduced number of errors in inhalation technique may account for this additional improvement.

Aerosol Bag for Administration of Bronchodilators to Young Asthmatic Children

Haesoon Lee and Hugh E. Evans (SUNY, Downstate Med. Center)
Pediatrics 73:230–232, February 1984   5–4

Some young children cannot be taught to inhale an aerosol properly from a canister nebulizer. The authors devised a rebreathing bag for aerosol administration and evaluated it in 20 asthmatic children aged 3 to 6 years. The bronchodilator efficacy of albuterol aerosol administered by bag was compared with that of canister administration in children aged 7 to 15 years. The bag (Fig 5–3) was made from a plastic freezer bag of 1-qt size by placing a mouthpiece in one corner. It was half-inflated with air before the mouthpiece was placed between the child's lips, and the parent then actuated the canister that was inside the bag and directed to the center of the lumen.

All the young child-parent pairs learned the aerosol bag technique within 5 minutes and performed it properly. The peak expiratory flow rate rose effectively after the inhalation of one puff of metaproterenol aerosol from the aerosol bag. The 15 clinically stable older asthmatics studied had substantial increases in FEV_1 after inhaling two puffs of albuterol from the aerosol bag. Differences between aerosol bag inhalation and use of a canister were not significant, and individual patients responded similarly to the two methods of treatment. Blood pressure and pulse rate did not change with either form of treatment.

The aerosol bag is effective for treatment of young asthmatic children with an aerosol bronchodilator at home. It precludes the need to purchase a jet nebulizer. The aerosol bag has been especially useful when sudden asthmatic attacks occur despite regular oral medication. Nocturnal attacks have been successfully treated with the bag technique. Parent-child teams have rapidly learned the proper method of aerosol inhalation from the bag.

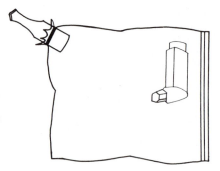

Fig 5–3.—Aerosol bag. Quart-size freezer bag was modified by snipping off corner of bag and inserting mouthpiece into opening and securing it with rubber band wound around it. Aerosol canister is placed inside bag by opening zippered end of bag. (Courtesy of Lee, H., and Evans, H.E.: Pediatrics 73:230–232, February 1984. Copyright American Academy of Pediatrics 1984.)

▶ This article and the preceding one both deal with alternatives to the use of aerosol preparations directly from the canister in the management of patients with asthma. Studies have demonstrated that less than 10% of the nebulized medication from a canister actually is deposited in the airway below the larynx. Most, nearly 80%, of the dose is impacted in the mouth and the posterior portion of the pharynx. This is under the best of circumstances. Despite the small amount of bronchodilator deposited in the lower airway, the bronchodilator effect is excellent. Some authors have advocated holding the aerosol container some distance from the mouth when it is actuated to minimize the dose that is deposited in the pharynx. This point, to my knowledge, has never been documented clearly. Even though inhaling aerosols from a canister nebulizer is a relatively easy procedure, one recent study demonstrated that nearly half of patients between ages 7 and 15 years failed to inhale aerosols correctly (*Clin. Pediatr.* 22:440, 1983). Imagine what trouble younger children must have! The incorrect techniques of most children can be identified by simply looking at what they are doing. In almost all instances, the correct technique can be learned easily once it is taught. Occasionally, patients who cannot master proper inhalation from a canister may need other approaches. The tube spacer should work for just about anybody. The principle of this most likely is based on the fact that the tube acts as a reservoir so that you have more leeway with the timing of pressing on the nebulizer before the inhalation process begins. Obviously, younger children may not even be able to use the tube spacer, and that is the point of the article by Lee and Evans, in which a simple freezer bag is used to inhale from. There seems to be no limit to the ingenuity of physicians and parents of children with asthma in coming up with offbeat but quite satisfactory solutions to unique problems.—J.A.S., III

The Usefulness of Chest Radiographs in First Asthma Attacks
Jeffrey C. Gershel, Harold S. Goldman, Ruth E. K. Stein, Steven P. Shelov, and Micha Ziprkowski (Albert Einstein College of Medicine, New York)
N. Engl. J. Med. 309:336–339, Aug. 11, 1983   5–5

Asthma is the most common chronic illness of childhood and remains a leading cause of morbidity. Chest radiography often is recommended for children having a first episode of wheezing.

The usefulness of this approach was examined in a series of 371 consecutive children older than age 1 year who came to a pediatric emergency room over a 1-year period with an initial episode of wheezing. Routine treatment included subcutaneous epinephrine therapy, up to 0.3 ml of 1:1000 solution. Up to three doses were given 20–30 minutes apart.

The chest x-ray study was considered compatible with uncomplicated asthma in 94.3% of cases, whereas 21 patients had findings not necessarily routinely seen in uncomplicated asthma, most commonly segmental atelectasis, alone or with pneumonia, and pneumonia alone. No pneumothoraces were seen, and no child was suspected of having a foreign body in the airway. The children with "positive" radiographs were significantly likelier than the others to have a pulse rate of 160 or greater or a respiratory rate of 60 or greater. They more often had localized rales or decreased breath sounds, and they had more localized rales and wheezing after emergency-room treatment. They were admitted much more often than children with uncomplicated asthma. Only 10 true positive x-ray studies were correctly identified in the emergency room, and in 22 instances x-ray studies were misinterpreted as indicating pneumonia.

These results fail to support routine chest roentgenography in children older than age 1 year who present with a first episode of wheezing. Careful clinical evaluation appears adequate for identifying patients whose treatment might be altered by positive radiographic findings. A selective approach would reduce unnecessary exposure for the large majority of patients whose care is not likely to be improved by radiographic examination.

▶ Quite a furor followed the publication of this study. You might have thought that Gershel et al. had attacked motherhood, the American flag, and apple pie all at one time. What they merely did was to show that chest x-ray studies performed solely because of a first episode of wheezing will have an extraordinarily low yield. Intuition should tell anyone that much. The question is whether or not a low yield means no yield worth looking for. That is the sticky issue, and it is around that point that divergent opinions arise. The 11th edition of *Nelson Textbook of Pediatrics* says that every child suspected of asthma should have a roentgenogram of the chest, with posteroanterior and lateral views. This is based on the dogma that was ingrained in all of us in medical school: "All that wheezes may not be asthma." Indeed, it is true that an aspirated foreign body, bronchiolitis, pneumonia, cystic fibrosis, congestive heart failure, and vascular rings, etc., all can cause wheezing. If, however, a child has a mild initial wheezing episode, has a clinical status normalizing with one dose of epinephrine, is afebrile, has no history of foreign body ingestion, and has no localizing findings on chest examination, how likely is it that you will find a chest x-ray film that will change your approach to the management of that particular patient? With these criteria, it must be extraordinarily rare to find a chest roentgenogram that would do anything to influence your approach to the management of the child. Certainly, there will be that one in whatever number of children who have aspirated a foreign body who might present this way, but as we all know; most foreign bodies aspirated by children are not radiologically dense. A standard chest x-ray examination would not be likely to pick these up. If you did want to exclude a foreign body, decubitus films, inspiration-expiration films, or chest fluoroscopy are the indicated procedures. Routine chest x-ray examinations do not reliably exclude the presence of inhaled foreign bodies in any way whatsoever.

Although I feel a bit uneasy about withdrawing from the concept of obtaining routine chest x-ray films with first episodes of wheezing, I believe I will do so after digesting and thinking about the information provided by this study. I also feel that honest differences of opinion can exist in this regard, and no one ought to be too dogmatic on either side. Hopefully, all the noise will settle down and time will be permitted to work this situation out. As Mark Twain once said, "Noise proves nothing. Often a hen that has merely laid an egg cackles as if she had laid an asteroid."—J.A.S., III

Inability to Predict Relapse in Acute Asthma

Robert M. Centor, Barry Yarbrough, and Judy P. Wood (Med. College of Virginia)

N. Engl. J. Med. 310:577–580, Mar. 1, 1984   5–6

In an attempt to validate the index developed by Fischl et al. to predict relapse in asthmatic patients, data were collected on 114 asthmatics seen in an emergency department. The components of the Fischl index are shown in the table, in which PEFR stands for peak expiratory flow rate. Thirty-seven patients were older than age 45 years. Twenty-eight patients, including 17 aged 45 and younger, were excluded from analysis because of incomplete data collection. An index score of 4 or above was 50% sensitive and 82% specific in predicting hospital admission. In predicting relapse, the index was 18% sensitive and 82% specific. Higher index scores did correlate with a greater chance of discharge with a prescription for an oral corticosteroid preparation. Relapsed patients could not be distinguished by logistic regression analysis from those successfully treated.

Although the Fischl index does correlate with the severity of asthma, it does not aid decision making in the emergency room. Physicians must continue to weigh many factors, some of them nonquantifiable, in deciding whether to admit asthmatic patients to the hospital. Asthmatics relapse for a variety of reasons, not all of which are related to the severity of asthma. The reasons may include poor compliance, reexposure to allergen, inability to afford expensive medication, and an inadequate discharge prescription. It is unlikely that any index will be able to predict relapse accurately in patients seen in a variety of settings.

▶ This report followed immediately after one that asked exactly the same question, "Are there predictable factors that can be observed during the management of an acute asthmatic attack that tells one that a patient is likely to relapse quickly?" (Rose, C. C., et al.: *N. Engl. J. Med.* 310:573, 1984). Both studies reached exactly the same conclusion. If you use the highly tauted Fischl index (see the table in the abstract, from the article of Fischl, M. A., et

	SCORING SYSTEM FOR PREDICTOR INDEX	
FACTOR *	VALUE FOR A SCORE OF 0	VALUE FOR A SCORE OF 1
Pulse	<120	≥120
Respirations	<30	≥30
Pulsus paradoxus	<18	≥18
PEFR	>120	≤120
Dyspnea	Absent or mild	Moderate or severe
Accessory muscle use	Absent or mild	Moderate or severe
Wheezing	Absent or mild	Moderate or severe

*Values for the seven factors are added to obtain index score.
(Courtesy of Centor, R.M., et al.: N. Engl. J. Med. 310:577–580, Mar. 1, 1984. Reprinted by permission of the New England Journal of Medicine.)

al.: *N. Engl. J. Med.* 305:783, 1981) you are as likely as not to be wrong in concluding that your patients will do okay when they leave the emergency room. The index looks at only seven variables in a predictive fashion. These studies that failed to show any value to the index focused largely on adult patients, but there were pediatric patients as well. The younger patients did no better than the older patients with respect to any predictive factors. I think if anyone among us was asked to sit down and write out a potential list of factors that would influence whether a patient with asthma was likely to re-lapse after treatment for an acute asthmatic episode, he or she could probably generate a list of variables that extends into several score of potential possibil-ities. These possibilities are even more numerous in children. I would not mind seeing a study done solely in the pediatric age group, but, frankly, such a study may not be feasible or even practical. A crystal ball, a spin of a bottle, a toss of a coin, or one's "gut" intuition is probably just as good as any predic-tive index. There just are too many variables to make such a weak study fly. It is obvious, you cannot fly like an eagle with the wings of a wren.—J.A.S., III

Parapneumonic Pleural Effusion and Empyema in Children
Tasnee Chonmaitree and Keith R. Powell (Univ. of Rochester, Rochester, N.Y.)
Clin. Pediatr. (Phila.) 22:414–418, June 1983   5–7

Since the introduction of antimicrobial agents effective against *Staph-ylococcus aureus,* pleural effusion and empyema associated with pneu-monia have become relatively uncommon diseases. The authors report the clinical, laboratory, and roentgenographic findings in 50 patients with parapneumonic pleural effusion or empyema who were among 3,248 chil-dren younger than age 19 years admitted to Strong Memorial Hospital, Rochester, New York, with pneumonia in 1962 through 1980.

Forty-two of the 50 cases were confirmed by chest films and thoracen-tesis. Twenty-one patients had parapneumonic effusion and another 21 had parapneumonic empyema; the other 8 had roentgenographic evidence of fluid in the pleural space, but did not undergo thoracentesis. Clinical signs in both groups included fever, tactile and vocal fremitus, respiratory difficulties, rales, intercostal space fullness, and cyanosis. Pleural friction rub was present in 2 patients with empyema (Table 1). Forty-eight percent of the patients with pleural effusion and 60% of those with empyema had a white blood cell count greater than 15,000 cells/cu mm. More than 10,000 mature neutrophils or more than 500 bands per cc mm, or both, were detected in 71% of patients with pleural effusion and in 80% of those with empyema.

Initial radiographic findings showed minimal effusion in 5% of patients with pleural effusion and in 24% of those with empyema, moderate ef-fusion in 57% and 38%, respectively, and massive effusion in 38% of patients in each group. Both effusion and empyema were seen predomi-nantly as unilateral diseases, without a tendency to involve a particular

TABLE 1.—FINDINGS OF PATIENTS WITH PARAPNEUMONIC PLEURAL EFFUSION AND EMPYEMA

	Effusion (n = 21)		Empyema (n = 21)	
	Number	(%)	Number	(%)
History of preceding respiratory illnesses	4	(19)	3	(14)
Signs				
Fever	17	(81)	20	(95)
Tactile and vocal fremitus	17	(81)	20	(95)
Respiratory difficulties	11	(52)	13	(62)
Rales	5	(24)	11	(52)
Intercostal space fullness	7	(33)	6	(29)
Pleural friction rub	0	(0)	2	(10)
Cyanosis	1	(5)	1	(5)
Laboratory findings WBC (mean)	16,542		20,040*	
WBC > 15,000	10	(48)	12	(60)*
Mature neutrophils >10,000 or bands >500	15	(71)	16	(80)*
X-rays				
Lobar infiltration	9	(43)	11	(52)
Segmental	6	(29)	7	(33)
Bilateral patchy	5	(24)	3	(14)
Interstitial	1	(5)	0	(0)

*Information available in only 20 patients.
(Courtesy of Chonmaitree, T., and Powell, K.R.: Clin. Pediatr. (Phila.) 22:414–418, June 1983.)

side. Clinical, laboratory, and roentgenographic findings did not differ significantly between the two groups. Thus the likelihood of obtaining purulent or nonpurulent fluid could not be predicted from these findings.

Bacteria in pleural fluid or blood were isolated in only 6 (29%) of the 21 patients with pleural effusion, but in 13 (62%) of the 21 patients with empyema (Table 2). An additional 6 patients with pleural effusion and another 3 with empyema had findings suggestive of an infectious process. *Staphylococcus aureus* was isolated in 35% of the cases, *Streptococcus pneumoniae* in 30%, and *Streptococcus pyogenes* in 20%.

Sixteen of the children with pleural effusion were treated with antibiotics and thoracentesis; only 5 required closed-chest drainage. Two patients with empyema died. Of the remaining 19, all were treated with antibiotics, thoracentesis, and closed-chest drainage. All patients with pleural effusion improved or were cured without complication, whereas 4 patients with empyema developed complications related to closed-chest drainage.

The pattern of parapneumonic effusion and empyema in children continues to evolve. Although a presumptive diagnosis of staphylococcal disease applied to more than 90% of the cases in the late 1950s and early 1960s, it now applies in only about one-third. Thus, tests such as the Gram

TABLE 2.—ETIOLOGY OF PARAPNEUMONIC EFFUSION
AND EMPYEMA

	Effusion (%)	Empyema (%)	Unclassified* (%)
Documented infection	6 (29)	13 (62)	1 (13)
Staphylococcal	3	4	0
Pneumococcal	2	4	0
Streptococcal			
(β hemolytic)	1	3	0
α Streptococcal	0	1	0
Enterococcal	0	1	0
Hemophilus influenzae	0	0	1
Probable infection	6 (29)	3 (14)	4 (50)
Staphylococcal	1	3	1
Pneumococcal	1	0	1
Streptococcal			
(β hemolytic)	2	0	1
Mycoplasma	0	0	1
Atypical measles	1	0	0
Viral	1	0	0
Etiology not identified	9 (43)	5 (24)	3 (38)
TOTAL	21	21	8

*Presence of fluid in pleural space was evidenced by chest films only; thoracentesis was not performed.
(Courtesy of Chonmaitree, T., and Powell, K.R.: Clin. Pediatr. (Phila.) 22:414–418, June 1983.)

stain, CIE, and latex agglutination may help identify a causative agent, especially if the patient has already received antibiotics.

Theophylline Disposition in Cystic Fibrosis
A. Isles, M. Spino, E. Tabachnik, H. Levison, J. Thiessen, and S. MacLeod
Am. Rev. Respir. Dis. 127:417–421, April 1983   5–8

Theophylline therapy improves lung function in patients with cystic fibrosis (CF). The drug disposition of theophylline, 12 mg/kg orally or 5.7 mg/kg intravenously, was assessed in 10 patients with CF and 10 healthy volunteers of similar age studied at The Hospital for Sick Children, Toronto, Ontario. Blood samples were obtained 2–24 hours after oral administration, and during the first 90 minutes and 2–8 hours after intravenous infusion.

Mean serum theophylline concentrations after intravenous infusion were consistently lower in patients with CF, with the concentration at 8 hours being approximately half of that in controls (Fig 5–4). Total body clearance (TBC) and volume distribution (VD) were significantly greater in patients with CF than in controls (Table 1). When TBC was related to total body surface area rather than to body weight, the twofold increase in TBC in patients with CF persisted ($P < .001$) (Fig 5–5). After oral administration

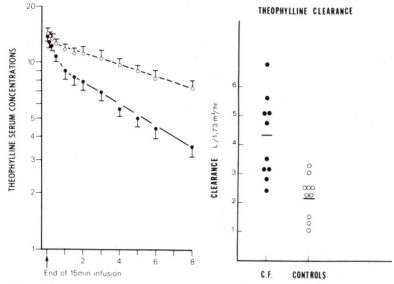

Fig 5–4 (left).—Mean (± SEM) serum theophylline concentrations after 6 mg of the drug per kilogram was administered intravenously in 10 patients with cystic fibrosis *(solid circles)* and 10 healthy controls *(open circles)*.

Fig 5–5 (right).—Mean and individual values for theophylline clearance in 10 cystic fibrosis *(C.F.)* patients *(solid circles)* and 10 healthy controls *(open circles)*.

(Courtesy of Isles, A., et al.: Am. Rev. Respir. Dis. 127:417–421, April 1983.)

of sustained-release theophylline, the maximal concentration in patients with CF was only 53% of that achieved in controls $(P < .001)$, despite equivalent doses and a similar bioavailability for the two groups (Fig 5–6 and Table 2). The fraction of the dose adsorbed over time did not differ significantly between groups. In patients with CF, 46% of the theophylline was present as free drug, compared with 36% in control subjects $(P < .01)$.

The results are consistent with those of other reports of increased drug elimination in patients with CF. Thus, if theophylline is to be used in these

TABLE 1.—Pharmacokinetic Results Obtained After Intravenously Administered Theophylline*

Group	n	K (min⁻¹)	t½ (min)	VD (L/kg)	TBC (ml/h/kg)	TBC (L/h/1.73 m²)
Patients with CF	10	0.0021 ± 0.0007	361 ± 123	0.59 ± 0.1	75.1 ± 27.9	4.3 ± 1.5
Control subjects	10	0.0013 ± 0.0004	568 ± 188	0.44 ± 0.05	35.4 ± 10.3	2.2 ± 0.7
p		< 0.01	< 0.05	< 0.005	< 0.001	< 0.001

Definition of abbreviations: K = elimination rate constant; t½ = elimination half-life; VD = volume of distribution; TBC = total body clearance.
*Values are mean ± SD.
(Courtesy of Isles, A., et al.: Am. Rev. Respir. Dis. 127:417–421, April 1983.)

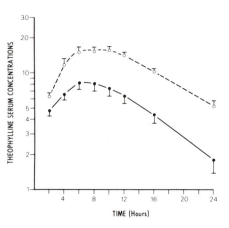

Fig 5–6.—Mean (± SEM) concentration time profile after administration of sustained-release theophylline, 12 mg/kg orally, in 10 cystic fibrosis patients *(solid circles)* and 10 healthy controls *(open circles)*. (Courtesy of Isles, A., et al.: Am. Rev. Respir. Dis. 127: 417–421, April 1983.)

patients, doses larger than those usually given to asthmatic patients may be required to maintain therapeutic serum concentrations.

▶ George Rodgers, Associate Professor of Pediatrics and Pharmacology/Toxicology, University of Louisville, comments:

"Now we know that drugs other than antibiotics are also cleared abnormally by cystic fibrosis (CF) patients. It is becoming clear that drug metabolism and elimination are probably abnormal in many, if not most, chronic diseases. It certainly behoves all of us who care for such patients to take care with the use of drugs in these patients and to be alert for signs of undermedication and overmedication.

"This article also points out our frequent lack of understanding about how disease affects drug metabolism. One might have anticipated that CF patients, most of whom have some degree of liver involvement, would have had decreased clearance of a hepatically cleared drug such as theophylline. The surprising finding of increased clearance implies that other factors, either endogenous or exogenous, are having a marked effect on the liver at the subcellular level. How many other drugs received by these patients are similarly affected? Are we seeing only a drug interactional effect, or is it the disease state that is causing the unexpected results? Obviously, further research is needed to an-

TABLE 2.—Pharmacokinetic Data After Orally Administered Sustained-Release Theophylline*

Group	n	Actual Dose (mg/kg)	Cmax (mg/L)	F
Patients with CF	10	11.5 ± 0.7	8.9 ± 3.5	0.89 ± 0.18
Control subjects	10	11.4 ± 1.4	16.6 ± 4.1	0.91 ± 0.18
t test		NS	< 0.001	NS

Definition of abbreviations: Cmax = maximal concentration achieved; F = fraction of dose absorbed (bioavailability).
*Values are mean ± SD.
(Courtesy of Isles, A., et al.: Am. Rev. Respir. Dis. 127:417–421, April 1983.)

swer these questions. In the meantime, those who care for CF patients receiving theophylline should monitor levels closely and recognize that higher than usual doses, and perhaps more frequent dosing, may be required to achieve efficacy. However, they may also find that with the decreased protein-binding found in these patients, adverse side efects may be more commonly seen at serum levels usually considered safe and therapeutic."

Relationship of Parental Smoking and Gas Cooking to Respiratory Disease in Children
Edem E. Ekwo, Miles M. Weinberger, Peter A. Lachenbruch, and William H. Huntley (Univ. of Iowa)
Chest 84:662–668, December 1983   5–9

Parental smoking has been related to an increased risk of respiratory illness in infants and to respiratory infections and breathlessness in older children. Similar relationships with gas cooking also have been described. These relationships were reassessed in a survey of 1,355 children aged 6 to 12 years in Iowa City. Most were from middle and upper social classes. The study group represented about two thirds of all children of this age group in the school district. Data on parental smoking was complete for 84% of children. Lung function was evaluated in 89 children whose parents did not smoke and 94 whose parents did.

The risk of hospitalization for respiratory illness in children younger than age 2 years was increased when gas was used for cooking or at least one parent smoked. The occurrence of coughing with colds in children was significantly more likely when one or both parents smoked. Small but significant increases in FEV_1 and forced expiratory flow after receiving isoproterenol were found in children of parents who smoked but not in children of nonsmokers. No such relationship with gas cooking was apparent. Height and weight were similar for the children of parents who smoked and those who did not. Initial lung function values before inhalation of isoproterenol did not differ significantly in the two groups of children.

Parental smoking appears to be associated with an increased risk of some respiratory disorders and symptoms in children. A similar but independent effect of gas cooking is a possibility. Children whose parents smoke at home have increased airway reactivity after bronchodilator therapy, but it is not clear whether these changes persist or are of clinical importance.

Longitudinal Study of Effects of Maternal Smoking on Pulmonary Function in Children
Ira B. Tager, Scott T. Weiss, Alvaro Mūnoz, Bernard Rosner, and Frank E. Speizer (Harvard Med. School)
N. Engl. J. Med. 309:699–703, Sept. 22, 1983   5–10

The effects of maternal smoking were studied in 1,156 white children, from 404 families, examined prospectively yearly for 7 years.

The percentage of children whose mothers were current smokers was highest among children with the lowest average levels of forced expiratory volume in 1 second (FEV_1) over the first 6 years. The trend toward decreasing frequency of maternal smoking with increasing mean level of FEV_1 in the child older than age 6 years was significant ($P < .001$). Maternal cigarette smoking lowered ($P = .015$) the expected average annual increase in FEV_1 after correction for previous FEV_1, age, height, change in height, and cigarette smoking in the child or adolescent. The effects of the smoking habits of the mother and the child on the change in FEV_1 in the child appeared to be additive, since no significant interaction was detected between these effects. Maternal smoking tended ($P = .174$) to have a similar effect on the forced expiratory flow between 25% and 75% of forced vital capacity.

It was estimated that if two children have the same initial FEV_1, age, height, increase in height, and personal cigarette-smoking history, but the mother of one has smoked throughout his life whereas the mother of the other has not, the difference in the change in FEV_1 over time in the exposed versus the unexposed child will be approximately 28, 51, and 101 ml after 1, 2, and 5 years, respectively, or a reduction of 10.7%, 9.5%, and 7.0%, respectively, in the expected increase (table). Socioeconomic status and exposure to gas cooking stoves did not appear to explain the observed association between maternal smoking habits and rate of growth of lung function in children.

The lungs of nonsmoking children with mothers who smoke apparently grow at only 93% of the rate seen in nonsmoking children with nonsmoking mothers. This, along with the smoking habits of the child himself,

EFFECT OF CHILD'S AND MOTHER'S CIGARETTE-SMOKING HABIT ON EXPECTED RATE OF GROWTH IN FEV_1 OVER A FIVE-YEAR PERIOD, BASED ON AUTOREGRESSIVE MODEL*

CHILD'S SMOKING †	MOTHER'S SMOKING ‡	EXPECTED RATE OF GROWTH IN FEV_1 (ML)		
		AFTER 1 YR	AFTER 2 YR	AFTER 5 YR
No	No	262	539	1436
Yes	No	168 (64.1)	366 (67.9)	1094 (76.2)
No	Yes	234 (89.3)	488 (90.5)	1335 (93.0)
Yes	Yes	140 (53.4)	315 (58.4)	993 (69.2)

*The projected growth rates for a male child who starts with population-median values for FEV_1 (1.93 L), height (146 cm), and change in height (5 cm per year). Figures in parenthesis indicate the percentage of increase to the level in a nonsmoking child of a currently nonsmoking mother.
†"No" denotes had never smoked, and "yes" had ever smoked.
‡"Yes" denotes former smokers or never smoked, and "yes" current smoker.
(Courtesy of Tager, I.B., et al.: N. Engl. J. Med. 309:699–703, Sept. 22, 1983. Reprinted by permission of the New England Journal of Medicine.)

may be important in the development of chronic obstructive airway disease in adulthood.

► Miles Weinberger, Professor of Pediatrics and Chairman, Pediatric Allergy and Pulmonary Division, University of Iowa Hospitals, comments:

" 'A custome lothesome to the eye, hateful to the nose, harmfull to the braine, dangerous to the Lungs, and in the black stinking fume thereof neerest resembling the horrible Stygian smoke of the pit that is bottomless.''—James I, from *Counterblaste to Tobacco,* 1604.

"Despite this early criticism, cigarette smoking became an accepted and cherished pastime in Western society, developed into a major industry in the United States employing over 400,000 people and with domestic sales of 20 billion dollars, produced federal, state, and municipal revenues from excise and sales taxes of over 7 billion dollars in 1981, and was practiced by as much as 50% of the population by the early 1960s when the Surgeon-General first reported the adverse effects of cigarette smoking on health (Whelan, E. M.: *A Smoking Gun: How the Tobacco Industry Gets Away with Murder,* Stickley Co., Philadelphia, 1984).

"Convincing epidemiologic data link cigarette smoking to bronchogenic carcinoma, cancer of the buccal cavity, larynx, and esophagus, cancer of the bladder, chronic obstructive pulmonary disease in adults, and various cardiovascular disorders. Cigarette smoking also contributes to asthmatic symptoms in patients with underlying hyperreactive airways and is, in fact, the major cause of pulmonary diseases in adults.

"Passive smoking has been reported to be associated with an increased frequency of lung cancer in spouses and progeny of smokers (Correa, P., et al.: *Lancet* 2:595, 1983), small airway dysfunction from exposure in the work environment (White, J. R., and Froeb, H. F.: *N. Engl. J. Med.* 302:742, 1980), increased IgE levels (Kjellman, N.-I. M.: *Lancet* 1:993, 1981), and increased permeability of the pulmonary epithelium (Hogg, J. C.: *Chest* 83:1, 1983). In the survey of 1355 school-age children by Ekwo et al., parental smoking was associated with a more than twofold increase in risk of hospitalization from respiratory disease during the first 2 years of life, and these data were consistent with findings of at least four previous reports. Moreover, asthma, when present, is more severe in children of smoking parents (Gortmaker, S. L., et al.: *Am. J. Public Health* 72:574, 1982).

"The study by Tager et al. demonstrates an association between a smoking mother and lower mean pulmonary function values over a 5-year period in school-age children. This study confirmed previous reports and is consistent with the bronchodilator responsiveness seen by Ekwo et al. in children from homes with smoking parents and the increased frequency of symptoms of obstructive airway disease, i.e., asthma, in such children.

"Smoking thus constitutes a major health hazard to those who actively smoke and additionally appears to cause an increased risk of illness to those who live with smokers, particularly children younger than age 2 years and those of all ages predisposed to have asthma. The Committee on Genetics and Environmental Hazards of the American Academy of Pediatrics has recommended that physicians increase their efforts to inform patients about the hazards of smoking and has encouraged support for legislation prohibiting smoking in public places frequented by children, particularly hospitals and other health facilities (*Pediatrics* 70:314, 1982). This would appear to be consistent with our traditional emphasis on preventative pediatrics."

Home Care for Children on Respirators
Barbara H. Burr, Bernard Guyer, I. David Todres, Barbara Abrahams, and Thomas Chiodo
N. Engl. J. Med. 309:1319–1324, Nov. 24, 1983   5–11

A study was conducted to document the experiences of 6 families who brought their ventilator-dependent children home from intensive care units. Cases for study were identified in late 1980 through a survey of 14 hospitals in Massachusetts that have the capability to care for newborns or children on ventilators. Fourteen families were identified; 8 had children on ventilators residing at home. Six families agreed to participate in the study. A structured interview was used to document the child's history and care requirements from the parents' point of view.

The 6 children had a wide diversity of problems. Their respiratory failure could be attributed to either intrinsic lung disease or a neuromuscular disorder. All were considered relatively stable or improving when discharged from the acute care hospital. Parental skills included gastrotomy feeding, tracheostomy care, chest physical therapy, cardiopulmonary resuscitation, and the teaching and supervision of nurses and other personnel. The experience of 2 families is described below.

CASE 1.—Girl, born in 1978 and aged 11 months when taken home, had respiratory arrest at birth and later had a diagnosis of myotubular myopathy. Hydrocephalus required shunting, and gastrostomy was necessary. Since she has been home, her strength has improved so that she can be taken off the respirator for 10 hours per day when awake. She has made steady developmental gains, especially in the area of communication. Assisting the family at home are two shifts of registered nurses each day, a physical therapist, an early-intervention team, and a supportive pediatrician.

CASE 2.—Girl, 7½, who went home at age 3 months, has become increasingly independent as she has grown despite a diagnosis of Ondine's syndrome. She was placed on an iron lung upon discharge for sleep and remained well until age 6 months when she developed severe pneumonia and seizures. She had frequent episodes of pneumonia until age 3½ years. She is currently on an Emerson volume respirator for 10 to 12 hours at night and is able to attach and detach it herself. She is currently in a regular first-grade class. Her speech is completely intelligible.

Without exception, the parents have reported that bringing their children home from the hospital has had a beneficial effect on family relations. But they have described their loss of privacy, their limited social lives, disruption of sleep patterns, and difficult schedules as part of their unusual situation. No family has felt in a position to have additional children. Summarized in the table are the detailed records most families have kept

HOSPITAL AND HOME CARE COSTS FOR SIX VENTILATOR-DEPENDENT CHILDREN, 1980*

CASE NO.	HOSPITAL CARE		HOME CARE		ANNUAL COST REDUCTION FROM HOSPITAL TO HOME CARE (%)
	ANNUAL COST	FUNDING SOURCE/ COVERAGE (%)	ANNUAL COST	FUNDING SOURCE COVERAGE (%)	
1	$336,000	Private insurance, 100	$45,000	Private insurance, $500,000 maximum will be exhausted; (projected) Medicaid, 85 Parents, 15	$291,000 (86)
2	$241,200	Private insurance, 100; SSI/Medicaid, 100, 1979 (after private insurance exhausted, 1979)	$74,500	Medicaid, 85 Parents, 15	$166,700 (69)
3	$245,000	SSI/Medicaid, 100	$1,000	SSI/Medicaid, 95 Parents, 5	$244,000 (100)
4	$192,000– $357,000	Private insurance, 100	$21,500	Private insurance, 80 Parents, 20 ($250,000 maximum)	$170,500– $335,500 (89–93)
5	$120,000– $219,000	Private insurance, 100	$29,000	Private insurance, 80 Parents, 20 ($250,000 maximum)	$91,000– $190,000 (76–87)
6	$109,500– $182,500	Private insurance, 100	$1,000	Private insurance, 80 Parents, 20 ($250,000 maximum)	$108,500– $181,500 (99)
				Total savings/year $1,071,700→1,408,700	

*SSI = Supplemental Security Income.
(Courtesy of Burr, B.H., et al.: N. Engl. J. Med. 309:1319–1324, Nov. 24, 1983. Reprinted by permission of the New England Journal of Medicine.)

of their child's medical expenses. These records show the important financial savings to be realized with home care. Despite these dramatic cost savings from home care, families were financially penalized for bringing their children home because when insurance benefits are exhausted, the hospitalized child is eligible for Supplemental Security Income and Medicaid benefits. However, unless the family's income is low enough, all benefits are lost when the child leaves the hospital. The authors contend these cost problems should be rectified because of the benefits of home care for children on ventilators.

▶ Allen I. Goldberg, Medical Director, Division of Respiratory Care, Children's Memorial Hospital, Chicago, comments:

"Children on respirators are bona fide intensive care unit candidates. Burr and associates are among selected professionals who have challenged this tradition as well as the health care delivery and reimbursement systems that are set up to deal with expensive acute care, but which are not designed to answer the question, 'What next?' This was inevitable, because intensive care costs for these children currently exceed $330,000 per year, and well-designed home care programs consistently save more than two thirds of acute care charges. Thirty years of experiences with polio survivors on respirators at home and more recent pediatric home care demonstrations have proved the limitless human potential of persons at home where they belong.

"Care for life-supported children at home represents complex issues for the primary physician. Each individual program has uniqueness that demands a well-organized, personalized, case-management approach. In the hospital, this can be done with the patient's interdisciplinary primary care team assisted by a core resource group available to explain the issues and facilitate the process. Each child must meet strict medical criteria based on the necessity of clinical stability that results from optimal ventilation and pharmacologic support. A properly selected home care candidate should need no major diagnostic or therapeutic intervention within a period of a month. The primary physician must understand and accept these criteria and translate them into a medical prescription that is the foundation of the home care plan.

"Resolving medical issues only begins the successful home care program. Developmental, social, organizational, and reimbursement criteria must also be met. A child on a respirator at home requires a family and community commitment demonstrated by involvement and extensive preparation. The home care program demands detailed planning and organization for nursing and respiratory care, provision and maintenance of equipment and supplies, emergency care, case monitoring, and follow-up reevaluation. Under current reimbursement policies, comprehensive funding for home care is not readily available. It is inappropriate to send a child home with less than 100% of required funding; there are always additional economic burdens on the family due to extra non-medically related expenses.

"The physician must be continually involved in the planning process of home care as a committed member of the home care team. There must be an assurance that, once at home, the child will be in a safe environment in which to grow and develop. Not all children on respirators can go or remain at home because of medical, social, developmental, or educational reasons. Other institutional options (intermediate care, respiratory rehabilitation, transitional care, respite care); community living alternatives (group homes, foster care, schools); and skilled nursing facilities are needed for temporary or permanent situations. The physician must assume leadership in guaranteeing the appropriate utilization and coordination of regional resources that can be made available for these children, a new disabled population dependent on technology."

Survival Rates in Cystic Fibrosis

R. W. Wilmott, S. L. Tyson, R. Dinwiddie, and D. J. Matthew (Hosp. for Sick Children, London)

Arch. Dis. Child. 58:835–836, October 1983   5–12

Life tables were calculated for 273 British children with cystic fibrosis for the period 1974–1979, in part to determine whether mortality was greater among girls and patients with meconium ileus (MI).

Children with MI had greater perinatal mortality, the first year mortality being 6.5% compared with 0% in non-MI children. Children between ages 10 and 13 years who had MI also had a slightly greater mortality rate than did the non-MI patients. Survival to 16 years was significantly less common in MI patients than in non-MI patients. If the 8 patients who died in the first year from surgical complications before referral to the cystic fibrosis center are excluded, the survival rates were not significantly different. Survival for girls was not significantly different from that for boys up to age 16 years. Girls had a slightly lower cumulative survival rate after age 8 years. Survival in the MI series improved appreciably (Fig

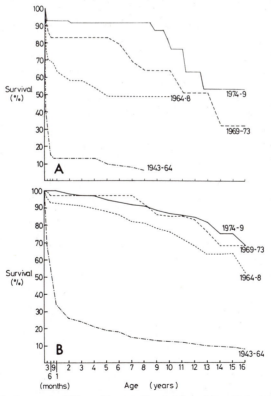

Fig 5–7.—Survival curves in children with cystic fibrosis followed from birth. **A,** children with meconium ileus; **B,** children without meconium ileus. (Courtesy of Wilmott, R.W., et al.: Arch. Dis. Child. 58:835–836, October 1983.)

5–7) over rates reported in earlier series. There was little change in survival rates in the non-MI patients compared with those in a series from 1969 to 1973. There was no significant difference in survival rates between boys and girls with cystic fibrosis before age 16 years.

▶ Judy Palmer and Nancy Huang, at St. Christopher's Hospital for Children, Philadelphia, comment on this important topic.

"Longer survival for patients with cystic fibrosis (CF) has been most impressive since the 1960s, largely due to better antibiotic control of pulmonary infection and the establishment of cystic fibrosis centers that offer an interdisciplinary approach to pulmonary, nutritional, and emotional care. Furthermore, improvement in surgical technique and postoperative nutritional support has improved the outlook of newborns with meconium ileus and older patients with major complications. These improvements are reflected in this article by Wilmott et al. showing a marked increase from period 1 (1969 to 1973) to period 2 (1974 to 1979) in the survival rates of the groups with meconium ileus. The authors observed little improvement in patients with CF diagnosed beyond neonatal age from period 1 to period 2 and no advantage for early diagnosis or for male patients. Unfortunately, the study did not extend beyond age 16, so that definitive comparison of survival rates was not possible. This is because many patients with advanced disease may live past the midteens and survival differences may not be apparent until the later years.

"Latest advances in antibiotic therapy include the development of more potent agents and greater understanding of the peculiar pharmacokinetic behavior of these agents in patients with CF. Comprehensive care programs are being developed for adults. Future gains in survival rate and quality of the life of patients with CF are anticipated with improvements in treatment and with new insights into the pathogenesis of the disease process."

Pregnancy in Patients With Cystic Fibrosis
Judy Palmer, Cindy Dillon-Baker, Jan S. Tecklin, Barbara Wolfson, Beth Rosenberg, Barbara Burroughs, Douglas S. Holsclaw, Jr., Thomas F. Scanlin, Nancy N. Huang, and Edward M. Sewell
Ann. Intern. Med. 99:597–600, November 1983   5–13

As more patients with cystic fibrosis reach adulthood, questions arise about the potential hazards of pregnancy. A review was made of the medical records of 8 women with cystic fibrosis who had a total of 11 completed pregnancies. They were evaluated within 1 year before conception between 1974 and 1981. In group 1 (5 patients), the woman's overall condition after pregnancy returned to the pregravid level. In group 2 (3 patients), the woman's condition deteriorated during pregnancy and did not return to pregravid condition postpartum.

The two groups were similar for age at diagnosis, age at pregnancy, and maternal height. Patients in group 1 had Shwachman-Kulczycki clinical scores of more than 74 and percent mean weight for height of more than 88%, whereas in group 2 patients, the corresponding figures were less than 66 and less than 84% respectively. Brasfield chest roentgenogram scores showed moderate to advanced disease in group 2 and were near normal levels in group 1. Pulmonary function studies in group 2 showed restrictive and obstructive disease, whereas in group 1 only mild to moderate airway obstruction and normal lung volumes were seen. The 5 women in group 1 had little change in their clinical status post partum and were able to assume full responsibility for infant care; 4 of these women had second pregnancies 2–4 years later. One patient in group 2 had post partum hemorrhage because of vitamin K deficiency and died 2 months post partum. The other 2 women in group 2 had poor health and required considerable assistance in caring for their infants; 1 died 24 months post partum. The birth weights, gestational ages, and head circumferences of infants of group 2 women were generally less than those of infants of group 1 women. None of the infants had positive sweat test results at 1–16 months of age.

Four factors are associated with a favorable outcome of pregnancy in the woman with cystic fibrosis and her infant: a good Shwachman-Kulczycki clinical score, good nutritional status, nearly normal findings on chest roentgenography, and good pulmonary function with normal lung volumes and only mild to moderate airway obstruction.

▶ As survivorship has improved in cystic fibrosis, it is not at all surprising now to see increasing numbers of reports of pregnancy in patients with the disease. For many years, the concept existed that pregnancy would not be likely in women with cystic fibrosis. Time has proved this to be wrong. This is not to say that women with cystic fibrosis conceive without difficulty. The age of menarche for the cystic fibrosis patient is 14.4 years in the United States, compared with 12.9 years for unaffected American girls. (Neinstein et al.: *J. Adolesc. Health Care* 4:153, 1983). In this study, the most important factor determining whether or not menarche would occur was the weight of the patient. Ninety-five percent of the patients with cystic fibrosis who achieve menarche weighed more than 82 lb., whereas 75% of the amenorrheic patients weighed less than 82 lb. Even if menarche is achieved, there is only about a 50% probability that normal menses will occur. About one half of patients have dysfunctional uterine bleeding or oligomenorrhea. In a survey of sexual activity among adolescent and young adult women with cystic fibrosis, 0 of 16 patients younger than age 18 years had had intercourse, while 9 of 16 patients older than age 18 years had been or were sexually active.

In order to find out how our patients eventually grow up and fare with pregnancy, we have to look to the internal medical literature (the article above was abstracted from *Annals of Internal Medicine*). As can be seen, young women with cystic fibrosis can do satisfactorily with pregnancy if they are in reasonably good medical condition prior to the onset of the pregnancy. If they have low Shwachman scores, poor nutrition, grossly abnormal chest roentgenograms, and severe pulmonary functional abnormalities, the pregnancy will only make the situation worse. Unfortunately, the adult medical literature has relatively little interest in the offspring of a pregnancy, so it is hard to come by specific data dealing with the products of the pregnancy. The data from the *Annals of*

Internal Medicine give us only a rough insight into what happens to the infants of women with cystic fibrosis. These data suggest that if the mother is in good condition prior to and during the pregnancy, the baby will do very well. In women who deteriorate during pregnancy, the likelihood is that the babies will be born with significantly low birth weights (the average birth weight in this group of infants was 1.8 kg). Long-term follow-up of the latter group of babies does not exist.

As more data accumulate, we, as pediatricians, will be able to advise teenagers more properly about the potential possibilities of conception and its inherent risks.—J.A.S., III

Diagnostic Delay in Cystic Fibrosis: Lessons From Newborn Screening
B. Wilcken, S. J. Towns, and C. M. Mellis (Camperdown, Australia)
Arch. Dis. Child. 58:863–866, November 1983   5–14

Screening neonates for cystic fibrosis (CF) using the dried blood spot immunoreactive trypsin (IRT) assay is now practical, but its value is disputed. The delay between the onset of symptoms and the clinical diagnosis of CF was examined in 33 infants seen in a CF clinic before institution of a screening program, as well as the natural history of the disease during the first weeks of life in 48 infants in whom CF was detected on newborn screening.

Of the 33 infants with CF diagnosed clinically, the disease was detected in 11 before age 2 months, in 9 between ages 2 and 12 months, and in 13 after age 12 months. Of the 11 infants with CF diagnosed before age 2 months, 5 had meconium ileus, 1 had meconium plug syndrome, and 3 had a close relative with CF; the possibility of CF was discussed with the parents of these children during the first week of life. The most common mode of presentation in infants with CF diagnosed between ages 2 and 12 months was failure to thrive, usually with obvious gastrointestinal tract symptoms. Most of the children with CF diagnosed after age 12 months had respiratory symptoms, usually in association with gastrointestinal tract symptoms (table). In the latter group, the mean delay between presentation and diagnosis was 2.6 years. In the 48 infants with positive screening test results, notification of an elevated IRT value on the second blood sample and request for a sweat test were usually made between ages 3 and 6 weeks; the mean age at diagnosis was 37 days. Eleven of these infants had meconium ileus, and 30 of the remaining 37 had gastrointestinal tract symptoms at the time of diagnosis. Pulmonary symptoms also were present in 14 of these 30 infants. Seven infants had no symptoms at the time of diagnosis. The diagnosis of CF was considered clinically in only 4 of the 30 infants with symptoms.

There are appreciable delays between the onset of symptoms and the diagnosis of CF without screening. Thus, screening for CF may be justified not only with regard to prophylactic treatment, but also to facilitate early and aggressive treatment of mild symptoms.

PATIENTS AGED 12 MONTHS AND OLDER AT THE TIME OF DIAGNOSIS

Case No	Age at diagnosis (yrs)	Age at first presentation	Symptoms at presentation	Visits to doctor before diagnosis (No)	Hospital admissions before diagnosis (No)
1	3·5	1·5 yrs	Rectal prolapse	5	—
2	1·3	1 yr	Rectal prolapse, resp	6	1
3	2·3	9 mths	GIT resp	12	2
4	2·5	4 mths	FTT, resp	14	—
5	1·3	Birth	FTT	10	—
6	1·1	3 mths	FTT/GIT, resp	14	1
7	4	5 mths	Resp	13	—
8	3	6 wks	Resp	26	3
9	2·5	3 mths	GIT, resp	6	4
10	3·5	2 mths	GIT, resp	10	8
11	4·2	1 yr	Relative with CF, GIT, resp	30	2
12	8	3 mths	Sibling with CF, GIT, resp	72	2
13	2·5	3 mths	Sibling with CF, GIT, resp	4	—

FTT = failure to thrive; GIT = gastrointestinal; Resp = respiratory.
(Courtesy of Wilcken, B., et al.: Arch. Dis. Child. 58:863–866, November 1983.)

▶ Although not everyone agrees with the value of neonatal screening for cystic fibrosis, the data included in this report from Australia and another report from Colorado (*Lancet* 1:42, 1984) provide useful and valuable information concerning dried blood spot immunoreactive trypsin assays in the newborn period. In both reports, most (presumably) cases of cystic fibrosis are able to be detected by this form of newborn dried blood screening assay. The data from Colorado that examined 90,000 infants found that 83% of all positive results of tests collected at ages 2 to 4 days were false positive. This, of course, is a high number, but probably not unacceptable if the test does pick up the large majority of patients with CF. The Colorado study also showed that if the test is still positive at age 4 to 6 weeks, it is 80% predictive of the disease. Of course, a sweat test performed in the usual way always is used as the confirmatory test. In Colorado, preliminary results indicate that the addition of a second test for immunoreactive pancreative lipase values provides additional information. Neonates with cystic fibrosis who have raised trypsinogen levels also have increased lipase levels, whereas most infants without cystic fibrosis with raised trypsinogen levels have normal lipase levels.

Legitimate debate still exists concerning the value of a newborn screening test for cystic fibrosis. Arguments for screening include improvement in clinical condition (specifically, lung function and nutrition), prevention of further births in the family by genetic counseling, and the possibility of instituting research programs to test new modes of treatment. One can flip the coin and look at these same questions differently. To date, there really are no unequivocal data that clearly document the role of early intervention in producing a better outlook for children with cystic fibrosis. This is not to say that early intervention does not produce a better outcome, just that it has never been documented clearly or proved. Likewise, there are no data whatsoever to suggest that early diagnosis will in any way affect the decision of parents to have another child. It has been estimated that up to 70% of parents whose first child was affected with cystic fibrosis decided to proceed with subsequent pregnancies after genetic counseling. Among families with at least two children, one of whom had cystic fibrosis, 25% of parents decide to attempt another pregnancy. These data are essentially no different than the population as a whole of parents who have no affected children with cystic fibrosis. This entire story would change, obviously, if there were some accurate prenatal test for cystic fibrosis, or at least one would think so. The major difficulty currently with screening for cystic fibrosis in the newborn period has to do with the anxiety that it can produce among parents who have a child with a positive screening test. You can tell such parents that there is only about a one in five chance that their child has cystic fibrosis, but that will probably do little to assuage their anxieties. Even if the child has cystic fibrosis, this may not be able to be documented very quickly because sweat testing may not give satisfactory results at the early age at which the screening test report comes back. Repeat testing of the immunoreactive trypsin level is of little value because the numbers fall off very quickly in patients with cystic fibrosis as the pancreas "burns out," so distinguishing these patients from normal is impossible with this test after a few weeks of age in many instances.

An Ad Hoc Committee Task Force on Neonatal Screening, formed by the Cystic Fibrosis Foundation, met in 1983 to review all of the currently available information. Their report appeared in the November 1983 issue of *Pediatrics* (p. 741). Their conclusion was: "Until sufficient information related to these and other issues can be obtained, the Task Force strongly recommends that no mass population screening for cystic fibrosis be implemented, even if a valid and reliable test is available." The Committee also urged strongly that all the issues involved, many of which are as discussed above, be evaluated by scientific methods. In other words, most of the unknowns can be studied appropriately, and a recommendation was strongly made to do this.

It seems apparent that we will be seeing, ever so slowly, some of these questions answered from other parts of the world as well as from isolated pockets of screening programs within the United States. If some of the answers are favorable or if a reliable prenatal screening test for cystic fibrosis comes along and is validated, then widespread screening will most likely proceed.—J.A.S., III

Amyloid-Related Serum Protein (SAA) as an Indicator of Lung Infection in Cystic Fibrosis
G. Marhaug, H. Permin, and G. Husby
Acta Paediatr. Scand. 72:861–866, November 1983   5–15

Chronic respiratory tract infection with progressive respiratory failure is the chief cause of death from cystic fibrosis (CF). Amyloid-related serum protein (SAA) was analyzed by radioimmunoassay in 32 patients with CF and the findings compared with levels of other acute-phase reactants and with lung function values. Amyloid-related serum protein (SAA) is a low molecular weight protein complexed to high-density lipoprotein in serum as one of its apoproteins. It probably is the precursor of the amyloid fibril protein AA found in secondary amyloidosis. Sixteen male and 16 female patients with a mean age of 13 years were studied. All but 4 patients had had chronic bronchopulmonary infection by mucoid strains of *Pseudomonas aeruginosa* for a mean of about 5 years. Ten of these patients were treated with tobramycin and ceftazidime intravenously for 2 weeks.

Levels of SAA correlated significantly with impaired lung function due to active *P. aeruginosa* infection, and also with C-reactive protein values. Both patients without pathogens in the sputum had normal SAA levels. Levels of SAA appeared to correlate better with bacteria in the sputum than did C-reactive protein. Levels of SAA also correlated with orosomucoid in the serum, but not as closely as with C-reactive protein. No correlation with serum IgG levels was noted. Falling serum SAA levels in treated patients paralleled the clinical responses to treatment.

Radioimmunoassay of serum SAA may prove useful both in selecting CF patients for antibiotic therapy and in evaluating the response to treatment. Elevation of SAA and other acute-phase proteins during infection presumably reflects the inflammatory response to the infecting agent. The reduction in serum SAA accompanying control of infection by adequate antibacterial therapy may help prevent secondary amyloidosis, although this complication is very infrequent in CF.

▶ At first I thought this report was for the birds, one of those "mynah" studies that ultimately never pans out. If these investigators are correct, however, they have described a powerful new tool to follow patients with cystic fibrosis. Amyloid-related serum protein is a low molecular weight protein in serum and is probably the precursor of amyloid fibril protein found in secondary amyloidosis. Only a very few cases of amyloidosis have been observed in cystic fibrosis, but this most probably relates to the short lifespan of patients with cystic fibrosis.

Keep your eyes open for more about amyloid-related serum protein. If these authors are correct, it has a far wider application in many other diseases, and this protein may well make it into the "big" leagues.—J.A.S., III

Importance of Viruses and *Legionella pneumophila* in Respiratory Exacerbations of Young Adults With Cystic Fibrosis
J. Efthimiou, Margaret E. Hodson, P. Taylor, A. G. Taylor, and J. C. Batten
Thorax 39:150–154, February 1984   5–16

About a fifth of respiratory exacerbations in patients with cystic fibrosis may not be associated with common bacteria or viruses, and *L. pneumophila*, which has a predilection for patients with chronic lung disease, is a plausible cause. The role of viruses and *L. pneumophila* in acute respiratory exacerbations in 25 male and 21 female patients with cystic fibrosis, aged 16 to 41 years, was examined. Twenty-four patients had respiratory symptoms and FEV_1 15% or more below baseline. The other 22 were in clinically and functionally stable condition. Thirty healthy subjects also were evaluated.

A fourfold rise in complement fixation antibody titer was found in 29% of the patients showing deterioration and in 1 patient in stable condition. Various viruses, *Mycoplasma pneumoniae*, and *Coxiella burnetii* were responsible for these antibody elevations. Another patient with respiratory illness consistent with Legionnaires' disease had a fourfold rise in *L. pneumophila* antibody in the indirect fluorescent antibody test. Eight patients in all (17%) had demonstrable antibody against *L. pneumophila*. All of them had moderate to severe disease with air flow limitation, but only 1 was receiving corticosteroid therapy. Titers were lower in all patients at follow-up 1 year later. Titers could not be related to pulmonary function or to the use of aerosol therapy. The deteriorated and stable groups did not differ significantly with regard to their chief sputum pathogens or respiratory symptoms before the study.

Bacteria, particularly *Pseudomonas aeruginosa,* are the chief pathogens in patients with cystic fibrosis, but viral, *Mycoplasma, Coxiella,* and *Legionella* infections may be associated with as many as a third of acute exacerbations of respiratory disease in young adult patients. These organisms should be sought as well as the usual bacteria and treatment begun where appropriate.

▶ Anywhere between one fourth and one third of respiratory infections that produce clinical decompensation in patients with cystic fibrosis may be the result of infections with organisms other than those we commonly think of. As this study suggests, viruses, *Mycoplasma,* and perhaps even *Legionella* may be the culprits. Indeed, this article reports what may be the first unequivocally documented seroconversion during active infection with *Legionella* in a patient with cystic fibrosis. The prevalence of positive antibody titers is about 5 times higher than that in age-matched controls, suggesting that many patients with cystic fibrosis have had prior contacts with this organism. Whether this is a result of an increased exposure or immune compromise is unexplained.

The dramatic change in survivorship of patients with cystic fibrosis (the median survivorship in the United States is now well into the third decade of life) largely reflects changing approaches toward pulmonary problems in these patients. General anesthesia is now used only with very great caution because of its documented potential to deteriorate lung function (Richardson et al.: *Acta Pediatr. Scand.* 73:75, 1984). One can get a rough handle on the rate of deterioration of pulmonary function by measuring the DNA content of sputum (Carswell et al.: *Eur. J. Respir. Dis.* 65:53, 1984). The effects of daily and regular chest physiotherapy are now without question (Zinman, R.: *Am. Rev. Respir. Dis.* 129:182, 1984; and Cerny, F., et al.: *Am. J. Dis. Child.* 138:261, 1984). A great deal more is understood about the pharmacology of antibiotics. Several antibiotics, such as methicillin, dicloxacillin, piperacillin, and gentamicin, are eliminated more rapidly in patients with cystic fibrosis, as is trimethoprim-sulfamethoxazole (Reed et al.: *J. Pediatr.* 104:303, 1984). Furthermore, even though antibiotic resistance is being noted, frequent regular hospitalizations for antibiotic therapy are commonplace in most centers that treat cystic fibrosis (Zaff, M., et al.: *Acta Paediatr. Scand.* 72:651, 1984).

Life was simpler a decade ago when all we had to worry about in patients with cystic fibrosis was *Staphylococcus* and *Pseudomonas*. Now we have to think about organisms that for all intents and purposes we didn't know existed before. In our mind, all this produces an alienation of infections. Despite this, all the new information that has come along has produced remarkable improvements in the quality of life of children and young adults with cystic fibrosis.—J.A.S., III

6 The Gastrointestinal Tract

Esophageal Replacement With Colon in Children: Functional Results and Long-term Growth
James P. Kelly, Gary D. Shackelford, and Charles L. Roper (Washington Univ., St. Louis)
Ann. Thorac. Surg. 36:634–643, December 1983   6–1

The results of colon interposition for esophageal replacement were reviewed in 23 consecutive children, 15 boys and 8 girls, operated on in 1959–1972. Fourteen children were treated for severe caustic burns of the esophagus and 9 were treated for long-segment esophageal atresia with or without tracheoesophageal fistula. Mean age of the 23 at the operation was 2.9 years.

A two-team approach generally was used. The esophagocolic and esophagogastric anastomoses are shown in Figure 6–1. A Heineke-Mikulicz pyloroplasty or pyloromyotomy is carried out unless a gastrostomy already has been done.

The 1 early death was due to intraoperative complications from an ischemic colon segment. Fourteen patients had early complications and 4

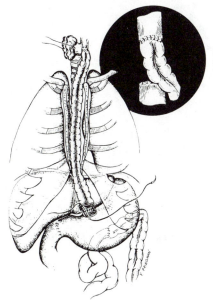

Fig 6–1.—Esophagocolic and esophagogastric anastomoses. Insert shows proximal esophagocolic anastomosis. (Courtesy of Kelly, J.P., et al.: Ann. Thorac. Surg. 36:634–643, December 1983.)

had late complications. Four of 18 patients who had barium swallows a mean of 10.4 years after surgery had redundancies of the colon segment, but only 1 was symptomatic as a result. Two patients had operative revision of the proximal anastomosis because of stricture or fistula. No patient had cervical dysphagia, and transit times were not abnormally prolonged.

All but 3 of 22 surviving patients have normal dietary habits and can eat relatively rapidly. Two patients report bloating after a large meal. Considerable "catch up" growth is evident in children who had esophageal atresia with or without tracheoesophageal fistula, but those with damage from lye have remained in the 50th growth percentile.

Nearly 90% of these children had excellent functional and radiographic findings on long-term follow-up after colon interposition surgery for esophageal replacement. The colon appears to provide an excellent conduit for esophageal substitution. The procedure is technically easy. Long-term growth has been excellent.

▶ Colon, jejunum, and stomach tubes have been used as substitutes for the esophagus in the pediatric population for some time now. The procedure generally is used either for esophageal atresia or for caustic damage to the esophagus. Way back in 1907, a Doctor Bircher was the first one to bypass the esophagus by using a skin tube. Since then, the procedure has been performed in selected cases over the years. However, long-term information on functional results in growth in children has been limited. What we see here, with a mean time of follow-up of 13 years after colon interposition, is that children are doing extraordinarily well. They are able to swallow adequately and grow along normal growth percentiles. How you could ever take something near where your bottom is and put it near where your mouth is and get it to work is beyond me, but I suppose it *does* work.

The prediction of the presence and severity of esophageal injury after the ingestion of a caustic substance is a major problem for us clinicians. Unfortunately, signs or symptoms cannot accurately predict the presence and severity of esophageal lesions in the development of esophageal strictures. In a study of the correlation between signs and symptoms of injury, including the presence of burns in the mouth and the severity of esophageal damage, Gaudreault et al. (*Pediatrics* 71:767, 1983) showed that only esophagoscopy appeared to be accurate in evaluating involvement of the esophagus after the ingestion of a caustic substance. The esophagus is not very forgiving in this regard. While normally time heals all wounds, where the esophagus is concerned time wounds all heals. The esophagus is a delicate organ that scars easily.—J.A.S., III

When Does Reflux Esophagitis Occur With Gastroesophageal Reflux in Infants? A Clinical and Endoscopic Study, and Correlation With Outcome
Patrick Ryan, Mervyn Lander, T. H. Ong, and Ross Shepherd (Royal Children's Hosp., Brisbane)
Aust. Paediatr. J. 19:90–93, June 1983   6–2

Clinical observations and investigations including cineradiography (90%), gastric scintiscans (25%), and acid reflux tests (20%) were used to diagnose gastroesophageal reflux (GOR) in infants. From 126 patients with symptomatic GOR, 62 (median age, 6.5 months) were selected for endoscopy for suspected esophagitis. Symptoms suggesting esophagitis were excessive crying due to suspected pain, irritability or sleep disturbance, or both (44%), feeding difficulties and dysphagia (44%), hematemesis (18%), and "torticollis" (8%). Patients were followed for 6–24 months until there either was improvement on medical management or antireflux operation was indicated.

Peptic esophagitis was observed in 34 (55%) of the 62 patients; 11 had severe changes, including 2 with strictures (1.6%); erythema or friability, or both, were observed in 23. Symptoms and signs of patients with gastroesophageal reflux with and without endoscopic esophagitis are compared in the table.

Satisfactory response to medical treatment was obtained in 41 (66%) symptomatic infants. The 2 patients with strictures required surgery after initial endoscopic dilatation and medical therapy. Of those with negative endoscopy results, 93% responded to conservative measures, compared to only 41% with esophagitis. Of the 11 patients with severe esophagitis, 9 (82%) required antireflux surgery, compared with 2 of 28 (7%) with no esophagitis and 11 of 23 (48%) with moderate esophagitis. Indications for surgery (22 cases) were persisting severe symptoms, recurrent aspiration, persisting severe esophagitis, continued failure to thrive, persisting frequent regurgitation with irritability and feeding difficulty.

Earlier studies have indicated that without active therapy approximately 60% of infants will be free of symptoms by age 18 months, with the greatest improvement when the child starts to sit upright. About 30% continue to have symptoms during childhood, approximately 5% develop

GASTROESOPHAGEAL REFLUX IN INFANTS AND CHILDREN WITH AND WITHOUT ENDOSCOPIC ESOPHAGITIS: COMPARISON OF ASSOCIATED SYMPTOMS AND SIGNS

Symptoms/Signs	Endoscopy +ve	Endoscopy -ve
Repeated regurgitation and/or rumination	34 (100%)	27 (96%)
Excessive crying "colic" and irritability*	29 (85%)	16 (58%)
Sleep disturbance*	27 (79%)	6 (21%)
Failure to thrive*	14 (41%)	3 (11%)
Haematemesis*	10 (29%)	1 (3%)
Recurrent respiratory disease	7 (21%)	9 (28%)
Sutcliffe-Sandifer Syndrome*	5 (15%)	0 (0%)
Neurological deficit*	4 (12%)	0 (0%)
Total	34	28

*Significant difference.
$P < .05$.
(Courtesy of Ryan, P., et al.: Aust. Paediatr. J. 19:90–93, June 1983.)

strictures, and 5% will die of pneumonia or malnutrition. Of those with esophagitis, 59% eventually require surgery. The importance of diagnostic endoscopy is emphasized to detect "pathologic" reflux, as cineradiology, scintiscan, motility studies, and pH monitoring detect only the presence or absence of GOR and are poor predictors of esophagitis.

When symptoms of GOR do not justify endoscopic evaluation, or where esophagitis is minimal, management should include postural therapy, thickening of feeds, antacids or antacid-alginate preparations.

When negative results of endoscopy do not correlate with symptoms, this may be due to reflux that causes heartburn in the absence of esophagitis. Positive results of endoscopy are an indication for aggressive medical management and are useful in predicting cases that are likely to require surgical intervention, or at least close follow-up.

Infant Seat as Treatment for Gastroesophageal Reflux
Susan R. Orenstein, Peter F. Whitington, and David M. Orenstein (Univ. of Tennessee, Memphis)
N. Engl. J. Med. 309:760–763, Sept. 29, 1983   6–3

The belief that use of an infant seat ("chalasia chair") aids in the prevention of gastroesophageal reflux was subjected to a prospective, controlled, crossover study. Nine infants, aged 0.5 to 4.2 months, with confirmed gastroesophageal reflux participated in 18 paired 2-hour postprandial trials at 60 degrees of elevation in an infant seat and in a prone position.

Positioning in an infant seat was associated with more gastroesophageal reflux than was prone positioning. The mean percentage of postprandial time with esophageal pH below 4.0 was 28.2% for seated and 12.8% for

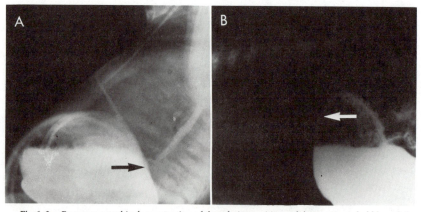

Fig 6–2.—Roentgenographic demonstration of the relative positions of the gastric air bubble and the gastroesophageal junction in an infant positioned in the infant seat at an elevation of 60 degrees (**A**) and prone (**B**). Arrows indicate locations of the gastroesophageal junction, which is submerged when a child is in the seat but not when he is prone. Of note is the spontaneous reflux of barium occurring while the infant is seated. (Courtesy of Orenstein, S.R., et al.: N. Engl. J. Med. 309:760–763, Sept. 29, 1983. Reprinted by permission of the New England Journal of Medicine.)

prone trials ($P = .023$). This difference was due largely to more episodes of reflux occurring in seated babies (16.0 vs 10.1 episodes; $P = .002$).

The infant seat is not therapeutic in gastroesophageal reflux in children younger than age 6 months; rather, it is detrimental when compared with simply placing the infant prone. One reason for this may be that the posterior entry of the esophagus into the stomach submerges the gastroesophageal junction in the 60-degree upright position of the infant seat (Fig 6–2).

▶ Judith Sondheimer, Associate Professor of Pediatrics, State University of New York Upstate Medical Center, comments:

"This study and the preceding one, both on gastroesophageal (GE) reflux, lead us to questions regarding therapy. The article by Orenstein et al. and its look-alike (*J. Pediatr.* 103:534, 1983) evaluate the hallowed 'upright position' commonly recommended for infants with GE reflux and find that it is not associated with a decrease in frequency or duration of reflux episodes when compared to the horizontal prone or prone upright position. She suggests that the supine upright position attained in the infant seat puts the GE junction under water in a pool of gastric contents, thus facilitating reflux during normal spontaneous relaxations of the lower esophageal sphincter (LES). Before discarding the infant seat in GE reflux therapy however, I would have two suggestions: (1) compare reflux frequency and duration in infants lying horizontal supine and lying 60 degrees upright supine in infant seats to see if there is *any* therapeutic advantage to the infant seat, and (2) try keeping an 8-month-old infant in a reflux harness. It is not simple, and I am not convinced the harness is entirely safe for home use. Older infants who might be able to crawl up the incline and roll over might entrap the neck in the harness straps. We need more studies like these to evaluate other 'time-honored' aspects of reflux therapy, e.g., thick feedings, small feedings, and frequent feedings, to see if any is worth the effort.

"The study by Ryan et al. concludes that patients with esophagitis are less responsive to 'medical management' than are those without symptoms suggesting esophagitis. This conclusion fits with my clinical experience, but leaves unanswered the important question of why these patients are so hard to treat. In the presence of esophagitis, the LES pressure usually is reduced. Does this lowered barrier allow for more frequent reflux? Is the LES of the patient with esophagitis more likely to relax spontaneously and allow reflux? Distal esophageal peristaltic activity may be feeble in the presence of esophagitis. Does this factor perpetuate GE reflux? Is the distal esophageal smooth muscle less responsive to cholinergics in the presence of esophagitis? Clearly, there is much to learn about therapy of GE reflux."

Oral Rehydration in Hypernatremic and Hyponatremic Diarrheal Dehydration: Treatment With Oral Glucose-Electrolyte Solution
Daniel Pizarro, Gloria Posada, Nora Villavicencio, Edgar Mohs (Natl. Children's Hosp., San Jose, Costa Rica) and Myron M. Levine (Univ. of Maryland)
Am. J. Dis. Child. 137:730–734, August 1983   6–4

The presence of hypernatremia or hyponatremia in infants with abnormal water losses caused by diarrhea and vomiting complicates the treatment of this condition. The safety and efficacy of oral rehydration were assessed in the treatment of 94 well-nourished, bottle-fed infants with hypernatremic (61 patients) or hyponatremic (33 patients) diarrheal dehydration.

All the hypernatremic infants and 25 of those who were hyponatremic received two thirds of the total fluid volume as glucose-electrolyte solution containing 90 mmol of sodium per liter and one third as plain water. The remaining 8 hyponatremic infants received glucose-electrolyte solution alone. Administration of the oral glucose-electrolyte solution rapidly and successfully rehydrated all 61 hypernatremic infants to a state of normal hydration (mean, 8.5 hours), as well as 31 of the 33 infants with hyponatremia (mean, 10 hours). However, 2 hypernatremic infants required intravenous fluids during the maintenance phase to keep up with continuing diarrheal losses and were considered treatment failures (failure rate, 3%). In addition to the 2 hyponatremic infants who were not successfully rehydrated, 1 of the successfully rehydrated infants could not keep pace with diarrheal fluid losses and required intravenous fluids, for a treatment failure rate of 9%.

Mean serum sodium levels decreased to normal in the hypernatremic infants and increased to normal in the hyponatremic infants. Net sodium gain in the hyponatremic infants who received no free water was greater than that in those who did. Overt convulsions occurred in 5 hypernatremic patients during the course of oral rehydration. This 8% rate of convulsions compared favorably with a 14% rate previously encountered when intravenous rehydration was used.

Infants with overt diarrheal dehydration and hypernatremia can be treated successfully with an oral rehydration regimen that uses a glucose-electrolyte solution containing 90 mmole of sodium per liter, alternating with plain water. In children with hyponatremia, administration of glucose-electrolyte solution alone, without extra water, gives superior results because of the higher sodium intake.

Differential Leukocyte Count in Acute Gastroenteritis: Aid to Early Diagnosis

Shai Ashkenazi, Yaakov Amir, Gabriel Dinari, Tommy Schonfeld, and Menachem Nitzan

Clin. Pediatr. (Phila.) 22:356–358, May 1983   6–5

Precise etiologic diagnosis is important in patients with acute gastroenteritis for which specific treatment is available, e.g., shigellosis. It has been suggested that 85% of these patients have more band than segmental neutrophils in peripheral blood smears. Total and differential leukocyte counts were evaluated as an aid in the differentiation of bacterial and nonbacterial infection in 238 infants with acute gastroenteritis seen at the Beilinson Medical Center in Petah Tikva, Israel.

TOTAL AND DIFFERENTIAL LEUKOCYTE COUNT IN 238 PATIENTS
WITH ACUTE GASTROENTERITIS

Etiologic Agent	Number of Patients	Age (Years)	WBC (10^3/cu mm)	B/N Ratio*	Absolute Band Count (/cu mm)	Patients with More Bands Than Neutrophils
"Nonbacterial"	46	5.03 ± 0.56†	8.43 ± 0.47†	0.08 ± 0.01†	383 ± 102†	—
E. Coli	12	0.86 ± 0.16	9.05 ± 0.77	0.09 ± 0.03	411 ± 181	—
Campylobacter	25	1.05 ± 0.60	10.30 ± 0.80	0.23 ± 0.04 $p < 0.001‡$	1352 ± 488 $p < 0.01‡$	6 (24%)
Salmonella	25	3.86 ± 0.71	9.32 ± 0.76	0.22 ± 0.05 $p < 0.01‡$	983 ± 244 $p < 0.05‡$	3 (12%)
Shigella	130	5.6 ± 0.29	8.85 ± 0.24	0.38 ± 0.02 $p < 0.001‡$	2021 ± 123 $p < 0.001‡$	42 (32%)

*B/N ratio = ratio between band and band plus mature neutrophil count.
†All results are expressed as mean ± SEM.
‡P values calculated as compared with the nonbacterial group. Significant differences in the absolute band count also were found between the *Shigella* compared with the *Campylobacter* ($P < .02$), *Salmonella* ($P < .01$), and *Escherichia coli* ($P < .001$) groups.
(Courtesy of Ashkenazi, S., et al.: Clin. Pediatr. (Phila.) 22:356–358, May 1983.)

Total white blood cell (WBC) counts were similar among the various etiologic groups, but variations in the differential counts were marked (table). Infants in the *Shigella, Salmonella,* and *Campylobacter* groups had significantly higher absolute band counts than those found in the *Escherichia coli* or nonbacterial groups. These differences were even more pronounced when the leftward shift was expressed as the ratio between band forms and the total neutrophil count (B/N ratio). Infants with shigellosis had the highest absolute band counts and the highest B/N ratio, and these were significantly higher than in infants with *Campylobacter* ($P < .02$), *Salmonella* ($P < .01$), and *E. coli* ($P < .001$) infections. A B/N ratio greater than 0.10 differentiated the *Shigella, Salmonella,* and *Campylobacter* groups from those with *E. coli* and nonbacterial gastroenteritis with a sensitivity of 84.3% and a specificity of 74.5%. The predictive value for shigellosis obtained from this ratio was 3.6. Serial leukocyte counts in 10 infants showed the leftward shift to disappear after 2 days, reflecting clinical improvement.

The results confirm the conclusion that the total WBC count is of little value in differentiating bacterial from nonbacterial gastroenteritis. However, a B/N ratio greater than 0.10 should lead one to suspect *Shigella, Salmonella,* or *Campylobacter* gastroenteritis until the results of stool culture are available.

Changing Incidence of Infantile Hypertrophic Pyloric Stenosis
E. G. Knox, E. Armstrong, and R. Haynes (Univ. of Birmingham)
Arch. Dis. Child. 58:582–585, August 1983   6–6

A report from Scotland had noted an unprecedented increase in infantile hypertrophic pyloric stenosis (IHPS) as 2.2/1,000 births in 1970–1977, 5.2/1,000 births in 1978, and 8.8/1,000 births in 1979. The present study considered the possibility of past underdiagnosis or present overdiagnosis, of demographic change (IHPS is more frequent in earlier than in later births), and of changing ethnic distribution, all factors that would influence outcome.

The incidence of IHPS per 1,000 live births in the West Midlands Health Region increased from 125 in 1974 to 210 in 1980, or from 1.88/1,000 to 3.11/1,000. The corresponding figures for boys increased from 2.85 to 5.01 between 1974 and 1980; for girls, they increased from 0.87 to 1.15. An analysis of treatment procedures indicated an increase in surgical cases from 1.46 in 1974 to 2.64 in 1980.

Looking for the causes of these changes, another study found that 22% of IHPS patients were being breast-fed at age 1 week compared with 15.9% of controls. It was suggested that some factor transmitted in the milk might contribute to the etiology of IHPS. In the area of the present study, incidence of breast-feeding increased from 48% in 1975 to 63% in 1980, a proportional increase of 31%.

▶ The rise in the incidence of pyloric stenosis in Great Britain appears to be a real phenomenon. This was first noted in Scotland 5 years ago. Shortly thereafter, Wales and then Manchester also noted an "unprecedented" rise in the incidence of hypertrophic pyloric stenosis (Walsworth-Bell, J. T.: *J. Epidemiol. Community Health* 37:149, 1983). This spread is heading our way, with Ireland now reporting a 450% increase in the incidence of pyloric stenosis between the years 1971 and 1983 (Grant et al.: *Lancet* 1:1177, 1984). If whatever is causing this leaks into the North Atlantic, it is liable to hit the United States with a tidal wave. Actually, many pediatric surgeons here have felt that they are seeing more and more cases of pyloric stenosis.

In the hands of experienced clinicians, the diagnosis of hypertrophic pyloric stenosis is fairly straightforward in most cases. The appropriate age, a history of projective vomiting, observation of peristaltic waves crossing the anterior abdominal wall, and palpation of the pyloric "olive" are sufficient indications for operation. When some of the clinical findings are unclear, however, we or the surgeons must resort to other more definitive tests. Until recently, the barium upper gastrointestinal tract series has been the radiologic diagnostic method of choice. Although accurate, the barium examination involves the use of radiation and the introduction of additional fluid into an already obstructed stomach. A few years back, we commented here in the YEAR BOOK on the role of ultrasound in the diagnosis of pyloric stenosis. For some reason it still has not caught on in many centers. I don't know why, because every report to date shows the usefulness of this procedure. A recent report (*Radiology* 147:499, 1983) strongly suggests that ultrasound be the initial diagnostic imaging procedure in patients suspected of having hypertrophic pyloric stenosis whose clinical features are atypical. If the results on ultrasound are positive, no other procedure (other than surgery) is necessary. If ultrasound findings are equivocal or normal, an upper gastrointestinal tract series should be performed to evaluate the cause of the vomiting further. It should be noted that normal electrolyte values do not exclude the diagnosis of pyloric stenosis. Some 40%

of all infants with documented hypertrophic pyloric stenosis are presenting now with normal serum electrolyte concentrations (Touloukian, R. J., et al.: *J. Pediatr. Surg.* 18:394, 1983).

Why there may be an increasing rise in the incidence of pyloric stenosis is puzzlesome. The report by Knox et al. suggests that the wider practice of breast-feeding may be related etiologically to this increased incidence. Breast milk contains very high concentrations of prostaglandins such as prostaglandin E_2, which is known to increase the frequency and strength of contractions of the pylorus. This really seems terribly far-fetched, and one would be willing to bet that the increased frequency of pyloric stenosis and the increased trends toward breast-feeding in Great Britain are coincidental phenomena. I will go out on a limb and actually say that if the point of all this is to revert back to the use of cow's milk, it will result in "udder" failure (pardon the pun).—J.A.S., III

Congenital Lactase Deficiency
E. Savilahti, K. Launiala, and P. Kuitunen
Arch. Dis. Child. 58:246–252, April 1983   6–7

Congenital lactase deficiency is one of at least 20 rare autosomal recessive disorders that are excessively common in Finland. The clinical and laboratory findings are reported on 16 infants with congenital lactase deficiency (CLD) who were treated at a university hospital in Helsinki (13 patients) or Kuopio, Finland (3), in the past 17 years.

The 16 patients came from 12 families; none of the parents exhibited symptoms after eating lactose. In each case, the mother noted watery diarrhea in the neonate, generally after the first feed of breast milk, and at the latest by age 10 days. Lactose malabsorption was verified at a mean age of 36 days (range, 3 to 90 days) by which time the infants were dehydrated and all but 1 weighed less than at birth. No infant was in vascular collapse.

Subsequent lactose removal stopped the watery diarrhea, and lactose-free feeding was begun. (Six infants received Nutramigen; 10 received a soy-based formula.) At that time mean weight (for age) was -2.8 SDs and mean height was -1.2 SDs. At age 1 year, mean weight was -1.0 SD and mean height was -0.8 SD. At age 2 (13 cases) mean weight was -0.5 SD and mean height was -0.5 SD. In 5 patients older than age 10 the catch-up growth has been complete.

Allergic symptoms developed in 1 infant in each of the dietary groups. When the infants were being breast-fed, thin-layer chromatography demonstrated a lactose concentration of 20 to 90 gm/L in feces. In 15 of 24 lactose tolerance tests performed on 13 infants, no significant increase in blood glucose levels was observed; the largest increase seen was 0.8 mmol/L at 40 minutes. Abnormal absorption was seen in only 2 infants when testing was carried out during lactose feeding or within 1 week of its elimination; in each of these infants, later absorption tests were normal.

Four early jejunal specimens showed slight to partial villous atrophy, but in later specimens villous height was normal. Compared with that of age-matched control subjects, mean height of epithelial cells was reduced, and there were significantly fewer intraepithelial lymphocytes.

Diagnosis of CLD, as opposed to acquired lactase deficiency, was based on the finding of lower lactase activities in jejunal biopsy specimens, although there was some overlap between those from patients with CLD and those with acquired lactase deficiency. Except in 1 case, values for maltase and sucrase activities were normal.

In this series, the diagnosis of CLD was based on the finding of a selective deficiency of lactase and a normal or near-normal morphology in jejunal biopsy specimens. The permanence of this deficiency can be followed by a lactose tolerance test.

▶ John N. Udall, Assistant Professor of Pediatrics, Harvard Medical School, and Assistant in Pediatrics, Pediatric Gastrointestinal and Nutrition Unit, Massachusetts General Hospital, comments:

"This interesting and provocative study once again raises the question of the frequency of congenital lactase deficiency. Some have doubted the existence of this disorder because secondary lactase deficiency occurs so commonly early in life with malnutrition, rotavirus enteritis, cow's milk protein allergy, and other diseases that cause small intestinal villous atrophy. It is difficult to separate primary from secondary lactase deficiency. Lebenthal and Rossi (*Textbook of Gastroenterology and Nutrition in Infancy,* Raven Press, New York, 1981, pp. 673–688) have suggested that diagnosis of the congenital deficiency be established on the basis of (1) a history of diarrhea the first few days of life following the introduction of breast milk or a lactose-containing formula; (2) lactose malabsorption documented by lactose absorption or breath-hydrogen tests, or by acid stools that contain reducing substances; (3) dramatic clinical improvement when lactose is eliminated from the diet; (4) little or no lactase in a biopsy specimen of small intestinal tissue obtained when the infant is thriving, and (5) normal morphology of the small intestine on microscopic examination.

"It is of concern that the authors noted villous atrophy in some biopsy specimens and that enterocolitis was present in one patient secondary to the soy-protein formula. Furthermore, full recovery was not attained for many months, because weight at age 1 year was 1.0 SD below controls. Finally, 2 of their subjects were reported elsewhere to have antibody to rotavirus (*J. Infect. Dis.* 148:1166–1167, 1983), a finding suggestive of an earlier viral infection. The authors, aware of these problems, state in the discussion that jejunal biopsy specimens were taken months later when children were thriving.

"Diagnosis of congenital lactase deficiency must be established after a thorough clinical and laboratory evaluation using accepted criteria. Only then can we hope to determine the frequency of this condition in various populations."

α_1-Antitrypsin Deficiency

Daniel Alagille (Univ. Paris-Sud)
Hepatology 4:(Suppl.)11S–14S, 1984

6–8

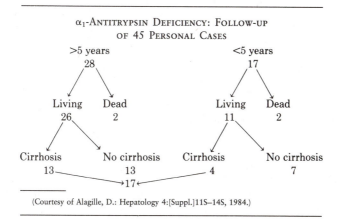

<small>α₁-ANTITRYPSIN DEFICIENCY: FOLLOW-UP
OF 45 PERSONAL CASES</small>

(Courtesy of Alagille, D.: Hepatology 4:[Suppl.]11S–14S, 1984.)

Liver disease from α_1-antitrypsin deficiency occurs only in Pi ZZ homozygous children. Eleven percent of such infants have prolonged neonatal cholestasis. Cholestasis is complete and permanent in about half the affected children. Nonspecific biochemical signs of obstructive jaundice are present, with no α_1-globulin peak on serum electrophoresis. The diagnosis is confirmed by determining serum antitrypsin activity and by genetic Pi typing. Typical, periodic acid-Schiff-positive granules are seen in periportal liver cells.

Spontaneous clinical regression is typical of this cholestatic syndrome and usually occurs before age 6 months. The later course of liver disease is variable. Twenty-five of the author's 45 Pi ZZ infants with prolonged neonatal cholestasis later developed cirrhosis. Poor prognostic factors included jaundice after age 6 months, early splenomegaly, persistent hard hepatomegaly, liver dysfunction, and early portal fibrosis. Infants with an early pattern of few interlobular bile ducts had the poorest outcome. Nineteen of 25 patients initially seen with cirrhosis had portal hypertension, and 8 of those with cirrhosis died in childhood (table). Six of the 8 deaths from progressive liver failure occurred before age 4 years. Seven of these patients had few interlobular bile ducts. The other patient died of intercurrent sepsis.

A protein-restricted diet and portosystemic shunting have been beneficial to children with cirrhosis, but the long-term course of such patients is unpredictable. A low-protein diet is especially indicated when signs of hepatic encephalopathy appear. Four of the author's patients underwent portacaval shunting after many severe episodes of gastrointestinal bleeding; 3 are survivors. The results must be compared with those obtainable by liver transplantation.

▶ It is not common for us to present four articles in a row dealing with the same topic. This past year, however, must be said to be the year of α_1-antitrypsin deficiency. More studies appeared dealing with the natural outcome from the results of liver transplantation and prenatal diagnosis than ever before.

You might question the value of taking up so much space with these reports. I believe there is some benefit in doing this. The most common form of the deficiency, which occurs in persons who are homozygous for a Pi phenotype of the protein, has a prevalence of 1 case per 2,000 in whites. This makes this disorder at least twice as common as cystic fibrosis, which takes up its fair share of the YEAR BOOK each year.

α_1-Antitrypsin deficiency is a genetic deficiency of the plasma protease inhibitor α_1-antitrypsin. We all know this leads to a degenerative lung disease and fatal cirrhosis of the liver. At the protein level, the deficiency is caused by the substitution of a glutamic acid for lysine at residue 342 in human α_1-antitrypsin. At the DNA level, the amino acid substitution is caused by a C to A transition at a corresponding location in the gene. All this results in production of a protein that is structurally abnormal and thus is functionally deficient.

α_1-Antitrypsin normally protects the body against enzymes that tend to destroy certain tissues. Its specificity is actually against released elastase. Curiously, α_1-antitrypsin and another plasma protease inhibitor, antithrombin III, share a similar structure, which has been estimated to have arisen by divergent evolution from a common ancestral protein some 500 million years ago. While α_1-antitrypsin protects the body against elastase, antithrombin III controls coagulation by inhibiting activation of clotting. The only reason for mentioning all this is that very recently a mutation in the DNA gene of α_1-antitrypsin was reported that converted this material in a 14-year-old boy to a substance that was virtually identical to antithrombin III. The boy died of a bleeding disorder (Owen, M. C., et al.: *N. Engl. J. Med.* 309:694, 1983).

What follows in the next three articles is a discussion of the outcome of α_1-antitrypsin deficiency. These studies are particularly timely because all this is a very tricky issue. The trickiness lies with the fact that if you can predict that someone is likely to do poorly with α_1-antitrypsin deficiency, there are at least two significant therapeutic options. In highly selected cases of patients in whom development of significant liver disease is likely, some patients will improve remarkably after portacaval shunt (Starzl, T. E., et al.: *Lancet* 2:424, 1983). The only definitive therapy currently, however, is liver transplantation, which will be discussed later on in this chapter. Just as important a reason for trying to determine as much as one can about the prognosis in α_1-antitrypsin deficiency is the fact that we now have a prenatal diagnostic tool in hand that can be done by simple amniocentesis. This technique, using DNA isolated from cultured amniotic cells, provides a safer method for prenatal diagnosis of α_1-antitrypsin deficiency than has been available before (*N. Engl. J. Med.* 310:639, 1984).

Thus, while this co-editor of the YEAR BOOK normally wouldn't give a duck a drink of water if he owned Lake Michigan, he has selected a series of articles dealing with one topic whose time has truly come. So read on. . . . —J.A.S., III

Early Assessment of Evolution of Liver Disease Associated With Antitrypsin Deficiency in Childhood

Gabriella Nebbia, Michèle Hadchouel, Michel Odievre, and Daniel Alagille (Univ. Paris-Sud)

J. Pediatr. 102:661–665, May 1983   6–9

Neonatal cholestasis usually subsides, but the further course of liver disease is variable; a bimodal evolution has been shown, either with development of cirrhosis or with a long-term favorable course. In a study in 45 children with neonatal cholestasis associated with α_1-antitrypsin (α_1-AT) deficiency (phenotype Pi type Z), certain hallmarks that enable early assessment of prognosis were identified.

Mean serum concentration of α_1-AT was 54.23 mg/100 ml. Pi type ZZ was found in 44 children and Pi type Z− was found in 1. Six siblings had Pi type ZZ but no history of neonatal cholestasis. In 38 patients a liver specimen was obtained by needle or surgical biopsy before age 6 months. Follow-up included laboratory investigations, serial liver biopsies, and, for some children, laparoscopy. Patients were divided into two groups.

Twenty-five children with cirrhosis diagnosed by 8 years of age (group 1) had at least two of the following characteristics: hard hepatomegaly, sometimes nodular; portal hypertension, assessed by direct measurement or evidenced by esophageal varices; nodules on the liver surface, detected by laparoscopy or laparotomy; or regeneration nodules on histologic examination. Group 2 included 20 children without the above characteristics and considered to be progressing favorably.

Nine of the 25 children in group 1 were small for gestational age. Jaundice was noted in 12 during the first week of life and in all 25 by the tenth week. Slightly firm hepatomegaly was present in all 25 and the spleen tip was palpable in 10. An early biopsy specimen from 19 patients showed cirrhosis in 3, significant portal fibrosis with ductular proliferation in 8, slight portal fibrosis in 2, and paucity of interlobular ducts in 6.

Serum bilirubin concentration returned to normal by the sixth month in 17 patients and by the eighth month in 2. Increasingly severe jaundice and a downhill course to liver failure and death occurred in the other 6 children by the fourth year. The liver remained large and firm in all children, and nodules were eventually palpable in 9. Gastroesophageal varices were found in 12 patients and hematemesis occurred in 6. Cirrhosis appeared to be well tolerated clinically. Liver function tests showed some degree of impairment in all patients, and a moderate elevation in level of serum glutamic pyruvic transaminase (SGPT) activity was constantly found in 21.

Four of the 20 patients in group 2 were small for gestational age. Jaundice began during the first week of life in 11 infants and in all 20 before the eighth week. Slightly firm hepatomegaly was present in all and the spleen tip was palpable in 6. Although some of the children in this group had only minimal abnormalities, histologic evidence of significant portal fibrosis in some cases made long-term prognosis less certain.

During the cholestatic phase, the only effective means of establishing prognosis is by liver biopsy. The amount of portal fibrosis and ductular proliferation are good criteria. Paucity of interlobular ducts and small size for gestational age seem to be characteristic of this condition. As the right hepatic lobe often shrinks and only a hard epigastric mass indicates continuing liver disease, careful clinical examination is of great importance. The level of SGPT activity proved to be the most sensitive liver function test. However, persistent normalization of liver function tests, although rare, constitutes the only clear-cut biochemical evidence of good outcome. Normalization of liver size and consistency was most important from a clinical point of view.

Prospective Study of Children With α_1-Antitrypsin Deficiency: Eight-Year-Old Follow-up
T. Sveger (Univ. of Lund)
J. Pediatr. 104:91–94, January 1984   6–10

Deficiency of α_1-antitrypsin predisposes patients to both juvenile liver disease and the early onset of emphysema. The results of screening for α_1-antitrypsin (α_1AT) deficiency in 200,000 Swedish infants in 1972–1974 were reviewed. A total of 183 affected children aged 4 years were followed up, and 169 were available for evaluation at age 8 years. There were 117 PiZ, 2 PiZ⁻, 49 PiSZ, and 1 PiS⁻ children in the study.

Severe physical abnormalities were found in 3 PiZ children and 1 PiSZ child. Seven PiZ children had atopic dermatitis. One with PiSZ had psoriasis. Mean height and weight were comparable to those of normal Swedish children. No child had clinical evidence of liver disease. Levels of γ-glutamyltransferase were elevated in 6% of PiZ children, and alanine aminotransferase values were abnormal in 29 of 79 PiZ children without neonatal cholestasis. Bronchitis lasting over a week occurred in 23 PiZ and 11 PiSZ subjects, 8 of whom also had asthma. Five patients had had uncomplicated pneumonia. Individual children had juvenile rheumatoid arthritis and gluten-induced enteropathy.

The prognosis for PiZ infants with neonatal liver disease is better than previously thought, but the chance of complete recovery remains uncertain. The pathophysiology of liver disease in α_1AT deficiency is poorly understood. New approaches to preventing both liver disease and emphysema may be developed in the near future. Children with α_1AT deficiency should be warned not to smoke.

Outcome of Liver Disease Associated With α_1-Antitrypsin Deficiency (PiZ): Implications for Genetic Counseling and Antenatal Diagnosis
H. T. Psacharopoulos, A. P. Mowat, P. J. L. Cook, P. A. Carlile, B. Portmann, and C. H. Rodeck
Arch. Dis. Child. 58:882–887, November 1983   6–11

Several studies confirm the association between genetic deficiency of α_1-antitrypsin (protease inhibitor phenotype, PiZ) and serious liver disease in children. Information concerning the frequency and prognosis of liver disease in the fetus with PiZ would be of obvious value to parents faced with the option of terminating a PiZ pregnancy. Hepatic features were reviewed in 136 children with PiZ, 82 of whom were studied prospectively. The pattern of liver disease also was studied in 27 observed families with more than 1 PiZ child and in 20 previously described families.

Of the 82 prospectively studied children, 74 had chronic liver disease; in 67, liver disease developed in infancy. Of the latter group, jaundice developed in 62. Life-threatening hemorrhage developed in 8 infants. All 67 infants had hepatomegaly, but only 50% had splenomegaly. Two had serious cerebral hemorrhage with permanent neurologic sequelae. Nineteen children died of liver disease at ages ranging from 7 months to 17 years; 19 have cirrhosis and 14 have persisting clinical or biochemical evidence of liver disease. Fifteen children have no clinical features of liver disease and now have normal results on liver function tests at ages ranging from 9 months to 11 years. Four children were seen initially at ages 5–7 years; 2 presenting with cirrhosis had hematemesis and ascites, respectively, and 2 had hepatosplenomegaly and moderate hepatic fibrosis. The child with ascites died of liver disease 18 months later. The 3 survivors have persistently abnormal results on liver function tests. Of 10 PiZ children aged 8 months to 14 years who were identified after liver disease developed in a sibling, 7 had no clinical or laboratory evidence of liver disease and 3 had elevated aspartate aminotransferase values; on liver biopsy, portal tract fibrosis, was found in 2 of the 3. The outcome of liver disease in 34 families with 2 affected children was similar in both children. Analysis of the families with 1 severely affected child indicated that if a first PiZ child of PiZ heterozygote parents has unresolved liver disease, there is a 78% likelihood that a second PiZ child will have similar liver disease.

The results confirm the frequent association of α_1-antitrypsin deficiency with serious liver disease in infancy and early childhood. Because the risk to any subsequent fetus before protease inhibitor phenotyping is about 20% when both parents are PiMZ, prenatal diagnosis by fetoscopy, fetal blood sampling, and protease inhibitor phenotyping is an option that should be considered. Skilled counseling and support are essential if the procedure is not to be followed by long-term morbidity.

▶ John D. Lloyd-Still, Chief of the Division of Gastroenterology, Children's Memorial Hospital, Chicago, comments on the three reports dealing with α_1-antitrypsin deficiency:

"α_1-Antitrypsin deficiency is the most common cause of 'medical' neonatal hepatitis syndromes (in contrast to biliary atresia that requires surgery). This study and the two preceding ones presented here provide much needed data on prognosis. Since the recognition of hepatic complications of this disorder in 1968, long-term follow-up has been limited. The Swedish study updates the 8-year follow-up on a prospective study of 200,000 newborns. The 4-year follow-up has been reported previously (*Acta Paediatr. Scand.* 70:171, 1981). By 8 years of age, 6 of the 183 α_1-antitrypsin-deficient children had died. However, 83% of the PiZ children had had no clinical signs of liver disease in infancy. The data on lung complications are too limited for comment. The optimistic findings on this prospective study are in marked contrast to the other two studies from large referral centers in Paris and London. When clinical manifestations of hepatic involvement (neonatal cholestasis, hepatosplenomegaly, or cirrhosis) lead to the diagnosis of α_1-antitrypsin deficiency, significant chronic liver disease will develop in approximately 75% of the patients. The persistence of hepatosplenomegaly and elevated liver enzymes identifies these patients. Infants small for gestational age seem to be more susceptible, perhaps because of deficiencies of serum inhibitors (*Pediatr. Res.* 18:215A, 1984). If a family has 1 child with chronic liver disease secondary to α_1-antitrypsin deficiency, there is a 78% chance that siblings with the same disorder will have a similar clinical picture.

"Other recent developments include the assignment of α_1-antitrypsin to chromosome 14 by somatic cell hybrid analysis (*Proc. Natl. Acad. Sci U.S.A.* 79:870, 1982) and the first report of the prenatal diagnosis of α_1-antitrypsin deficiency by direct analysis of the mutation site in the gene (*N. Engl. J. Med.* 310:639, 1984). Transplantation offers the only method of returning the level of α_1-antitrypsin to normal (ibid. 302:272, 1980). Some preliminary evidence suggests that breast-feeding may lessen some of the adverse effects of this disease by supplying antiprotease activity (*Pediatr. Res.* 18:216A, 1984). This seems yet another advantage for breast-feeding."

Human Liver Transplantation: Analysis of Data on 540 Patients From Four Centers

Bruce F. Scharschmidt (Univ. of California, San Francisco)
Hepatology 4:(Suppl.)95S–101S, 1984   6–12

Data were reviewed on liver transplantation in 540 patients from four centers in the United States and Western Europe (Table 1). A total of 33 different diagnoses were represented. One fourth of the transplants were done for neoplastic disease, 43.5% for cirrhosis of all types, and 17% for neonatal cholestasis. The overall 1- and 3-year survival rates for patients with neoplastic disease were 26% and 12%, respectively, and differed little

TABLE 1.—Transplant Centers Providing Data
for This Analysis

Location	Corresponding surgeon	Total no. of patients
University of Pittsburgh Pittsburgh, Pa.	Dr. Thomas E. Starzl	296
University Hospital Groningen Groningen, The Netherlands	Dr. Rudd A. F. Krom	26
University of Hannover Hannover, West Germany	Dr. Rudolf Pichlmayr	81
University of Cambridge Cambridge, England	Dr. Keith Rolles	137

(Courtesy of Scharschmidt, B.F.: Hepatology 4:[Suppl.]95S–101S, 1984.)

TABLE 2.—SURVIVAL ANALYSIS BY DISEASE AND DATE OF TRANSPLANT FOR ALL FOUR CENTERS*

Disease	All patients					Transplant before January 1, 1980					Transplant after January 1, 1980				
	No.	Median survival (months)	Survival probability at intervals (%)			No.	Median survival (months)	Survival probability at intervals (%)			No.	Median survival (months)	Survival probability at intervals (%)		
			≥3 mos	≥1 yr	≥3 yr			≥3 mos	≥1 yr	≥3 yr			≥3 mos	≥1 yr	≥3 yr
Tumors (all types)	139	4.1	50.3	25.8	12.5	77	2.9	46.8	20.8	11.7	62	5.9	54.7	32.8	—
Hepatocellular carcinoma	88	5.4	55.7	32.9	16.7	47	4.8	55.3	29.8	17.0	41	8.1	56.0	37.0	—
Cholangiocarcinoma	36	2.6	47.0	17.4	7.0	22	1.7	31.8	9.1	4.6	14	9.7	71.4	31.8	—
Cirrhosis (all types)	235	2.2	45.9	36.5	28.6	116	1.7	40.5	29.3	21.6	119	5.2	51.6	44.9	40.8
Alcoholic	25	1.1	24.0	20.0	20.0	20	1.3	25.0	20.0	20.0	5	0.6	20.0	20.0	—
Nonalcoholic (all types)	210	2.9	48.6	38.5	29.4	96	1.9	43.8	31.2	21.9	114	5.8	53.0	46.0	41.7
Primary biliary	62	5.3	51.1	41.6	37.6	18	2.0	38.9	33.3	27.8	44	6.4	56.4	45.0	45.0
Postnecrotic/chronic active	48	1.1	43.8	41.2	30.0	13	1.2	38.5	30.8	23.1	35	1.0	46.1	46.1	39.5
Biliary atresia/neonatal cholestasis	90	4.2	50.3	39.1	28.2	52	2.0	38.5	25.0	15.4	38	—	69.2	63.9	—
Sclerosing cholangitis	19	2.0	33.6	20.2	20.2	7	2.5	28.6	14.3	14.3	12	1.8	37.3	24.8	24.8
Metabolic disorders (all types)	35	28.2	55.1	51.8	44.4	16	3.0	43.8	37.8	31.2	19	—	65.5	65.5	65.5
α₁-antitrypsin deficiency	24	28.2	56.5	51.6	41.3	10	4.0	50.0	40.0	30.0	14	—	61.3	61.3	61.3
Wilson's disease	5	—	80.0	80.0	80.0	2	—	100	100	100	3	—	66.6	66.6	—
Miscellaneous															
Budd-Chiari	14	—	71.4	71.4	54.0	5	—	60.0	60.0	60.0	9	19.9	77.8	77.8	47.7
Acute hepatic failure	2	—	0	—	—	1	—	9	—	—	1	—	0	—	—
Caroli's disease	2	—	0	—	—	1	—	0	—	—	1	—	0	—	—
Congenital hepatic fibrosis	2	—	50	50	50	1	—	0	—	—	1	—	100	100	100
Nodular transformation	1	—	100	100	100	1	—	100	100	100	0	—	—	—	—

*Dashes indicate insufficient data.
(Courtesy of Scharschmidt, B.F.: Hepatology 4:[Suppl.]95S–101S, 1984.)

in patients receiving transplants before and after 1980 (Table 2). Among cirrhotic patients, those with alcoholic cirrhosis had the poorest 3-year survival (20%). Survival of patients with nonalcoholic cirrhosis increased after 1980. Patients with biliary atresia, sclerosing cholangitis, metabolic disease, and miscellaneous disorders had 3-year survival rates of 20% to 44% and showed a consistent trend toward better survival after 1980. Fewer than 40% of the 52 patients given a second liver transplant after the first failed survived to 1 year, and none survived beyond 3 years. Fewer than 10% of evaluable deaths were due to rejection; causes that were not necessarily directly liver related predominated.

Liver transplantation has had a better outcome in patients with non-neoplastic liver diseases than in those with liver tumors, and survival of the former has improved in recent years. This improvement may not be entirely attributable to the use of cyclosporine. The quality of life of transplant recipients who have survived for at least 4 months, judged from limited data on hospital time and functional status appears to be good. All but 5 of 184 such patients were considered to be fully rehabilitated; 3 were in fair and 2 were in poor condition. A survey of transplant recipients at one center indicated that more than 80% of patients who lived longer than a year had resumed their former work or activities.

▶ The history of liver transplantation dates back to the immediate post-World War II years when early experiments, largely in dogs, showed the technical feasibility of transplanting livers. The first human liver transplantation was performed in 1963 by Starzl and his associates, then at the University of Colorado in Denver. The first and several subsequent patients survived for only a short time. Although survival improved in the following years, the 1-year survival reported by the Starzl team prior to the use of cyclosporine (from 1963 to the late 1970s) ranged from only 24% to 33% in children. Because of these relatively discouraging results, liver transplantation during the first decade was performed almost exclusively by the Denver center, although small numbers of transplantations were reported from other parts of the world as well. The real turn-around in liver transplantation came with the introduction of cyclosporine as an immunosuppressive to help prevent rejection. In June of 1983, the National Institutes of Health held a Consensus Development Conference dealing with liver transplantation. The entire proceedings of that conference are contained in the journal *Hepatology* (4:[Suppl.], 1984). This article by Scharschmidt, which was, in fact, a presentation at that conference, reviews the world's literature and summarizes the results of transplantation in over 540 such operations carried out through the world as well as the several centers that are now doing this in the United States. In the past 3 to 4 years, a noticeable increase in the number of transplant recipients with 1-year survival has been achieved. One-year survival now approaches 70% in selected groups. At the time of the Consensus Conference, the longest survival after liver transplantation was over 13 years, and 6 patients had lived for more than a decade after this procedure. All these transplantations were performed during childhood. When decisions are made about the need for transplantation, two things must be held in the balance. Is the natural history of the problem with which the patient presents such that medical management is no longer likely to produce reasonable survivorship? Is transplantation likely to? It is not possible to review here each of the pros and cons regarding transplantation for the wide variety of pediatric disorders that it is capable of being used in. Some of these include extrahepatic biliary atresia, chronic active hepatitis, primary biliary cirrhosis, α_1-antitrypsin deficiency, Wilson's disease, Crigler-Najjar syndrome, tyrosinemia, Byler's disease, Wolman's disease, glycogen storage diseases, hereditary defects of urea cycle enzymes, disorders of lactate-pyruvate or amino acid metabolism, hepatic vein thrombosis, and primary sclerosing cholangitis. Additionally, transplantations have been done for malignancies involving the liver, but the outlook here has not been overwhelmingly encouraging. The YEAR BOOK reader is referred to the summary statement of the National Institutes of Health Consensus Development Conference for details concerning who are currently thought to be eligible candidates for transplantation.

No transplantation program will be successful without physicians and the public alike being more acutely aware of the need for organs. The event of death in a previously healthy child is such a devastating blow to the family and to the health care team that it is often difficult to broach the subject of organ donation at the time of such sorrow. This reason alone probably accounts for much of the shortage of organ donors in the pediatric age group. Nonetheless, numerous potential liver recipients have died while awaiting a new liver despite the fact that a national search was being conducted. Starzl et al. have put forth a plea in this regard (*Pediatrics* 71:856, 1983) and remind us how to contact the nearest organ procurement program via a nationwide transplant hotline operated by the North American Transplant Coordinators Organization (NAPCO). The national hotline for this is the following number: 800-24-ALERT.

Finally, one cannot provide enough kudos for Thomas Starzl. Obviously, many centers are now involved with liver transplantation and all seem to be doing a good job. Normally, however, it is not the first person to perform a procedure that receives the acclaim. It usually goes to the person who popularizes it. In the case of liver transplantation, Doctor Starzl is all at one time the same man.—J.A.S., III

Extrahepatic Biliary Atresia
Daniel Alagille (Univ. Paris-Sud)
Hepatology 4:(Suppl.)7S–10S, 1984   6–13

Extrahepatic biliary atresia (EHBA), the partial or total absence of permeable bile ducts between the porta hepatis and the duodenum, is the most common cause of extrahepatic cholestasis in infants. The reported incidence ranges from 1 in 8,000 to 1 in 10,000. Most cases can be diagnosed by ^{131}I-rose bengal testing and needle biopsy of the liver. The diagnosis is confirmed at exploration by complete dissection of the fibrous remnants and exploration of the porta hepatis.

All patients died before age 2 years until Kasai's operation was described in 1959. Presently 30% to 35% of patients are operated on successfully by hepatoportoenterostomy in some form. A total of 248 infants were

EHBA—Histologic Findings at Open Liver Biopsy
5 Years After Operation

Cirrhosis	
Micronodular	13
Macronodular	7
Biliary structures in portal areas	
Absent	8
Few	9
Present	3
Cell infiltration	
Absent	3
Moderate	13
Marked	14
Normal liver cells	20
No cholestasis	20

(Courtesy of Alagille, D.: Hepatology 4:[Suppl.]7S–10S, 1984.)

operated on at the author's center, 121 of them before 1977, and 37% were alive 5 years or more after operation. Ten of the 44 surviving patients have mild chronic icterus. The oldest is aged 14 years. The type of operation did not appear to influence long-term survival. Growth and general health are normal in all children but 1, including those who initially had severe growth retardation before closure of the jejunal external fistula. The histologic findings 5 years after operation are given in the table. The most impressive change apart from cirrhosis was the absence of bile ducts or ductules, but no histologic bile stasis was evident. Four patients underwent portosystemic shunting for variceal bleeding.

Surviving patients who were operated on for EHBA have for the most part led nearly normal lives despite the persistently abnormal appearance of the intrahepatic bile ducts and the presence of cirrhosis with portal hypertension. The effect of the liver damage on long-term survival remains to be determined. How bile is excreted in patients with absent intrahepatic bile ducts is uncertain; the role of lymphatic drainage is unclear.

▶ Extrahepatic biliary atresia is the most common cause of bile duct obstruction in the young infant. Biliary enteric anastomosis (the Kasai procedure) performed in the first 2 months of life provides significant improvement for at least 5 years in one third of patients, although cirrhosis and disappearance of the intrahepatic bile ducts occur with increasing age. While the success of this procedure cannot be predicted for the individual patient, it should be used as initial therapy for extrahepatic biliary atresia. The current concepts regarding liver transplantation are that in the absence of severe hepatic decompensation in these children, liver transplantation is being delayed as long as possible to permit the child to achieve maximum growth. In children with successful Kasai's procedures, liver transplantation is being deferred until progressive cholestasis, hepatocellular decompensation, or severe portal hypertension supervene. Multiple attempts at the Kasai procedure render eventual transplantation technically more difficult and operationally more dangerous and therefore should be avoided in favor of liver transplantation. The status of liver transplantation for biliary atresia has been reviewed recently by Iwatuski et al. (*J. Surg.* 8:51, 1984) and by Ascher et al. (ibid., p. 57). Their data seem to imply that survival after liver transplantation of children with biliary atresia has been inferior to that of children with liver-based inborn metabolic errors. This seems to be partly due to the fact that previous major surgical procedures such as the Kasai procedure make the transplant operation more difficult. In addition, anatomical anomalies, such as hypoplastic, sclerotic, sometimes thrombosed portal veins, are more common in children with advanced biliary atresia. Nonetheless, in the cyclosporine era the survival of children who undergo liver transplantation for biliary atresia has increased almost to the level of overall survival in the pediatric cases as a whole.

If any of the readers of the YEAR BOOK are interested in a follow-up of reovirus type 3 infection and its relationship to biliary atresia, the data seem to continue to accumulate incriminating this virus in at least some cases of this disorder. In 1982, Morecki et al. (*N. Engl. J. Med.* 307:481, 1982) published results in which reovirus type 3 could be linked serologically to neonatal cholestatic syndromes. They showed that 68% of infants with biliary atresia had reovirus antibody, whereas only 8% of control infants did. This group has updated their data, which appear to be showing the same sorts of results (*Hepatology* 3:877, 1983). Unfortunately, not everybody in the world has been able to reproduce these findings. Some have found equal numbers of positive serologies in infants with biliary atresia and in control infants. The story of reovirus infection and biliary atresia just doesn't seem to want to settle down. Perhaps we should all go to Rio and enjoy ourselves while the protagonists fight it out.—J.A.S., III

Hepatic Fibrosis in Fetal Alcohol Syndrome: Pathologic Similarities to Adult Alcoholic Liver Disease
Jay H. Lefkowitch, Alan R. Rushton, and Kuo-Ching Feng-Chen
Gastroenterology 85:951–957, October 1983   6–14

The nature and pathogenesis of the hepatic injury in fetal alcohol syndrome (FAS) remain unclear, but the portal tract fibrosis described in recent cases resembles the changes found in adult alcohol-induced liver injury. The authors report the histologic findings in a liver biopsy specimen obtained from a girl aged 17 months with FAS. The mother acknowledged frequent alcohol abuse during the 38-week pregnancy.

Girl, aged 1 year, was diffusely hypotonic and could not sit without support. Delayed physical and motor development had been noted in the early months of life. Height and weight were below the third percentiles. Serum transaminase levels were twice normal. An EEG showed increased posterior rhythmic activity and hypersynchronous and slow drowsing rhythm. Hepatomegaly persisted at age 17 months, and the serum transaminase concentrations were markedly elevated. A liver biopsy specimen showed parenchymal fat with portal and perisinusoidal fibrosis. On electron microscopy, the perisinusoidal spaces contained deposits of intermediate and large collagen fibers, myofibroblasts, and subendothelial basement membrane-like material, as well as occasional Ito cells. When last seen at age 5½ years, the child exhibited continued growth retardation, was mentally dull, and had physical findings characteristic of FAS. Hepatosplenomegaly was absent. Truncal and limb ataxia was noted, without nystagmus.

The liver changes in this case of FAS resemble those seen in adult human alcoholic liver disease and in baboons. The accumulation of secretory material in the hepatocyte endoplasmic reticulum cisternae may reflect a chronic effect of ethanol in inhibiting glycoprotein secretion. The changes in hepatic collagen, lipid, and protein metabolism induced by alcohol in the fetal period may persist for some time after birth.

▶ This report and a few others that have shown essentially the same thing are truly sobering. Investigations of the fetal alcohol syndrome have clearly established a risk of multiple congenital anomalies, neurologic deficits, and growth retardation in the offspring of mothers drinking heavily during pregnancy. While these effects are believed to result from the toxic effects of ethanol or its metabolites (such as acetaldehyde), or both, and possible nutritional deficiencies, it is also possible that ethanol induces an impairment of umbilical circulation resulting in fetal hypoxia and acidosis. To make matters even worse alcohol can get out into breast milk and can affect an infant even after birth.

The only effective way of addressing the problem of the fetal alcohol syndrome is through appropriate education. Thus far, we have seen no apparent results, however. For people who abuse themselves, nature has neither rewards nor punishments. There are only consequences. In this case, unfortunately, the consequences are to the newborn infant.

Quiz: Can you name the top three alcohol-selling places in the United States? Answer: Nevada, District of Columbia, and New Hampshire. In Nevada, for example, the average volume in gallons drunk per person in the drinking-age population (age 14 years and older) for distilled spirits, wine, and beer was 8.9, 6.6, and 49.6 gallons, respectively. The reference for this staggering observation is from M. M. Hyman et al.: *Drinking, Drinkers, and Alcohol-Related Mortality and Hospitalizations* (Rutgers University Center of Alcohol Studies, New Brunswick, N. J., 1980). Utah is the state in the union with the least alcohol consumption, with 1.5 gallons of distilled spirits, 1.0 gallons of wine, and 21 gallons of beer per drinking-age person per year.—J.A.S., III

Portal Obstruction in Children: I. Clinical Investigation and Hemorrhage Risk

F. Alvarez, O. Bernard, F. Brunelle, P. Hadchouel, M. Odièvre, and D. Alagille (Hôp. de Bicêtre, Bicêtre, France)
J. Pediatr. 103:696–701, November 1983   6–15

One hundred eight children with obstruction of the portal vein were examined between 1958 and 1980. Symptoms included splenomegaly and gastrointestinal tract hemorrhage. On admission, liver function tests were

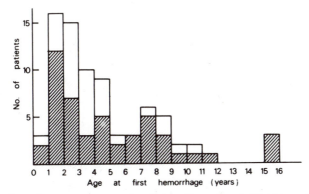

Fig 6–3.—Age at first spontaneous gastrointestinal tract hemorrhage in 78 children with portal vein obstruction. Grey area is idiopathic and white area is nonidiopathic. (Courtesy of Alvarez, F., et al.: J. Pediatr. 103:696–701, November 1983.)

normal in most children. The factor V value was most frequently abnormal in the coagulation tests.

Ultrasonography was performed in 37 children, and two direct signs of obstruction were present in all but 1. There was no normal portal vein on a scan through its axis. Angiograms included splenoportography in 50 children and superior mesenteric arteriography in 28 of these 50. No complication was reported. Eighty-six children (79%) experienced at least one episode of gastrointestinal tract bleeding. One or more episodes of spontaneous gastrointestinal tract bleeding occurred in 78 patients, in 45 before the age of 4 years (Fig 6–3). No difference in risk was found between the idiopathic and nonidiopathic groups. Two of the 108 children died, 1 during an episode of gastrointestinal tract bleeding and the other of heart disease; both had severe congenital heart disease. Fiberoptic endoscopy of the esophagus, performed in 81, showed varices in 79. Gastric varices were found in 16 of the 56 (28%) children examined.

The authors suggest from this study that intravascular coagulation occurs within the veins of the portal system, outside or inside the liver, and that it may reflect an ongoing obstructive process. They conclude that their data confirm that thrombocytopenia is a principal sign of hypersplenism. Although they think that ultrasonography is a reliable noninvasive means of correctly diagnosing portal vein obstruction in children, it may fail when obstruction is limited to a segment of the extrahepatic portal system.

▶ This study by Alvarez et al. was accompanied in the same issue of the *Journal of Pediatrics* by their report dealing with the results of portosystemic shunt surgery for portal vein obstruction. Portal hypertension in children must be considered in two groups: those with primary intrahepatic disease in which the underlying liver disease determines the prognosis and those with portal vein obstruction and normal liver function in whom variceal hemorrhage is the major problem that can lead to death. Portal vein thrombosis, the topic of the studies, is either idiopathic or the result of some injury to the portal vein. The latter most frequently results from umbilical vein catheterization in the newborn period. Whatever the cause, eventually most children are diagnosed because they either bleed from esophageal varices or are found to have markedly enlarged spleens on a routine physical examination. What to do about this problem is what the two studies by Alvarez et al. are about. I am glad that I wasn't one of the reviewers of these studies in the *Journal of Pediatrics*. They have created more furor among pediatric surgeons than one possibly could imagine.

The reports of the Alvarez group are in contrast to most other reports concerning the management of extrahepatic portal vein thrombosis in childhood. Pediatric surgeons in the United States (unlike in France, where these reports originated from) feel that the initial bleeding episode in patients with portal vein thrombosis rarely, if ever, causes death and that subsequent bleeding episodes during the next 5 to 10 years of life are associated with very low morbidity (Fonkalsrud, E. W.: *J. Pediatr.* 103:742, 1983). There are additional considerations when one is thinking about doing a portal diversion. An effective portosystemic shunt "steals" blood flow from the liver. Some patients who have undergone this procedure for portal vein thrombosis have developed hepatic encephalopathy long after shunt surgery was performed (*Ann. Surg.* 192:341, 1980). Patients in the series from France did not have this problem on the short haul. Additionally, portacaval shunts cause a wide range of metabolic alterations of the liver. Hepatocytes undergo atrophy, fatty infiltration, and drastic changes on electron microscopy. These changes are caused by the diversion around the liver of the so-called hepatotrophic factors in venous blood, of which insulin is the most important. This might, in fact, result in severe depressions in lipid and bile acids synthesis (Starzl, T. E., et al.: *J. Pediatr.* 103:741, 1983).

Despite all these potential objections to shunt surgery, the data from France indeed are most impressive and present the largest number of pediatric cases ever recorded in the medical literature having shunt surgery for this purpose. One would hope that colleagues in the United States and in France would get together and hash all this out and make peace with one another. If they don't, the debate may spead over into the lay community and someone might suggest that we send France a bill for the repairs to the Statue of Liberty. Stranger things have happened out of little quarrels.—J.A.S., III

Steatohepatitis in Obese Children: Cause of Chronic Liver Dysfunction
J. Roberto Moran, Fayez K. Ghishan, Susan A. Halter, and Harry L. Greene (Vanderbilt Univ.)
Am. J. Gastroenterol. 78:374–377, June 1983   6–16

Hepatic abnormalities including fatty hepatitis, fibrosis, and cirrhosis have been described in obese adults. Three obese children recently seen for nonspecific abdominal pain and abnormal liver function were found to have steatohepatitis.

Boy, 10, had had right upper quadrant tenderness and persistently elevated serum

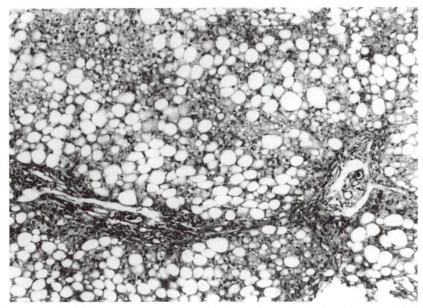

Fig 6–4.—Fibrosis extending from one portal tract of liver to another. Hematoxylin-eosin; original magnification × 200. (Courtesy of Moran, J.R., et al.: Am. J. Gastroenterol. 78:374–377, June 1983.)

glutamic oxaloacetic transaminase (SGOT) activity for 6 months. There was no history of jaundice or of exposure to drugs or hepatotoxic agents. The boy weighed 76 kg, over the 95th percentile for age, and was 151 cm tall. The liver was palpated 1 cm below the costal margin and was slightly tender. The SGOT activity was 110 IU/L, the serum glutamic pyruvic transaminase (SGPT) 121 IU/L, and the alkaline phosphatase 316 IU/L. The total bilirubin concentration was 0.3 mg/dl. Antinuclear and anti-DNA antibody tests were negative. The total cholesterol concentration was 208 mg/dl and the serum triglyceride concentration, 195 mg/dl. The lipoprotein pattern was consistent with type IIB hyperlipidemia. An inappropriately high insulin value was found during the rise in serum glucose concentration on tolerance testing. Liver biopsy showed prominent hepatocellular distention by fat, scattered foci of acute inflammation, and a moderate increase in connective tissue extending between the portal tracts (Fig 6–4). An exercise program was begun, and a diet designed to meet lean tissue growth requirements was prescribed. Liver tenderness was absent 6 months later, when the SGOT activity was 56 IU/L and the SGPT, 61 IU/L.

There is substantial evidence for an increase in collagen content with the development of fatty liver. The histologic findings in overweight patients resemble those of alcoholic hepatitis and also those seen after jejunoileal bypass for obesity. Obese children with hepatomegaly, abnormal liver function, or both should have a liver biopsy after other common causes of chronic liver dysfunction are ruled out. Nonalcoholic steatohepatitis probably can progress to cirrhosis. Obese patients without conditions such as diabetes or hyperlipidemia may benefit from dietary modification, but protein malnutrition must be avoided. Progression to more severe liver disease probably can be avoided by proper dietary management.

▶ Prior to this report, diminished self-esteem, ostracism by peers, reduced physical activity and exercise tolerance, increased stress on weight-bearing joints, and the possibility of the pickwickian syndrome were the only significant morbidities associated with childhood obesity. The present study, however, shows that overweight children can present with nonspecific abdominal pain, laboratory evidence of liver dysfunction, and histopathologic findings compatible with steatohepatitis. Even worse, this looks as if it can progress to cirrhosis. This is unfortunate, because no specific treatment is available for nonalcoholic steatohepatitis except weight reduction, and that, as we all know, is a difficult task to pull off at any age.

I thought being overweight was simply a matter of living beyond your seams, but as this study suggests, being overweight is really no laughing matter. Because of the apparent progression to more severe forms of liver disease, one can postulate that weight control is an absolutely essential aspect of the care of these children.—J.A.S., III

Biliary Tree in Cystic Fibrosis: Biliary Tract Abnormalities in Cystic Fibrosis Demonstrated by Endoscopic Retrograde Cholangiography
S. Bass, J. J. Connon, and C. S. Ho (Mount Sinai Hosp., Toronto)
Gastroenterology 84:1592–1596, June 1983   6–17

Two female adolescents with cystic fibrosis were investigated by endoscopic retrograde cholangiography (ERCP) for recurrent abdominal pain.

CASE 1.—Girl, 13, with cystic fibrosis, was seen in 1978 for jaundice. She had experienced crampy abdominal pains frequently for 12 years. In 1979, she was readmitted after 3 weeks of almost daily epigastric pain. An ERCP revealed multiple irregular filling defects throughout the biliary tree with dilatation of the ducts. The cystic duct and gallbladder were not seen. An endoscopic papillotomy was performed, and several small stones, thickened bile, and mucus were drained. One week later, a repeat ERCP revealed persistence of many of the filling defects. Pain recurred 1 month later. A third ERCP showed small stones in the intrahepatic bile ducts. In October 1981 she presented with severe right upper quadrant pain and fever of 1 day's duration. The gallbladder contained several stones; histology was consistent with acute and chronic cholecystitis.

CASE 2.—Girl, 19, with cystic fibrosis, presented in 1981 with abdominal pain; episodes of burning epigastric pain, which first began in 1978, had been diagnosed as cholelithiasis. An ERCP (Fig 6–5) showed cystic dilatation of the intrahepatic ducts and marked irregularities of the smaller proximal ductules. Numerous small, rounded filling defects were noted. On endoscopic papillotomy, a stone, along with thickened bile and mucus, was removed. Patient was asymptomatic for 1 week and then pain recurred. An ERCP was repeated and showed a marked reduction in the number of intrahepatic ductules. In January 1982 the patient

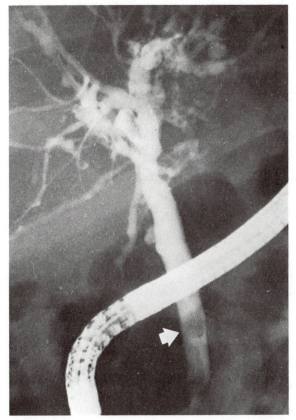

Fig 6–5.—Endoscopic retrograde cholangiography shows cystic dilatation of some intraheptic bile ducts as well as segmental narrowing and irregularity in others. In addition, there are multiple small filling defects in many branches, including the common bile duct where a large stone is present *(arrow)*. (Courtesy of Bass, S., et al.: Gastroenterology 84:1592–1596, June 1983.)

developed high fever, jaundice, rising alkaline phosphatase, and leukocytosis. The jaundice cleared but the patient continues to have almost daily episodes of abdominal pain.

The authors propose that the use of ERCP be strongly considered when noninvasive tests are nondiagnostic in the clinical setting of suspected biliary tract disease in cystic fibrosis patients. They have not encountered any complications in more than 20 children who have undergone this procedure.

Cholelithiasis in Children With Immunoglobulin A Deficiency: A New Gastroenterologic Syndrome

Yehuda L. Danon, Gabriel Dinari, Ben-Zion Garty, Charlotte Horodniceanu, Menachem Nitzan, and Michael Grunebaum (Tel Aviv Univ.)
J. Pediatr. Gastroenterol. Nutr. 2:663–666, November 1983   6–18

Ultrasonography was performed in 13 consecutive pediatric patients to determine the prevalence of gallstones in selective IgA deficiency. Criteria for diagnosis of selective IgA deficiency included extremely low or undetectable IgA levels, with normal or increased concentrations of other immunoglobulins. There were 5 girls, 8 boys, aged 1–18 years, with a mean of 6.5 years. No patient had symptoms related to the biliary tract.

Three girls and 5 boys demonstrated abnormal biliary sonograms. Four had cholelithiasis, while the presence of biliary sludge was diagnosed in the other 4. One patient with gallstones had associated celiac disease. Repeated episodes of diarrhea were present in 1 of the 4 patients in each group. Extensive examination failed to reveal the cause of the diarrhea. No evidence of hemolysis, family history of gallstones, or obesity was found in any patient.

The role of IgA in local defense of the biliary tract and gut led the authors to speculate that in IgA deficiency, local changes in biliary structure or function may occur to predispose to the formation of gallstones. It is suggested that the association of cholelithiasis with selective IgA deficiency has not been previously described and constitutes a new gastrointestinal manifestation of this relatively common immunodeficiency disorder. It also is suggested that all patients with selective IgA deficiency be screened for the presence of gallstones.

▶ Selective immunoglobulin (IgA) deficiency is the most common form of immunodeficiency. Not only is it the most common form, but it also appears to be very common in general throughout the world. About 1 in 500 individuals has IgA deficiency. While many patients with selective IgA deficiency may be asymptomatic, a number show an increased incidence of associated diseases. Collagen vascular diseases, autoimmune disorders, inflammatory bowel disease, respiratory infections, allergy, lambliasis, celiac disease, intestinal nodular lymphoid hyperplasia, diarrhea, and hepatitis are among the disorders described in association with IgA deficiency. It was the suspicion that IgA played some role in the local defense of the biliary tract that led these Israeli investigators to perform ultrasound in their population of 13 patients with IgA deficiency. About two-thirds showed stones even though the mean age of the children was only 6½ years. The authors speculate that lack of IgA in the bile may predispose to biliary infection. Bacteria in the gallbladder then would provide enzyme activity to break down bilirubin products and cause precipitation of pigment stones. Unfortunately, no data were able to be presented to tell us whether or not the stones were cholesterol or pigment in origin. In any event, the importance of this study is that it informs us of a newly described association: that of IgA deficiency and cholelithiasis.

Roslyn et al. tell us that we also should be aware of an increased risk of gallstones in children receiving total parenteral nutrition (TPN). The association between gallstones and administration of TPN has been reported anecdotally before. What Roslyn et al. have done is to review data on all of the patients receiving TPN at one institution in order to determine the exact incidence of gallstones (*Pediatrics* 71:74, 1983). With ultrasonography, 43% of children receiving TPN had cholelithiasis. The highest incidence of cholelithiasis was seen when TPN was being administered to patients who had ileal resections (64% incidence). These are staggering figures, because about half of the patients with stones ultimately were operated on. The implications here are pretty clear. Any patient receiving TPN over a long period should have routine gallbladder sonography.

Is sonography of the gallbladder adequate to pick up gallbladder disease? Maybe yes, maybe no. H. B. Patriquin et al. (*AJR* 141:57, 1983) asked the question, "Is thickening of the gallbladder a predictor of cholecystitis?" They found 23 patients who had a gallbladder wall more than 3 mm thick. The diseases associated with this were hypoalbuminemia, ascites, and venous hypertension. None of 26 patients with gallstones had thickened gallbladder walls. Five children with surgically proved acute cholecystitis had normal gallbladder wall thickness on ultrasound. Thus, it may be concluded that ultrasound evidence of thickening of the gallbladder wall is not associated with acute cholecystitis and in and of itself is not an indication for cholecystectomy. This is important and valuable information, because it is somewhat contrary to what most adult gastroenterologists have taught us. de Lacey et al. asked the question, "Should cholecystography or ultrasound be the primary investigation for gallbladder disease?" (*Lancet* 1:205, 1984). They found that both procedures were highly effective in detecting stones, with false negative rates of only 1%. However, because some stones and some instances of acalculous disease will be missed by either technique, serious consideration should be given to further investigation of all gallbladders considered normal by either examination. Remember, the one advantage of the cholecystogram is that it does give you some evidence of function of the gallbladder. In the final analysis, however, I think everyone would conclude that ultrasound is the first procedure of choice in this day and age whenever the gallbladder is being evaluated. Unfortunately, ultrasound is so easy to do that it is being severely abused in many institutions. Practically every child with unexplained abdominal pain has suddenly become a candidate for ultrasound of the gallbladder. It may be time to call a moratorium on use of this instrument unless there are hard and fast clinical signs to suggest that something is wrong. There is nothing so useless as doing efficiently that which should not be done at all.—J.A.S., III

Idiopathic Disorders of Fecal Continence in Children
Pierre Arhan, Ghislain Devroede, Bertrand Jehannin, Claude Faverdin, Yann Révillon, Daniel Lefevre, and Denys Pellerin
Pediatrics 71:774–778, May 1983   6–19

Constipation is associated with encopresis in many children. However, constipation of psychogenic origin is often postulated when the underlying pathophysiology is poorly understood. The authors assessed anorectal motility and colorectal transit of radiopaque markers in 176 consecutive patients aged 2 to 15 years, who were examined at the Hôpital des Enfants-Malades, Paris, for idiopathic disorders of bowel function other than Hirschsprung's disease.

Seventy (42%) of the 167 children for whom the age of onset was known had become constipated by age 1 month. However, peak age at first clinical examination was 6 years, with the older the patient at the time of onset, the earlier the consultation. Referral diagnosis was aganglionosis in 34 patients (19%), idiopathic constipation in 115 (65%), encopresis in 14 (8%), and surgical symptoms in 13 (8%), of whom 6 had intestinal obstruction and 7 were believed to have an abdominal tumor. The rectal ampulla was empty in 12% of patients and filled with normal stools in 37%; a fecaloma was present in 50%. In addition to fecaloma, plain films showed marked air distention of the bowel in 5 patients (3%), air-fluid levels in 6 (3%), and spina bifida occulta in 56 (31%).

Anorectal motility studies showed that resting pressure in the rectal ampulla and upper anal canal was significantly greater in constipated patients than in normal control subjects. Involuntary fluctuations in rectal pressure were observed in 47% of constipated patients. These spontaneous variations were observed more often in the upper anal canal. The activity coefficient in the upper anal canal did not differ significantly among patients with or without spina bifida occulta. The higher the activity coefficient in the upper anal canal, the greater the variations of pressure in the rectum at rest. All patients exhibited a rectoanal inhibitory reflex.

Colorectal motility studies showed retardation of transit time of a radiopaque marker in the proximal or distal large bowel, or both, in 61% of the constipated children. Transit times were similar in patients with or without spina bifida occulta. Of the children who had a normal transit time in all parts of the digestive tract, 50% had at least 1 abnormal measurement at anorectal manometry: 18% showed an increased anal activity coefficient, 3% had increased rectal pressure, 14.3% had increased anal pressure, 3% had increased marginal pressure, and 18% showed an increased threshold distending volume.

This study demonstrates that functional abnormalities do exist in the colon, rectum, and anus of most children who have idiopathic disorders of fecal continence but do not have Hirschsprung's disease. The cause of these abnormalities remains to be determined.

▶ This study makes at least four observations: (1) that the anus is hypertonic in chronically constipated children; (2) that the threshold for rectoanal inhibitory reflex is raised; (3) that instability and antagonism of pressures in the rectum and anal canal are similar to those present in children with meningomyelocele; and (4) that chronic constipation is associated with decreased rectal sensitivity, as demonstrated by a raised conscious threshold. The obvious unanswered question is whether these findings are the cause of the constipation or whether some underlying psychologic factor acts to cause constipation that then produces the secondary physiologic abnormalities. The authors of this study seem to favor the former explanation. A subsequent study (*Pediatrics* 73:199, 1984) found similar abnormalities but concluded that the hypomotility in untreated patients is the result of chronic fecal impaction and rectal distention, not the cause. This was based on the observation that vigorous management of the constipation improved bowel motility. Although rectal and sigmoid hypomotility did not appear to be the cause of the constipation, the authors of the latter article indicated that it might have contributed to its severity. One could even speculate that if there is some organic cause for chronic constipation in children, impairment of defecation conceivably could alter the personality of those children. This then enters into the issue of what came first, the hen or the egg. As with most of these issues, it is truly impossible to sort it out and one simply is left with the conclusion that a hen is only an egg's way of making another egg.

If you really want to try something novel in managing a chronically constipated patient, you might look to the report of Kreek et al. (*Lancet* 1:261, 1983). These investigators from Cornell University hypothesized that motility disorders leading to chronic constipation might result in part from relative or absolute excess of one or more of the endogenous opioids or from abnormal binding of these opioids by their specific receptors in the intestine. It has been shown that naturally occurring opioids, such as endorphins, do bind to intestinal walls. Recall that it has been known for over 2,000 years that natural opiates, such as paregoric, promptly reverse both acute and chronic diarrhea. Why not try the opposite, by giving specific narcotic antagonists such as naloxone to patients with chronic constipation? This is exactly what the investigators from Cornell University did, and—low and behold!—the patients so treated had a marked increase in passage of "number twos." That certainly is a nifty (if not practical) way of treating constipation. Quite seriously, however, this particular study does provide immense insights into what may be going on on a physiologic basis in patients with chronic constipation.

In closing this particular commentary, it should be mentioned that one other cause of constipation has surfaced in the past year. This was the report of an 11-year-old girl who presented with abdominal pain and inability to defecate. On rectal examination, a "crunchy" rectal mass was felt. It turned out that this young lady had downed three packages of unshelled sunflower seeds 1 week previously. Under general anesthesia, a mass of macerated sunflower seeds was dislodged manually. The sordid details of all this may be found in the *New England Journal of Medicine* (310:748, 1984). The importance of this case is that it is the second reported one of colonic obstruction from a phytobezoar. The other reported case was not from sunflower seeds, but from bubble gum (*South. Med. J.* 75:775, 1982).—J.A.S., III

Sigmoidoscopy, Colonoscopy, and Radiology in Evaluation of Children With Rectal Bleeding
S. Cucchiara, S. Guandalini, A. Staiano, B. Devizia, G. Capano, G. Romaniello, V. Poggi, O. Tamburrini, A. Settimi, and G. de Ritis (Univ. of Naples)
J. Pediatr. Gastroenterol. Nutr. 2:667–671, October 1983   6–20

The diagnostic roles of sigmoidoscopy, colonoscopy, and double-contrast radiology were evaluated in 103 children (mean age, 44 months; range, 1 month to 12 years) with rectal bleeding, with or without other gastrointestinal tract symptoms. Results are shown in the table. Twelve children had anal fissures revealed by anal inspection. In 20 children, aged 2–10 years, single polyps were diagnosed; 14 were localized at the rec-

DIAGNOSTIC PROCEDURES AND DIAGNOSIS IN 103* CHILDREN REFERRED
BECAUSE OF RECTAL BLEEDING

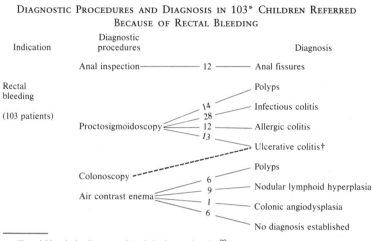

*Two children had a diagnosis of Meckel's diverticulosis by ⁹⁹Tc scanning.
†Colonoscopy and air-contrast enema allowed definitive assessment of the disease.
(Courtesy of Cucchiara, S., et al.: J. Pediatr. Gastroenterol. Nutr. 2:667–671, October 1983.)

tosigmoid level and were identified by proctosigmoidoscopy. Infectious colitis was diagnosed in 28 children aged 1 month to 5 years who had diarrhea with fresh blood or guaiac-positive stool with mucus and leukocytes. In 12 children, aged 2–16 months, colitis due to cow's milk allergy was diagnosed. Thirteen others, aged 2–12 years, had ulcerative colitis. After initial proctosigmoidoscopy that allowed histologic diagnosis, all of the children underwent colonoscopy and double contrast radiography. Lymphoid nodular hyperplasia was documented in 9 children. In 1 child, angiodysplasia of the left colon was diagnosed at colonoscopy; findings on both sigmoidoscopy and radiology were negative. In 2 children with rectal bleeding, ⁹⁹Tc scanning led to the diagnosis of Meckel's diverticulosis; findings on endoscopy and radiology, however, were normal.

These results indicate that the first two diagnostic steps, i.e., examination of the anal region and rectosigmoidoscopy, can disclose the source of bleeding in most children with rectal bleeding, with or without other gastrointestinal tract symptoms. Colonoscopy, a more stressful procedure that is not without potential complications, should be limited to use in patients with normal or nondiagnostic findings on sigmoidoscopy; for patients with recurrent bleeding after removal of rectal polyps; for the diagnosis and follow-up of inflammatory bowel disease, for polypectomy of proximal polyps; and for further investigation of abnormal findings on barium enema roentgenography.

▶ The approaches outlined in this report nicely provide guidelines for the evaluation of children who have rectal bleeding. The schema in the table will guide us through a series of diagnostic procedures from the most innocuous to the more complex. "Scopic" procedures certainly have come of age.

One should not forget that rapid upper gastrointestinal tract bleeding may present with what looks like rectal bleeding, so that if the outline above fails to reveal an answer, more thorough evaluation is in order. While we are on the topic of gastrointestinal tract bleeding, it should be mentioned that the Hemoccult test, while perfectly satisfactory for stool examination for blood, is inappropriate for testing blood from the upper gastrointestinal tract (*N. Engl. J. Med.* 310:125, 1984). The manufacturers of Hemoccult have determined that tests for fecal occult blood cannot be used to detect blood in gastric aspirates or vomitus because the low pH in these fluids frequently causes false negative results. Finally, add to the list of things that cause "pseudomelena" chocolate cookies. Life was quite simple when all we had to remember as causes of nonheme black stools were iron, bismuth (such as in Pepto-Bismol), charcoal, licorice, and certain fruits. Steven Sulkes, from Rochester, New York, now tells us that if you ingest one-half to one pound of chocolate sandwich cookies, it will be productive of black stools (ibid., p. 52). Even though variation in the brand of chocolate cookies did not change the character of the black stool, Sulkes has forever saddled us with this phenomenon being called "Hydrox fecalis." The author of this brief report and several volunteers were the study subjects who gobbled down all the Oreos. The by-line for the report was from the Monroe Developmental Disabilities Service Office (forever hereafter known as "the home of the cookie monsters").—J.A.S., III

7 The Genitourinary Tract

Proteinuria in Children With Insulin-Dependent Diabetes: Relationship to Duration of Disease, Metabolic Control, and Retinal Changes
Demetrius Ellis, Dorothy J. Becker, Denis Daneman, Louis Lobes, Jr., and Allan L. Drash (Univ. of Pittsburgh)
J. Pediatr. 102:673–679, May 1983   7–1

Renal insufficiency is a most important complication of long-standing insulin-dependent diabetes (IDD). Proteinuria is the single most consistent abnormality and usually occurs 14 to 17 years after diagnosis of IDD. It is an ominous sign that antedates the onset of renal failure by 4 to 5 years. The authors examined the relationship between early retinopathy and subclinical proteinuria in 67 children (mean age 14.3 years). Mean duration of disease was 6.2 years. None of the patients had suspected urinary tract infection or other disorders besides IDD, and results of physical examinations were normal with the exception of the fundoscopic findings.

Concentrations of serum and urinary β_2-microglobulin (β_2-M) were measured by radioimmunoassay, as were serum and urinary concentrations of albumin, transferrin, and IgG. Interassay coefficient of variation of urinary assays ranged from 17.6% for albumin to 4.5% for IgG and less than 3.4% for all serum protein assays. Concentrations of serum and urinary creatinine were measured as well as glycosylated hemoglobin (GHb). Fluorescein and photographic studies were performed with standard and stereo fields. Retinopathy was defined by presence of one or more of the following: intraretinal lipid deposition or hemorrhage, microaneurysms, intraretinal microangiopathic changes, capillary occlusions, intraretinal leakage of fluorescein, and infarction of nerve fiber layers.

Mean GHb concentration in these patients 1 to 3 years prior to this study was 11.9; at the time of the study, mean GHb value was 12.4. In the group as a whole, more patients had a mean GHb value greater than 11% (63%) than a mean value of 11% or less (37%). The study group had a significantly higher level of creatinine clearance than that in normal children. The level of creatinine clearance did not change with increasing duration of illness. Clearance and fractional excretion of β_2-M were significantly above normal in the study population. No correlation between urinary excretion of β_2-M and creatinine clearance existed. Mean 24-hour urinary excretion of albumin, transferrin, and IgG was significantly elevated above normal values. Protein selectivity index of the 55 patients older than age 10 years was 1.03, and the ratio of albumin, transferrin, and IgG excreted was similar to that in healthy children.

Twenty-five (37%) patients had retinopathy. Although this condition was rare during the first 5 years of illness, 52% of patients with illness for 5 to 10 years and 70% of patients with illness longer than 10 years had retinopathy. Large molecular weight proteinuria was present in 31 (46%) patients, of whom 10 had the disease for less than 5 years. Only 18 (27%) patients had both proteinuria and retinopathy, whereas 10% had retinopathy alone and 19% had microproteinuria alone. Presence of one of these conditions predicts a small but significant risk of the other.

Frequency of serious complications of IDD remains high and greatly influences the quality of life and longevity. Patients with onset of IDD during childhood are particularly prone to development of microvascular disease, most evident in retinal and glomerular capillaries.

Long-term follow-up may provide answers as to the risk of developing more serious retinopathy or nephropathy and whether good glycemic control may protect against complications of IDD.

▶ John I. Malone, Professor of Pediatrics and Co-Director of the University of South Florida Diabetes Center in Tampa, comments:

"Ellis and colleagues at the University of Pittsburgh report the relationship between retinopathy and nephropathy in a group of children with diabetes ranging in duration from 0.6 year to 17 years (mean, 6.2 years). The influence of metabolic control was assessed by a retrospective analysis of glycosylated hemoglobin measured during the 1 to 3 years before evaluation of the retina and renal function. The retina was evaluated by fluorescein anginography, and renal function was evaluated by the urinary excretion of one or more large molecular weight proteins. The authors were able to demonstrate evidence of retinal abnormalities in 37% of the group and increased urinary macroproteins in 46%. The microvascular disease seen in the eye increased from 4% of children with diabetes less than 5 years, to 52% with diabetes less than 10 years and 70% with diabetes less than 17 years. Macroproteinura was found in 15% of those with diabetes less than 5 years, 19% with diabetes less than 10 years, and 12% with diabetes less than 17 years. The major clinical importance of these observations is that microvascular abnormalities are occurring in children with diabetes of short duration. The pediatrician must be aware and should be concerned about appropriate methods for preventing this process.

"The question remains: 'What is the proper method of intervention?' The glycosylated hemoglobin levels in those with retinopathy did not differ from the levels in those without retinopathy. Blood and urine glucose concentrations did not affect the urinary excretion of macroproteins. Does this mean that blood glucose concentration does not play a role in the microvascular disease of diabetes? I believe not. The reports of Robinson et al. (*Science* 221:1177, 1983) and Engerman and Kern (*Diabetes* 33:97, 1984) that elevated concentrations of another sugar galactose in the rat and dog result in microvascular abnormalities identical to diabetes indicate that elevated "sugar" concentrations in addition to glucose play a role in the pathogenesis of the microvascular disease associated with diabetes. The report of Abouna and associates (*Lancet* 2:1274, 1983) that shows improvement in the renal vascular pathology of a kidney transplanted from a diabetic to a nondiabetic subject goes further to indicate that correction of the diabetic state will result in reversal of the microangiopathy.

"There is little question that the retinopathy and nephropathy of diabetes occur only in those individuals who have some degree of hyperglycemia. The toxic level of glucose, however, seems to be variable from one individual to another. Although we must encourage our patients to seek physiologic levels of blood glucose control, we have no way to prescribe this treatment today. Our present treatment modalities make these efforts dangerous for most children. It seems that our current time and money would be better spent developing methods (none presently exists) to normalize the metabolism in children with diabetes rather than embarking on another study to determine if good glycemic control will prevent the secondary microvascular complications."

Randomized Clinical Trial of Cyclosporine in Cadaveric Renal Transplantation

Canadian Multicenter Transplant Study Group, chaired by C. R. Stiller (Univ. Hosp., London. Ont.)
N. Engl. J. Med. 309:809–815, Oct. 6, 1983   7–2

Initial results were analyzed of a randomized, nonblinded, multicenter trial of cyclosporine in 209 patients, aged 12 years or older, who received cadaveric renal transplants and were followed for 1 to 17 months (median, 8 months). Patients were treated either with cyclosporine and prednisone or with standard therapy that included azathioprine and prednisone. Cyclosporine recipients received a loading dose of 20 mg/kg orally within 12 hours before surgery and 10 mg/kg every 12 hours thereafter. The dose was adjusted to achieve trough levels between 100 and 400 ng/ml. After 30 days, the dose was reduced by 2 mg/kg if trough levels were above 100 ng/ml. It was then reduced monthly when possible.

Predicted 1-year graft survival (Fig 7–1) was 80.4% in patients receiving cyclosporine and 64.0% in those receiving standard therapy ($P = .003$). Predicted 1-year patient survival was 96.6% in patients given cyclosporine and 86.4% in those given standard therapy. A detrimental effect on 1-year graft survival was seen in cyclosporine recipients if they received kidneys that were perfused by machine for longer than 24 hours (70% vs. 88%; $P = .005$) or if the time used to perform the surgical anastomosis was longer than 45 minutes (60% vs. 89%; $P = .002$). In the control group, graft survival was better in patients who had had 5 or more blood transfusions than in those who had had 2 to 4 transfusions (77% vs. 55%; $P = .05$); the number of transfusions was not a risk factor in the cyclosporine group.

The incidence of graft rejection episodes was not significantly different in the two groups. Serum levels of creatinine and blood urea nitrogen were higher in the cyclosporine than in the control group of 30 days after transplantation and thereafter. At day 90, mean serum creatinine level was 2.6 mg/dl in the cyclosporine group and 2.0 mg/dl in controls ($P = .03$). Posttransplantation acute tubular necrosis (i.e., need for dialysis because

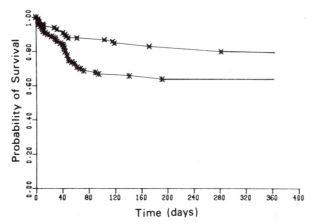

Fig 7–1.—Product-limit estimates for graft survival in cyclosporine-treated patients *(upper curve)* and patients given standard therapy *(lower curve)*. Estimate of 1-year graft survival was 80.4% in cyclosporine-treated patients and 64% in the standard-treatment group (*P* = .003). Each graft loss is noted; observation continued for 17 months, but the last graft loss occurred at day 281 in the cyclosporine group and at day 192 in the standard treatment group. (Courtesy of Canadian Multicenter Transplant Study Group: N. Engl. J. Med. 309:809–815, Oct. 6, 1983. Reprinted by permission of the New England Journal of Medicine.)

of uremia or a serum creatinine level more than 10 mg/dl) occurred in 52% of the cyclosporine group and 39% of controls (*P* = .081).

Three patients receiving cyclosporine and 11 receiving standard treatments died. Lymphoma developed in 1 patient receiving cyclosporine. There were 81 infectious complications in the cyclosporine group and 99 in the control group. Aside from drug-induced nephrotoxicity, the frequency of noninfectious complications was similar in the two groups except for renal artery thrombosis or stenosis, which occurred more often in the cyclosporine group. Severe leukopenia occurred in 12 patients given standard therapy and in 1 given cyclosporine.

Cyclosporine rather than azathioprine is probably the immunosuppressive agent of choice in cadaveric renal transplantation. It is not known whether prednisone is required together with cyclosporine. Patients receiving a kidney given more than 24 hours of pulsatile machine perfusion, or patients who had a difficult surgical anastomosis that required a rewarming time exceeding 45 minutes, may require a modification in immunosuppressive therapy, such as using alternative therapy at least until normal graft function is established.

▶ The immunosuppressive properties of cyclosporine have been known now for about 9 years. Beginning about that time, individual transplant centers began to experiment with the use of this immunosuppressive in patients who were about to undergo renal transplantation. Control studies have been very few in number, and what is presented here is about the largest series reported to date using cyclosporine. Cyclosporine is a metabolic product of certain types of fungi. It was approved in 1983 by the Food and Drug Administration for general use in transplantation. Currently, it is being used for all sorts of transplants, including liver, heart-lung, and bone marrow. The Canadian Multicentre Transplant Group has attempted to probe the real role of cyclosporine in kidney transplants. Their findings are rather interesting. First off, cyclosporine is a terrific immunosuppressant significantly influencing graft survival. As noted, it helps and works best when the kidneys are relatively fresh and when the actual surgical procedure can be done quite speedily. The major problem with cyclosporine is that it is a known nephrotoxic agent. Thus, renal function must be monitored carefully after transplantation, and it may be necessary to measure drug levels and adjust the dose of the immunosuppressant accordingly. Cyclosporine is such a potent immunosuppressive agent that it has been reported to be associated with the development of malignancy in a very small percentage of patients. Other problems related to the drug, such as hepatotoxicity, have not been major. The findings of the Canadian group have been reproduced more recently in a slightly smaller series of patients from Canada (Merion, R. M., et al.: *N. Engl. J. Med.* 310:148, 1984).

An interesting spinoff from the use of cyclosporine is the potential that transplant recipients may no longer need pretransplantation multiple transfusions. As has been mentioned in prior YEAR BOOKS, all transplantation centers have accepted the concept that donor organ rejection is diminished if a transplant recipient has had multiple transfusions prior to surgery. The exact reasons for the ability of multiple transfusions to prevent graft rejection is still not known, but there is no question concerning the efficacy of this approach. In the Canadian study involving cyclosporine, there appeared to be no additive benefit of pretransplantation transfusion. The European Multicenter Trial Group also found no evidence for a beneficial effect of pregraft blood transfusion in renal transplant recipients treated with cyclosporine (*Lancet* 2:186, 1983). It should be noted that in neither study was this question being directly controlled for. A prospective trial would now be difficult because it might be considered unethical to withhold transfusion from transplantation candidates. I think we probably will see such control trials, but only after animal studies have been performed. One such animal control study to date has supported the concept that pretransplantation transfusions are no longer necessary when such powerful immunosuppressants as cyclosporine are used (Niessen, G. J. C. M., et al.: ibid. 1:339, 1984). The whole concept of how transfusions may be of benefit in kidney transplantation has been reviewed recently by Paul Terasaki (*Transplantation* 37:119, 1984).

Whereas chronic peritoneal dialysis previously was considered a second choice to hemodialysis except in special circumstances such as for small infants, children without vascular access, or patients unstable while receiving hemodialysis, this situation has turned around 180 degrees. Now, wherever possible, continuous ambulatory peritoneal dialysis (CAPD) is the treatment of choice for medical, psychologic, and economic reasons. This has been discussed previously in the YEAR BOOK. Despite the real value of CAPD, transplantation remains the procedure of choice in everybody's mind for definitive correction of renal failure. The need to move this down as a procedure to be used even in very young children also has become apparent. H. W. Schnaper et al. (*Am. J. Kidney Dis.* 2:645, 1983) have described remarkable cerebral cortical atrophy in pediatric patients with end-stage renal disease who are being dialyzed. In a series of 15 children with end-stage renal disease, 8 had cortical atrophy on computed tomography scanning and 2 showed ventricular enlargement. Although these changes were not necessarily associated with any clinical signs or symptoms, they do suggest that something associated with the uremic state results in damage to central nervous system tissue. R. S. Trompeter et al. have shown that renal transplantation can be done in very young children (*Lancet* 1:373, 1983). They successfully operated on children weighing less than 10 kg and found acceptable rates of engraftment. Even though growth is improved markedly in children undergoing CAPD, some do have problems in this regard, and many still have difficulties with renal osteodystrophy (*J. Pediatr.* 103:729, 1983). These also lend credence to the concept of early transplantation.

If you didn't have a chance to read the brief report from San Francisco dealing with the use of "grocery store baking soda" in the management of chronic metabolic acidosis, it is well worth your time (*Clin. Pediatr.* 23:94, 1984). Arm and Hammer Baking Soda is USP grade sodium bicarbonate. When appropriately mixed with distilled water, it forms a pharmacologic grade of sodium bicarbonate solution that costs only 3% of the cost of pharmacy-prepared solutions. For example, the average patient with renal tubular acidosis can be appropriately treated for acidosis with baking soda costing only 29 cents a month. This is the best bargain in the world at a time when the only way to buy four suits for less than a dollar is to purchase a deck of playing cards.—J.A.S., III

Growth in Children With Various Therapies for End-Stage Renal Disease
Robert S. Fennell III, John K. Orak, Terry Hudson, Eduardo H. Garin, Abdollah Iravani, Wayne J. Van Deusen, Richard Howard, William W. Pfaff, R. Dixon Walter III, and George A. Richard (Univ. of Florida)
Am. J. Dis. Child. 138:28–31, January 1984   7–3

Growth failure is a major problem in children with end-stage renal disease. The growth of children younger than age 15½ years who were undergoing continuous ambulatory peritoneal dialysis (CAPD) for end-stage renal disease was compared with the growth of children undergoing hemodialysis and others having successful renal transplantation. Nine children on CAPD with a mean age of 8 years were followed for a mean of 16 months, and 15 hemodialysis patients with a mean age of 9½ years were followed for 15 months. Thirty-four children with a mean age of 10 years who had kidney transplants were followed for 20 months. The most common cause of end-stage renal disease was chronic glomerulonephritis. The transplant recipients received an average daily prednisone dose of 0.34 mg/kg 18–24 months postoperatively.

More patients on CAPD and more of those who were operated on grew at 80% or more of predicted velocity, compared with the hemodialysis group. The former groups did not differ significantly in growth rate. The difference was significant only for children younger than age 11 years in the hemodialysis and transplant groups. In terms of percent of predicted growth rate, the children on CAPD grew better than those on hemodialysis and as well as the transplanted patients. Some correlation was found between growth and allograft function. The children on CAPD were less acidotic than those on hemodialysis and were likelier to show improvement in renal osteodystrophy during follow-up. There were no significant differences between the two groups in reported caloric intake.

Renal transplantation in children with a serum creatinine below 2.5 mg/dl is associated with an average growth velocity of about 80% of that predicted by the bone age, and those on CAPD can do as well. Children on hemodialysis have grown less well than the other groups, for reasons that remain unclear. The differences cannot be attributed entirely to acidosis and osteodystrophy.

▶ Donald E. Potter, of Children's Renal Center, University of California Hospitals and Clinics, San Francisco, comments:

"The design and results of this study are very similar to those of a previous study from Toronto (*J. Pediatr.* 102:681, 1983). Growth was considered to be normal or good if it was >80% of the growth rate of normal children. Good growth was achieved in 44% of children receiving CAPD, 0% of children receiving hemodialysis, and 53% of children after transplantation in this study and 59% of children receiving CAPD, 11% of children receiving hemodialysis, and 65% of children after transplantation in the Toronto study. This is rather convincing evidence that growth is better with CAPD than with hemodialysis, although a previous study with smaller numbers failed to show a difference (*N. Engl. J. Med.* 307:1537, 1982).

"The authors had difficulty determining the reasons for the better growth achieved with CAPD. Growth retardation in uremic children is influenced by a number of factors, including poor calorie intake, acidosis, osteodystrophy, and, perhaps, high blood urea nitrogen levels. As the authors acknowledge, there is no satisfactory way of comparing blood urea nitrogen and serum carbon dioxide levels in CAPD and hemodialysis patients, because the levels fluctuate with each hemodialysis but are kept constant with CAPD. Indeed, the authors conjecture that the stability of blood biochemical levels may be more important than the magnitude of the levels in determining growth. Regardless of the mechanisms involved, improved growth has been demonstrated as another advantage of CAPD. This form of dialysis is now being used in more than 75% of the patients in some pediatric programs and is even considered preferable to renal transplantation under some circumstances."

Acquired Renal Scars in Children
A. Leo Winter, Brian E. Hardy, Douglas J. Alton, Gerald S. Arbus, and Bernard M. Churchill (Hosp. for Sick Children, Toronto)
J. Urol. 129:1190–1194, June 1983   7–4

The records of some 4,000 children seen between 1965 and 1980 with urinary tract infections were reviewed. Of these, 36 girls and 1 boy, aged

1 to 16 years (average, 5.7 years), showed 41 kidneys with acquired scarring (i.e., loss of at least 3 mm of renal parenchymal thickness between two successive intravenous pyelograms) and without neurogenic bladder or structural defects other than reflux. At the start of the follow-up period, 27 kidneys were normal and 14 were minimally scarred. Scars were graded in increasing severity as focal, polar, or diffuse (Fig 7–2).

Before the development of renal scars, all children had had confirmed episodes of pyelonephritis (34) or unexplained pyrexia (3); 78% of these episodes had been treated inappropriately. Of 26 children who began the study with normal kidneys, 13 had had appropriately treated episodes of pyelonephritis that did not lead to renal scarring.

Voiding cystourethrography, performed in 36 children, showed 55% of kidneys without ureteral reflux on initial studies; 43% never demonstrated vesicoureteral reflux during the follow-up period. In kidneys with ureteral reflux, a positive correlation ($P < .05$) was noted between grade of reflux and severity of renal scarring. No kidney demonstrated intrarenal reflux

Fig 7–2—Scars were graded in increasing severity as diffuse, polar, or focal. (Courtesy of Winter, A.L., et al.: J. Urol. 129:1190–1194, June 1983.)

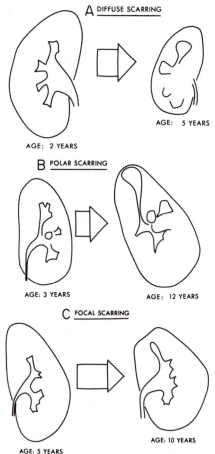

at any time. The apparent competence of the ureterovesical valve mechanism and severity of renal scarring were not related.

The use of prophylactic antibiotics tended to limit the extent of renal scarring ($P < .2$, $< .1$). Of the 37 children, 15 underwent reimplantation surgery from 0 to 3.7 years after renal scars were first noted (average, 1.4 years). Of these, 7 showed further progression of scars and 8 did not. Only 1 child became hypertensive, and none showed any deterioration of renal function.

Episodes of acute pyelonephritis should be treated early and aggressively to prevent renal scarring. Prophylactic antibiotic therapy should be instituted in all children with intrarenal reflux and in children without reflux who have severe or prolonged episodes of pyelonephritis because these episodes may be followed by development of renal scars. Children with high grades of reflux (grades IV and V) in whom renal scars have not developed should undergo early reimplantation, because reflux is unlikely to stop spontaneously and the kidneys are at risk of severe scarring.

Treatment of Ruptured Kidney by Gluing With Highly Concentrated Human Fibrinogen
W. Brands, J. Haselberger, C. Mennicken, and M. Hoerst (Univ. of Heidelberg Clinic, Mannheim, West Germany)
J. Pediatr. Surg. 18:611–613, October 1983   7–5

In blunt abdominal trauma in childhood, the kidney is involved in 50% of instances of organ damage.

Girl, 11, fell with the right flank onto a bicycle stand. Macrohematuria developed, with increasing pressure sensitivity of the right flank and right kidney bed. An intravenous pyelogram showed a normal excretory urogram on the left side and marked extravasation of contrast material on the right. A median transverse kidney rupture with dislocation of the two kidney portions was suspected. Selective renal angiography demonstrated the presence of this condition, without injury to the vascular system. Immediate operation via a flank incision on the right side was performed. After removal of a wedge-shaped detached parenchymal fragment, the two halves of the kidney were adapted and firmly fixed together over a large surface after the fibrin glue had been previously applied to the parenchymal surfaces. A small tear in the renal pelvis was firmly closed with catgut single-button sutures. On the 17th postoperative day, the right renal space system appeared completely normal, with smooth flow of the contrast medium.

The following materials were used in the gluing procedure: human coagulable plasma protein (Immuno Ltd., Heidelberg), 90 mg/ml; thrombin (Topostasin, Roche), 3000 NIH, dissolved in Ringer's solution with double concentration of calcium ions; factor XIII concentrate (Fibrogamin, Behringwerke, Marburg), 250 units. Aprotinin (Antogosan, Behringwerke) was used for inhibition of local fibrinolytic activity.

The procedure is comparable to the use of an industrial two-component glue. Fibrinogen is applied first and then coated with a solution of factor XIII, aprotinin, calcium chloride, and thrombin (Fig 7–3). The tissue por-

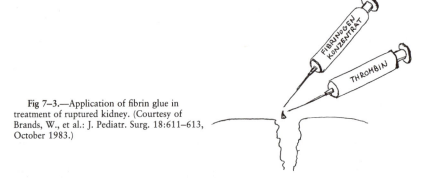

Fig 7–3.—Application of fibrin glue in treatment of ruptured kidney. (Courtesy of Brands, W., et al.: J. Pediatr. Surg. 18:611–613, October 1983.)

tions must be pressed together immediately because the glue solidifies in a few seconds; fibrinogen is transformed by thrombin into unpolymerized fibrin, and then factor XIII is transformed into factor XIIIa, which results in progressive polymerization of fibrin in the presence of calcium chloride and increasing mechanical strength of the glued parts.

Only operation can finally establish the possibility of an attempt at conservation. Early preoperative angiography is of greatest importance. Without knowledge of the uninjured vessels as shown in the angiogram, nephrectomy would have been performed because of the massive hemorrhage found intraoperatively.

Besides the excellent hemostatic effect of the glue, the adaptation of the tissue surfaces without a foreign body reaction is striking.

Ocular Histopathologic and Biochemical Studies of Cerebrohepatorenal Syndrome (Zellweger's Syndrome) and Its Relationship to Neonatal Adrenoleukodystrophy

Sander M. Z. Cohen, Frank R. Brown III, Lois Martyn, Hugo W. Moser, Winston Chen, Mildred Kistenmacher, Hope Punnett, Warren Grover, Zenaida C. de la Cruz, Nongnart R. Chan, and W. Richard Green
Am. J. Ophthalmol. 96:488–501, October 1983   7–6

The eyes of three infants with cerebrohepatorenal disease who died were examined. The findings included ganglion cell loss, gliosis of the nerve fiber layer and optic nerve, optic atrophy, and retinal and pigment epithelial changes resembling those of retinitis pigmentosa. Bileaflet inclusions identical with those characterizing neonatal adrenoleukodystrophy were seen in the pigment epithelium and in pigmented macrophages, but not in the cornea. An excess of very-long-chain fatty acids was found in the ocular tissues, as in adrenoleukodystrophy. A greater than fivefold increase in these fatty acids was found in the cholesterol ester fraction, compared with a control specimen.

The cerebrohepatorenal syndrome and neonatal adrenoleukodystrophy share similar ocular abnormalities and the presence in the ocular tissues of saturated very-long-chain fatty acids. Condensations of paired, electron-dense leaflets were seen in pigment epithelial cells and in macrophages in the subretinal space in all three of these cases of cerebrohepatorenal syndrome. Changes resembling those of retinitis pigmentosa are found in both disorders. Such changes are found in a variety of diseases, including metabolic storage diseases. Increased amounts of very-long-chain fatty acids also have been found in fibroblasts, brain, and adrenal tissue from patients with cerebrohepatorenal syndrome.

▶ "Zellweger's syndrome," you say. What is Zellweger's syndrome? Perhaps it is better known by another term, "cerebrohepatorenal syndrome." If that still doesn't mean a great deal, suffice it to say that Zellweger's syndrome is now considered to be the most thoroughly documented example of a recently formulated group of diseases, namely, peroxisomal disorders. Perhaps a more thorough explanation is in order.

The infant with hypotonia and severe neurologic dysfunction or seizures presents a difficult and important problem in differential diagnosis. These signs and symptoms can be associated with multiple things. However we now must include Zellweger's syndrome in the differential diagnosis. This disorder was first described 21 years ago. Diagnostic features include an abnormal skull shape and facial appearance, enlargement and impaired function of the liver, renal cortical cysts, and stippled irregular calcifications of the patellae. Eye abnormalities are as described in this article by Cohen et al. The eyes may show Brushfield's spots, as in Down's syndrome. In fact, some children with Zellweger's syndrome have been diagnosed mistakenly as having mongolism. The incidence of this disorder is about 1 per 100,000 births. It is transmitted as an autosomal recessive disease and thus mandates precise diagnosis and genetic counseling because the disease is invariably fatal, with most children rarely surviving beyond age 4 months. In 1973, Goldfischer et al. (*Science* 182:62, 1973) found that patients with Zellweger's syndrome lack peroxisomes. Peroxisomes are single-membrane-limited cytoplasmic organelles that contain oxidases, which produce hydrogen peroxide, and catalase, which reduces hydrogen peroxide to water. Peroxisomes have additional multiple other functions involved with fatty acids and bile acids.

A. E. Mosher et al. (*N. Engl. J. Med.* 310:1141, 1984) have shown that one of the results of this peroxisomal disorder is the production of very-long-chain fatty acids. In fact, the presence of such fatty acids in the blood of patients with Zellweger's syndrome allows prompt diagnosis. Indeed, these investigators have speculated that using cultured amniocytes and examining the production of the types of fatty acids made should be able to establish a prenatal diagnosis of Zellweger's syndrome. This report had only been out about 1 month when investigators from Norway and Sweden (*Lancet* 1:1234, 1984) in fact did make a prenatal diagnosis of Zellweger's syndrome retrospectively. This all came about in a curious way. The mother of an infant with Zellweger's syndrome had a healthy child in 1976, and in 1978 she had a boy who died at age 1 week of an ill-defined disorder. Because of this, the next pregnancy in 1983 was studied with amniocentesis. No specific abnormal findings were found on karyotype or in α-fetoprotein levels. The child born of this pregnancy had all the characteristics of Zellweger's syndrome, which was documented and proved by long-chain fatty acid studies. The child died at age 6 months. Fortunately, a centrifuged sample of amniotic fluid had been stored, and 11 months later the cells were thawed and examined for fatty acid synthesis. Indeed, the diagnosis could have been made prenatally in the affected child.

Reading this commentary might strike you as a bit like eating an artichoke, you had to go through so much to get so little. Suffice it to say that Zellweger's syndrome is an interesting disorder that we will be hearing more about in the future.—J.A.S., III

Comparison of Aortography, Renal Vein Renin Sampling, Radionuclide Scans, Ultrasound, and the IVU in the Investigation of Childhood Renovascular Hypertension

D. A. Stringer, P. de Bruyn, M. J. Dillon, and I. Gordon (Hosp. for Sick Children, London)

Br. J. Radiol. 57:111–121, February 1984   7–7

The findings in 17 children who underwent renal angiography between 1977 and 1980 and had a diagnosis of primary renovascular disease causing hypertension were reviewed. Twelve angiograms showed bilateral involvement. A significant renal venous renin ratio was found in 14 patients. Segmental renal venous sampling yielded significant findings in all but 1 of 13 patients. Five patients had definite or probable neurofibromatosis. The chief angiographic findings in these patients were main renal artery stenosis and collaterals. Ten patients had definite or probable fibromuscular dysplasia. The most common angiographic abnormality in this group was segmental renal artery stenosis. Eight patients had intrarenal and extrarenal collaterals, and 5 had cutoff peripheral vessels. Only 2 had main renal artery stenosis. A "string of beads" appearance was seen in only 2 cases of fibromuscular dysplasia. Hypertension was cured in 3 of the 6 patients who were operated on, and management was made much easier in the other 3. Only 1 patient had an intrarenal operation.

Most children in this study had normal findings on both intravenous urography (IVU) and abdominal ultrasonography. Radionuclide studies with ^{99m}Tc-dimercaptosuccinic acid (DMSA) were helpful in showing photon-deficient areas due to intrarenal vascular anomalies. Renal venous renin ratios were valuable in demonstrating abnormalities. The best angiographic approach is macroroentgenography, with both anteroposterior and oblique views. Initial renal screening by ultrasonography and DMSA scanning is recommended. The urogram should be omitted, or done after the other studies are completed. Renal venous renin ratios may be normal in angiographically abnormal cases, emphasizing the need for complete segmental renal venous renin estimates.

Effect of Captopril on the Renin-Angiotensin System in Hypertensive Children

Aaron L. Friedman and Russell W. Chesney (Univ. of Wisconsin)
J. Pediatr. 103:806–810, November 1983   7–8

The effects of captopril on the renin-angiotensin-aldosterone (RAA) system was evaluated in 9 children, aged 6–18 years, with severe hypertension. Three had end-stage renal disease and were receiving hemodialysis, 2 developed severe hypertension after kidney transplantation, and the other 4 had systemic lupus erythematosus, hemolytic uremic syndrome, essential hypertension, and segmental renal artery stenosis with renal hypoplasia, respectively. In all patients, captopril produced a reduction in blood pressure and permitted the elimination or a decreased dosage of other antihypertensive agents. In 4 patients, treatment with captopril was stopped, but not as a consequence of adverse drug effect. In all patients, plasma renin activity (PRA) and angiotensin I (A-I) levels remained high or increased after captopril therapy. Values for angiotensin II (A-II) decreased after captopril treatment in 5 of the 6 patients in whom valid comparisons were obtained. Captopril intervenes in the RAA system by inhibiting angiotensin-converting enzyme, thereby diminishing the conversion of A-I to A-II (Fig 7–4).

The authors conclude that their findings on children receiving captopril are much like those described for adults. The major effects on the RAA

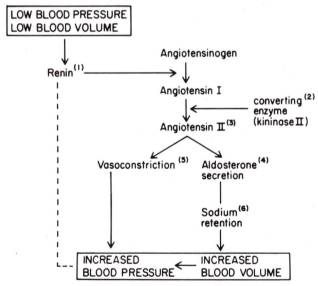

Fig 7–4.—Role of renin-angiotensin-aldosterone axis in blood volume and blood pressure homeostasis. Sites at which specific pharmacologic agents exert their action: *(1)*, β-adrenergic blockers (inhibit renin release); *(2)*, converting enzyme inhibitors; *(3)*, competitive antagonist A-11; *(4)*, aldosterone antagonist; *(5)*, vasodilators; *(6)*, diuretics. (Courtesy of Friedman, A.L., and Chesney, R.W.: J. Pediatr. 103:806–810, November 1983.)

system include a persistent elevation in PRA and A-I, with a concomitant fall in circulating A-II and aldosterone.

▶ Trying to make a diagnosis of renovascular hypertension can be as difficult as trying to sew buttons onto a custard pie. The preceding article shows us an approach to the diagnosis of childhood renovascular hypertension; the investigators from the Hospital for Sick Children, Great Ormond Street, London, tell us that the high incidence of intrarenovascular anomalies in children with renovascular disease emphasizes the need for angiographic techniques that will identify these often subtle findings. A child with systemic hypertension, an increased peripheral venous renin level, and two normal kidneys on ultrasound raises the real possiblity of renovascular disease as the cause of the hypertension. At the beginning of an investigation, it would be helpful to choose an imaging technique that will pick up the more common renal causes of hypertension, e.g., the pyelonephritic scar or the small kidney, as well as most of the children suffering from renovascular disease. When seen in this overall perspective, it is strongly recommended that the initial renal screening of children with systemic hypertension should be an ultrasound study and a radionuclide scan. An intravenous pyelogram is no longer considered necessary as part of this evaluation except under unusual circumstances. Ultimately, angiograms will be necessary in most cases, and as the authors from England suggest, one must be prepared to look for subtle intrarenal findings.

What to do about hypertension is the topic of this study by Friedman and Chesney. It seems clear that captopril is an effective antihypertensive agent in children. This drug works by intervening in the renin-angiotensin system by inhibiting angiotensin-converting enzyme, thereby diminishing the conversion of angiotensin I to angiotensin II. A block at this level may cause a rise in peripheral renin activity but also will cause a decline in plasma aldosterone levels (see Fig 7–4, in that article). Coinciding with the fall in plasma aldosterone values, plasma potassium concentrations increase, although there is rarely symptomatic hyperkalemia. Most patients using captopril and diuretics do not experience significant diuretic-induced hypokalemia. Thus, one of the nice effects of captopril when used in conjunction with diuretics is the little change in potassium caused by this combination. Even though it seems logical that captopril would be most effective in patients with hyperrenin hypertension, all forms of hypertension in children seem to respond to captopril. There are many theories as to why this is true, but it is true, and captopril thus is an effective agent for just about any kind of hypertension in children. This has been borne out by other studies as well (*J. Pediatr.* 103:799, 1983).

Captopril has entered the pediatric market with great caution because of the known observation that 50% of adults will develop adverse side effects as a result of this drug. Side effects in children seem to be much fewer, and in the reference just cited the only significant side effect was neutropenia, which did not require discontinuation of the drug.

Obviously, if a child with hypertension is documented to have renovascular hypertension, consideration for surgery will be in order. If, however, the renal vessel abnormality is sufficiently discrete, percutaneous transluminal renal angioplasty might obviate the need for surgery. This has now been used on a number of occasions.—J.A.S., III

Hyperammonemia in a Boy With Obstructive Ureterocele and *Proteus* Infection
Binod Sinha and Ricardo Gonzalez (Univ. of Minnesota)
J. Urol. 131:330–331, February 1984   7–9

The hyperammonemia associated with urinary stasis and infection by urea-splitting organisms can cause encephalopathy even if liver function is normal. The authors describe an infant with ureteroceles obstructing the ureters and bladder outlet who had sepsis and hyperammonemia despite normal liver function.

Boy, aged 10 months, had developed fever 4 days before being seen, followed by melena and gross hematuria with clots. He became lethargic and unresponsive and had seizures. Examination showed hyperactive tendon reflexes and episodes of motor activity with tonic extension of the arms. The rectal temperature was 38.2 C and the pulse, 160 beats per minute. The boy was generally unresponsive but withdrew from painful stimuli. A left upper quadrant mass was felt, and the right kidney was enlarged. Blood-tinged urine was expressed from the urethra. The hemoglobin concentration was 9.6 gm/dl. The white blood cell count was 33,000/cu mm, with 90% neutrophils. The blood urea nitrogen concentration was 106 mg/dl, and the blood ammonia concentration, 185 μmole/L. There was evidence of metabolic acidosis. Liver enzyme activities were normal. The urine contained red and white blood cells, bacteria, and 2+ protein, and culture yielded *Proteus mirabilis*. Ultrasonography showed dilatation of both renal collecting systems, and cystography indicated a filling defect at the base of the large, trabeculated bladder. An EEG suggested diffuse cerebral dysfunction of toxic or metabolic origin. Percutaneous nephrostomy tubes were placed bilaterally after 4 hours of hemodialysis and tracheal intubation. Antegrade pyelography showed massive bilateral hydroureteronephrosis. Cystoscopy revealed a large ectopic ureterocele on the right, obstructing the bladder. The blood ammonia concentration fell to normal. On hospital day 12 a duplicated collecting system with a ureterocele from the upper pole ureter was removed on the right side. Another ureterocele was removed on the left, and the ureters were reimplanted. Cental nervous system dysfunction has not recurred, and renal and liver functions have remained normal.

Hyperammonemia can occur in a patient with urinary stasis and infection by a urea-splitting organism. Encephalopathy can result when ammonia is transferred to the systemic venous circulation rather than diffusing back into the urine. Urinary drainage and antibiotic therapy lead to clinical improvement as the blood ammonia concentration declines.

▶ This observation is a very important one that all of us should attempt to remember. As discussed in Chapter 6, Gastroenterology, in this YEAR BOOK, children who have portacaval shunts as part of the management of portal hypertension are unusually susceptible to the development of hyperammonemia.

These types of urinary infections could be fatal for such children, and a word to the wise should be sufficient.—J.A.S., III

Desmopressin Response of Enuretic Children: Effects of Age and Frequency of Enuresis
Ernest M. Post, Robert A. Richman (SUNY Upstate Med. Center), Piers R. Blackett, Paul Duncan (Univ. of Oklahoma), and Kenneth Miller (Lutheran Genl. Hosp., Park Ridge, Ill.)
Am. J. Dis. Child. 137:962–963, October 1983   7–10

A three-center, double–blind crossover study of effectiveness, dose dependency, and side effects of desmopressin in children with enuresis was designed. The study was carried out over four 2-week periods: pretreatment baseline, administration of drug A, administration of drug B, and posttreatment observation. Desmopressin acetate (0.1 mg/ml) was randomly assigned to be either drug A or B. Fifty-two children, aged 6–16, who had a history of severe primary or secondary nocturnal enuresis participated. After conclusion of the baseline period, parents were instructed to administer the drug, 0.2 ml (equivalent to 40 μg of desmopressin acetate) at 8 P.M. each night in each nostril. Drinking was prohibited until the morning. At Syracuse, the same group had participated 3 months earlier in an identical study using a lower dose of desmopressin (20 gm night).

Forty-four children had fewer than 5 dry nights during the base period, and 8 had 5–7 dry nights; 39 (75%) had a reduction in the frequency of enuresis while taking desmopressin. None had significant adverse effects. There was no difference in the mean number of dry nights with desmopressin between those taking it before (mean ± SEM, 7.3 ± 0.9 nights) and after the placebo (mean ± SEM, 5.4 ± 0.9 nights; t = 1.53). The mean number of dry nights was significantly increased during the desmopressin period in comparison with either the pretreatment or placebo period. During the desmopressin period, 6 children (12%) had a good response (13–14 dry nights) and 15 children (29%) had 8–12 dry nights.

Among the 17 children aged 9 years or older, with 4–7 dry nights during the base period, 12 (71%) responded to desmopressin (8–14 dry nights); the 6 children with a good response were also older than age 9. In contrast, none of the 15 children younger than age 9 with fewer than 3 dry nights before therapy responded to the drug.

Desmopressin is proposed as treatment of enuresis because of its antidiuretic action. It is safe and sometimes effective, especially in children older than age 9 years. The higher dose (40 μg) is recommended for 2-week trials as it is more likely to be effective than the lower dose.

▶ Enuresis remains a common disorder of childhood. One of every 5 children is nocturnally enuretic at the time he or she begins school and approximately 1% to 2% of this population continues to be enuretic at the time of graduation from high school. We still don't seem to have any greater insight into the reasons for enuresis in most children. We also seem to be willing to hang our hats on practically anything that tells us why this problem occurs or gives us some clue as to what might be a terrific therapy. Take, for example, the observation of Booth et al. (*Br. J. Urol.* 55:367, 1983). These investigators biopsied the bladders of a number of children with enuresis and showed histologically that the bladder of these children had trabeculation and collagen infiltration similar to the bladders of adults with obstructive uropathy. Some have seized on this report to swing the tide back to organic causes of enuresis. It probably just isn't so, however. Such histologic findings could just as well be an effect rather than the cause of enuresis.

This study by Post et al. is one of the few controlled investigations that have looked at desmopressin for the treatment of enuretic children. This nicely controlled report answers some questions but leaves us a bit ignorant with respect to others. Desmopressin can work, but the overall success rate was just 41%. It seemed to work best in older children and in those with less significant problems with enuresis. Unfortunately, these investigators did not examine the persistence of the effects of desmopressin beyond 3 months of treatment. Thus, we have no insights whatsoever regarding the potential long-term benefits of this drug. As we all know, the way desmopressin works when given just before bedtime is simply to decrease the amount of urine in the bladder. Everyone has hoped for long-term benefits via some sort of conditioning that might be the result of being free of bedwetting for some time as a result of this drug. The latter point has never really been documented clearly. Despite this weakness, the investigators reporting this study conclude with the statement that desmopressin seems to be a reasonable alternative to other pharmacologic agents, alarm systems, and hypnosis for treating the child with enuresis. While I agree that anyone who goes to a psychiatrist or psychologist probably ought to have his or her head examined, I do not necessarily agree that desmopressin is more useful than the alarm approach. Trials with the alarm have shown short-term benefits of up to 80%, success rates and long-term benefits that most likely will surpass the use of desmopressin. Desmopressin thus seems to be relegated to adjunctive therapy or as a "quick fix" for children who want to be guaranteed an enuresis-free night on special occasions.—J.A.S., III

Urinary Tract Abnormalities in Children With Supernumerary Nipples
Izhak B. Varsano, Lutfi Jaber, Ben-Zion Garty, Masza M. Mukamel, and Michael Grünebaum (Tel-Aviv Univ.)
Pediatrics 73:103–105, January 1984   7–11

Conflicting data have been reported on the association between renal abnormalities and supernumerary nipples. Urinary tract abnormalities were sought in 26 children with supernumerary nipples, found during a 1-year survey of patients referred to an emergency room and a general pediatric outpatient clinic. The 16 boys and 10 girls had a mean age of 3 years. Intravenous urography was done in all cases, and ultrasonography was done in the last few patients. Anomalies were discovered in 5 of the

16 boys and in 1 girl. Two children had a double excretory system, and 1 each had bilateral polycystic kidneys, hydronephrosis with ureteropelvic junctional stenosis, junctional stenosis alone, and ureteral prolapse. Four children with normal urographic findings had a history of urinary tract infections. No subect had clinical evidence of genitourinary pathology. The only other anomaly was mild hypospadias in 1 subject. One child had Niemann-Pick disease.

Urinary tract abnormalities were present in about one fourth of children with supernumerary nipples in this survey, compared with the 5%–10% expected in an unselected newborn population. The association was especially prominent in male patients. Three of the 6 children with abnormalities are at an increased risk of renal infection, insufficiency, or both. Children with supernumerary nipples, particularly boys, should be examined for urinary tract abnormality. Radiologic study is necessary on the first suspicion of urinary tract pathology.

▶ The controversy over supernumerary nipples just doesn't seem to die. The authors of this article suggest, ". . .[C]hildren with supernumerary nipples, especially male children, should be evaluated to exclude urinary tract abnormalities" because of a 25% incidence of the same. Curiously, this report followed by only 3 months a study reported from the very same institution (Mimouni, F., et al.: *Am. J. Dis. Child.* 137:952, 1983) that, while showing an incidence of supernumerary nipples of 1 in 40 infants, concluded, "It would not seem justifiable to do invasive exploratory investigations in every infant with this minor anomaly." The latter study was based on examination of almost 1,700 infants, but did not include ultrasound examination of all infants with supernumerary nipples. Even though both of these reports were from the same institution, different investigators were involved in each study. I suppose what is necessary is for routine sonography to be done when such extra nipples are found to see what a wider experience might be in other people's hands.—J.A.S., III

Diagnosis of Testicular Torsion
Bruce E. Haynes, Howard A. Bessen (Los Angeles County Harbor-UCLA Med. Center, Torrance), and Vital E. Haynes (Sharp-Cabrillo Med. Center, San Diago, Calif.)
JAMA 249:2522–2527, May 13, 1983   7–12

Torsion of the spermatic cord or a testicular appendage occurs in 1 of every 160 men by the age of 25; 65% of these torsions occur between the ages of 12 and 18 years. In a review of the literature, the authors discuss the diagnosis of testicular torsion and present guidelines for physicians examining patients with acute scrotal pain and swelling.

The testis is extremely sensitive to any impairment of blood flow through the spermatic cord. The normal testis is surrounded by tunica vaginalis, except where the testis attaches to the epididymis and posterior scrotal wall (Fig 7–5). In "bell-clapper" deformities, the tunica vaginalis com-

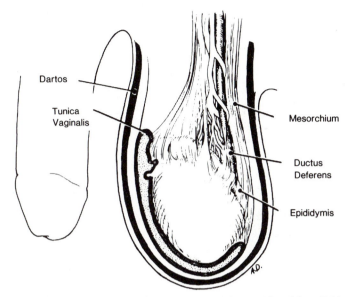

Fig 7–5.—Relationship of tunica vaginalis to testis in normal state. Adapted from Holder, L.E., et al.: Radiology 125:739–752, 1977. (Courtesy of Haynes, B.E., et al.: JAMA 249:2522–2527, May 13, 1983; copyright 1983; American Medical Association.)

pletely surrounds the testicle and extends above it, thereby allowing the testicle to move freely on the spermatic cord (Fig 7–6). Torsion usually occurs spontaneously when the testis, lacking its normal attachment to the scrotal wall, twists one or more times on the spermatic cord. Undescended testes are more prone to these abnormalities. The four testicular appendages are pedunculated and also may undergo torsion.

Testicular torsion is a surgical emergency, with salvage rates typically reflecting the interval between onset of symptoms and operation. Although the causes of scrotal swelling are well known, the clinician often must distinguish torsion from epididymitis (table). This differentiation, however, is complicated by overlapping ages of peak incidence, shared symptoms, and the urgency to make the correct diagnosis. Radionuclide blood flow scans have an accuracy of 95% in the diagnosis of testicular torsion, but delays in arranging for a scan could have serious consequences. Doppler blood flow studies, including a funicular compression test, are reasonably accurate (88%), but correct technique is essential and indeterminate results are not uncommon.

Immediate surgery is indicated in any patient in whom torsion is strongly suspected and in any patient in whom there is a suspicion of torsion who will have to wait more than 1 hour for a nuclear scan. Nuclear scans are recommended in patients younger than age 35 years when evidence of torsion is not compelling enough to warrant immediate exploration and evidence of epididymitis or another lesion is equivocal. Doppler studies may be most useful in the confirmation of blood flow in patients in whom

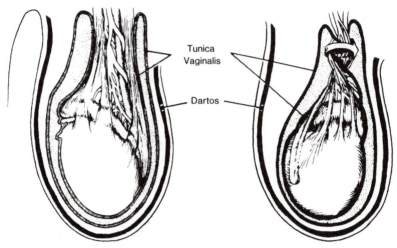

Fig 7–6.—"Bell-clapper" malformation resulting in torsion. Adapted from Holder, L.E., et al.: Radiology 125:739–752, 1977. (Courtesy of Haynes, B.E., et al.: JAMA 249:2522–2527, May 13, 1983; copyright 1983, American Medical Association.)

epididymitis is strongly suspected. The diagnosis of epididymitis in men younger than age 35 should be made cautiously; those older than age 35 with epididymitis may be treated conservatively.

Micturition Studies and Sexual Function in Operated Hypospadiacs
J. Svensson and R. Berg (Karolinska Hosp., Stockholm)
Br. J. Urol. 55:422–426, August 1983   7–13

The most common complication after hypospadias surgery is fistula formation. The authors investigated micturition patterns in 33 male patients, aged 15–34, operated on during early childhood for hypospadias of varying degree. All patients underwent urethral reconstruction, with or without previous correction of chordee. The mean interval between urethral reconstruction and voiding studies was 19 years.

In all patients, the meatus was on the undersurface of the glans or in the sulcus coronarius. A small fistula 1 cm proximal to the meatus in the sulcus coronarius was seen in 1 patient. Another patient with 45XO/46XY karyotype had the testes removed because of the increased risk of testicular cancer. The most common complaint was spraying during micturition (13 patients). Two patients reported that voiding in the standing position was impossible, another 2 had difficulty in starting micturition, and 1 reported postmicturition dribbling. Thirteen patients believed that the penis was too small at erection, and 5 complained of persistent curvature of the penis at erection, although only 1 reported that sexual intercourse was impossible. Two patients had weak or painful ejaculation. Eight patients had

DIFFERENTIAL DIAGNOSIS OF TORSION

Characteristics	Torsion of Spermatic Cord	Epididymoorchitis	Torsion of Appendage
Age, yr	<35 (perinatal, peripubertal peaks)	>16 (unless urinary tract infection or urinary tract abnormality)	<16 (adolescent peak)
Pain			
Onset	Acute	Gradual	Acute or gradual
Location	Testis; radiates to groin, abdomen	Epididymis; then testis, groin, abdomen	Appendage, then testis
History of similar pain	Common	Uncommon (unless prior epididymitis)	Occasional
Vomiting	Common	Uncommon	Uncommon
Dysuria, urethral discharge	Rare	Common	Rare
Fever	Unusual	Common (low grade)	Unusual
Involved testis			
Position	High-riding	Dependent	Normal; "blue-dot" sign early
Tenderness	Diffuse	Epididymal, becomes diffuse	Appendage, becomes diffuse
Contralateral testis	Possible horizontal lie	Normal (vertical)	Normal
Ipsilateral spermatic cord	Normal	Thickened, tender	Normal
Prostatic tenderness	Rare	Occasional	Rare
Pyuria	Unusual	Common	Unusual
Blood flow (Doppler studies, technetium Tc 99m scan)	Decreased	Increased	Normal, increased

(Courtesy of Haynes, B.E., et al.: JAMA 249:2522–2527, May 13, 1983; copyright 1983, American Medical Association.)

no problems with regard to micturition, penile size, erection, or ejaculation. Neither mean maximum flow nor the voided volume in the hypospadiacs differed significantly from these values in controls. Micturition time, however, was significantly longer in the hypospadiacs $(P < .05)$.

The irregular form of the reconstructed meatus probably accounts for some of the complaints of urinary stream spraying. Persistent curvature of the penis may be prevented by the injection of saline into the corpora during operation. Measurement of urinary flow may be the best way to diagnose lower urinary tract obstruction. Long-term follow-up studies appear to indicate that the Denis Browne procedure results in an adequate urethra.

▶ Max Maizels, Assistant Professor of Urology, Northwestern University Medical School, and Director, Urological Research and Center to Assist the Regulation of Enuresis, Children's Memorial Hospital, comments:

"The authors attempt to assess long-term results of surgical correction of hypospadias in childhood, emphasizing the quality of micturition. Thirty-three boys had correction of hypospadias during childhood or adolescence using the technique of Denis Browne (staged urethroplasty). Evaluation of the boys 1–28 years later disclosed about 10% complained of spraying of the urinary stream and fewer complained that voiding in the standing position was impossible. Postvoid dribbling, a perception of the small penis or curvature of the penis, and a recessed meatus also were noted. By physical examination, the urethral meatus resided on the undersurface of the glans or in the coronal sulcus. Objective evaluation of the parameters of voiding was attempted by a measurement of urinary flow rates. The authors compared the results of urodynamic testing in the study group with surgically corrected hypospadias against urodynamic testing of controls. The only difference noted was that the time to void was statistically significantly longer in persons with hypospadias than in controls. The authors conclude that the Denis Browne urethroplasty seems to provide adequate urethras as judged by long-term urodynamic follow-up studies. A considerable number of patients, however, complain of spraying of the urinary stream.

"It is difficult to assess surgical procedures performed almost 30 years ago without imposing the standards of modern hypospadias surgery. The Denis Browne urethroplasty is an acceptable technique to reconstruct the hypospadiac urethra; however, it is notorious for the problems mentioned. Current technology emphasizes the correction of hypospadias as a *single*-staged procedure along with placing the urethral meatus on the glans. Intraoperatively, complete correction of chordee is verified by the installation of fluid into the corpora to simulate an erection. Persistence of penile curvature can be remedied by further excision of chordee tissue ventrally or perhaps by excising portions of tunica albuginea of the corpora dorsally to compensate for atresia of the ventral penile shaft. Follow-up results of the duration presented in this article are not available for single-stage procedures; however, early follow-ups suggest that complete correction of chordee and attainment of a funneled stream capable of being directed by the children are routine. Thus, although, the Denis Browne urethroplasty may have been the gold standard 30 years ago, it is not today."

Endocrine Studies in Patients With Advanced Hypospadias

Terry D. Allen and James E. Griffin (Univ. of Texas, Dallas)
J. Urol. 131:310–314, February 1984   7–14

Hypospadias no longer appears to be solely a local dysmorphic disorder. Fifteen boys, aged 4 years and younger, who had perineal or deep penoscrotal hypospadias and a scrotal cleft were evaluated. Fourteen major abnormalities of potential endocrinologic significance were found in 11 of the patients. A poor testosterone response to human chorionic gonadotropin was seen in 7. In several instances it improved over time, and 2 patients gained normal responses. Five of the 8 patients given testosterone had phallic enlargement and increased scrotal rugation, but 2 did not respond; the latter patients had the highest androgen receptor numbers in the series. One child had been exposed to progesterone in the first trimester.

One had an abnormal karyotype, and 1 had an absent gonad on one side. One patient with a family history of Reifenstein's syndrome had low receptor numbers.

The findings suggest that hypospadias is a local manifestation of an endocrinopathy, rather than a local dysmorphic problem. One major cause may be delayed maturation of the hypothalamic-pituitary-testicular axis. The most striking abnormality in these cases was in the testosterone response to chorionic gonadotropin injection. Clinical responses to testosterone administration suggested that long-range decisions relating to sex assignment should not be based solely on initial examination of the external genitalia.

▶ This study is certainly well written. However, the worst possible thing is to write something well and be absolutely wrong. Only time truly will tell if these authors are barking up the wrong tree. Although theoretically it seems reasonable to consider that hypospadias may be a local manifestation of some underlying systemic endocrinopathy, efforts to confirm this in numerous studies have yielded only mixed results. While the authors of this article have observed that subjects with hypospadias have a higher than expected probability of not responding with an increase in testosterone to human chorionic gonadotropin injections, other investigators have focused on the penis itself as being at fault. Coulam et al. (Proceedings of the Annual Meeting of the American Urologic Association, abstract no. 6, 1983) concluded that most of the hypospadias patients they studied exhibited either defective conversion of testosterone to dihydrotesterone or some qualitative defect of the androgen receptor in the penis. This latter concept is an interesting one, because androgen insensitivity is described in at least one other disorder (the testicular femininization syndrome). Most subjects with hypospadias do not show decreased sensitivity to testosterone upon closer examination (*Am. J. Obstet. Gynecol.* 147:513, 1983). I think it will be a long time before we can ever be certain of the exact reason why some boys have hypospadias at birth.

Before leaving the penis to go on to other urologic matters, some mention should be made of the micropenis. D. M. Salisbury et al. caution us that any time we see a newborn with a small penis we should consider that that infant may have had prenatal gonadotropin deficiency. The male external genitalia are formed as a result of androgen secreted by the fetal testis under the influence of placental human chorionic gonadotropin. This process is over with by the end of the first trimester, and any growth of the penis after that is due to testosterone stimulation by the infant's pituitary luteinizing hormone. Consequently, prenatal gonadotropin deficiency of any cause may result in a small but normally formed penis—the micropenis. Thus, the micropenis may be physical evidence of hypopituitarism. Whereas we pediatricians recognize the significance of virilization of female genitalia as occurs in congenital adrenal hyperplasia, the importance of underdevelopment of male external genitalia is often not appreciated. Obviously, a newborn with hypopituitarism may suffer disastrous consequences as a result of lack of ACTH, with resultant adrenal failure under stress. So, the next time you see a small penis, look it up on the charts to see whether it is indeed small (*J. Pediatr.* 87:663, 1975) and, if it is, think of hypopituitarism. The report by Salisbury et al. appeared in the *British Medical Journal* (288:621, 1984).—J.A.S., III

Congenital Abnormalities and Growth Patterns Among Cryptorchidic Boys
K. Bjøro Jr. and T. Dybvik (Gjøvik, Norway)
Ann. Chir. Gynaecol. 72:342–346, 1983   7–15

Associations of various congenital abnormalities with cryptorchidism are unclear. Inadequate pituitary hormone secretion in early life could alter growth in cryptorchid children. The relationships among congenital abnormalities, birth weight, and gestational age in 165 boys operated on between 1977 and 1982 for cryptorchidism were examined. Cases of retractile testes were excluded. Thirty-two patients had bilaterally undescended testes.

The rate of prematurity in 144 evaluable cases was 11.8%, and the rate of postmaturity was 7.6%. Congenital abnormalities were detected in 9% of patients; they covered a wide range. More than half these patients had bilaterally undescended testes. Patients were taller than their brothers at all ages up to 10 to 11 years, and a similar but less marked tendency was observed for body weight. Height and weight at age 18 and subsequently differed little from measurements of brothers at the same age or of fathers. Testicular maldescent in the father was reported in 4% of cases, and in 6.5% of cases a brother was reported to be cryptorchid.

A high rate of premature birth and a high incidence of congenital abnormalities was found in this series of cryptorchid boys. Patients appeared to be somewhat taller and slenderer than their brothers prepuberally, suggesting a hypogonadal pattern of growth. Final height did not differ from that of the patients' brothers or fathers. The degree of genetic influence in cryptorchidism remains unclear.

▶ Incomplete descent of one or both testes into the scrotum represents the most common congenital defect. Single or bilateral failure of descent occurs in about 3% of male infants overall. Slightly over one half of these will show descent in the first month of life and only 1% of boys will have undescended testes at age 1 year. There have been multiple observations associating cryptorchidism with other congenital anomalies. The most common of these are those of the urogenital tract. Even so, the frequency is sufficiently low that no one recommends routine study of the urinary tract in uncomplex, undescended testes. This article from Norway is much more ominous in some respects. It suggests that a small percentage (about 10%) of boys with cryptorchidism will have a wide variety of congenital anomalies. What association is occurring here is beyond me. But the data are there and require pursuit.

This past 1½ years has been a banner time with regard to the controversies over circumcision in the United States (Thompson, H. C.: *Am. J. Dis. Child.* 137:939, 1983; Maisels, N. J., et al.: *Pediatrics* 71:453, 1983; Wallerstein,

E.: ibid. 72:750, 1983; and Halve, R. L., et al.: *Clin. Pediatr.* 22:813, 1983). These reports involve things such as the "humane" circumcision using regional anesthesia, despite the fact that the most humane thing would be not to perform the circumcision to begin with. The report by Maisels et al. indicates that printed literature stating all of the reasons why circumcision is not necessary does not dissuade parents from going ahead with the procedure for their infant sons. There is probably only one thing that will significantly reduce the circumcision rate in the United States. It is the same thing that had the most impact in Great Britain—and that is to have no third-party coverage for the procedure if it is being done on a "routine" basis.

(Since this is the last commentary in the chapter "The Genitourinary Tract," I thought I might take some editorial privileges to indicate that we who coedit serve not only to punctuate. As an example of this, because this chapter was written during a period of time off at home, I asked my wife what it was like to have a man around the house. Her reply: "It makes a vas deferens." Such is life.)—J.A.S., III

8 The Heart and Blood Vessels

Hypomastia and Mitral Valve Prolapse: Evidence of a Linked Embryologic and Mesenchymal Dysplasia
Carol A. Rosenberg, Gordon H. Derman, William C. Grabb, and Andrew J. Buda (Univ. of Michigan)
N. Engl. J. Med. 309:1230–1232, Nov. 17, 1983   8–1

Because both the breast and the mitral valve are of mesenchymal origin, an association may exist between development of breast size and mitral valve prolapse. The authors studied the prevalence of mitral valve prolapse in patients with primary hypomastia and examined the prevalence of hypomastia in a population with known mitral valve prolapse. Three groups of subjects were studied: 27 women aged 22–58 with hypomastia (group A), 33 control women aged 21–60 (group B) and 28 women aged 16–65 with mitral valve prolapse (group C).

Results showed that of the 27 (48%) patients with hypomastia, 13 met echocardiographic criteria for mitral valve prolapse. In contrast, only 2 (6%) of the 33 control women had prolapse. Of the 28 patients with prolapse, 17 had hypomastia, compared with 8 of the controls. All associations are statistically significant. In group C, 13 (46%) of the patients had one or more thoracoskeletal abnormalities as compared with 2 (6%) of the control women; this result was statistically significant. In group A, 11 (40%) had at least one thoracoskeletal abnormality, which was also significantly greater than in controls. Embryologic data derived from 5 human embryos confirmed the simultaneous presence of breast and mitral value mesenchymal proliferation, active chondrification of the ribs and vertebral column, and development of sternal bars.

Hypomastia is described as an additional nonauscultatory characteristic associated with mitral valve prolapse. This clinical finding may strengthen a diagnostic impression or arouse suspicion that prolapse is present. Identification is important, because patients with this disorder may be predisposed to bacterial endocarditis and require antibiotic prophylaxis; may experience symptomatic arrhythmias, transient ischemic attacks, or stroke; and often may present with cardiac symptoms.

▶ The associations with mitral valve prolapse just do not seem to ever end. It was not enough that patients with mitral valve prolapse tended to have pectus excavatum, scoliosis, straight back, and other miscellaneous skeletal abnormalities. Now, young ladies with this disorder also have a greater than 50% probability of demonstrating hypomastia. This cannot be found in boys, because they have no "mastia" worth speaking about. You might ask how the investigators in this study were able to come up with 27 women with hypomastia. They simply went to a plastic surgery practice and evaluated all women who had a desire for breast augmentation procedures and who had a breast size of under 200 cc. We are not told how the breast size was determined, whether this was by best guess, nonfilling of a 6-oz drinking cup, or water displacement. Whatever technique was used, there was general agreement that the breast size was small.

Exactly what causes the complex associations seen with mitral valve prolapse is not known. It has been postulated that mitral valve prolapse may represent a forme fruste of Marfan's syndrome, in which a basic connective tissue disorder leads to myxomatous changes in the mitral valve and the associated skeletal abnormalities. It has been postulated that the association of mitral valve prolapse and von Willebrand's disease may represent a dysplasia that resembles other inherited disorders of connective tissue. The data presented in this study indicate an association between primary hypomastia and mitral valve prolapse and could provide evidence that a linked embryologic and mesenchymal dysplasia may be the unifying concept explaining many of the associated conditions seen with mitral valve prolapse. There is a high prevalence of this disorder in patients with von Willebrand's disease, Ehlers-Danlos syndrome, and pseudoxanthoma elasticum, as well as those with Marfan's syndrome. Additionally, the platelet, a mesenchymally derived cell, has a high incidence of hyperactivity in patients with prolapse, which may predispose them to transient ischemic attacks and stroke (*Circulation* 63:552, 1981).

Identification of patients with mitral valve prolapse is probably quite important because such patients may be predisposed to bacterial endocarditis and therefore may require antibiotic prophylaxis. In any event, if I were a plastic surgeon seeing a young lady for a breast augmentation procedure, I probably would think twice about going ahead and operating without doing some further studies. Some feel that all patients with mitral valve prolapse should have complete coagulation studies prior to surgery. This would seem to be especially appropriate where cosmetic results are imperative. If a plastic surgeon is not careful, he could wind up being a plastic sturgeon on some malpractice lawyer's wall.—J.A.S., III

Management of Critical Aortic Stenosis in Infancy

James D. Sink, Jeffrey F. Smallhorn, Fergus J. Macartney, James F. N. Taylor, Jaroslav Stark, and Marc R. de Leval (Hosp. for Sick Children, London)

J. Thorac. Cardiovasc. Surg. 87:82–86, January 1984   8–2

Aortic valvular stenosis that produces left ventricular failure in infancy carries a high mortality. A review was done of the management of 8 infants suspected of having critical aortic stenosis, 6 boys and 2 girls aged 2 days to 7 months at admission. All patients underwent valvotomy, 6 at age 2 weeks or younger. Six infants presented with congestive heart failure. Cross-sectional echocardiography showed hypertrophy of the left ventricular free wall and interventricular septum in all cases. Aortic valvotomy was carried out under inflow occlusion without invasive studies being done.

The valves were seen to be bicuspid and dysplastic and primitive in nature and are often thickened and gelatinous. One extremely ill infant died at operation when the heart fibrillated; severe endocardial fibroelastosis was found at autopsy. Another infant with severe fibroelastosis and mitral stenosis died 5 weeks postoperatively. Four surviving patients were asymptomatic at follow-up 6–28 months after operation. One infant became asymptomatic after ligation of a persistent ductus that had not been patent at initial evaluation. Three patients with continued evidence of left ventricular hypertrophy had a second valvotomy; the postoperative course was uneventful in all instances.

Aortic stenosis can be diagnosed accurately in infants by cross-sectional echocardiography. Cardiac catheterization can be avoided in most cases (Fig 8–1). Inflow occlusion is a safe and reliable operative approach in infants without associated intracardiac lesions. Mortality compares fa-

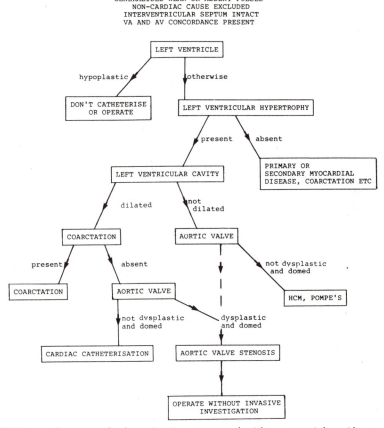

Fig 8–1.—A decision tree for the noninvasive assessment of a sick neonate or infant with suspected critical aortic stenosis. *HCM*, hypertrophic cardiomyopathy. (Courtesy of Sink, J.D., et al.: J. Thorac. Cardiovasc. Surg. 87:82–86, January 1984.)

vorably with that of operations using cardiopulmonary bypass. Several infants have required early reoperation, possibly because of aggressive follow-up evaluation. Two patients were asymptomatic at the time of reoperation.

▶ Although uncommon, aortic valvular stenosis of such severity as to produce left ventricular failure in infancy is associated with high mortality. In those infants presenting with congestive heart failure, medical treatment is only rarely effective on the long haul, and early surgical intervention is mandatory for survival. As the investigators demonstrate in this report, if the only abnormality present is valvular stenosis, cardiac catheterization is not requried. Echocardiography will give all the information that is needed. The operation itself can be done without cardiopulmonary bypass. Whether or not balloon catheter dilatation of the aortic valve would work in such infants is not commented on in this article. Presumably, percutaneous transluminal balloon valvuloplasty has not reached the immediate newborn period as far as aortic valves are concerned in this report. It certainly has been used in older children with aortic stenosis (Lababidi, Z., et al.: *Am. J. Cardiol.* 53:194, 1984). This same technique has been used in the dilatation of coarctation of the aorta in young infants (Finley, J. P.: *Br. Heart J.* 50:411, 1983).

The first trip to the operating room for infants with critical aortic stenosis is usually not the last. Many infants require early reoperation. The long-term outlook and need for valve replacement require further follow-up. If anyone is interested in reading about the present status of prosthetic cardiac valves, there is an excellent summary of this in the *Archives of Internal Medicine* (143:1965, 1983).—J.A.S., III

Spontaneous Closure of Secundum Atrial Septal Defect in Infants and Young Children

John T. Cockerham, Thomas C. Martin, Fernando R. Gutierrez, Alexis F. Hartmann, Jr., David Goldring, and Arnold W. Strauss (St. Louis)
Am. J. Cardiol. 52:1267–1271, Dec. 1, 1983   8–3

Ostium secundum atrial septal defects (ASD) account for about 7% of congenital heart disease diagnoses in children. Although these defects generally are not regarded as a significant problem in infancy or early childhood, ASD in children younger than age 1 year has been associated with a mortality of approximately 9% when managed medically. The defect may close spontaneously, even in symptomatic patients, but it also may cause a significant problem in infancy. The records of 264 children with uncomplicated ostium secundum ASD were reviewed to assess its significance in early childhood.

Secundum ASD was diagnosed in 264 (5%) of more than 5,000 patients who underwent cardiac catheterization between 1958 and 1983. Of these 264 patients, 87 (33%) were younger than age 4 years. Subnormal weight gain and frequent episodes of pneumonia, cyanosis, or tachypnea were present in 26 patients (30%), including 16 (18%) of 87 with congestive heart failure. These findings were more common in children seen in the first year of life. Four patients died, but only 1 death was directly attributable to the ASD. Overall, 21 patients underwent a second cardiac catheterization; 15 of these had no evidence of a left-to-right atrial shunt. Spontaneous closure occurred more frequently in patients seen initially in the first 2 years of life, but occurred in patients up to age 4 years. Mean right atrial pressures, left atrial pressures, and the difference between mean left and right atrial pressures did not differ significantly between patients with and without spontaneous closure. There was a significant difference in the Qp:Qs (shunt size calculated from oximetry data), with shunt size tending to be smaller in those with spontaneous closure (1.9 ± 0.4 vs. 2.6 ± 1.1; $P < .02$). Analysis of hemodynamic data did not reveal any statistically significant differences between patients with an ASD who were younger than age 4 years and those who were older at the time of diagnosis. Significant differences were observed between patients with ASD that closed spontaneously and patients with atrial valve shunting secondary to a valve-incompetent foramen ovale. These included significant differences in age at the initial study (11 months vs. 2 months; $P < .001$), mean left atrial pressure (7.7 mm Hg vs 12.3 mm Hg; $P < .02$), and difference between mean right and left atrial pressures (1.0 mm Hg vs. 4.2 mm Hg; $P < .01$).

In light of the high incidence of spontaneous closure of ASD, even in symptomatic patients, intensive medical management rather than surgery is recommended for those with ASD who are aged 2 years or younger. In patients older than age 4 years with ASD, elective surgical correction is recommended because of the likelihood that spontaneous closure will not occur.

Vasodilator Therapy in Children: Acute and Chronic Effects in Children With Left Ventricular Dysfunction or Mitral Regurgitation
Robert H. Beekman, Albert P. Rocchini, Macdonald Dick II, Dennis C. Crowley, and Amnon Rosenthal (Univ. of Michigan)
Pediatrics 73:43–51, January 1984   8–4

The acute and chronic effects of vasodilator therapy were evaluated in 13 children aged 14½ years or younger with severe left ventricular dysfunction or mitral regurgitation. Eleven initially were treated with digoxin and diuretics for congestive heart failure. The 7 patients with the highest ventricular filling pressures received nitroprusside by infusion at a rate of 2 µg/kg/minute during cardiac catheterization. The others received an intravenous bolus of hydralazine, 0.25 mg/kg. One patient received captopril orally. Ten children then received chronic oral vasodilator therapy as well as digoxin and diuretic therapy. The patients who responded to nitroprusside received prazosin, 0.05–0.1 mg/kg 4 times daily, and the others received hydralazine, 0.25–0.5 mg/kg 4 times daily. One patient received 37.5 mg of captopril 3 times daily. The mean follow-up was 5.7 months.

Acute hemodynamic improvement occurred in all nitroprusside-treated patients. All patients but 1 with a normal cardiac index improved when given hydralazine intravenously. All children improved while receiving chronic oral vasodilator therapy, with a reduction in symptoms of heart failure and, in 5 cases, the resolution of all symptoms. Physical findings of heart failure also improved, and growth velocity increased (Fig 8–2). There was no consistent improvement in echographic estimates of left ventricular function. Two patients had recurrent congestive failure that did not respond to altered vasodilator therapy. Overall improvement was not sustained during follow-up, and only half the children lived for 6 months or longer after the start of vasodilator therapy.

Vasodilator therapy may benefit children with congestive heart failure due to severe left ventricular dysfunction or mitral regurgitation, but it cannot be expected to alter the underlying disease state. Orally administered prazosin or captopril can be used in children with elevated ventricular filling pressures who respond to a trial of nitroprusside. Others may benefit from hydralazine therapy. Another drug can be tried if the child deteriorates after an initially good clinical response.

▶ Traditional medical therapy for congestive heart failure consists of the administration of digoxin and diuretics. In recent years, however, vasodilators have emerged as important additional agents in the management of heart failure due to a number of cardiac causes. Vasodilators decrease smooth muscle tone in

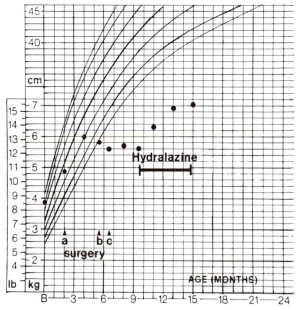

Fig 8–2.—Growth chart of a patient demonstrating improved weight gain in response to oral hydralazine therapy. Patient had severe left ventricular dysfunction and previously had undergone three surgical procedures for anomalous pulmonary venous return. (Courtesy of Beekman, R.H., et al.: Pediatrics 73:43–51, January 1984. Copyright American Academy of Pediatrics 1984.)

arteriolar and venous capacitance vessels, thereby decreasing ventricular afterload, preload, or both. This promotes more complete ventricular emptying, thus increasing the patient's cardiac output. This effect has proved to be beneficial in patients with mitral regurgitation, aortic regurgitation, and primary or ischemic cardiomyopathy. The drugs such as the ones discussed in this article have been used now for a fair amount of time in many pediatric intensive care unit-type settings, but there are few reports of any long-term clinical trials with the use of oral vasodilator therapy. This is the value of this study. It shows that, on the short haul, the effect of vasodilation can be spectacular. Unfortunately, long-term results are variable. Many children die with recurrence of heart failure. Such poor long-term results, in the face of early improvement with vasodilators, can be due to a number of factors. It simply may reflect the natural history of severe cardiac disease. It also could be a manifestation that drug tolerance to the use of vasodilators eventually occurs in these types of patients. The remarkable thing to me about hydralazine and drugs that work like it is that it may sustain the life of a child with cardiomyopathy sufficiently long that the underlying disease process eventually burns out on its own. I sense that many people use these types of drugs only as last-ditch efforts. Maybe this is their real role, but no child with congestive heart failure should probably die without being afforded the benefit of afterload-reducing agents.

Since we've been talking about agents that treat congestive heart failure, here are the latest updates on digoxin, which include two interesting observations. One is that newborn infants frequently produce a substance that gets into the plasma and has digoxin-like immunoreactive properties. No one knows where this material is from, but it is produced endogenously. Several infants have been described who have such sufficient amounts of this material that it causes false positive digoxin values. This makes the use of digoxin measurements in this age group quite complex (Valdes, R., et al.: *J. Pediatr.* 102:947, 1983). A second important observation is the fact that the new antiarrhythmic drug amidorone changes the half-life of digoxin clearance. The addition of amidorone to digoxin therapy can increase digoxin serum levels as much as 800%. If you are not familiar with amidorone, it was originally used as an antianginal agent but soon was found to be highly effective in controlling most of the supraventricular as well as ventricular arrhythmias. It is particularly helpful in patients with Wolff-Parkinson-White syndrome. The recent review of this apparently spectacular drug may be found in *Pediatrics* (72:813, 1983).—J.A.S., III

Incidence of Acute Rheumatic Fever: A Suburban Community Hospital Experience During the 1970s
Richard H. Schwartz, Seymour I. Hepner, and Mohsen Ziai
Clin. Pediatr. (Phila.) 22:798–801, December 1983   8–5

The incidence of acute rheumatic fever has declined remarkably in the past 3 decades, but the disease has not been eradicated. The authors report data on 23 cases seen in middle-class children from Fairfax County, Virginia, in 1970 through 1980. All the children had private primary-care physicians. Parents of 1 child were from Saudi Arabia, 1 child had an American Indian father, and the other 21 were white children of European ethnic background. Diagnosis of acute rheumatic fever was based on modified Jones' criteria except for 2 children with Sydenham's chorea.

The 12 girls and 11 boys were aged 5 to 18 years. All were admitted to the hospital with a diagnosis of acute rheumatic fever, 19 of them (83%) betweeen 1970 and 1974 and only 2 (7%) between 1976 and 1980. The table summarizes the criteria used to diagnose acute rheumatic fever. Hospital stay was 2 to 30 days. Eighteen patients treated with aspirin alone improved dramatically within 3 days after starting salicylate therapy. Two children in this series had visited their pediatrician for a sore throat 2 to 3 weeks prior to hospital admission. Throat culture for both was positive for group A streptococci, and penicillin was prescribed for 10 days. The parents of 10 children recalled the child had had a sore throat within 1 month of onset of rheumatic fever. Annual age-adjusted incidence rate of initial attacks of acute rheumatic fever per 100,000 children in Fairfax County declined from 3.0 in 1970 to 0.5 in 1980.

DIAGNOSTIC CRITERIA FOR 23 CHILDREN WITH
ACUTE RHEUMATIC FEVER ADMITTED TO FAIRFAX
HOSPITAL IN 1970–1980

Diagnostic Criteria	Number of children	Percent
Major criteria		
Migratory polyarthritis	10	43
Rheumatic carditis	6	26
Polyarthritis plus carditis	7	30
Sydenham's chorea	2	9
Erythema marginatum	0	0
Subcutaneous nodules	0	0
Minor criteria		
Clinical		
Fever	17	74
Arthralgias	18	78
Laboratory and electrocardiographic		
Leukocytosis	11	48
Erythrocyte sedimentation rate		
≥ 20 mm/hr	22	96
C-reactive protein	10	43
Prolonged P-R interval	8	35
Evidence of preceding streptococcal infection		
Antistreptolysin O titer ≥ 333		
Todd units	20*	87
Scarlet fever	2	9
Throat culture positive for group A streptococcis	5	22

*Two patients without elevated ASO titer had Sydenham's chorea and another had carditis, arthralgia, and elevated erythrocyte sedimentation rate.

(Courtesy of Schwartz, R.H., et al.: Clin. Pediatr. (Phila.) 22:798–801, December 1983.)

▶ Where has all the rheumatic fever gone? For speculations on the answers to this question, see the commentary of Alan Bisno that appeared in the same issue of *Clinical Pediatrics* as the article presented here. Everyone's presumption, including Bisno's, is that there has been a decline in the rheumatogenic potential of currently prevalent group A streptococci. Unfortunately, there is no way to prove this point.—J.A.S., III

Autoantibodies to SS-A/Ro in Infants With Congenital Heart Block
Barbara R. Reed, Lela A. Lee, Catherine Harmon, Robert Wolfe, James Wiggins, Carol Peebles, and William L. Weston
J. Pediatr. 103:889–891, December 1983   8–6

Neonatal lupus erythematosus is a rare syndrome characterized by congenital heart block (CHB) or transient cutaneous lupus. The mothers of these neonates may have connective tissue disease, but consistently have circulating antibodies to SS-A/Ro antigen. The prevalence of serum SS-A/Ro autoantibodies were assessed in 12 unselected children with CHB, 6 of whom were studied with their mothers in the neonatal period and 6 retrospectively.

Seven of the 12 infants were boys. Complete atrioventricular dissociation was present in 10 infants and 2:1 atrioventricular block in 2. Two children had annular, erythematous, scaly plaques on sun-exposed skin that were histologically typical of lupus erythematosus. Six of the mothers were without symptoms, 1 was photosensitive, 2 had arthralgias, 2 had sicca syndrome, and 1 had systemic lupus erythematosus. All of the 6 children studied during the neonatal period and their mothers had circulating antibodies to SS-A/Ro. Three of these infants followed serologically for 1 year were seronegative at 1 year, but their mothers remained seropositive with the same antibody specificities. Of the 6 families studied retrospectively, 3 mothers had SS-A/Ro autoantibodies, 1 had RANA antibodies only, and 2 had no evidence of antinuclear antibodies on immunofluorescence and immunoprecipitation studies. Autoantibody status was not determined in the children of these mothers. Of the 6 infants with SS-A/Ro antibodies, 1 also had SS-B/La antibodies and 1 had RANA antibodies. Of the 9 mothers with SS-A/Ro antibodies, 3 also had SS-B/La antibodies, 2 had RANA antibodies, and 1 had antinative DNA antibodies.

The findings suggest that CHB may be related to transplacental passage of maternal SS-A/Ro antibodies and that neonatal lupus may be the most common etiologic factor in CHB.

Cardiac Pacing in Children and Young Adults
Deborah G. Wampler, Cathleen Shannon, Gina V. Burns, and Paul C. Gillette (Baylor College of Medicine)
Am. J. Dis. Child. 137:1098–1100, November 1983   8–7

Pacemakers are being used with increasing frequency in children. New pacemakers are smaller, more sophisticated, can be programmed, have output telemetry, are more reliable, and are longer lasting. Implant techniques have been modified, so that they are less traumatic to the patient and result in better electric measurements. Transvenous implants seem to be the preferred method in children who weigh 13.5 kg or more. Physiologic dual-chamber pacemakers make the patients feel better. The authors attempted to determine if these new techniques and technology have led to improved results in pediatric pacing by reviewing the records of 143 pediatric and young adults followed up in the Texas Children's Hospital Pacemaker Clinic in Houston during a 15-year period between November 1967 and June 1982. The 143 patients had follow-up of 171 pacemakers. Patients were newborn to age 40 years (mean, 9.5 years).

The electrophysiologic indications for pacemaker implantation were third-degree atrioventricular block (81 patients), sick sinus syndrome (53), and other dysrhythmias (9). In 116 patients, the pacemaker was implanted by a cardiac surgeon in the operating room with the patient under general anesthesia. Twenty-seven had pacemakers implanted by a pediatric cardiologist using sedation and local anesthesia. Of the 12 patients (8%) who died during follow-up, 1 died because of pacemaker malfunction. At the end of the study, the average interval between hospitalizations was 22 months. Causes for pacemaker-related reoperation included electric malfunction (10 patients), infection (2), and premature battery depletion (9). The 14 patients with lithium batteries had depletion at an average of 2.31 years. Endocardial leads clearly have a lower voltage threshold than do epicardial leads.

The authors believe, based on their review, that patients should be considered for pacemaker implantation if they are symptomatic, are likely to become symptomatic, or are severely limited by bradycardia. Patients should receive pacemakers to allow as nearly normal and active a life as possible.

▶ Craig Byrum, Professor of Pediatrics, State University of New York Upstate Medical Center, comments:

"Cardiac pacing in children has changed considerably in recent years, mostly as a consequence of rapid advancements in pacing technology. As this article by Wampler et al. nicely demonstrates, the rates of pacemaker failure and pacemaker-related complications have diminished dramatically. Our own pacing experience in children at the Upstate Medical Center in Syracuse mirrors the Houston experience, demonstrating a significant increase in the interval between initial implant and follow-up pacer-related operations. Not surprisingly however, the operation interval correlates to the age at implant in that earlier age at implant is associated with an earlier need for reoperation (0.9 years for implant at age ≤2 years vs. 2.3 years for implant at age >2 years. In light of the continued need for reoperation in patients who have been committed to pacemaker therapy, the indications for initial implantation must be strictly adhered to; they include surgical heart block (a decreasing phenomenon in our institution to a level of 0.2% for all open heart operations over the past 4 years), nonsurgical bradydysrhythmias (sick sinus syndrome, congenital block, etc.) with either unacceptable low rates for age or frank symptoms of syncope, and other dysrhythmias as alluded to by Wampler et al. We believe that the level of sophistication of evaluation of patients considered for implant must rise to the level of sophistication of pacemaker technology and should include, in addition to stress testing and ambulatory ECG monitoring, complete catheter electrophysiologic evaluation. This approach allows the pacemaker mode to be tailored to the specific strengths and weaknesses of the child's conduction system, avoids potential pacemaker complications such as pacemaker-induced arrhythmias and pacemaker syndrome, and deters placement of unnecessary hardware in the patient. Goals for the future in pacemaker therapy for children should include, in addition to producing longer-lived pacemaker sources, reduction in pulse generator size for cosmetic purposes in our smaller patients and attempts to develop pacemakers that respond to metabolic and temperature changes in the body. In other words: There's nothing like the real thing!"

Experience With Iatrogenic Pediatric Vascular Injuries: Incidence, Etiology, Management, and Results
D. Preston Flanigan, Teresa J. Keifer, James J. Schuler, Timothy J. Ryan, and John J. Castronuovo (Univ. of Illinois, Chicago)
Ann. Surg. 198:430–442, October 1983   8–8

The authors evaluated 76 children for iatrogenic arterial injuries in 79 lower extremities in a 32-month period. Forty-two of the children were followed prospectively after cardiac catheterization, and 10 of them sustained vascular injuries. The other 34 children were referred with 35 vascular injuries resulting from transfemoral cardiac catheterization in 20, umbilical artery catheterization in 10, and recent operation in 5 (Table 1). All injuries were evaluated by segmental Doppler pressure recording. An ankle-brachial pressure index (ABI) of less than 0.9 was considered to be abnormal.

Thirty injuries involved the common femoral artery and 10, distal vessels. There were 2 aortic injuries. Mean patient age was 31 months; 84% of patients were aged 4 years and younger. Twelve operations were carried out. Fourteen of the 22 patients followed during medical management received heparin, and 2 received urokinase also. The other 8 patients had contraindications to anticoagulant therapy. The mean ABI after injury was

TABLE 1.—SOURCES OF PEDIATRIC ARTERIAL INJURIES

Etiology	No. of Injuries
Transfemoral cardiac catheterization	30
Umbilical artery catheters	10
Surgical procedures	5
Total	45

(Courtesy of Flanigan, D.P., et al.: Ann. Surg. 198:430–442, October 1983.)

0.34, but initial values were unrelated to clinical outcome. The ABI returned to normal in more than 90% of heparin-treated patients and in more than 60% of patients who were observed. Limb length discrepancies exceeding 0.5 cm developed in 1 patient who was operated on and in 5 who were managed medically (Table 2). They represented one third of patients with ischemia lasting longer than 30 days. No patient had tissue loss or required amputation.

Iatrogenic arterial occlusion is usually evident from the history and physical findings. The presence or absence of a palpable femoral pulse is a key factor in deciding on management. Immediate limb-threatening ischemia is infrequent after iatrogenic arterial injury, but it does occur and calls for early revascularization where feasible. Many patients, however, are poor surgical risks. Most children who have not been operated on have eventually had a normal ABI, although retarded limb growth has been a problem. Operation usually is required for aortic thrombosis. Other children with pulse loss should be heparinized if possible and observed for 6 hours before reconstruction is undertaken. Operation may be indicated for older patients with distal occlusions. The role of thrombolytic therapy should be studied further.

▶ The fact that 76 children were evaluated for iatrogenic vascular injuries in just 32 months in one institution highlights the common nature of this problem everywhere. Children may experience arterial occlusion from multiple sources. Embolization from cardiac sources and spontaneous arterial thrombosis secondary to dehydration, polycythemia, infection, and congestive heart failure account for most nontraumatic etiologies. It would seem that these events are rare compared to the incidence of iatrogenic traumatic arterial occlusions. Most arterial injuries occur after arteriography, cardiac catheterization, umbilical artery catheterization, and needling procedures for arterial blood samples. A high incidence of complications after these procedures is not surprising because the vessels are extremely small and many of these children are severely ill with decreased cardiac output, polycythemia, and dehydration. At particularly high risk are older children with the nephrotic syndrome (Sullivan et al.: *South. Med. J.* 76:1011, 1983). It is well known that the peripheral arteries of younger children tend to go into spasm much more readily. One staggering observation

TABLE 2.—CHILDREN DEVELOPING LEG LENGTH DISCREPANCIES

Patient	Age* (Mo)	Length of Ischemia (Mo)	ABI†	Leg Length Discrepancy (cm)
1	1	5	0	0.50
2	2	2	.6	0.75
3	48	7	.78	2.25
4	3	14	.58	3.00
5	NB‡	20	0	1.00
6	13	13	.2	0.50

(Courtesy of Flanigan, D.P., et al.: Ann. Surg. 198:430–442, October 1983.)

from this study was that 25% of patients undergoing femoral catheterization show evidence of iatrogenic vascular injury. Obviously, not all these by any means require surgical intervention, but careful observation along with determination of blood flow via the Doppler technique and perhaps heparinization are necessary for these types of patients. A few conclusions can be made from this report and others like it (Klein, M. D., et al.: *J. Pediatr. Surg.* 17:933, 1982). The pediatric cardiologist must work closely with the surgeon interested in vascular surgery if identification of injuries that might otherwise be overlooked is to be done and prevention of complications initiated. Secondly, the follow-up of patients with complications should be indefinite. Thus far, no one has been able to predict which patients are going to develop limb-growth discrepancies. The duration of ischemia and the degree of occlusion by Doppler technique are not predictive. The role of thrombolytic therapy in very young children is also something that has not been evaluated thoroughly. All surgeons seem to agree on one thing, and that is that conservative therapy with very careful monitoring seems to produce the best results. Early surgery seems to be indicated most frequently in cases of large aortic thrombi.—J.A.S., III

Level, Trend, and Variability of Blood Pressure During Childhood: The Muscatine Study
Ronald M. Lauer, William R. Clarke, and Robert Beaglehole
Circulation 69:242–249, February 1984   8–9

The predictive value of childhood blood pressure measurements for the development of hypertension and other disorders in adult life is unknown. The findings were reviewed in a longitudinal study of schoolchildren in Muscatine, Iowa, in whom blood pressure was measured in alternate years from 1970 to 1981. A total of 4,313 children were examined three to six times, starting at ages 5 to 14 years. Each reading was expressed as a percentile rank, and the average percentile rank, trend in rank, and variability over time were calculated for each subject.

The relation between average blood pressure rank and average rank of body size was significant, as was that between trend of blood pressure and trend of body size percentiles. Height, weight, relative weight, and triceps skinfold thickness were assessed. A subgroup of 5.4% of the children had systolic pressure levels in the upper quintile with either a flat or a rising trend and low variability and appeared to be consistently tracking toward future hypertension (Fig 8–3). Six percent of the children had pressure levels in the lower four quintiles with a high trend and low variability. A group of 7.4% of the children had mean systolic pressure levels in the upper quintile with high variability; they resembled adults with labile hypertension.

There appear to be important relationships among body size, growth, and blood pressure in childhood. The final rank order of blood pressure may not be totally established until full body size is reached, but groups of children can be distinguished that consistently maintain a high rank order or that consistently increase or decrease their rank order of blood

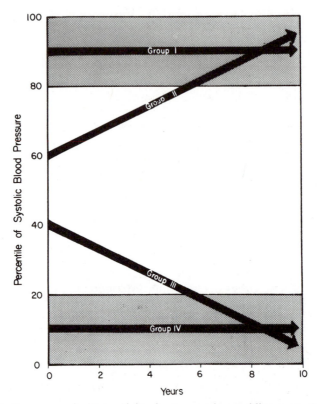

Fig 8–3.—Four groups of subjects with blood pressure tracking in different ways. Stippled areas indicate upper and lower quintiles of blood pressure. Group I (consistently high) maintains blood pressure in upper quintile; group II (increasing high) tracks upward over time to upper quintile, and average percentile over time was in upper quintile; group III (decreasing low) tracks downward to lowest quintile, and average percentile over time was in lowest quintile; and group IV (consistently low) maintains blood pressure in lowest quintile. All groups have low variability. (Courtesy of Lauer, R.M., et al.: Circulation 69:242–249, February 1984; by permission of the American Heart Association, Inc.)

pressure. Further studies of these children could help elucidate the early roles of genetic, environmental, and nutritional factors that contribute to essential hypertension in adult life.

Validity of Mass Blood Pressure Screening in Children
David E. Fixler and W. Pennock Laird (Univ. of Texas, Dallas)
Pediatrics 72:459–463, October 1983   8–10

A mass blood pressure screening program was carried out on Dallas high-school students between 1976 and 1980. Initially, 10,641 eighth graders were screened. The screenings were repeated 2 and 4 years later as this student body progressed to twelfth grade.

Students with initial systolic or diastolic blood pressures at or above the

95th percentile (Table 1) were recalled for second and third examinations (Table 2). Prevalence of initially elevated systolic or diastolic pressure, or both, ranged from 8.9% to 13%. Prevalence of persistent blood pressure elevation was 1.6% for eighth graders, 1.7% for tenth graders, and 1.9% for twelfth graders. Of those with persistent elevations in the eighth grade, approximately 40% had persistent elevations in the tenth grade.

The validity of the test is expressed in quantitative terms as sensitivity, specificity, and predictive value. Sensitivity may be defined as the proportion of true positives correctly identified; in the tenth-grade survey, sensitivity was 72%. Specificity is defined as the ability to give a negative finding in the absence of the condition; specificity in this survey was 91%. Predictive value of a positive test is the likelihood that a subject with a positive test has the condition; predictive value was only 17% due to the tendency of youths with elevated blood pressure to have normal pressure on reexamination.

The cost of the examinations was $5.53 per student. Also to be consid-

TABLE 1.—BLOOD PRESSURE LEVELS AT 95TH PERCENTILE

Group by Race	8th Grade		10th Grade		12th Grade	
	Girls	Boys	Girls	Boys	Girls	Boys
Systolic (mm Hg)						
Black	130	130	128	134	126	136
White	126	132	128	138	124	138
Mexican-American	128	132	128	136	128	136
Diastolic (K$_5$, disappearance)						
Black	76	74	76	78	76	78
White	74	72	76	80	74	78
Mexican-American	74	74	76	78	77	78

(Courtesy of Fixler, D.E., and Laird, W.P.: Pediatrics 72:459–463, October 1983. Copyright American Academy of Pediatrics 1983.)

TABLE 2.— PREVALENCE OF SUSTAINED BLOOD PRESSURE ELEVATIONS*

	8th Grade Survey (1976–1977)	10th Grade Survey (1978–1979)	12th Grade Survey (1980–1981)
No. initial screened	10,641	9,017	6,542
2nd examination	947 (8.9%)	900 (10.0%)	850 (13.0%)
3rd examination	277 (2.6%)	306(3.4%)	301 (4.6%)
Persistent blood pressure elevation	170 (1.6%)	153 (1.7%)	124 (1.9%)

*Sensitivity = (true positives, correctly identified)/(true positives) = 152/211 × 100 = 72%. Specificity = (true negatives, correctly identified)/(true negatives) = 8,058/8,806 × 100 = 91%.

†Estimated from a 10% sample of those with negative findings on initial screening.

(Courtesy of Fixler, D.E., and Laird, W.P.: Pediatrics 72:469–463, October 1983. Copyright American Academy of Pediatrics 1983).

ered is the potential for psychologic morbidity due to being labeled as hypertensive, for the initial misclassification of children with transient blood pressure elevations may cause unnecessary anxiety. Close communication with parents to alleviate misunderstandings regarding the implications of a single high reading in a child is imperative.

A mass screening program must be evaluated in terms of its yield, the number of cases identified in which prognosis is improved as a result of earlier detection. Drug therapy should be started only after salt restriction or weight reduction have proved unsuccessful. Drugs should be used only in children with persistent hypertension (greater than 90 mm Hg before age 12 years and greater than 100 mm Hg after age 12 years). No cases of persistent hypertension were found among the 10,641 eighth graders of the Dallas survey.

Results of the present study support the recommendations of The Task Force on Blood Pressure Control in Children that mass community screening programs not be instituted for children and adolescents, as there is potential for psychologic damage by misclassifying a child as hypertensive. Measurement of blood pressure should be a routine procedure in office practice where the significance of positive findings can be discussed with parents.

▶ The rationale for mass blood pressure screening is based on the presumption that once high-risk children are identified, the hypertensive process may be halted in its early stages in instituting preventive measures. Hypertension is a well-known risk factor for the later development of heart disease, stroke, and renovascular disease. Several studies have suggested that essential hypertension in adults may have its origins in youth. Because prevention is preferable to cure, it may seem reasonable to advocate mass screening programs for high blood pressure in children to determine those youngsters with established hypertension as well as those who appear to be at risk for developing hypertension. The validity of this concept is what this article and the preceding one are about.

The report from Muscatine, Iowa, seems to imply that trends are established among certain groups of children with respect to blood pressure. Some children who track in the highest percentiles will continue to track in those percentiles. Some who are in the lowest percentiles tend to stay in those low percentiles. Children in between can go up or down with time. The results from the Bogalusa Heart Study likewise appear to suggest that some trends are established in childhood with respect to blood pressure (Webber, L. S.: *J. Chronic Dis.* 36:647, 1983). In this study, systolic blood pressure remained high on second examination in 35% of children with initially high systolic pressures and remained high on third examination in 30%. Diastolic blood pressures were more difficult to interpret.

The exact usefulness of this information is the topic of this article from Dallas. There, only 152 of 900 students with blood pressures initially above the 95th percentile were subsequently found to have sustained elevation. This produced a predictive result of only 17%. In fact, the prevalence of persistent hypertension was only between 1% and 2% of all children overall. Most importantly, among the 10,000+ 8th graders who were examined as part of the mass screening program in Dallas, no cases of hypertension were found that required treatment. The study from Dallas supports the recommendations of the Task Force on Blood Pressure Control in children, namely, that mass community blood pressure screening programs should not be instituted for children and adolescents. As there is potential for psychologic damage by misclassifying a child as hypertensive, the recommendation was made that the measurement or blood pressure should be a routine procedure in the office practice of pediatrics where explanations and follow-up can be accomplished easily. Whether the recommendations of the Task Force are correct requires more time to sort out. There are enough longitudinal studies underway to answer the important questions, and until those answers are firmly in hand, we probably should stick with the current recommendations. Until more information is in, this commentator will keep a low profile on this topic and keep his comments to himself, following the dictum that until necessary one should, "See no upheaval, hear no upheaval, and speak no upheaval."—J.A.S., III

Concurrent Validity Studies of Blood Pressure Instrumentation: The Philadelphia Blood Pressure Project
William F. Barker, Mary L. Hediger, Solomon H. Katz, and Evelyn J. Bowers
Hypertension 6:85–91, Jan.–Feb. 1984   8–11

There is increasing evidence that blood pressure screening in adolescence may detect early hypertension, but the use of proper instrumentation is important in maximizing the interpretive value of serial readings. Two studies in adolescents were undertaken to compare auscultatory blood pressure measurements with the Baumanometer and Random-zero sphygmomanometer, ultrasonic measurements with the Arteriosonde 1216, and infrasonic measurements with the Physiometrics SR-2 device. The Baumanometer is a conventional mercury-gravity sphygmomanometer. The Random-zero device minimizes terminal digit preference and examiner bias. The instruments were compared serially in 48 older adolescents, and all but the Random-zero device were compared both serially and simultaneously in 24 older and younger adolescents.

Reliability estimates in the first study were high except for the Arteriosonde 1216 diastolic readings. The Physiometrics SR-2 yielded lower mean diastolic pressure readings than the other devices. Diastolic phase V readings made with the Random-zero device were higher when it was used at the end of the sequence of instrument presentations. The Arteriosonde 1216 also proved to be unreliable in recording diastolic pressure in the second study. The Physiometrics SR-2 gave diastolic readings significantly lower than simultaneous and serial diastolic phase IV readings. The rigid, oversized cuff used with the Physiometrics SR-2 gave reduced systolic pressure readings when the subject's arm circumference was small.

There is at present no definitely acceptable alternative to the conventional manual mercury sphygmomanometer for screening adolescents for high blood pressure. Screening is best done by a well-trained examiner using a conventional mercury manometer in a standardized manner.

▶ You might feel a little "underwhelmed" by this article. The reason for including it in the YEAR BOOK is based on the anecdotal observation of several of my friends in practice who say they are being requested by parents to do blood pressure checks on their child after the child dropped a quarter in the automatic blood pressure-taking machine in the local shopping mall and the results suggested that he or she was hypertensive. The spread of automated blood pressure-taking devices in these types of settings has reached epidemic proportions.

Measuring blood pressure indirectly using automated devices should offer significant advantages, i.e., less examiner training and minimization of errors and bias in examiner perception. Automated devices may offer greater sensitivity in measuring the diastolic sounds that can be barely audible by auscultation. This is especially important in measuring the blood pressure of children and adolescents because there is a greater likelihood that these sounds will be faint or tend to persist to near 0 mm Hg. Although there is general agreement that ultrasonic instruments facilitate the measurement of blood pressure in newborns, use of these instruments for older children and adults for routine blood pressure checks has never been investigated accurately. The purpose of this study by Barker et al. was to compare several different types of newer instruments with a routine mercury sphygmomanometer (the Baumanometer). The Random-zero sphygmomanometer is essentially the same as a Baumanometer except that in order to minimize an examiner's bias toward thinking what a normal blood pressure would be, the Random-zero allows for random and blind resetting of the zero level on the instrument within a range of 0 to 60 mm Hg. For this reason, the blood pressure cuff must be inflated some 80 to 100 mm above the expected diastolic level because the instrument's zero set is unknown. The Arteriosonde 1216 measures systolic blood pressure by recording the pressure at which the arterial wall vibrations cause a Doppler shift, which is picked up by ultrasonic waves emitted by a transducer installed within the blood pressure cuff. Diastolic blood pressure is recorded when the arterial wall vibrations are sensed by the transducer to stop. This instrument is equipped with an automatic timed inflation and deflation system. The final instrument examined was the Physiometrics SR-2. This instrument does not measure Korotkoff sounds directly, but infrasonically detects the oscillations in the arterial walls that have been shown to produce the blood pressure sounds. This instrument can be operated manually or automatically. It comes with an oversized, rigid cuff that is recommended for use when subjects are ambulatory. From my experience in shopping malls, it is the latter instrument that I have run across most frequently.

How well do all of these instruments work compared to the old-fashioned mercury sphygmomanometer? Not very well, at least in adolescents. As Barker et al. indicate, at present there is no definitely acceptable alternative to the conventional manual mercury sphygmomanometer for screening adolescents for high blood pressure. This is best done by a well-trained examiner using a conventional instrument in a standardized manner.

One place where routine blood pressure monitoring may be worthwhile is in the video arcade. Gwinup et al. (*Postgrad. Med.* 74:245, 1983) examined the cardiovascular changes produced in a group of young men. This study was begun when a video-game machine was installed in the medical students' lounge at the University of California, Irvine Medical Center. In order to understand the results of this study, you have to understand what video-game machine was installed. The game was called "Berserk." In this game, a character appears on the left side of the screen and moves toward the right side. The vertical movement of the character, as well as the firing of rockets by the character, is controlled by the player. As the character advances to the right, rockets are fired at it by a number of robots that also appear on the screen. The player scores points by shooting and destroying robots and avoiding the shots fired by robots as the character advances toward the right side of the screen. Presumably this instrument is quite a challenge for the average medical student, at least in California. The reason for saying this is that the systolic blood pressure of the average medical student went up 36 mm Hg during the game. The heart rate increased by 18 beats per minute. The only cure for these physiologic responses was to become good at the game, because expert players had little cardiovascular changes. Now to the long list of problems related to video machines that currently includes psychologic disturbances, Space Invaders' wrist, Pac-Man thumb, and Space Invaders' epilepsy (Ed note: I've never seen a case of this, and until I do I consider this a "myth fit"), we must add medical student "Berserk" hypertension. When I was a medical student, if we had any free time at all we usually just sat around the fraternity house watching "Mission Impossible" and never seemed to suffer any untoward problems from it even though we knew that television was nothing more than chewing gum for the eyes.—J.A.S., III

Hypertension in Children With Neurogenic Tumors
Mark E. Weinblatt, Margaret A. Heisel, and Stuart E. Siegel
Pediatrics 71:947–951, June 1983   8–12

Hypertension has been related to excessive catecholamine production and commonly is associated with pheochromocytoma, a catecholamine-secreting tumor. The incidence of hypertension was assessed in 59 children with neurogenic tumors seen at Children's Hospital of Los Angeles or North Shore University Hospital, Manhasset, New York, in 1974 to 1981. Details of 4 cases are presented.

Eleven (19%) of the 59 children were found to be hypertensive at the time of diagnosis or with progression of disease. All 11 had primary abdominal tumors and 10 had abnormal findings on intravenous pyelograms. Neuroblastoma was found in 9 patients, 6 of whom had stage IV disease. Of the remaining 2 children, 1 had a stage III ganglioneuroblastoma and the other had a primary adrenal ganglioneuroma with lymph node involvement. No patient showed evidence of renal failure, all had normal creatinine and blood urea nitrogen levels, and none had a history of preexisting hypertension.

In 8 patients antihypertensive therapy, including different combinations of diuretics, vasodilators, selective α-blockers and β-blockers, and an angiotensin-converting enzyme inhibitor, had a variable but generally poor effect. All blood pressure values returned to normal after excision of the tumor or administration of effective antitumor therapy. Two patients required vasopressive agents to correct transient hypotensive episodes after tumor excision. There was no correlation between elevated blood pressure levels and levels of urinary catecholamine metabolites.

Hypertension was found more frequently in these children with neurogenic tumors than has previously been reported. Blood pressure in patients with newly diagnosed neurogenic tumors should be monitored carefully until definitive therapy has begun to produce a beneficial effect on the tumors.

Nifedipine in Hypertensive Emergencies of Children
Uğur Dilmen, M. Kazim Çağlar, D. Ali Şenses, and Erol Kinik (Hacettepe Children's Hosp., Ankara, Turkey)
Am. J. Dis. Child. 137:1162–1165, December 1983   8–13

The acute antihypertensive effect of sublingually administered nifedipine was studied in 21 patients with different clinical diagnoses. The 13 girls and 8 boys were aged 8 to 16 years and were seen between November 1, 1982 and April 30, 1983. Levels of serum urea nitrogen and serum creatinine were tabulated (Table 1). Nifedipine, 0.25 to 0.50 mg/kg, was administered during an acute hypertensive attack only once, after which the patient was observed for 6 hours for signs of flushing.

Sublingual administration of nifedipine lowered mean systolic blood pressure (BP) from 181 to 132 mm Hg and mean diastolic BP from 136 to 98 mm Hg after 30 minutes (Table 2 and Figs 8–4 and 8–5). There was no significant decrease between the systolic and diastolic BP 1 hour before and just before administration of nifedipine. The antihypertensive effect was maximal after 30 minutes and continued for 360 minutes. Heart rate increased significantly 30 minutes after nifedipine was given. Postural hypotension was not observed in any patient and flushing was observed only in 4 with acute poststreptococcal glomerulonephritis.

This study provides evidence that nifedipine given sublingually is a safe and effective drug for controlling BP in hypertensive emergencies in children.

▶ Nifedipine sounds better than hot apple cider on a cold winter afternoon. When this article was published, it appeared to report the first documented administration of nifedipine for hypertension in children. The results were terrific.

Nifedipine is a calcium-channel blocking agent whose main action in man is a reduction of peripheral resistance. Calcium antagonists prevent the entry of calcium from the extracellular fluid into the intracellular medium via selective channels. Because of this effect, these drugs have become known as calcium-channel blockers. Indeed, the contraction of vascular smooth muscle is depen-

TABLE 1.—LABORATORY VALUES, SYMPTOMS, AND NIFEDIPINE DOSE

Patient	Weight, kg	Serum Urea Nitrogen, mg/dL	Creatinine, mg/dL	Nifedipine, mg/kg	Hypertensive Symptoms
1*	23	110	3.2	0.5	Convulsion
2*	30	85	4.0	0.3	Severe headache, vomiting
3	22	18	0.8	0.4	Drowsiness, severe headache
4*	25	90	4.0	0.4	Drowsiness, vomiting
5*†	22	175	10.0	0.35	Unconsciousness, epistaxis
6*†	25	220	3.5	0.4	Unconsciousness, vomiting
7*	40	140	4.0	0.25	Headache, disorientation, vomiting
8	30	90	2.5	0.35	Severe headache
9*†	25	170	5.5	0.4	Mucosal bleeding, drowsiness
10*†	21	210	6.0	0.5	Mucosal bleeding, drowsiness
11	36	50	1.4	0.3	Convulsion
12*	34	110	3.2	0.3	Severe headache, vomiting
13	30	45	1.3	0.3	Headache, convulsion
14*	30	125	3.0	0.3	Severe headache, vomiting
15	29	20	1.2	0.3	Convulsion
16	24	35	1.1	0.25	Convulsion
17	27	30	1.2	0.3	Severe headache, vomiting, drowsiness
18	30	90	1.8	0.3	Severe headache
19*†	24	240	6.0	0.4	Unconsciousness, mucosal bleeding
20	25	55	1.0	0.3	Convulsion
21*	20	90	2.5	0.4	Drowsiness, vomiting

*Patient had end-stage chronic renal failure.
†Patient was undergoing peritoneal dialysis.
(Courtesy of Dilmen, U., et al.: Am. J. Dis. Child. 137:1162–1165, December 1983; copyright 1983, American Medical Association.)

TABLE 2.—SYSTOLIC/DIASTOLIC BLOOD PRESSURE READINGS*

Patient	Before Nifedipine 1 hr	Immediately	After Nifedipine, min 30	60	120	180	240	300	360
1	220/170	200/170	160/120	160/120	155/125	155/120	150/115	155/115	155/120
2	210/170	200/180	165/120	160/120	155/115	155/115	155/120	155/120	155/120
3	200/160	210/160	165/150	165/150	165/150	160/145	165/150	165/150	165/150
4	200/160	190/150	140/100	140/100	140/100	145/105	145/105	145/105	150/105
5	200/155	200/150	140/100	140/100	145/100	145/100	145/105	145/105	140/105
6	200/150	200/150	130/100	135/100	135/105	135/105	130/100	130/100	140/100
7	200/140	200/140	135/100	135/100	140/100	140/100	145/100	145/100	140/100
8	180/135	180/130	130/100	130/100	130/100	135/100	135/100	135/100	130/100
9	180/130	170/130	130/100	135/100	135/100	130/95	130/95	130/100	135/100
10	180/135	170/135	120/85	120/85	125/90	130/95	130/95	135/100	135/100
11	160/135	160/130	110/70	115/75	115/75	115/75	110/80	110/80	110/80
12	160/130	160/130	125/100	125/100	125/90	130/95	130/95	130/100	130/95
13	160/125	160/120	120/80	120/80	125/85	125/80	120/80	120/80	120/80
14	160/120	160/120	125/100	125/100	125/95	130/95	130/95	130/95	130/95
15	160/100	155/100	125/100	125/100	125/100	120/100	125/100	130/100	130/100
16	165/110	160/110	120/80	120/80	120/80	125/85	125/80	125/80	125/90
17	160/100	165/100	115/80	115/80	115/80	110/85	110/90	110/90	110/95
18	200/150	205/145	130/90	130/90	135/90	130/90	130/90	130/90	120/90
19	190/140	190/145	130/90	130/90	135/95	130/90	130/95	135/95	140/100
20	185/140	190/140	135/100	135/100	135/95	130/95	130/95	130/90	130/90
21	180/120	180/120	125/85	125/85	125/85	130/90	130/85	125/85	125/85

*In mm Hg.
(Courtesy of Dilmen, U., et al.: Am. J. Dis. Child. 137:1162–1165, December 1983; copyright 1983, American Medical Association.)

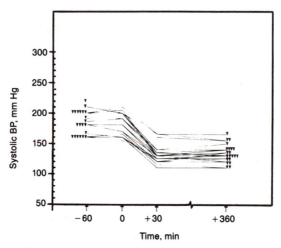

Fig 8–4.—Systolic blood pressure before and after administration of nifedipine. Triangles represent individual patients. (Courtesy of Dilmen, U., et al.: Am. J. Dis. Child. 137:1162–1165, December 1983; copyright 1983, American Medical Association.)

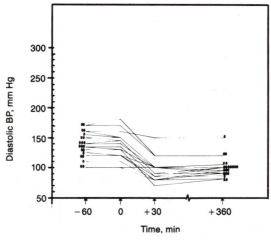

Fig 8–5.—Diastolic blood pressure before and after administration of nifedipine. Dots represent individual patients. (Courtesy of Dilmen, U., et al.: Am. J. Dis. Child. 137:1162–1165, December 1983; copyright 1983, American Medical Association.)

dent on the flow of extracellular calcium. Verapamil and nifedipine are the two most popular calcium-channel blockers that have been used as coronary dilators in adults. Verapamil in pediatrics is used almost exclusively for the management of supraventricular tachycardia. Nifedipine does not have this effect. It does lower the blood pressure quickly and can be given under the tongue—hence, its usefulness in the management of hypertensive emergencies. The drug has been used successfully as part of the management of systemic hypertension in adults. Its use in children clearly will require more evaluation.

Double-blinded trials with appropriate controls matched with other agents will ultimately determine what nitch this drug will have in the pediatric armamentarium. I like to define double-blinded controls as "the study that is so designed as to tell the good guise from the bad." I think nifedipine will either fare well or farewell.—J.A.S., III

Portacaval Shunt in Patients With Familial Hypercholesterolemia

Thomas E. Starzl, H. Peter Chase, Edward H. Ahrens, Jr., Donald J. Mc-Namara, David W. Bilheimer, Ernst J. Schaeffer, Jean Rey, Kendrick A. Porter, Evan Stein, Antonio Francavilla, and Leland N. Benson (Univ. Health Center of Pittsburgh)
Ann. Surg. 198:273–283, September 1983   8–14

Portacaval shunt was performed in 10 patients with homozygous and 2 with heterozygous familial hypercholesterolemia (FH). Follow-up ranged from 14 months to nearly 9 years. Eight of the 12 were children. Nine of the 10 homozygous patients were low-density lipoprotein (LDL) receptor negative and the other was receptor defective. One of the 2 heterozygous patients was from a kindred in which FH homozygous relatives were receptor negative.

Recovery after portacaval shunt was prompt and uncomplicated. One patient died of heart disease after 4 months, 1 after 18½ months, and 1 after 30 months. The other 9 are alive after 14 to 103 months. Total serum cholesterol concentration was lowered by 20% to 55.4% during follow-up, with commensurate decreases in level of LDL cholesterol. The effect on levels of high-density lipoprotein (HDL) cholesterol and triglyceride was variable. Tendinocutaneous xanthomas diminished or disappeared. Growth and development in children proceeded or accelerated. There was no detectable emotional or intellectual deterioration. Hepatic failure did not occur, although concentrations of blood ammonia and levels of serum alkaline phosphatase increased relative to preoperative values. Cardiac symptoms were often improved, but evidence of reversal of cardiovascular lesions was inconclusive.

Portacaval shunt, with or without supplementary treatment, provides palliation only for patients with FH. Restoration of normal serum cholesterol values has not been achieved in any patient with homozygous disease. Because the portacaval shunt has been effective therapy for those with FH who were refractory or intolerant to medical treatment, it is recommended that it be performed before development of irreversible cardiovascular damage.

▶ Most children with familial hypercholesterolemia do not do exceptionally well on medical treatment. Medical management of hypercholesterolemia by dietary manipulation and by administration of agents that are given orally is a very rigorous approach with less than optimal results in most cases. This is the reason why the findings of Starzl et al. utilizing surgery for this problem are so impressive. Portacaval shunts clearly lower cholesterol levels in children with familial hypercholesterolemia. The operation works best for those who are heterozygotes, although there is significant lowering in homozygotes as well.

The mechanism by which portacaval shunting causes a lowering of cholesterol is by inhibition of hepatic synthesis. In Chapter 6, "Gastroenterology," there is a brief discussion of all the physiologic consequences of diverting blood flow from the liver. Basically, many enzyme systems are decreased in their synthesis rates, presumably because of the fact the liver is deprived of first-pass exposure to hormones (especially insulin) and other putative hepatotropic factors from splanchnic viscera. These metabolic abnormalities have been worrisome to many investigators. There is a small but definite risk of hepatic encephalopathy after shunting procedures. Some investigators also have been concerned about the long-term effects of elevated blood ammonia levels on intellectual functioning. Starzl has seen neither of these two complications in his group of patients. If medical management and portacaval shunting do not work for patients with familial hypercholesterolemia, there are only a few other relatively mediocre procedures that can be tried, including ileal diversion which presumably interferes with cholesterol recycling. At the conclusion of this article, Starzl makes the ultimate speculation that because the liver is the major organ regulating metabolism in the body, perhaps all the metabolic abnormalities associated with familial hypercholesterolemia could be rectified by the use of liver transplantation. It remains to be seen whether any therapeutic approach that lowers blood cholesterol levels really affects morbidity and longevity. The whole issue of whether reduction of cholesterol is effective in prevention of vascular disease has been reviewed recently (*Lancet* 1:317, 1984).

The amount of information that has become available recently regarding cholesterol and its management in children has been almost encyclopedic. Although the beauty of an encyclopedia is that it knows what we needn't, when it comes to cholesterol we should be as knowledgable as possible. What is some of this new information? First off, cholesterol screening in childhood does accurately predict adult cholesterol levels (Orchard, T. J., et al.: *J. Pediatr.* 103:687, 1983). In Beaver County, Pennsylvania, 611 children had cholesterol level determinations done at age 12 and at age 21. About 50% of the top 20% of cholesterol levels remained in the top quintile after 9 years. Seventy percent remained in the top two quintiles. Besides transplantation, one way to lessen the cardiovascular risk of cholesterol is to attempt to lower the cholesterol level by diet modification. The fact that diet can work is easily seen among adolescents who are Seventh-Day Adventists. The Seventh-Day Adventist Church prohibits smoking among its members and encourages them to adopt a lacto-ovo-vegetarian diet. The average diet only contains 34% of calories as fat, with 11% derived from saturated fats. Among adolescents at one Seventh-Day Adventist boarding school, the mean cholesterol level was only 138 mg/dl. Mean blood pressures were also low (104 for systolic and 65 for diastolic). None of the adolescents smoked. Much to the dismay of the egg industry, a study from Seattle and Amhurst, Massachusetts, demonstrated that an egg a day would cause your low-density lipoprotein cholesterol level to be 12% higher than eating no eggs a day (Sacks, F. M., et al.: *Lancet* 1:647, 1984).

It has been demonstrated unequivocally that all societies are made up of four types: the lovers, the ambitious, the observers, and the overweight fools. It also has been demonstrated unequivocally that the latter group are the happiest.

(For a magnificent review of childhood obesity, see the article by William Dietz, "Childhood Obesity: Susceptibility, Cause, and Management," in the *Journal of Pediatrics* [103:676, 1983]).—J.A.S., III

Pediatric Cardiopulmonary Resuscitation: Review of 130 Cases
Stephen Ludwig, Robert G. Kettrick, and Margot Parker (Univ. of Pennsylvania)
Clin. Pediatr. (Phila.) 23:71–75, February 1984   8–15

The cardiopulmonary resuscitation (CPR) records of 130 pediatric patients who had a cardiac arrest were reviewed. Ninety-six resuscitations were done on hospitalized patients and 34 on patients in the emergency department. The age distribution of the patients is given in the table. Two thirds of the patients were younger than age 1 year when arrest occurred. The most common diagnoses involved the respiratory system. Airway management alone sufficed in 30% of hospital cases and in 2 emergency department cases. External cardiac compression was used in 60% and 94% of cases, respectively. The mean numbers of drugs used were 2.45 in hospital cases and 4.25 in emergency department cases.

The outcome is shown in Figure 8–6. Ninety percent of the hospitalized patients were initial survivors. Three of the 9 who failed to respond were terminally ill. Overall survival was 65%. Only 56% of emergency department patients were initial survivors. Six of the 15 deaths were diagnosed as being due to sudden infant death syndrome. Four patients had been dead for some time before arrival at the hospital. Overall survival was 29%. The initial survival rate for both groups was 82%, and the final survival rate was 55%.

Pediatric CPR can be approached with an optimistic attitude as regards immediate survival. Separate courses in pediatric resuscitation are appro-

AGE DISTRIBUTION OF CHILDREN REQUIRING CPR

Age Range	Hospitalized Patients (%)	Emergency Department Patients (%)	Total (%)
0–28 days	32(33)	8(24)	40(31)
1 month–1 year	35(36)	8(24)	43(34)
1 year–4 years	19(20)	9(26)	28(22)
5 years–9 years	4(4)	7(20)	11(7)
10 years–16 years	6(6)	2(6)	8(7)
Median	3 months	1 year	5 months
Mean	1.54 years	2.88 years	1.98 years

(Courtesy of Ludwig, S., et al.: Clin. Pediatr. [Phila.] 23:71–75, February 1984.)

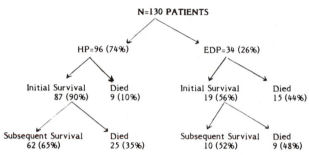

Fig 8–6.—Outcome of pediatric CPR. *HP*, hospitalized patients; *EDP*, emergency department patients. Percentages indicate percent of subgroup, not entire patient group studied. (Courtesy of Ludwig, S., et al.: Clin. Pediatr. [Phila.] 23:71–75, February 1984.)

priate because of differences from adults in airway, breathing, cardiac function, and drug management.

▶ David Jaffee, Attending Physician, Division of Ambulatory Services, Children's Memorial Hospital, and Associate in Pediatrics, Northwestern University Medical School, comments:

"Pediatric resuscitation has been relatively neglected as an area for scientific investigation. Ludwig et al. point out that pediatric CPR has developed from the adult model. The advent and maturation of Emergency Medicine as a subspecialty have begun to produce research on many aspects of resuscitation of adults. Topics of current controversies include: open versus closed cardiac massage; use of calcium versus calcium-channel blockers in arrest protocols; use of pneumatic antishock garment, etc. This study by Ludwig et al. adds to the relatively few studies of outcome of pediatric resuscitation as it is currently practiced and helps to provide a foundation for subsequent research.

"This study also highlights several important points:

"1. *Age.*—Children requiring resuscitation are generally young (median age, 5 months). By analogy to adults, the extremes of the age spectrum are overrepresented among patients requiring resuscitation.

"2. *Pathophysiology.*—It is now well established that the underlying pathologic conditions leading to arrest in children are more variable than in adults and that respiratory illnesses lead the list, followed by cardiac, neurologic, and then gastrointestinal disorders.

"3. *Airway.*—The fact that 30% of hospitalized patients were resuscitated solely with airway maneuvers indicates the importance of prompt and meticulous airway care at an arrest scene. In addition, early and frequent evaluation of all patients with compromised airway and especially young infants with any significant respiratory diseases may preclude the need for resuscitation in some cases.

"4. *Outcome.*—The overall survival of 55% reported by Ludwig et al. is higher than in any of four previous studies in this field, in which survival to discharge ranged from 7% to 47%.

"The data of Ludwig et al. also provide a clue to understanding the wide disparities in survival. Those children resuscitated as inpatients had 65% survival, whereas survival among patients resuscitated in the emergency department was only 29%. Monitored or witnessed arrests, therefore, are associated with a better prognosis than unmonitored arrests, presumably because of shorter delay to institution of resuscitation. Also, those previous studies that reported the lowest survival included only patients who had complete cardiac arrests, whereas this series by Ludwig and his associates included some patients who suffered respiratory arrests without full cardiac arrests. As in any clinical research, the characteristics of the patient population selected for study can markedly affect the outcomes.

"During the next decade we can anticipate an expansion of research on specific techniques of resuscitation and their effect on coronary and brain perfusion. This research certainly will result in modifications in advanced life-support protocols for children that hopefully will improve both the quantity and quality of survival."

9 Blood

Developmental Changes in Serum Ferritin and Erythrocyte Protoporphyrin in Normal (Nonanemic) Children
Amos S. Deinard, Samuel Schwartz, and Ray Yip (Minneapolis)
Am. J. Clin. Nutr. 38:71–76, July 1983   9–1

The authors studied 4,039 children aged 6 months to 12 years to characterize developmental variations of serum ferritin and erythrocyte protoporphyrin (EP). Hematocrit values, EP values, and serum ferritin levels were measured. Evidence of undue lead absorption excluded 37 children from the study; 183 others were excluded due to low hematocrit values (90% of the 183 had low serum ferritin or elevated EP values, or both).

Mean values of ferritin and EP for male and female subjects of each age group were similar, and there was no statistically significant difference among whites, blacks, and American Indians in age-matched samples. Even though iron status was comparable among the three racial groups, hematocrit values were 0.7% lower in blacks.

An approximately 50% increase in mean ferritin concentration and a 25% decrease in mean EP concentration were found at age 6 to 12 years, compared to age six months to 2 years. The -2 SD value for serum ferritin increased from 12 to 21 µg/L with increasing age (Fig 9–1), whereas the $+2$ SD value of EP decreased from 65 to 42 µg/dl in whole blood with increasing age (Fig 9–2). Serum ferritin values were found to rise throughout the first 12 years of life; EP values were highest at age 1–2 years, then fell to constant levels after age 4–6. The rise of hematocrit value with age appears to be associated with improving storage and availability of iron for heme synthesis.

The low EP values observed in early infancy and the upward trend in the next 12 months are due to the fact that infants are born with adequate iron stores that are maintained at least until age 6 months, when depletion develops as a consequence of rapid growth. Then they rise and peak between ages 1 and 2 years. This time of highest mean EP value coincides with the highest prevalence of anemia in childhood. After age 2 years a progressive fall in mean EP value to near adult level after age 6 is consistent with reaccumulation of adequate iron stores, a concept that is supported by the low prevalence of anemia (2%) in the group aged 6–12 years.

▶ The tests most commonly used to confirm the diagnosis of iron deficiency have been the serum iron and transferrin saturation assays. In recent years, the erythrocyte protoporphyrin (EP) and serum ferritin assays have been shown to correlate well with iron status and are also useful in diagnosing iron deficiency. The unfortunate problem is that none of these tests when taken alone is fully diagnostic of iron deficiency. This has resulted in the need for reliance

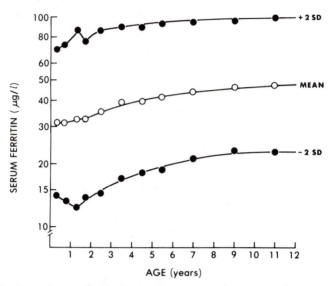

Fig 9–1.—Increase in serum ferritin concentrations, age 6 months to 12 years. Mean values ± 2 SD. (Courtesy of Deinard, A.S., et al.: Am. J. Clin. Nutr. 38:71–76, July 1983.)

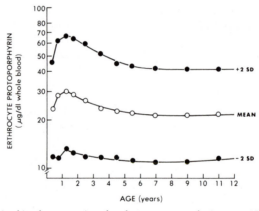

Fig 9–2.—Relationship of concentration of erythrocyte protoporphyrin to age. (Courtesy of Deinard, A.S., et al.: Am. J. Clin. Nutr. 38:71–76, July 1983.)

on multiple assays in order to increase one's confidence that one is dealing with an iron-deficient individual. Compounding all this is the wide range of variation of normal that occurs in healthy children with respect to each of these diagnostic tests, and the same may be true of the hemoglobin concentration itself. The value of this study by Deinard et al. is that it has attempted to establish extremely specific age-related "normal" ranges throughout the first 12 years of life.

While I like this study in the abstract, I find many problems with it in the concrete. The age-old issue with iron deficiency and the tests to diagnose it always comes down to the question of "who judges the judge." For example, although none of the infants and children in this study was judged to be anemic by "standard criteria," there was a sharp decline in serum ferritin values between ages 1 and 2 years, at which time the EP values tended to increase. Now, one can understand the fall in ferritin values because, more likely than not, this is an age at which total body stores of iron are diminished as an infant is rapidly growing. Does not, however, the increase in EP value manifest evidence of limitation of iron supply to the bone marrow? The only way of answering this question is to see if all of these variations are totally ablated by the true judge, that is, the administration of iron and observation of what these numbers would do in a "truly iron-sufficient" population of children. Basically, what I am saying is that one cannot take a group of children who are not anemic and do all of these studies for iron deficiency and truly be able to interpret them with absolute confidence. Even children who are not anemic but who are below the mean for hemoglobin level may well have a rise in the hemoglobin value if they are treated with iron. This has been shown time and time again.

In an article very similar to this one, the same investigators evaluated the role of EP as a screening test for iron deficiency (*Pediatrics* 72:214, 1983). If the relationship of EP to serum ferritin is compared and a serum ferritin value less than or equal to 15 μg/L is used as the criterion of iron deficiency, the optimal cutoff for EP appears to be 35 μg/dl of whole blood. At this level, 88% of subjects with low levels of serum ferritin can be detected (sensitivity), in contrast to 53% detected at a higher cutoff of equal to or greater than 50 μg/dl, which is the value commonly used to screen for lead poisoning. At an EP screening level of 35 μg/dl of whole blood, 90% of the subjects with normal serum ferritin levels are correctly determined to be screen negative (specificity). The predictive value of low levels of serum ferritin for all subjects above the screening level is 38%. The conclusion of this report was that, in general, an elevated EP level by itself represents inadequate iron delivery for hematopoiesis and signals iron deficiency regardless of whether the serum ferritin value is below the diagnostic level or not. A trial course of orally administered iron is suggested for children who are found to have an elevated EP value, with an increase in hemoglobin or hematocrit serving retrospectively as a confirmation of prior iron deficiency. This approach seems to make more sense. It should be noted that if ferritin concentrations are used as a test for iron deficiency, there will be a difference between ferritin values obtained by venous and capillary techniques. Capillary ferritin values will run almost 20% higher than venous values. Apparently this is an artifact of the way in which the plasma or serum is separated from whole blood. Spinning blood in a small capillary tube apparently squeezes or leaches out ferritin from white blood cell elements, elevating the serum or plasma ferritin value. Spinning venous blood in a larger tube does not cause this phenomenon and results in lower (truer) ferritin values. One must be wary of ferritin value obtained by capillary techniques (Majia, L. A., et al.: *Clin. Chem.* 29:871, 1983).

By now, I think most people in practice are becoming a bit leery of seeing more and more written about the role of this, that, or the other thing in diagnosing iron deficiency. There seems to be a tendency to try to fit some preconceived notion of the developmental processes that are going on in iron deficiency into a rigid set of laboratory developmental changes. There seems to be too much variation between children to make this have sensible rhyme and reason in all cases. It is on this basis that if there is any suspicion, either based on history or any single piece of laboratory data, that a child is iron deficient, going to the ultimate judge is the best answer. And as we all know, the ultimate judge is a trial of iron.—J.A.S., III.

Elevated Erythrocyte Adenosine Deaminase Activity in Congenital Hypoplastic Anemia

Bertil E. Glader, Karen Backer, and Louis K. Diamond
N. Engl. J. Med. 309:1486–1490, Dec. 15, 1983   9–2

Congenital hypoplastic anemia, or Diamond-Blackfan syndrome, is characterized by hypoplastic macrocytic anemia in early infancy and a variable subsequent course. Some patients continue to be dependent on steroids or transfusions, and the risk of leukemia may be increased. The authors document an increase in the activity of adenosine deaminase, a critical enzyme in the purine salvage pathway, in patients with congenital hypoplastic anemia. Samples of whole blood were obtained from 12 patients with congenital hypoplastic anemia, 18 with hemolytic anemia, 3 with steroid-dependent nephrosis, and 50 normal control subjects. Fourteen samples of cord blood also were analyzed.

Mean adenosine deaminase activity in red blood cells from patients with congenital hypoplastic anemia was 2.2 IU/gm of hemoglobin, compared with a control mean of 0.6 IU/gm. Activity in samples from study patients was greater than in cord blood or in red blood cells from patients with hemolytic anemia, acquired aplastic anemia, Fanconi's hypoplastic anemia, acquired pure red blood cell aplasia, or transient erythroblastopenia of childhood. Two of 6 families of study patients included at least 1 parent with elevated activity of red blood cell adenosine deaminase. Twin brothers in 1 family both had congenital hypoplastic anemia.

Increased adenosine deaminase activity in erythrocytes is a unique feature of congenital hypoplastic anemia and may prove to be a useful marker of the disorder. Whether the purine metabolic abnormality in this disease is causally related to altered function of the stem cells is unclear. Adenosine deaminase activity also is elevated in leukemic blast cells, and 5 cases of leukemia have been described in about 200 patients known to have congenital hypoplastic anemia.

▶ "Why," you ask, "is red blood cell adenosine deaminase activity (ADA) increased in patients with congenital hypoplastic anemia (the Diamond-Blackfan syndrome)?" Even the investigators of this study are not giving us a good clue as to the reason for this association. They presume that the increased ADA is secondary to some primary derangement of nucleic acid metabolism in the Diamond-Blackfan syndrome. They cautiously speculate that there could be some relationship between ADA and the genetic nature of the Diamond-Blackfan syndrome. In most cases, Diamond-Blackfan syndrome does not appear to be inherited, although familial cases have been reported. Production of adenosine deaminase is regulated by chromosome 20. If there is any relationship here, the speculation would be that the gene responsible for failure of erythropoiesis in the Diamond-Blackfan syndrome could also be located on chromosome 20.

The real importance of this study is the fact that it shows that increased ADA is useful in diagnosing the Diamond-Blackfan syndrome. We pediatricians occasionally encounter children with anemia and reticulocytopenia in whom the major differential diagnosis is between transient erythroblastopenia (TEC) of childhood and the Diamond-Blackfan syndrome. It is important to differentiate between these entities because one is benign and self-limited, whereas the other is a lifelong condition that may lead to a variety of more serious complications. In general, congenital hypoplastic anemia presents in children younger than age 1 year and is characterized by red blood cells that have fetal characteristics and are macrocytic for the patient's age. In contrast, TEC commonly occurs after age 1 year, usually follows a viral infection, and is characterized by erythrocytes that lack fetal features and are normocytic for the patient's age. Unfortunately, during the period of recovery from TEC, erythropoiesis of the fetal type may be a prominent feature and some patients with TEC will show up with elevations of the fetal hemoglobin level and mean corpuscular volume. In these cases, elevations of ADA should serve to distinguish between the Diamond-Blackfan syndrome and TEC. Thus, this specific enzyme measurement of red blood cells should be extremely useful in the differential diagnosis of these two red blood cell hypoplastic disorders. Some diseases in certain years just seem to be very popular. This past year has been an extremely popular one for TEC. We seem to be up to our chins in articles about it. Unfortunately, most of the reports do not provide us with information that is very useful to our clinical practices. It's sort of like the man with a B.A., M.A., and Ph.D., but no J.O.B.—J.A.S., III

Diagnosis of Hereditary Spherocytosis in Newborn Infants
Werner Schröter and Elke Kahsnitz (Univ. of Göttingen, Göttingen, West Germany)
J. Pediatr. 103:460–463, September 1983   9–3

Normal range of osmotic fragility of red blood cells (RBC) and autohemolysis was determined in venous blood of 32 healthy infants aged 1 to 28 days. Hyperbilirubinemia with bilirubin concentrations of less than 8 mg/dl developed in 11 infants. Twenty-one had maximal serum bilirubin concentrations between 8 and 18.3 mg/dl and were treated with phototherapy. Hereditary spherocytosis (HS) was diagnosed in 5 infants during the first week of life; in 3 a family history of HS was already known and in 2 it was detected during the study.

In addition to studies of the 32 newborn infants, osmotic fragility of fresh and 24-hour incubated RBC was determined and autohemolysis tests were performed on 50 healthy children and adults. Normal range was

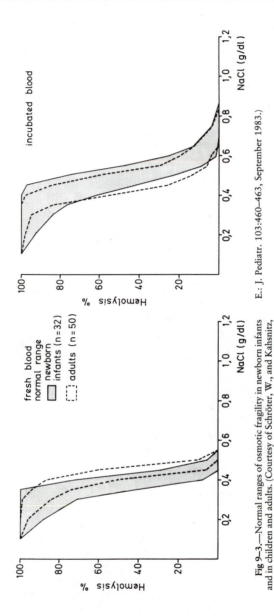

Fig 9–3.—Normal ranges of osmotic fragility in newborn infants and in children and adults. (Courtesy of Schröter, W., and Kahsnitz, E.: J. Pediatr. 103:460–463, September 1983.)

determined by graphic presentation of mean value of hemolysis at the given concentration of sodium chloride. Osmotic fragility of fresh RBC of newborn infants was lower than that of adults (Fig 9–3). At sodium chloride concentrations of 0.2, 0.35, 0.4, 0.45, and 0.5 gm/dl the difference between the two groups was statistically significant at the 0.05% level. After 24 hours' incubation, however, osmotic fragility of erythrocytes of newborn infants was increased when compared with those of children and adults at sodium chloride concentrations greater than 0.35 gm/dl. At sodium chloride concentrations less than 0.35 gm/dl, erythrocytes of neonates had a lower osmotic fragility than those of children and adults.

The degree of autohemolysis of erythrocytes of normal adults and newborn infants did not differ significantly. In both groups, addition of glucose reduced autohemolysis by 40% to 50%. The increase in autohemolysis was less pronounced in the 5 infants with HS than in older children.

Hyperbilirubinemia developed in the 5 infants with HS; 3 were given phototherapy, and an exchange transfusion was necessary in 1. Reticulocyte counts were significantly increased in only 2 infants, to 15.2% and 17%, respectively.

The preliminary conclusion from this limited study is that despite the lack of clinical signs, increased osmotic fragility and increased autohemolysis of RBC made the diagnosis of HS possible in newborn infants when venous blood was used for examination.

In HS the osmotic fragility of fresh and incubated erythrocytes is increased if the normal range of values for newborn infants is used for reference. The autohemolysis test shows essentially the same pattern as in adults with typical HS, but the rate of autohemolysis is not increased to the same extent in newborn infants as in adults.

Human Serum "Parvovirus": A Specific Cause of Aplastic Crisis in Children With Hereditary Spherocytosis

John F. Kelleher, Naomi L. C. Luban, Philip P. Mortimer, and Tomoteru Kamimura
J. Pediatr. 102:720–722, May 1983   9–4

Acute serum parvovirus-like virus (SPVL) infection was seen in a brother and sister and their mother; severe aplastic crises developed in these children who had hereditary spherocytosis. One case is described here.

Boy, 8, complained of vomiting and headache of 3 days' duration. Hereditary spherocytosis had been diagnosed 5 years earlier; the father was known to have hereditary spherocytosis. Physical examination of the boy revealed temperature of 38.4 C, shotty cervical adenopathy, and a spleen palpable 2 cm below the left costal margin. Hemoglobin level was 8.2 gm/dl; hematocrit value was 25.3%; leukocyte count was 4,200/cu mm, with 63% segmented neutrophils, 1% bands, 11% monocytes, 22% lymphocytes, and 1% atypical lymphocytes; reticulocyte count was 0%.

Five days later, the patient complained of increasing fatigue and was pale and lethargic. Temperature was 38.4 C, and the spleen was palpable 3.5 cm below the left costal margin. Hemoglobin level was 5.5 gm/dl, hematocrit value was 14.7%, and reticulocyte count was 0.1%. Leukocyte count was 18,800/cu mm, with 60% segmented neutrophils, 6% bands, 4% metamyelocytes, 23% mature lymphocytes, 1% atypical lymphocytes, 4% monocytes, and 3 nucleated red blood cells per 100 white cells. Platelet count was 426,000/cu mm. After admission to the hospital, the patient received gradual transfusion of washed red blood cells over 3 days. He recovered rapidly and when seen 5 weeks later the hemoglobin level was 10.3 gm/dl, hematocrit value was 38.9%, and reticulocyte count was 10.2%. Leukocyte count was 9,500/cu mm with normal differential; platelet count was normal.

Serum samples were tested by countercurrent immunoelectrophoresis (CIE). Human serum (Pi) with a high titer of antibody to SPLV was used to detect viremia, and serum (Pr) containing SPLV was used to detect antibody. The CIE tests showed SPLV in the serum of this boy, which was confirmed by electron microscopy. In all 3 patients, serologic evidence of SPLV was found.

In both of these children with hereditary spherocytosis, SPLV is believed to have caused aplastic crises. Commonly, crises of this type arise within a few days of a febrile illness and are characterized by a rapid fall in hemoglobin concentration, absolute reticulocytopenia, and transient leukopenia. They usually last for 7 to 10 days; recovery is heralded by normoblastemia, reticulocytosis, and thrombocytosis. The otherwise healthy mother had only reticulocytopenia and mild leukopenia, whereas the children with hereditary spherocytosis became severely anemic.

▶ This article was selected as a typical example of one of many that have shown that human serum parvovirus is capable of causing bone marrow aplasia in children with congenital hemolytic anemias. That parvovirus might be the culprit in aplastic crises was first suggested when antibody to parvovirus B19, better known as serum parvovirus-like virus (SPLV), was serendipitously detected in serum taken during an aplastic crisis in a child with sickle cell anemia (*Lancet* 1:664, 1981). Confirmation soon came from Jamaica, where during a 2-year period, some 10% of children in a long-term follow-up study of sickle cell anemia had aplastic crises. Evidence of infection with SPLV was found in 24 of 28 of these children (Serjeant, G. R., et al.: *Lancet* 2:595, 1981). Serum parvovirus-like virus is a ubiquitous human virus that suppresses the growth of bone marrow stem cells in vitro. In addition to sickle cell anemia, infection with SPLV has been reported to cause aplastic crises in hereditary spherocytosis, pyruvate kinase deficiency, and untransfused thalassemia intermedia (*Br. J. Haematol.* 55:391, 1983). With regard to hereditary spherocytosis, a retrospective study of published reports of aplastic crises in this disorder occurring between 1935 and 1964 concluded that they might all have been manifestations of infections by a single agent that could have been SPLV (Mortimer, P.: *J. Clin. Pathol.* 36:445, 1983). This virus does not seem to be transmitted in transfused blood, but can be passed on via clotting factor concentrates (*Lancet* 2:482, 1983).

Wouldn't it be attractive if SPLV was the cause of aplasia in other states, such as aplastic anemia, the Blackfan-Diamond syndrome, transient erythroblastopenia of childhood, or paroxysmal nocturnal hemoglobinuria? Not so, say Neal Young and others (*J. Clin. Invest.* 73:224, 1984). No connection could be established between these disorders and the presence of SPLV antigen or antibody in the serum of affected patients. Evans et al. (*Br. Med. J.* 228:681, 1984) suggest that immune globulin administered to patients at risk from aplasia from parvovirus might be helpful. They recognize, however, that this would have to be given indefinitely if it works at all. I don't think it would work and I hope no one does a study to try to prove it. It's better to be an unknown failure than a known one.—J.A.S., III

Anemia of Acute Inflammation in Children
Thomas C. Abshire and Jerry D. Reeves (David Grant USAF Med. Center, Travis AFB, California)
J. Pediatr. 103:868–871, December 1983   9–5

Sequential changes in hemoglobin concentration and erythrocyte sedimentation rate were measured in 27 previously healthy children hospitalized for a variety of moderately severe acute inflammatory processes. Eighteen of these 27 were retrospectively evaluated by review (9 boys and 9 girls, aged 7 months to 18 years). Nine previously healthy children, 5 girls and 4 boys aged 20 months to 10 years, were then prospectively evaluated over 4 months.

Eleven (61%) retrospectively studied children had mild anemia for age on admission, and the hemoglobin (Hgb) level dropped at least 0.8 gm/dl in 15 (83%) during active inflammation. Average number of days between initial and lowest Hgb value was 5.5 days. This change in Hgb level could not be accounted for by iatrogenic blood loss, clinical bleeding, or abnormal hydration. At peak of inflammation, 8 (44%) children had moderate anemia for age. Seven of 9 (78%) prospectively studied children manifested mild anemia for age on admission. The mean Hgb level dropped 1.8 gm/dl, and later mean Hgb level rose 2.4 gm/dl. Average interval between initial and lowest Hgb value was 5.6 days. No evidence of hemolysis was noted in most patients.

When data of both the retrospective and prospective studies were combined, mean decrease in the Hgb value during active inflammation was 1.8 gm/dl in an average of 5 days. Mean rise in the Hgb level during resolving inflammation for both groups was 2.0 gm/dl in an average of 5 days. Both results are statistically significant (Fig 9–4).

These findings indicate that most children with moderately severe acute inflammation experience a significant drop in Hgb concentration within 1 week of onset of illness. The more than 100 ml of noniatrogenic blood loss usually represented by this change appears to occur regardless of the specific cause of inflammation. In most children, mild to moderate anemia resolves without hematinic therapy. Causes of this acute anemia of inflammation remain unknown.

▶ This study is about "buoys and gulls" who develop anemia during the course of an acute inflammatory disease. If you get the sense that I think parts of this

INFLAMMATION

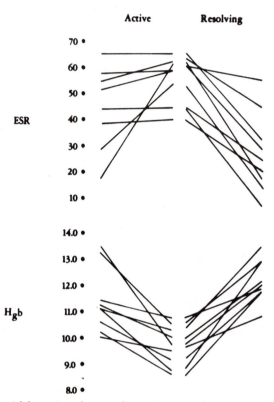

Fig 9–4.—Sequential changes in erythrocyte sedimentation rates and venous hemoglobin concentration in 9 children during active and resolving inflammation. (Courtesy of Abshire, T.C., and Reeves, J.D.: J. Pediatr. 103:868–871, December 1983.)

article are for the birds, you are correct. It is not that this is not a well-done study, for it is; it is just that attempting to put so many different diagnoses under the classification of acute inflammation in one article makes interpretation of the results a bit difficult. It is well known, as the authors point out, that *Hemophilus influenzae* infections very commonly will produce brisk falls in the hemoglobin level. This has been commented on previously in the YEAR BOOK and may be the result of some unknown hemolytic factor associated with this particular organism. You will note that the average fall in the hemoglobin level in this article was about 1.8 gm/dl. This is slightly to modestly in excess of the fall in the hemoglobin level that would be associated with complete cessation of bone marrow function in a 1-week period. These investigators could not find any evidence for hemolysis, although if hemolysis were occurring it would probably be at a low level that might not be detectable.

We have all seen this kind of anemia develop in patients who are admitted to the hospital with significant inflammatory disorders. We know enough about it not to treat it, which is the most important thing. This is different from the anemia of chronic disorders seen in certain states such as juvenile rheumatoid arthritis or cystic fibrosis. In these states, the anemia may not be due just to the chronic disorder. It could be due to iron deficiency, because earlier reports have suggested that one half to three fourths of all patients with juvenile rheumatoid arthritis who are anemic will have some rise in the hemoglobin level after administration of iron. An investigation of 39 clinically stable patients with cystic fibrosis showed that many of these patients were also relatively iron deficient (Ater, J. L., et al.: *Pediatrics* 71:810, 1983). When you see a child who has the anemia of chronic disorders and you can't be certain of whether or not they are iron deficient, you really don't have many options to tell what is going on. The most precise way is by bone marrow examination, but that is painful. Determination of the serum ferritin level can be helpful. One must recognize, however, that serum ferritin is an acute-phase reactant and tends to be elevated in chronic disease states associated with anemia in which there is inflammation. If you use a serum ferritin determination to attempt a diagnosis of iron deficiency, you must use a higher cutoff value of about 60 μg/ml because of this phenomenon (Blake, D. R., et al.: *Br. Med. J.* 283:1147, 1981). Sometimes you can never be sure based on all these laboratory tests whether or not a patient with the anemia of chronic disorders is or is not iron deficient. Treatment with iron is then your only alternative, and not a bad one at that.— J.A.S., III

Autoimmune Pancytopenia of Childhood Associated With Multisystem Disease Manifestations

Barbara A. Miller and Diana Schultz Beardsley (Boston)
J. Pediatr. 103:877–881, December 1983   9–6

Immune thrombocytopenia is a relatively common and usually self-limiting childhood disease that is only rarely associated with neutropenia and hemolytic anemia. The clinical and laboratory findings in 5 children with immune thrombocytopenia and neutropenia, 3 of whom had autoimmune hemolytic anemia, are described; none of the children had an identifiable underlying disease.

No child had associated specific immune deficiency disease, lupus erythematosus, or other identifiable collagen vascular disease, malignancy, or infectious disease. Autoantibodies against more than one hematopoietic cell line were detected in all 5 children. The results of bone marrow aspiration, done at presentation, were normal except for normal to increased megakaryocyte values in 2 children. Two others had hypoerythroid, hypocellular bone marrow with a hemolytic episode and low reticulocyte count; erythroid hyperplasia developed during an episode of hemolysis in the fifth child. Immunoglobulin eluted from red blood cells from 2 children yielded positive Coombs' test results. Evaluation of these eluates for binding to platelet proteins failed to identify any cross-reacting antiplatelet antibody. However, antibody eluted from platelets did bind to a 100,000-dalton platelet protein. These platelet eluates were negative against each child's own red blood cells in the Coombs' test, indicating that the antiplatelet and antierythrocyte antibodies were distinct in these 2 patients. In all 5 children, the disease followed a chronic, relapsing course over a period of 2½ to 6 years, and all had nonhematologic disease manifestations. Splenectomy was performed in 2 children because of bleeding and refractoriness to prednisone therapy.

These findings show that, even in the absence of identifiable underlying illness, autoimmune hematologic disease as a result of the production of antibodies against red blood cells, white blood cells, and platelets often involves a generalized disorder of immune function, with multisystem disease manifestations and a prolonged course.

Improved Classification of Anemias by MCV and RDW
J. David Bessman, P. Ridgway Gilmer, Jr., and Frank H. Gardner (Univ. of Texas, Galveston)
Am. J. Clin. Pathol. 80:322–326, September 1983   9–7

The two traditional principal parameters for the initial classification of anemic disorders are mean corpuscular volume (MCV) and reticulocyte count. New automated blood cell analyzers provide a measure of red blood cell volume distribution width (RDW) and a histogram of red blood cell volume distribution. Blood samples from 683 normal persons and 587 anemic patients were analyzed to evaluate how RDW complements the MCV to improve the classification of anemias from the blood sample alone.

The RDW was normal in patients with chronic disease, or aplastic anemia with no transfusion in the previous 4 months, or heterozygous alpha-thalassemia or beta-thalassemia. Also, the RDW was normal in patients with acute leukemia, solid tumors, multiple myeloma, or lymphoma before and during chemotherapy if unaccompanied by macrocytosis; those with macrocytosis had an elevated RDW. Patients with iron, folate, or vitamin B_{12} deficiency had a high RDW, even when both MCV and hemoglobin values were in the normal range. Similarly, all patients with hemoglobin SS, SC, or S-B thalassemia had an increased RDW. Further, RDW was normal in patients with acute hemorrhage if there was not a concomitant iron deficiency. From these findings, a classification of anemic disorders was derived based on red blood cell mean (MCV) and heterogeneity (RDW) (table).

Classification of patients by MCV category alone (high, normal, or low) was less than 90% sensitive in patients with chronic disease, chronic liver disease, sickle cell anemia, heterozygous thalassemia, and iron, folate, or mixed nutritional deficiency. Classification by RDW category alone (normal or high) was less than 90% sensitive in patients with chronic liver disease or chronic myelogenous leukemia, and in those given a transfusion. Normal individuals were accurately predicted by both MCV and RDW. Four types of artifactual patterns were found in 15 patients. Those with chronic lymphocytic leukemia had a normal RDW, except when the lymphocyte count was more than 150×10^9/L. In the latter case, the peak of erythrocytes was joined by a second peak of the lymphocytes. Counted

PROPOSED CLASSIFICATION OF ANEMIC DISORDERS BASED ON RED BLOOD CELL
MEAN (MCV) AND HETEROGENEITY (RDW)

MCV low RDW normal (Microcytic homogeneous)	MCV low RDW high (Microcytic heterogeneous)	MCV normal RDW normal (Normocytic homogeneous)	MCV normal RDW high (Normocytic heterogeneous)	MCV high RDW normal (Macrocytic homogeneous)	MCV high RDW high (Macrocytic heterogeneous)
Heterozygous thalassemia*	Iron deficiency*	Normal	Mixed deficiency*	Aplastic anemia	Folate deficiency*
Chronic disease*	S β-thalassemia	Chronic disease* chronic liver disease*·†	Early iron or folate deficiency*	Preleukemia†	Vitamin B$_{12}$ deficiency
	Hemoglobin H	Nonanemic hemoglobinopathy (*e.g.*, AS, AC)	Anemic hemoglobinopathy (*e.g.*, SS, SC)*		Immune hemolytic anemia
	Red cell fragmentation	Transfusion†	Myelofibrosis		Cold agglutinins
		Chemotherapy	Sideroblastic*		Chronic lymphocytic leukemia, high count
		Chronic lymphocytic leukemia			
		Chronic myelocytic leukemia†			
		Hemorrhage			
		Hereditary spherocytosis			

*MCV alone, less than 90% sensitive.
†RDW alone, less than 90% sensitive.
(Courtesy of Bessman, J.D., et al.: Am. J. Clin. Pathol. 80:322–326, September 1983.)

as red blood cells, lymphocytes caused an artifactually high RDW that was greatly disproportionate to their effect on the red blood cell count or indices (Fig 9–5, A). All of these patients had a hemoglobin value greater than 12 gm/dl and normal MCV when measured by the red blood cell peak alone. In patients with chronic myelogenous leukemia, however, RDW was slightly increased and MCV was normal. After transfusion, 4 patients with iron deficiency and 5 with aplastic anemia had striking bimodal histograms that resulted in a high RDW (Fig 9–5, B and C); thus, RDW reflected the difference between the MCV of recipient and donor cells. All but 1 of 10 patients with valvular prostheses had a normal RDW; the tenth patient, who had a markedly increased RDW, had red blood cell fragmentation detectable on examination of the smear and a prominent subpopulation of red blood cell fragments on the histogram (Fig 9–5, D). One patient with cold agglutinin disease had a bimodal red blood cell distribution and high RDW.

The findings indicate that the initial classification of anemia can be improved considerably by including RDW and histograms of red blood cell volume as part of the routine blood count.

▶ It took a long time for this type of study finally to be reported. For years now, most of us have been seeing a number on the complete blood count slip known as the "RDW." This number means "red blood cell distribution width," and it is a measure of the heterogeneity of distribution of red blood cell size (the equivalent of anisocytosis in analysis of the peripheral blood smear). Most of us know that if this number were large, a review of the peripheral blood

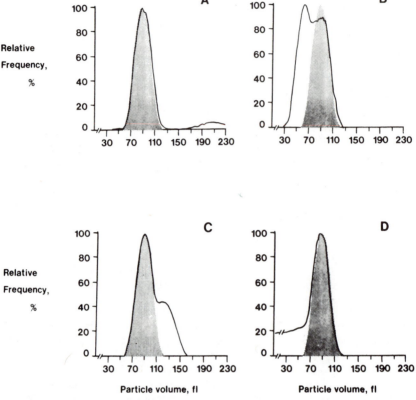

Fig 9–5.—Histograms of dimorphic populations. The shaded area represents a reference normal histogram, MCV 90 fL, RDW 13.2%. A, chronic lymphocytic leukemia, RBC 4.31 × 10¹²/L, lymphocytes 176 × 10⁹/L. Whole blood, MCV 93 fL, RDW 18.9%; red blood cell peak alone, MCV 91 fL, RDW 13.6%. B, patient with iron deficiency given transfusion: MCV 75 fL, RDW 20.3%. Patient's cells have MCV of 61 fL and RDW of 17.2%. C, patient with aplastic anemia given transfusion: MCV of 97 fL, RDW 18.9%. The patient's cells have MCV of 121 fL and RDW of 13.2%. D, red blood cell fragmentation resulting from prosthetic valve. Fragments are, at all sizes, smaller than whole cells; MCV 81 fL, RDW 19.4%. (Courtesy of Bessman, J.D., et al.: Am. J. Clin. Pathol. 80:322–326, September 1983.)

smear would show assorted sizes and shapes of red blood cells. What we did not know was how to interpret this number in light of the mean corpuscular volume (MCV). What Bessman et al. did was to examine the MCV and RDW in a wide range of clinical disorders and attempt to pigeonhole the diagnosis of each of these by examining these two numbers (see the table). I must caution that this article is one of the rare ones from the adult medical literature that make the YEAR BOOK. Most of the data are derived from adults, and we can only infer that the information will be correct for pediatric patients. I am quite certain that some smart young investigator will whip through a variety of pediatric patients using the MCV and RDW in a fashion similar to that in this study.

I would cut out the table from this manuscript and varnish it onto your office wall; I think you will find it that useful. I hope that when the pediatric numbers come along, that they will validate the classification system. Otherwise you may have to go back and have the table varnished from sight.—J.A.S., III

Significance of Nucleated Red Blood Cells in Peripheral Blood of Children
Richard H. Sills and Raymond A. R. Hadley
Am. J. Pediatr. Hematol. Oncol. 5:173–177, Summer 1983   9–8

The peripheral blood of 400 well children was examined to determine if normoblastemia is a normal finding, and 100 children with normoblastemia were evaluated prospectively to determine the significance of normoblastemia in a pediatric population. Studies were performed at Children's Hospital of Buffalo.

The 400 children in the control group were aged 3 months to 18 years. None demonstrated normoblastemia even though 1,000 white blood cells (WBC) were carefully examined in each subject. Patients younger than age 3 months or older than age 18 years were also excluded from the study of the 100 children with normoblastemia. Normoblastemia was confirmed and quantitated by counting 1,000 WBC and noting the number of nucleated red blood cells (NRBC). Hematologic studies performed on all patients included hemoglobin and red blood cell indices, as well as platelet, total white blood cell, and white blood cell differential counts.

No child with NRBC was perfectly well. Obvious episodes of hypoxia were associated with normoblastemia in 49 patients. Hematologic disorders were newly diagnosed in 22. Clinically obvious underlying disorders reported to be associated with normoblastemia were found in 88 of the 100 patients. The incidence of bone marrow replacement among patients without easily recognized etiology for normoblastemia was statistically significantly greater than the incidence among those with obvious etiology (incidence, 4 of 12 versus 4 of 88, respectively).

Failure to identify normoblastemia in any of the 400 children who served as controls suggests that NRBC are not a normal finding in the peripheral blood of children. Hypoxic disorders were the most common cause of NRBC in the 100 patients; anemia unrelated to bone marrow replacement was the second most common etiology. Malignancies occurred in only 8% of these patients, whereas they are the most common cause of normoblastemia in adults, accounting for 25% to 63% of cases.

Of the 12 children with normoblastemia of initially unknown origin, 4 had life-threatening disorders associated with bone marrow replacement. Total white blood cell count and the hemoglobin value were the only hematologic parameters that helped differentiate patients with or without bone marrow replacement.

Normoblastemia is rarely, if ever, a normal finding in children; hypoxia or anemia account for this finding in most patients. Incidence of bone marrow replacement is low in these children and definitely less than that found in an adult population. Bone marrow examination should be considered strongly in any ill patient with unexplained normoblastemia to rule out underlying, unrecognized malignancy.

▶ This must have been a very tedious study to do, reviewing the peripheral smear findings in over 500 children to determine the frequency and implications of the presence of nucleated red blood cells. The rewards of a job well done in many instances is simply to have the job done. This is a job that was well done and shows us that nucleated red blood cells are not a normal finding in the peripheral smear of any child. An interesting finding was that only 8% of pediatric patients with normoblastemia had malignancies in bone marrow. The more common etiologies were those of acute hypoxia and hemolytic anemias. Causes other than bone marrow infiltration are usually detectable on the basis of a history, a physical examination, and a modicum of other laboratory data. Thus, whenever nucleated red blood cells are found and no apparent cause is easily determined on the basis of a history, physical examination, or other studies, a bone marrow examination is in order to exclude malignancy.— J.A.S., III

Autoerythrocyte Sensitization
A. N. Campbell, Melvin H. Freedman, and P. D. McClure (Toronto)
J. Pediatr. 103:157–160, July 1983   9–9

Autoerythrocyte sensitization predominantly affects women, but the syndrome has been reported in men and a few children. The findings in 6 girls seen at The Hospital for Sick Children with various manifestations of autoerythrocyte sensitization are reported here and 1 case is presented.

Girl, 12, had an accessory navicular bone removed from the right foot and suffered a fracture of the navicular tubercle 2 years later. She subsequently incurred a painful swollen bruise of the left knee, which resolved slowly. One year later she sprained the right ankle. Within 3 months a painful, discolored swelling of that foot developed and a diagnosis of "sympathetic dystrophy" was made. The foot remained painful and she was admitted for investigation. Results of tests for platelet aggregation to adenosine diphosphate, collagen, and epinephrine and availability of platelet factor 3 were normal (Table 1).

A diagnosis of juvenile rheumatoid arthritis was considered and 2 months of aspirin therapy produced some relief of symptoms. Three months later she was placed in a volar cast after falling on the left wrist. Pain and swelling of the hand developed rapidly, with altered sensation in distribution of the median nerve. Swelling and ecchymosis of the entire forearm was observed after removal of the cast, but no abnormality of the carpal tunnel was found. Additional painful bruises of the left upper arm and face developed 1 month after resolution of the previous episode. Venographic study revealed no vascular malformations.

Intradermal injection of 0.1 ml of autologous red blood cells resulted in a tender bruise 2.5 cm in diameter within 12 hours, which was regarded as a positive reaction. Study of a specimen skin biopsy from one of the lesions revealed a perivascular lymphocytic infiltrate associated with hemosiderotic granules, indicating previous hemorrhage.

TABLE 1.—Clinical Data*

Patient	ESR	PC (×10³/μl)	PT (sec)	PTT (sec)	BT (min)	PA	PF₃A	LE cells	THC	Skin biopsy	Intradermal red cell test
1 (index case)	7	279	11.7	34.1	4	Normal response	Normal	Negative	1:24	Perivascular lymphocytic infiltration	Positive
2	3	260	11.8	32.3	5	Normal response	Normal	Negative	1:32	Red cell extravasation around dermal vessels	Positive
3	2	300	11.6	34.8	4	—	—	Negative	1:24	No biopsy	Negative
4	4	279	10.7	28.4	5	Normal response	Normal	—	—	No biopsy	Positive
5	4	310	11.5	35.5	7	Normal response	Normal	Negative	1:24	Normal	Negative
6	3	281	11.4	31.9	4	—	—	Negative	—	No biopsy	Positive

*BT = bleeding time; ESR = erythrocyte sedimentation rate; PA = platelet aggregation to ADP, collagen, and epinephrine; PC = platelet count; PF3A = platelet factor 3 availability; PT = prothrombin time; PTT = partial thromboplastin time; THC = total hemolytic complement (normal > 1:12).
(Courtesy of Campbell, A.N., et al.: J. Pediatr. 103:157–160, July 1983.)

TABLE 2.—SUMMARY OF CASE REPORTS

Patient	Age (yr)	History of previous injury	Sites of bruises and duration	Psychiatric history	Other disease manifestations	Treatment
2	12	None	Lateral aspect left knee; intermittent episodes for 6 mo	Blind mother, hard-working father, poor social life; lonely and sad child	None	Psychotherapy ongoing
3	14	None	Right arm, legs, chest wall; intermittent episodes for 2 yr	Adopted child; father's death by myocardial infarct witnessed by patient; mother had porphyria; patient depressed	Abdominal pain, nausea, vomiting	Psychotherapy, with good results
4	14	Right index finger	Right hand, forearm, upper arm over 2 mo	Frightened girl; dislike of male physicians; home life conflict	Abdominal pain, bloody diarrhea	Psychotherapy, with good results
		Right foot	Right leg			
5	15	Basketball injury to right eye	Eye, face, forehead	None sought	Blood-stained tears	No specific therapy given
		Right foot	Right leg			
6	12	Minor injury to forehead	Forehead and face; left hand and knee; left foot; episodes for 2 yr	Sexual abuse at 5 and 12 years; popular, attractive younger sister	None	Psychotherapy ongoing

(Courtesy of Campbell, A.N., et al.: J. Pediatr. 103:157–160, July 1983.)

Psychiatric examination revealed an unhappy home life with family conflicts and a preoccupation with the illness. Six months of psychotherapy brought about complete resolution of the symptoms.

The cardinal clinical feature of autoerythrocyte sensitization is a painful erythematous bruise. Erythema, tenderness, and swelling may spread to involve an entire limb. The extremities are most commonly involved, and lesions on the back are rare (Table 2). The skin manifestations often are associated with somatic symptoms. Many patients will have a marked psychologic disturbance, although the causal relation is uncertain. These patients may appear to be quiet and well adjusted, but often they are found to have extremely abnormal backgrounds. Hostility may be directed toward members of the opposite sex, especially attending male physicians.

Although there is no pathognomonic test, intradermal injection of autologous red blood cells can be useful. The differential diagnosis of this syndrome can be difficult. Younger patients seem to respond well to psychotherapy, which often is the only effective form of treatment.

It is believed that autoerythrocyte sensitization is more common in children or young adolescents than previously reported. Early diagnosis should be based on history, characteristic skin lesions, and psychologic evaluation. Multiple investigations only prolong the symptoms.

Role of Splenectomy in Homozygous Sickle Cell Disease in Childhood
A. M. Emond, P. Morais, S. Venugopal, R. G. Carpenter, and G. R. Serjeant (Univ. of the West Indies, Kingston, Jamaica)
Lancet 1:88–90, Jan. 14, 1984   9–10

Postsplenectomy syndrome and a tendency to spontaneous splenic atrophy have favored a conservative approach to children with sickle cell (SS) disease, but splenic complications are becoming more prominent, and prophylaxis against postsplenectomy septicemia has improved. A review was done of data on 60 Jamaican children with homozygous SS disease who underwent splenectomy, 46 because of sustained hypersplenism and 14 to prevent recurrent acute splenic sequestration. The age and sex distribution and indications for operation are given in the table. Presently, prophylaxis against postsplenectomy infection consists of benzyl penicillin before op-

Age and Sex Distribution and Indications for Splenectomy

Age (yr)	M	F	ASS	CHS	Totals
<1	2	0	2	0	2
1–<2	7	5	10	2	12
2–5	8	9	2	15	17
6–9	3	8	0	11	11
≥10	6	12	0	18	18
Total	26	34	14	46	60

(Courtesy of Emond, A.M., et al.: Lancet 1:88–90, Jan. 14, 1984.)

eration and during hospitalization, followed by depot benzathine penicillin monthly until age 7 years. Both 14-valent pneumococcal and *Hemophilus influenzae* B vaccines are given preoperatively.

Median follow-up has been 6 years, with a total of 369 patient-years of observation. Overwhelming sepsis was possible in 2 of the 3 deaths; the other was due to chronic renal failure. None of these 3 patients had received prophylaxis against infection. No confirmed case of pneumococcal septicemia or meningitis followed splenectomy. There was no perioperative mortality. The most common form of morbidity was acute chest syndrome, which was comparably frequent in the children given prophylaxis and the others. Both *H. influenzae* B and β-hemolytic streptococci were isolated from the sputum during attacks of acute chest syndrome in children not receiving prophylaxis.

Splenectomy can be an important part of the management of children with SS disease and life-threatening episodes of acute splenic sequestration and those who are limited by hypersplenism. The chief disadvantage of splenectomy is loss of the ability to respond immunologically to intravenous antigen. Penicillin prophylaxis is indicated, but its duration is controversial. The first 3 years after splenectomy appear to constitute the most critical period.

▶ No one that I know of likes taking out the spleen of a patient with homozygous sickle cell disease. We all know that such patients are already at high risk for septicemia from the types of organisms that children with no spleens have difficulty with. Removal of the spleen prematurely (before it autoinvolutes) in a patient with sickle cell disease may add fuel to the infectious fire because the child is having splenectomy at an extremely young age when he or she may not have gained very much immunologic experience with the *Pneumococcus* or *Hemophilus influenzae* organisms. Nonetheless, if an infant or child with sickle cell disease does show evidence of acute splenic sequestration or chronic hypersplenism, a legitimate reason for splenectomy may exist. In both of these cases the decision to perform splenectomy must be made after assessment of the advantages and disadvantages of the procedure, availability of alternative methods of treatment, and the natural history of the complication. Recurrence of acute splenic sequestration becomes less likely after age 5 and the tendency to spontaneous atrophy in sickle cell disease has favored a conservative approach for the child with hypersplenism who is a little bit older. We have tended to favor conservative prophylactic approaches consisting of a chronic transfusion program until a child is at least older than age 2 years. Such programs do prevent episodes of acute splenic sequestration (or at least none has been documented while children are on such programs) but they also prevent splenic involution that is the final natural act of stopping such sequestration crises. Thus, attacks of sequestration could occur after termination of a transfusion program. Therefore, many people who start a prophylactic transfusion program after a single episode of splenic sequestration do so with the full intent of ultimately removing the spleen when a child is "immunologically older." Although children older than age 2 with sickle cell disease have an apparently normal antibody response to pneumococcal vaccination given pre-operatively, there is still sufficient doubt concerning the efficacy of the vaccine that the use of prophylactic penicillin does seem justified. The duration of such penicillin prophylaxis is controversial, but this study by Emond et al. suggests that the most important period for sepsis occurs in the first 3 years after sple-nectomy. Opponents of the use of routine penicillin prophylaxis in children with sickle cell anemia state that there is no controlled evidence that this form of prophylaxis works. This is probably true, but it also reflects the fact that appro-priately designed studies have not been well performed in this regard. Anglin et al. have shown that patients with sickle cell anemia have fewer positive nasopharyngeal cultures for *Pneumococcus* when they are on prophylactic pen-icillin therapy (*J. Pediatr.* 104:18, 1984). Furthermore, penicillin prophylaxis did not result in emergence of penicillin-resistant organisms or in an increased rate of *H. influenzae* infection. Previous studies have been unable to demonstrate any effect of penicillin prophylaxis on the carriage rate of *Pneumococcus*. There is no question that children with sickle cell disease also should be given the pneumococcal vaccine prophylactically. This is best given after age 2 because of poor responses prior to that. This is also the reason for many individuals' choice of prophylactic hypertransfusions in children with sequestration prior to age 2. In addition to the use of the pneumococcal vaccine, data from Finland on normal children seems to indicate that prevention of *H. influenzae* type B bacteremia can be accomplished with an *H. influenzae* capsular polysaccharide vaccine (*N. Engl. J. Med.* 310:1561, 1984). That latter vaccine is not the be-all and end-all in normal children, and the same probably will hold true of patients with sickle cell anemia once they undergo clinical trials with this vaccine.

In summary, there probably is a role for splenectomy in children with sickle cell disease who have certain complications of the disease. If at all possible, the spleen should not be removed until after age 2 years even if this requires carrying the patient along on a hypertransfusion program until that age. If the spleen must come out, the pneumococcal vaccine should be given prior to splenectomy (and we soon may be also using the *H. influenzae* vaccine), and penicillin prophylaxis seems appropriate after the splenectomy as well. My per-sonal feeling is that it also should be used in any patient with sickle cell anemia who is old enough to have had functional asplenia develop. Above all, no form of prophylaxis, either vaccine or antibiotic, will prevent every episode of sep-sis. This has been documented clearly with several case reports. The same level of awareness of bacteremic complications must be held.

Finally, the hopes that were expressed in the 1984 YEAR BOOK (p. 237) con-cerning 5-azacytidine have been bashed. You will recall that this drug, which selectively increases fetal hemoglobin synthesis, was being tried in a few pa-tients. Specifically, it was being used in patients with thalassemia major to see if it would decrease transfusion requirements. It also was hoped that this drug, if it panned out in thalassemic patients, might be used for patients with sickle cell disease because a rise in fetal hemoglobin levels presumably would help sickling (Ley, T. J., et al.: *N. Engl. J. Med.* 307:1469, 1982). Apparently during the clinical trial in subjects with thalassemia, the drug proved not to be all that helpful relative to its toxicity. We are not likely to see it being further explored very extensively, except perhaps in a laboratory setting. Unfortunately, nothing fails like last year's success and nothing is so defeated as yesterday's triumphant cause.—J.A.S., III

Acute Chest Syndrome in Sickle Cell Disease
S. C. Davies, P. J. Luce, A. A. Win, J. F. Riordan, and M. Brozovic (Central Middlesex Hosp., London)
Lancet I:36–38, Jan. 7, 1984   9–11

It may be difficult to determine whether chest pain, fever, and radiographic shadowing are due to infection or to infarction in patients with sickle cell disease. The authors reviewed 25 consecutive episodes of acute chest syndrome occurring in 13 adults with sickle cell disease in a 5-year period. Nine patients had SS disease and 3, SC disease. The mean age was 23 years. Seven patients had single episodes of acute chest syndrome. Twelve patients had nonchest crises during the review period. Chest pain was present in all but two episodes, but usually was not pleuritic in nature. Nine patients coughed. The x-ray study abnormalities included patchy basal infiltrates, linear atelectasis, florid consolidation, and small pleural effusions. Nine episodes were bilateral. The fall in hemoglobin was greatest in patients with bilateral changes in x-ray studies. Leukocytosis was always present. Microbiologic studies were positive in only two episodes.

Treatment was with crystalloid fluid, fresh-frozen plasma, analgesia on demand, and antibiotic coverage, usually with amoxicillin. Patients who continued to deteriorate received exchange transfusion. Twelve patients underwent exchange transfusion. Those with bilateral abnormalities generally required more intensive exchange. Two patients, both with lateral involvement, died; both had platelet counts below $100 \times 10^9/L$.

Intravascular sickling in the lungs may account for much of the clinical picture in patients with sickle cell disease and acute chest syndrome. More severely affected patients have had significant decreases in hemoglobin and platelets and have responded rapidly to exchange transfusion. A prospective study with ventilation-perfusion lung scanning and detailed assessments of pulmonary gas exchange would help clarify the pathogenesis of acute chest syndrome.

Pitfalls in Diagnosis of Osteomyelitis in Children With Sickle Cell Disease
Doris L. Wethers and Ranjeet Grover (St. Lukes-Roosevelt Hosp. Center, New York)
Clin. Pediatr. (Phila.) 22:614–618, September 1983   9–12

Nine cases of osteomyelitis in children with sickle cell disease have been diagnosed since 1965. Data on 3 of these cases that illustrate problems in diagnosis or management are presented.

Girl, 5, with sickle cell disease had a 1-day history of fever and pain in the right upper arm. Roentgenography of the right arm and shoulder showed no abnormality. Blood was drawn for culture, and treatment was started with intravenous administration of ampicillin (300 mg/kg/day, divided every 6 hours). The culture showed *Salmonella* group B sensitive to ampicillin. A bone scan with ^{99m}Tc-diphosphonate on day 4 showed increased uptake consistent with a diagnosis of osteomyelitis, but films of the arm were still normal. A film taken during the second week of hospitalization showed irregularity of cortex and new bone formation consistent with osteomyelitis (Fig 9–6). The girl was discharged in good condition after 6 weeks of intravenous therapy. She was readmitted 21 months later with fever and pain in the same arm and was given ampicillin (200 mg/kg/day) and chloramphenicol (100 mg/kg/day) intravenously for 4 days. Chloramphenicol was discontinued when blood cultures showed ampicillin-sensitive *Salmonella* group B. She became afebrile in 4 days, but bone aspiration on day 9 was positive for *Salmonella*. Open surgical drainage of the distal third of the humerus on day 16 was positive for *Salmonella*. Intravenous injection of ampicillin was continued for a total of 8 weeks. The patient has been symptom free for 2 years.

The second patient had osteomyelitis caused by *Salmonella* and a bone scan that was normal despite verified disease. The third patient had *Staphylococcus aureus* infection, extensive asymptomatic involvement of the radius, and an abnormal bone scan.

The possibility of osteomyelitis should be considered in any febrile child with sickle cell disease and symptoms or signs referable to bone. Differentiation between infarct and osteomyelitis may be difficult. Blood should be cultured immediately and the child followed closely before antibiotics are given. If there are signs of severe local inflammation or if symptoms persist unabated, a direct aspirate for culture is obtained from the affected area, followed by repeat blood cultures. A bone scan using ^{99m}Tc-diphos-

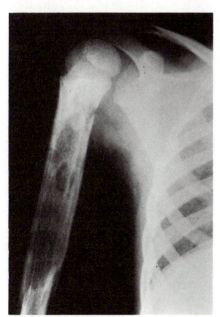

Fig 9–6.—Irregularity of cortex and new bone formation in girl aged 5 years. (Courtesy of Wethers, D.L., and Grover, R.: Clin. Pediatr. (Phila.) 22:614–618, September 1983.)

phonate is obtained as soon as possible and definitely within a week of onset of symptoms. If it is normal and osteomyelitis is still strongly suspected, a gallium scan is obtained.

If treatment is started prior to receiving results of culture study, antibiotics that will cover infections caused by *Salmonella, S. aureus,* and *Streptococcus pneumoniae* are used. Intravenous therapy for gram-positive osteomyelitis is given for 2 to 3 weeks, followed by oral therapy to complete a 6- to 8-week course. A longer total course of therapy probably is indicated for osteomyelitis caused by *Salmonella,* particularly if there is sequestrum and involucrum formation, suggesting chronicity. Serial bactericidal assays are done to determine appropriate dose and adequate serum levels of antibiotics.

Is There Increased Risk of *Hemophilus influenzae* Septicemia in Children With Sickle Cell Anemia?

Darleen Powars, Gary Overturf, and Ernest Turner (Univ. of Southern California, Los Angeles)
Pediatrics 71:927–931, June 1983   9–13

Children with sickle cell anemia have a considerably greater risk of disease due to *Streptococcus pneumoniae* than normal children. However, there is conflicting evidence regarding the risk of serious disease due to *Hemophilus influenzae* in these children. The incidence of *H. influenzae* septicemia-meningitis in children with sickle cell anemia was assessed retrospectively and the clinical findings were reviewed in 354 children younger than age 5 years with sickle cell anemia (645 person-years) and an additional 224 children aged 5 to 9 (824 person-years).

Ten cases of *H. influenzae* septicemia were identified, 2 in children younger than age 18 months, 6 in children aged 18 to 59 months, and 2 in children older than age 5 years. There were 3 deaths, all preventable; 2 were in children older than age 5 years. Two children had persistent or recurrent infection. All 10 had a prodrome ranging from 1 to 21 days in duration, which often was associated with upper respiratory tract infections, otitis symptomatology, and a low-grade fever that eventually exceeded 102 F. All patients had hemoglobinopathy. A decrease in hemoglobin concentration greater than 2 gm/dl and massive reticulocytosis were found in 4 patients. Two children had small fibrotic spleens at autopsy; both were severely anemic at the time of death.

Severe disease caused by *H. influenzae* is not rare among children with sickle cell anemia. The use of antibiotics in the febrile child with sickle cell anemia should be based on the 400-fold increased risk of pneumococcal septicemia in patients younger than age 5 years and the four-fold increased risk of *H. influenzae* septicemia in patients younger than age 9.

► Jeanne Lusher, Professor of Pediatrics, and Director, Division of Hematology-Oncology at the Children's Hospital of Michigan, in Detroit, comments on this article and the two preceding it:

"These three articles, each dealing with a different complication of sickle cell disease, underscore the difficulties in arriving at the proper diagnosis—and thus in selecting the most appropriate therapy. The first, by S. C. Davies and colleagues, concerns the etiology and pathogenesis of what is referred to as the "acute chest syndrome" in adults with sickle cell disease. While the authors' retrospective analysis deals with patients ranging in age from 12 to 45 years, and with several forms of S hemoglobinopathy (9 with SS, 3 with SC disease, and 1 with S-thalassemia), it nonetheless emphasizes the difficulties in evaluating and managing adolescent and adult patients with sickle cell disease who present with chest pain and fever. Although it is not completely clear how thorough the search for viral and bacterial pathogens was in these patients, it is stated that microbiologic studies were negative in 23 of 25 episodes. The authors thus conclude that infection is rarely the cause of the acute chest syndrome in adults. One might take issue with this conclusion, especially without a more detailed discussion of the attempts made to identify infectious agents in these patients. Because pneumonia and intravascular sickling in the lungs may occur concurrently, the authors' concluding statement concerning the need for a more detailed prospective study should perhaps have included the need for a more thorough search for viral and bacterial pathogens.

"The article by Wethers and Grover emphasizes the need for thinking about osteomyelitis in any child with sickle cell disease who has symptoms or objective findings referable to bone. While the vast majority of bone infarcts are aseptic, resulting from vaso-occlusion alone, one always must consider the possibility of bacterial osteomyelitis. Wethers and Grover provide an excellent review of this subject and point out the virtues and limitations of various diagnostic tests when bacterial osteomyelitis is suspected. Clearly the one most likely to provide the correct diagnosis is a direct aspirate of the affected area for culture; however, radionuclide scans may be useful if done early in the course of symptoms.

"The third article, by Powars, Overturf, and Turner, provides documentation of a small but definite increased incidence of *Hemophilus influenzae* septicemia/meningitis in children with sickle cell anemia (SS) as compared to published reports of incidence in normal children. While the risk appears to be of the order of two to four times normal (in contrast to the 400-fold increased risk of pneumonoccal septicemia in children of comparable age), the authors' data indicate that children with SS between ages 5 and 9 years and those younger than age 5 years may be at similar risk. Thus, in evaluating a febrile child with this hemoglobinopathy, one must consider the possibility of *H. influenzae* as an etiologic agent not only in those younger than age 2 years but in somewhat older children as well. The authors also point out that there is a clear distinction in the clinical presentation of SS patients with *H. influenzae* septicemia as compared to those with pneumonoccal septicemia—a distinction that we should all keep in mind."

Chloramphenicol-Responsive Chronic Neutropenia

Gene R. Adams and Howard A. Pearson (Yale Univ.)

N. Engl. J. Med. 309:1039–1041, Oct. 27, 1983   9–14

The neutropenias of childhood feature neutropenia and increased frequency of bacterial infections. A patient with severe, lifelong neutropenia who had many bacterial infections was encountered. Chloramphenicol administration in a repeated and reproducible fashion effected neutrophil maturation and maintained normal numbers of circulating neutrophils over an extended period.

Boy, 14, developed skin and middle ear infections at age 5 months. At age 18 months, he had "severe neutropenia." At age 3 years, white blood cell count was 2600/cu mm with 1% neutrophils. Bone marrow aspiration revealed a hypercellular marrow with granulocytic hyperplasia. He had delayed mental development, spasticity, and choreoathetoid movements consistent with spastic cerebral palsy. Treatment with prednisone (2 mg per kg of body weight per day) for 1 month produced no increase in neutrophil count. Between ages 3 and 7 years, the patient had multiple severe infections treated with various antibiotics. At age 8 years, with progressive pneumonia despite antibiotic therapy, he was given ampicillin, oxacillin, and chloramphenicol intravenously. Fourteen days after admission, total white cell count and absolute neutrophil count increased sharply. The pneumonitis resolved. One and 2 months later, the absolute neutrophil count had fallen to 25—150/cu mm. The patient responded positively to monilial and mumps intradermal antigens. On three separate occasions after treatment with orally administered chloramphenicol for skin infections, the absolute neutrophil count was noted to be within the normal range. At age 13, he was readmitted to the hospital and received chloramphenicol, 1.5 gm/day, orally. Ten days later the absolute neutrophil count rose sharply to 18,600/cm mm. He was later treated for 3 weeks with 2.0 gm thiamphenicol per day, but did not respond to this therapy. Chloramphenicol was reinstituted, and the hematologic condition improved. However, there has been no change in mental retardation, hyperactivity, choreoathetosis, or spasticity.

The authors note that chloramphenicol uniquely facilitated neutrophil maturation and has maintained normal levels of circulating neutrophils in this patient for more than 12 months. A predictable 10–12 days of treatment were necessary to produce the response, and 10–12 days after discontinuation of treatment, the absolute neutrophil count regularly fell. Although physicians are reluctant to use chloramphenicol in patients with blood dyscrasias, the authors suggest that a therapeutic trial with this drug might be considered in patients with severe congenital neutropenia.

▶ Laurence Boxer, Professor of Pediatrics, and Director of Pediatric Hematology/Oncology, C. S. Mott Children's Hospital, Ann Arbor, Michigan, comments on this curious but intriguing study:

"Although clinical descriptions of neutropenia in infection began to appear in the first quarter of the 20th century, the understanding of mechanisms of chronic neutropenia have been hampered because of inadequate methods for precisely measuring neutrophil production and utilization and the relative rarity of chronic neutropenic patients. Names that have evolved for the various forms of chronic neutropenia have not served to clarify either the pathophysiology or prognosis of this disorder. In general, cases that have been called "benign neutropenias" have been in patients with at least a few hundred neutrophils/ per cubic millimeter with cellular or hypercellular bone marrows and with little morbidity from infection. Patients with more serious problems with infections have been infants or individuals with extremely low blood neutrophil counts below 200/cu mm.

"The bone marrow in chronic neutropenia usually shows a rather distinctive abnormality. Late neutrophilic forms generally are reduced, but early neutrophil precursors often appear to be quantitatively and morphologically normal, as was the case with the present patient. In other words, this abnormality, which has been called 'maturation arrest' by hematologists, apparently can affect granulocytic cells at any level in the maturation process. Marrow neutrophil cell labeling indices and tritiated thymidine suicide studies utilizing the in vitro bone marrow culture have shown that the mitotic activity of neutrophilic precursor cells is not arrested. In many cases the study of bone marrow in patients with chronic neutropenia in in vitro suspension culture also suggests that the neutrophil precursors in these patients are capable of maturing to morphologically and functioning normal cells. The basis of the bone marrow defect in most cases of chronic neutropenia remains unknown. As with this patient, more monocytes appear to be generated relative to the production of neutrophils. It is known that monocytes and neutrophils appear to rise from the same cell clone. It is conceivable, therefore, that the bone marrow is diverted to monocytopoiesis by an abnormal regulation mechanism affecting cells differentiating into neutrophils.

"Lately, there has been much interest in attempts to induce cellular differentiation, especially of neoplastic cell lines, as potential means of ameliorating blood cytopenias. The factors regulating normal hematopoietic cell maturation and the effect of certain chemical 'inducers' on cell lines have been studied extensively in cell culture systems. Proliferation and differentiation seem to be independent facets of cellular maturation, although common controls exist. Normal myeloid precursors require protein inducers for viability and maturation in vitro. These proteins may be produced constitutively or secreted by various cell types, including lymphocytes and macrophages. Besides protein, certain chemicals and naturally occurring substances, such as retinoic acid and metabolites of vitamin D, also have been shown to induce cellular differentiation. Similarly, cytarabine will induce differentiation in a specific clone of mouse leukemia cells and HL60 human promyelocytic leukemia cells. Cytarabine may induce differentiation in leukemia cells of a particular genotype that express specific receptor cites on cell surfaces or perhaps by promoting a protein inducer that itself causes differentiation. Chloramphenicol similarly may be acting in this patient either by directly affecting the differentiated stem cells themselves or by altering production of protein inducers by other types of cells. Answers to questions regarding the mechanism by which chloramphenicol affected this patient might be surmised by performing in vitro studies to evaluate its effect on myeloid differentiation. It also would be of interest to know whether other chemicals might have the same beneficial effect. We now await reports from other laboratories to establish the utility of chloramphenicol treatment in patients with severe congenital neutropenias."

Homozygous Protein C Deficiency Manifested by Massive Venous Thrombosis in the Newborn
Uri Seligsohn, Anna Berger, Martha Abend, Lisa Rubin, Dina Attias, Ariela Zivelin, and Samuel I. Rapaport
N. Engl. J. Med. 310:559–562, Mar. 1, 1984   9–15

Activated protein C functions as a potent anticoagulant that inactivates activated factors V and VIII and also may stimulate fibrinolysis. Even a moderate reduction in the plasma protein C concentration may be associated with an increased risk of thrombosis. A family was encountered in which 2 infants died shortly after birth with massive venous thrombosis and in which concentrations of protein C antigen were reduced. The antigen was virtually absent from the plasma of 1 infant. Both parents and 12 other family members had reduced antigen values consistent with the heterozygous state.

The proposita received the diagnosis of bilateral renal vein thrombosis the day after birth. Protein C antigen was virtually undetectable in the blood. The infant died at age 34 days with extensive thrombosis involving the inferior vena cava and both renal and iliac veins. Multiple renal cortical infarcts and pulmonary infarcts were present. Another infant died with renal vein thrombosis, and 2 other siblings of the proposita had died neonatally. Both parents, who were first cousins, had partial protein C deficiency. Protein C reductions were found in 12 of 25 other family members aged 4 to 70 years, none of whom had had thrombotic episodes. Concentrations of all other vitamin K-dependent clotting factors were normal, as were the values for factors V:C, VIII:C, and antithrombin III. The proposita had reduced concentrations of vitamin K-dependent clotting factors and antithrombin III, but this is not infrequent in newborn infants.

Protein C deficiency is transmitted as an autosomal disorder in this family. The homozygous state may be manifested by the virtual absence of plasma protein C and fatal neonatal thrombosis. The risk of thrombosis in asymptomatic heterozygotes is unknown. More families will have to be studied before recommendations can be made for prophylactic anticoagulant therapy in asymptomatic heterozygotes.

Inherited Protein C Deficiency and Coumarin-Responsive Chronic Relapsing Purpura Fulminans in a Newborn Infant
Herman E. Branson, Richard Marble, Jacob Katz, and John H. Griffin
Lancet 2:1165–1168, Nov. 19, 1983   9–16

Protein C, a zygomen of a vitamin K-dependent serine protease, inhibits prothrombin activation and destroys platelet prothrombinase activity when activated. A case of coumarin-responsive chronic relapsing purpura fulminans syndrome in a protein C-deficient newborn is described.

Boy was born at full term to a preeclamptic mother without overt consumption coagulopathy by emergency cesarean section because of fetal bradycardia. Three hours after transfer to the neonatal intensive care unit because of hypotonia, the first of several ecchymomas were noted, with ultimate involvement of the buttocks, lower extremities, lower abdomen, scalp, and ears. The skin lesions progressed to form bullae and became necrotic. Therapy with ampicillin and kanamycin was begun. Coagulation test results were consistent with acute disseminated intravascular coagulation (DIC). Fresh-frozen plasma transfusion (10–30 ml/kg) had a transient (24–72 hours) palliative effect on coagulation and reversed progression of the skin lesions. Another 2 months of daily fresh-frozen plasma transfusion were required to stabilize the chronic purpura fulminans syndrome. During this period, repeated thrombotic and hemorrhagic episodes occurred resulting in hydrocephalus, blindness, and developmental delay. Platelet concentrations and blood coagulation factor levels were extremely low. Administration of fresh-frozen plasma immediately changed the acute consumptive clinical picture into one of chronic compensated DIC. Microangiopathic red blood cell fragmentation was noted during both active and quiescent phases of consumption coagulopathy. The infant was discharged after 3 months, well controlled on a regimen of daily fresh-frozen plasma transfusions (10 ml/kg). There were many rehospitalizations, primarily for review of possible venous access sites. Another means of supportive therapy was sought at age 28 months because of progressive deterioration with the use of peripheral routes of plasma administration. Cryoprecipitate and cryoprecipitate-poor plasma sustained the biochemical and clinical remission from acute DIC as well as fresh-frozen plasma did. The combination of aspirin-dipyridamole-heparin failed to control the clinical signs of purpura fulminans. The child was given a loading-dose protocol of coumarin therapy, 7.5 mg/24 hours for 5 days, after which he was maintained with doses in the therapeutic range of 3.75 mg/24 hours. They were no clinical signs of acute exacerbation of DIC during 19 days of treatment with coumarin. Biochemical test results during this time were consistent with a chronic consumptive state. After a sharp initial drop, the fibrinogen concentration stabilized between 150 and 200 mg/dl, the fibrin degradation product titer remained between 10 and 40 μg/ml, and the platelet count was consistently in the high-normal range. Plasma protein C levels during therapy were consistently less than or equal to 6%. The infant was discharged in remission; with oral anticoagulant therapy, he was symptom-free for 3 months until a fatal massive subarachnoid and intracerebral hemorrhage occurred. There was no evidence of neoplasia, hemangiomata, or organ malformation.

The only consistent abnormality in this child was a marked deficiency in the plasma protein C level, which led to identification of 3 symptom-free kin with low levels (31% to 40%) of plasma protein C. This is the first report of purpura fulminans in a patient with low plasma protein C levels in whom plasma protein deficiency was implicated as the cause of increased susceptibility to DIC.

▶ J. Paul Scott, Assistant Professor of Pediatrics, Northwestern University and Children's Memorial Hospital, Chicago, tells us about protein C:

"Protein C is a vitamin K-dependent protein that is activated in vitro by the action of thrombin on an endothelial cell cofactor called 'thrombomodulin.' After activation, protein C inactivates factors V and VIII; in addition, activated protein

C also may stimulate fibrinolysis. From this description, it is apparent that protein C is a potent modulator of the coagulation mechanism. Activated protein C joins antithrombin III and plasminogen and its activators as vitally important inhibitors of coagulation. These proteins protect against thrombosis. One would expect that a deficiency of protein C should result in a profound thrombotic tendency. Conversely, a deficiency of the inhibitor of protein C has been reported to be a cause of the rare combined deficiency of factors V and VIII. This article and the preceding one, in addition to several other abstracts that have been published, now demonstrate that a severe deficiency of protein C results in a profound disruption of the coagulation mechanism that presents in the neonatal period. This deficiency may be manifested as either multiple, deep venous thromboses or recurring episodes of purpura fulminans in the newborn. Other reports also suggest that the heterozygous state may predispose to deep venous thrombosis in young adults. The inheritance pattern of protein C deficiency appears to be autosomal and probably recessive.

"These reports underscore the need of practitioners to consider the possibility of an inherited, deficient, or dysfunctional protein as the etiology of thrombotic disease when it presents in children or young adults. Assays for protein C are not commonly available at this time but will become increasingly available at centers with a strong research interest in thrombosis and hemostasis. Therapy for the affected neonate includes replacement with a plasma product, of which prothrombin complex concentrates seem most logical, and possibly long-term anticoagulation. These clinical reports add to our knowledge of a protein that appeared to have enormous impact on the coagulation mechanism in the laboratory but initially lacked clinical evidence of its in vitro importance."

Danazol Increases Factor VIII and Factor IX in Classic Hemophilia and Christmas Disease
Harvey R. Gralnick and Margaret E. Rick (Natl. Inst. of Health)
N. Engl. J. Med. 308:1393–1395, June 9, 1983   9–17

To determine whether there was an increase in the level of factor VIII or factor IX, to assess how long it took for that increase to occur, and to evaluate how long the factor remained elevated after therapy (danazol, 600 mg/day) was discontinued, 5 patients with a lifelong history of hemorrhage all older than age 18, were studied; 4 had classic hemophilia and 1 had Christmas disease.

All patients previously had been receiving infusions, principally when pain in the area of a joint occurred. During the period of danazol trial, levels of the deficient coagulation factor rose markedly, usually within 5–6 days after initiation of therapy. Levels of factor VIII in patients with classic hemophilia rose from 1%–3% before treatment to 3%–8% during treatment. Level of factor IX in the patient with Christmas disease rose from 5% to 14%. After withdrawal of the drug at 14 days, there was a gradual drop in the activity of the deficient factor. Danazol therapy had no untoward effects. During the 70 patient-days of therapy, no patient required infusion of plasma products after the first day of trial.

Results of the present studies are similar to previously reported studies of danazol in hereditary angioedema and in α_1-antitrypsin deficiency. After withdrawal of the drug, infusions were required twice within 6 days, when the deficient coagulation factor had returned to levels near the base line.

Danazol therapy may decrease hemorrhagic tendency and reduce the need for transfusions of plasma products in classic hemophilia and Christmas disease. Controlled clinical trials will be required to establish its value in these applications.

▶ Danazol is a synthetic androgenic hormone. The investigators in this study decided to try danazol in hemophiliacs because of the agent's known ability to elevate levels of deficient proteins in two congenital disorders—the pulmonary emphysema that occurs in patients with α_1-antitrypsin deficiency and the angioedema that occurs in patients with a deficiency of the inhibitor (C1 esterase) of the first component of complement. Because hemophilia A and hemophilia B also result from deficiencies in normally structured protein, the investigators postulated that danazol might also be effective in increasing the activity of these clotting factors. This turned out to be the case. During the time patients with hemophilia A were receiving danazol, the number of infusions of factor VIII could be reduced to an average of less than half of the previous requirements. As can be seen in the details of this report, all the patients studied fit into the moderate, rather than the severe, range of hemophilia. If it turns out that danazol has no effectiveness in the severe variety of hemophilia (less than 1% factor VIII activity), the usefulness of danazol will turn out to be somewhat limited, because the majority of all factor VIII replacement is used in the severe category.

If danazol does find a nitch in the management of hemophiliacs it will be along side the use of arginine vasopressin (DDAVP). Arginine vasopressin will increase the level of factor VIII activity as much as sixfold in mild to moderate hemophiliacs and patients with von Willebrand's disease (J. Pediatr. 102:288, 1983). It does not work in severe hemophiliacs. Not only does DDAVP increase the factor VIII level of patients with von Willebrand's disease, it also shortens their bleeding time (*Lancet* 1:1145, 1984).

Danazol, when it hit the market as an androgen, did not find much acceptance as an anabolic steroid, given the wide variety of other similar agents. Now we see it being used in an extremely innovative fashion for management of patients with bleeding disorders. Curiously, it has been reported to increase the platelet count in some patients with idiopathic thrombocytopenic purpura as well (Ahn, Y. S., et al.: *N. Engl. J. Med.* 308:1396, 1983). All this seems a little bit like Star Wars medicine, but if danazol works it will be a welcome blessing to patients with these disorders.—J.A.S., III

High-Dose Intravenous γ-Globulin Therapy for Passive Immune Thrombocytopenia in the Neonate
Gaetano Chirico, Marzia Duse, Alberto G. Ugazio, and Giorgio Rondini (Univ. of Pavia, Pavia, Italy)
J. Pediatr. 103:654–655, October 1983   9–18

Passively acquired immune neonatal thrombocytopenia secondary to maternal idiopathic thrombocytopenic purpura (ITP) is a transient disorder that may persist for 1 to 4 months. It is usually treated with exchange transfusion followed by platelet transfusion. The case of one such infant in whom treatment with γ-globulin was followed by dramatic correction of thrombocytopenia without side effects is reported. The mother had acute ITP (platelet count, 5,000/cu mm) during the fifth month of pregnancy. Corticosteroid therapy was unsuccessful. Splenectomy, performed 1 month before delivery, resulted in an increase in the platelet count to 90,000/cu mm.

Female infant, born at 36 weeks' gestational age, and weighing 2,330 gm at birth, had petechiae on the trunk. Platelet count was 76,000/cu mm. It decreased gradually to 43,000/cu mm during the next 4 days, and new petechiae appeared. Intravenous administration of intact γ-globulin (0.4 gm/kg/day) for 5 days caused a sharp increase in serum IgG levels and platelet count (Fig 9–7). At age 19 days, another dose of γ-globulin was given because the platelet count and IgG levels had decreased. The platelet count increased gradually thereafter, with no further bleeding manifestations. At age 6 months, the infant had normal platelet count, growth, and development.

High doses of intact γ-globulin have a beneficial but temporary effect in children and adults with ITP. Because neonatal passive immune thrombocytopenia is transient, the effect of γ-globulin, although also transient, may be sufficient to improve the condition until spontaneous correction occurs. However, platelet transfusion should probably be performed when thrombocytopenia is severe and bleeding is life-threatening.

▶ It was a natural for someone eventually to do what was done in this report. Mori et al. (*Arch. Dis. Child.* 58:851, 1983), as have previous investigators, observed that as many as 80% of children with chronic idiopathic thrombocytopenic purpura (ITP) would respond with elevation of platelet counts after intravenous administration of γ-globulin. Commercial intravenous immunoglobu-

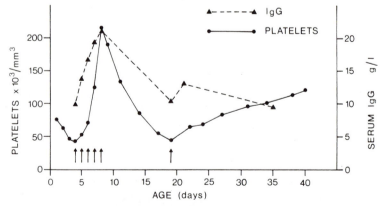

Fig 9–7.—Platelet counts and serum IgG concentrations in a neonate with passive immune thrombocytopenia given high doses (0.4 gm/kg/day) of γ-globulin intravenously. Arrows indicate γ-globulin injections. (Courtesy of Chirico, G., et al.: J. Pediatr. 103:654–655, October 1983.)

lin preparations may interfere with phagocyte Fc-receptor-mediated immune clearance (Fehr, J.: *N. Engl. J. Med.* 306:1254, 1982). The data in adults are far less impressive than those in children. The data looked so good in children, in fact, that the use of γ-globulin intravenously has been extended to a variety of other immune cytopenias. It has been used in the management of immune neutropenia and autoimmune hemolytic anemia (Bussel, J. B.: *Br. J. Haematol.* 56:1, 1984). In the study by Chirico et al., intravenous γ-globulin administration was used to treat a newborn born of a mother with ITP who passively transferred platelet-associated antibody to her infant in utero. Presumably, the same response would be seen with isoimmune thrombocytopenia in which the mother makes a specific antibody against antigens not present on her platelets but found on the surface of a baby's platelets. The data on the use of intravenous immunoglobulin therapy in the management of ITP are sufficiently impressive that most clinicians are using it prior to making a decision for splenectomy in patients who are not having natural resolution of the disease process on their own. The problem with immunoglobulin is that its effect is very often a transient one. There are not many alternatives, however, to splenectomy in children or adults with chronic ITP. Certainly, patients who fail splenectomy and who are having life-threatening episodes of bleeding deserve use of γ-globulin at least once to see if it works. You may ask, "What ever happened to vinca-loaded platelets?" A few years back, many people were using platelets that had been "loaded" with vinblastine to treat patients with refractory ITP. The idea here was to deliver an immunotherapeutic agent directly to a receptor cell that was destroying the platelets. The idea sounded wonderful at the time, but subsequently many failures have been noted. The use of such "loaded" platelets recently has been reviewed by W. F. Rosse (*N. Engl. J. Med.* 310:1051, 1984).

In case you have not heard enough about intravenously administered γ-globulin, some people are using it to treat childhood epilepsy and myasthenia gravis (*Lancet* 2:406, 1984). How this would work is beyond me, but once a bandwagon starts rolling, it is difficult to stop people from jumping on board. We will just have to wait for this tune to play itself out before we understand exactly what is going on.—J.A.S., III

10 Oncology

Childhood Cancer: Medical Costs
Shirley B. Lansky, Janet L. Black, and Nancy U. Cairns
Cancer 52:762–766, Aug. 15, 1983   10–1

The costs of cancer treatment are a major burden on families of affected children. A previous study indicated that nonmedical, out-of-pocket costs incurred because of the illness consumed about one fourth of the weekly budget.

In this study, medical charges for 64 families of children being treated for cancer on an outpatient basis were sampled for a 1-month period. The mean patient age was 9½ years. Mean family yearly income was $19,000. Leukemia was the most common diagnosis. Families of 10 patients who had died also participated in the study. The mean age of these patients at diagnosis was 8½ years and the mean age at death, 10½ years.

Monthly charges for living patients varied widely with the diagnosis and ranged from $100 to $1,800. Total cancer center charges throughout the illness for the patients who died ranged from $8,000 to $53,000, the mean being $34,558. Over half the charges were incurred in the diagnostic and terminal stages of illness. The mean outstanding debt 30 months after death of the child was $624. Medical costs amounted to an average of 5.8% of the weekly budget.

Medical costs to the families of children with cancer are much less than the nonmedical costs incurred during treatment. In addition, most families have long-term outstanding medical debts, which are particularly stressful for families whose child has died. An increase in available information on the high costs of cancer treatment may eventually benefit the families of children with cancer, as has been the case with chronic renal disease.

▶ As one would expect, medical charges for the total course of disease in a child with cancer are great. The medical charge from the cancer treatment center alone was more than 2 years' annual salary for most of the families. Fortunately, the vast majority of these medical charges were covered by third-party carriers. On the average, the part not covered by insurance companies, state aid, and similar sources amounted to about 5% of the monthly average income of a family. Even so, 75% of families in which the child had died still had outstanding medical debts to the cancer treatment center up to 3½ years after the death. As this study points out, what is more important than the 5% of the family budget that is going toward medical expenses is the additional 25% of the budget that goes toward nonmedical expenses related to the extra costs of going back and forth to the treatment center, staying overnight in lodgings away from home, etc. The final blow to these families comes with the death of a child and just trying to pay off funeral expenses, which averaged over $2,000 in this study.

One of the ways of dealing with these less than obvious costs is to recognize them for what they are and attempt to provide coverage. In many regards this has happened with kidney disease. Another way of dealing with the problem is continuously to do as has been done to date. That is to improve survival rates and curability of the disease being treated. In the 30-year period between 1950 and 1980, much has been accomplished. Deaths among children younger than age 15 years have decreased 50% for leukemia, 32% for non-Hodgkin's lymphoma, 80% for Hodgkin's disease, 50% for bone sarcomas, 68% for kidney cancer, and 31% for all other forms of cancer (*JAMA* 251:1567, 1984). Another approach toward minimizing the costs of cancer care is to do everything possible to prevent the development of cancer in children. Unfortunately, most cancers cannot be specifically localized to an etiology, and such approaches will have no major impact (presumably) on rates of cancer. Anything, however, is an improvement. This past year has seen more concern than any other prior year regarding environmental carcinogens. Take, for example, nitrosamines in rubber baby bottle nipples. These are potent carcinogens in animal test systems. They also have been present in baby bottle nipples for years. The only way of getting rid of significant amounts of these carcinogens is to boil them at least 5 to 6 times before their initial use (*Fed. Register* 48:57014, 1983). We also have heard a great deal recently about genetic damage possibly being related to ultrasound use prenatally. This story is far from clear, but in many other parts of the world ultrasound is used for virtually all pregnancies on a routine basis. This recommendation has not been accepted in the United States because of concerns over the effects on DNA (*J. Clin. Ultrasound* 12:11, 1984).

We doctors in the United States have been major sources of radiation exposure to neonates, especially those requiring intensive care. There is so much unknown in this area that any comment is difficult at this point. One very thoughtful review of the topic (Robinson, A.: *Br. J. Radiol.* 56:937, 1983) seems to indicate that despite the numerous x-ray studies performed in neonatal intensive care units, radiation exposure gives a neonate only a 1 in 10,000 chance for the subsequent development of malignancy, a figure not very different from background figures. These data may not even be very different from the effects of phototherapy on DNA. The amount of energy produced by routine phototherapy lights can induce strand breaks in the DNA of cultured human fibroblasts. Matters are made even more difficult if these same cells are irradiated in the presence of low concentrations of bilirubin. This will increase DNA breaks by some 30- to 40-fold, according to Rosenstein et al. (*Pediatr. Res.* 18:3, 1984). With all the other problems that occur in neonatal units as part of the need to provide intensive management and support for critically ill newborns, it's no wonder that I've heard some students comment that they felt like they were entering a woes garden when they walked in the nursery door for the first time.—J.A.S., III

Radiation Exposure and Estimate of Late Effects of Chest Roentgen Examination in Children

M. Gustafsson and W. Mortensson (Univ. Hosp., Lund, Sweden)
Acta Radiol. [Diagn.] (Stockh.) 24:309–314, 1983   10–2

Determinations were made of radiation doses to children from chest examinations done using current screen-film combinations. Thirty-eight patients aged 1 month to 11 years were included in the study; median age was 5.2 years. Frontal and lateral films were exposed. Five young infants were examined lying prone at exposures of 2–4 mamp. Thirteen patients aged 4 months to 6½ years were also examined while lying prone but with the cassette placed in a potter with a grid with a ratio of 12, making the focus-film distance 150 cm rather than 140 cm. Twenty patients aged 2½–11 years were examined erect at a focus-film distance of 150 cm. Tube voltage was 100 kV in the young infants and 120 kV in the other groups.

Radiation doses to the lungs, breasts, thyroid, and bone marrow corresponded to 5%–30% of yearly background radiation. The energy delivered per kilogram of body weight was lower in erect patients than in comparable patients examined while lying prone. The lateral projection accounted for about two thirds of the total energy delivered. Estimations of the risk of late stochastic effects suggested that the greatest risk to infants of both sexes and to older boys is radiation-induced leukemia and thyroid cancer. After infancy, girls are at risk of developing breast cancer. The risk of breast cancer generally is a greater problem than leukemia. Reversing the beam direction from posteroanterior to anteroposterior increases this risk, but the risk of leukemia is unchanged. Modification of the examination to reduce the number of exposures also can be helpful, but this must be done judiciously so as not to lose needed diagnostic information.

▶ Andrew K. Poznanski, Radiologist-in-Chief, Children's Memorial Hospital, Chicago, comments:

"There has been a considerable lack of understanding and a certain amount of hysteria among the public regarding the risk of diagnostic x-ray films. Information contained in this article will help to put some perspective into this whole subject, as it evaluates the doses to various organs and the potential risks from a chest x-ray examination. The figures that the authors use are projected from known effects of higher-dose radiation. This is necessary, as we have no evidence that any harmful effect occurs at the very low doses that are used in most diagnostic x-ray examinations. To err on the side of safety, we assume that some effect occurs at low dose. The risk estimates in this article are probably higher by a factor of more than 10, compared to what is considered likely in many departments, because the grid techniques that the authors used give several times the dose that can be given for similar-quality radiograms. Also, their estimates are based on the linear and no-threshold approach, while most authors now feel that it is likely that at very low doses a different relationship occurs and that the effect, if any, will be one half to one tenth of that predicted by the linear hypothesis. Even with their risk estimates, the overall risk is really minute. For example, they calculate the risk of death trom malignancy from a chest x-ray study (anteroposterior and lateral) to be 1 to 34 additional deaths if 10 million children were irradiated. According to the newer calculations, it would be only one tenth of those figures. This is a very tiny risk. It is approximately the same risk as being killed in an automobile accident when driving 0.5 to 15 miles. The 0.1 to 3.4 additional cancer deaths also would be a very small portion of the 1.6 million in the same 10 million children who will normally die from cancer within their lifetime.

"Another way to look at the problem is to consider radiation from x-ray studies in terms of background. The authors calculated that the doses to the various organs were 5% to 30% of the background radiation per year. This figure is a relatively small percentage of background, particularly since variations in background are often quite large. For example, the radiation dose from background in Denver is approximately 50% larger than in Chicago. Also, there is considerable variability even in one city. In a recent report of the National Council on Radiation Protection, it is apparent that the radiation dose to the bronchi from radon in houses that are not ventilated may be more than 100% greater than that of background in a well-ventilated home, whereas in some countries, radiation doses from radon may have been 10 to 50 times greater than the usual background dose.

"From these data, one can conclude that the risks of simple radiologic examinations, such as a chest x-ray study, are indeed minute and should not be considered in the decision making of whether the study should be done. Doses from more complex examinations can be considerably greater. For example, in angiography the organ doses can be a thousand times as great as that from a chest roentgenogram or, in computed tomography, a few hundred times greater, but even in those situations the risks are not very great. Certainly, one should not obtain a chest x-ray study or any other radiograph for frivolous reasons, but it seems that the other risks associated with a chest x-ray examination, such as earning the money to pay for the study or driving to the department of radiology to obtain the study, are probably greater than the study itself.

"For more detailed information on the risk of low-dose radiation, see Webster in the *American Journal of Roentgenology* (137:647, 1981)."

Postsepsis Prophylaxis in Cancer Patients
Walter T. Hughes and Gayle Patterson (Memphis, Tenn.)
Cancer 53:137–141, Jan. 1, 1984   10–3

The course following the withdrawal of antibiotic therapy in cancer patients treated for bacterial sepsis remains uncertain. The authors followed 100 children having cancer and documented bacterial sepsis for a month after the completion of adequate antibiotic therapy. Treatment was given intravenously for sepsis due to *Staphylococcus aureus, Escherichia coli, Pseudomonas aeruginosa,* or *Klebsiella pneumoniae.* Thirty-eight patients considered to be at high risk of *Pneumocystis carinii* pneumonitis were maintained on 5 mg of trimethoprim (TMP) and 25 mg of sulfamethoxazole (SMZ) per kilogram daily. The most common primary diagnosis was acute lymphocytic leukemia. Forty-five patients were in relapse

ETIOLOGY OF INITIAL SEPSIS: RECURRENT EPISODES WITH AND
WITHOUT PROPHYLAXIS

Organism	Received TMP–SMZ		No TMP–SMZ	
	No. of patients	No. (%) with recurrent episode*	No. of patients	No. (%) with recurrent episode*
S. aureus	12	1 (8.3%)	13	8 (61.5%)
E. coli	14	3 (21.4%)	11	7 (63.6%)
P. aeruginosa	3	0 (0%)	22	12 (54.5%)
K. pneumoniae	9	3 (33%)	16	12 (75%)
Total	38	7 (18.4%)	62	36 (62.9%)
			$\chi^2 = P < 0.001$	

*Recurrent episode: febrile episode requiring antibiotics during 1 month postsepsis.
(Courtesy of Hughes, W.T., and Patterson, G.: Cancer 53:137–141, Jan. 1, 1984.)

at the time sepsis was diagnosed. A large majority of patients was neutropenic. The distribution of TMP-SMZ prophylaxis according to the cause of sepsis is shown in the table. Forty-one patients were in relapse at the end of antibiotic therapy for sepsis, and 37 were neutropenic.

Recurrent infection or reinfection occurred in 23 of 26 neutropenic patients not maintained on prophylaxis and in 4 of 11 given TMP-SMZ. A comparable difference was seen in nonneutropenic patients; 11% of treated patients and 44% of those not treated had infection during follow-up. The differences in both groups were highly significant. Children in relapse were infected twice as often when not given TMP-SMZ. None of 19 patients who died during the study period had received prophylaxis. Fifty-four percent of neutropenic patients not given prophylaxis died.

There is a significant risk of infection in the month after bacterial sepsis is treated in children with cancer, despite presumably adequate treatment. Maintenance of treatment with TMP-SMZ appears to prevent recurrent episodes of infection in this setting. In patients who are not neutropenic and are in remission, the only benefit from TMP-SMZ is the prevention of *P. carinii* pneumonitis. A relatively low dose of TMP-SMZ proved effective in the present study.

Antimicrobial Therapy of Febrile Children With Malignancies and Possible Sepsis
Johnnie P. Frazier, William G. Kramer, Larry K. Pickering, Steve Culbert, Keith Brandt, and Lawrence S. Frankel
Pediatr. Infect. Dis. 3:40–45, January 1984   10–4

Various types of antimicrobial therapy have been used in febrile children with malignancy and neutropenia, because death can result from severe infection before a pathogen is isolated and identified. Netilmicin and gentamicin were compared as to efficacy and safety in a prospective series of 100 pediatric patients with malignancies and fever who were suspected of having infection or who had physical signs of infection. Empirical therapy with ticarcillin and either netilmicin or gentamicin was begun. Ticarcillin was given in a dosage of 300 mg/kg daily and gentamicin and netilmicin in dosages of 8 mg/kg daily. The most common diagnoses were acute lymphocytic leukemia and osteosarcoma. Infections were caused by a wide range of microorganisms.

About three fourths of the children were leukopenic at the outset and more than half at the end of treatment. The outcome is related to the microbiologic findings in the table. All but 2 of 40 children with microbiologically documented infection responded to treatment. Serum drug half-lives, volumes of distribution, and total body clearance rates were comparable in the netilmicin and gentamicin groups. Renal function deteriorated during antibiotic therapy in 1 patient in each treatment group, and other factors may have been responsible in both. No ototoxicity related to antibiotic therapy was observed. Superinfection occurred in 5 children, 3 of whom died.

Gentamicin or netilmicin, in combination with a β-lactam antibiotic, were equally effective and relatively nontoxic in these neutropenic children seen at M.D. Anderson Hospital and Tumor Institute, Houston, with fever and malignancy. It is unlikely that third-generation penicillin and cephalosporin antibiotics will improve response rates in such patients until microbiologic resistance develops against current drugs. The new agents, however, may reduce the side effects associated with presently used drug combinations.

▶ If you think the life of an oncologist is simple and uncomplex, just think about the issues involved with the management of fever and neutropenia in the child with cancer. This study gives only a slight insight into this problem. It suggests that approaches using limited numbers of drugs are the best ways to start off until the situation clarifies itself. Would that life would be that simple!

PATHOGENS ISOLATED FROM CHILDREN WITH
MICROBIOLOGICALLY DOCUMENTED INFECTIONS AND RESPONSE

Organism	With Bacteremia	Without Bacteremia	Clinical and/or Bacteriologic Cures*
Pseudomonas aeruginosa	7	1	8 (100)
Escherichia coli	4	3	7 (100)
Klebsiella pneumoniae	3	2	5 (100)
Other Gram-negative bacilli	6	0	5 (83)
Staphylococcus aureus	3	2	5 (100)
Other Gram-positive cocci	6	2	8 (100)
Total	29	10	38 (97)

*Numbers in parentheses indicate percent.
(Courtesy of Frazier, J.P., et al.: Pediatr. Infect. Dis. 3:40–45, January 1984.)

Pizzo et al. (*Am. J. Med.* 76:436, 1984) have reviewed the principles for the management of infectious complications in cancer patients. Each of the following questions was asked and then the controversies concerning management discussed: What are the risk factors associated with infection in granulocytopenic patients? Is it possible to identify patients who will become infected? Are body surveillance cultures useful in clinical management of granulocytopenia? What constitutes empiric antibiotic therapy for granulocytopenic patients? When should the initial empiric antibiotic regimen be modified? How should foreign bodies (such as central intravenous catheters) be managed in granulocytopenic patients? What is the best management in approaching the patient with pulmonary infiltrates? What is the best approach to unexplained fever in granulocytopenia? If you think this paper might ask more questions than it provides answers, you are quite correct. In this regard, the paper should have been titled "Serutan" because it is a bit backward from the way most papers are written. It is, however, an honest approach addressing a very difficult area.—J.A.S., III

Open Lung Biopsy in Immunocompromised Children With Pulmonary Infiltrates
Charles G. Prober, Hilary Whyte, and Charles R. Smith (Hosp. for Sick Children, Toronto)
Am. J. Dis. Child. 138:60–63, January 1984   10–5

Acute pulmonary infiltration is a common problem in immunocompromised patients. A review was made of experience with 44 immuno-

PATHOLOGIC AND MICROBIOLOGIC
DIAGNOSES

Diagnosis	No. (%) of Infections
Pneumocystis carinii infection	15 (33)
Viral pneumonia	21 (46)
Cytomegalovirus	8
Paramyxovirus	3
Other	2
Histologically only	8
Bacterial pneumonia	3 (7)
Fungal pneumonia	2 (4)
Malignancy	2 (4)
Interstitial pneumonitis	11 (24)

(Courtesy of Prober, C.G., et al.: Am. J. Dis. Child. 138:60–63, January 1984; copyright 1984, American Medical Association.)

compromised children who had acute pulmonary infiltrates and underwent 46 open lung biopsies between November 1976 and April 1982. Mean age of patients was 8½ years. Twenty-six had malignant disorders and 15 were immunodeficient. All patients were acutely ill with a pneumonic process at the time of thoracotomy. Four fifths of the patients had received antibiotic therapy before lung biopsy.

At least one infectious agent was found in 72% of biopsy specimens (table). Nonspecific interstitial pneumonitis was diagnosed in 24% of cases. Two biopsy specimens showed relapse of malignancy. Treatment was altered after surgery in 30 (65%) cases. Specific treatment was initiated in 12 cases, and preoperative broad-spectrum therapy was discontinued in 20 cases. Complications directly attributable to the biopsy procedure were minimal. There was no clinical bleeding at operative sites or wound infection. No patient required catheter insertion for pneumothorax. One patient had a bronchopleural fistula that closed spontaneously.

It is concluded that open lung biopsy is a valuable diagnostic procedure in immunocompromised children with acute pulmonary infiltration. A histologic diagnosis was made in all the present patients. Empirical treatment was altered in two thirds of the cases. The diverse conditions diagnosed would have precluded successful empirical management in many instances. Open lung biopsy is safe in these patients.

▶ Robert L. Baehner, Professor of Pediatrics and Clinical Pathology, Indiana University, and Director, Pediatric Hematology/Oncology, James Whitcomb Riley Hospital for Children, comments:

"A systematic aggressive approach to the immunocompromised child with respiratory symptoms was used in this study with beneficial results, confirming again the value of obtaining lung tissue for diagnostic studies in these patients. Most patients develop a predictable chronology of respiratory findings, including lethargy, fever greater than 38.5 C, nonproductive cough, and tachypnea of greater than 35 breaths per minute without abnormal pulmonary auscultatory findings. Chest radiographs often show dramatic changes and arterial Po_2 is usually less than 70 mm Hg. Because of a myriad of etiologies for such a clinical picture (even when the patient has been receiving prophylactic antiprotozoan, antibacterial, and/or antifungal treatment), preparations should be made as soon as possible for open lung biopsy and appropriate laboratory personnel notified. Preoperative coagulation studies, complete blood count, blood cultures, type and cross match, blood chemistries, and serologic studies are obtained. Platelet and packed red blood cell transfusions should be administered to patients with platelet counts of less than 50,000/cu mm and hemoglobin values less than 10.0 gm/100 ml, respectively. Under general anesthesia, approximately 3 gm of lung tissue is removed, and one portion is submitted for frozen and permanent sections to be stained with hematoxylin and eosin, methenamine silver nitrate, Gram-Weigert, fluorochrome acid-fast and other stains as indicated. Gram-Weigert and Giemsa stains of both frozen sections and impression smears are examined for the presence of bacteria, fungi, and/or protozoan cyst structures indicative of *Pneumocystis carinii*. The remaining portions of lung tissue are cultured for aerobic and anaerobic bacteria, fungi, mycobacteria, and viruses.

"Our own experiences as well as those of others confirm that the complication rate for open lung biopsy is low. The procedure is the preferred method to obtain sufficient tissue for establishing the correct diagnosis in the immuno-compromised child with pulmonary infiltrates."

Indwelling Venous Access Catheters in Patients With Acute Leukemia
James J. Reilly, Jr., David L. Steed, and Pamela S. Ritter (Univ. of Pittsburgh)
Cancer 53:219–223, Jan. 15, 1984   10–6

Venipunctures can become a painful ordeal for patients with acute leukemia. The authors have used surgically implanted indwelling venous access Hickman catheters in such patients. The double-lumen Hickman catheter is shown in Figure 10–1. Twenty-six catheters were placed in 25 patients (mean age, 43 years) with acute leukemia. The catheter usually was placed before combination chemotherapy was started. All catheters were inserted in the operating room with an anesthesiologist in attendance. The patient was lightly sedated and given local Xylocaine-epinephrine anesthesia. The external jugular or cephalic vein was used. After the vein was ligated distally, a subcutaneous tunnel was made from an upper abdominal stab wound. The catheter was drawn through this tunnel into the vein cutdown wound and then passed through a transverse venotomy into the mediastinum. The catheter tip was placed in the superior vena cava.

Patients received an average of 12 courses of combination chemotherapy, 11.5 units of packed red blood cells, 48 units of platelets, 4 units of fresh frozen plasma, and numerous doses of antibiotics via the catheters, which were in place for a mean of 101 days. Eight catheters remain functional

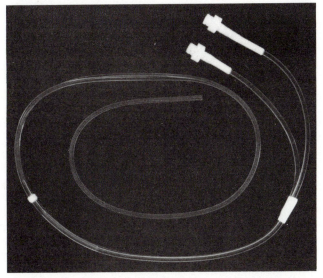

Fig 10–1.—The indwelling double-lumen Hickman catheter. (Courtesy of Reilly, J.J., Jr., et al.: Cancer 53:219–223, Jan. 15, 1984.)

an average of 225 days after insertion. Complications included early hemorrhage in 2 cases and catheter occlusion in 6 cases. Six catheters were removed because of persistent sepsis. Fourteen patients in all had bacteremia, predominantly from gram-negative organisms. Patient acceptance of the catheters was excellent. Several patients successfully have managed their catheters outside of the hospital.

The Hickman catheter has proved useful for gaining prolonged venous access in leukemic patients. Complications include hemorrhage, catheter occlusion, and sepsis; sepsis has been the most serious problem. Overall experience with the Hickman catheter has been satisfactory. Hemorrhagic complications can be minimized by platelet transfusions where appropriate. Heparin irrigation can prevent intraluminal thrombosis, and streptokinase infusion can dissolve an extraluminal fibrin sheath.

▶ The Hickman catheter has proved a useful method for gaining prolonged venous access in patients with acute leukemia. Its use has been extended to a variety of malignancies in children. In fact, it has been reported to be useful in tiny babies for hemodialysis when peripheral routes are not possible. It has been so successful in the cancer patient that its spread into nononcology cases is rapidly expanding. Patient acceptance is excellent. Despite this, central intravenous catheters brought out through the skin are not totally without risk. Complications are of three types: hemorrhage, occlusion, and sepsis. Regular heparin flushing is generally effective in preventing clotting within the lumen of the catheter, but will not keep fibrin from being deposited on the outside of the catheter. This eventually can build up and cause a nidus for infection or for embolization. Many catheters now have been left in place with this complication and have been treated with streptokinase to produce lysis of the thrombus. Bacteremia is the major reason why these catheters have to be removed. We have gained enough confidence with infection in the presence of catheters that they are not removed automatically every time a blood culture becomes positive. Generally, only if a patient is not responding to antibiotic therapy must a decision be made to remove the catheters. This is somewhat different from the concept, prevalent not that long ago, that all intravenous lines had to be changed in patients who were documented to be bacteremic or septic.

In many centers, the overall experience with Hickman catheters has been quite satisfactory. They should not be advocated for every oncology patient. They are reserved for patients who have difficulties with venous access and also for patients who are likely to have protracted hospitalizations, frequent blood work, and many episodes of neutropenia. Certainly, patients can be allowed to go home with such catheters after careful instruction. I would dare say that if there is any one thing that has improved the quality of life in some children with malignancy, it has been the introduction of one simple semipermanent intravenous line in the form of a Hickman catheter.—J.A.S., III

Superficial Lumps in Children: What, When, and Why?
Philip J. Knight and Charles B. Reiner
Pediatrics 72:147–153, August 1983

Superficial unexplained lumps in children, although of serious import in only about 1% of cases, can be a source of anxiety to parents. The clinical and histologic findings were reviewed in all children younger than age 16 who underwent excisional or dermatologic punch biopsy of a visible or palpable superficial lump at Columbus Children's Hospital, Columbus, Ohio, between January 1970 and December 1980. Children with certain lesions recognizable by their anatomical location and clinical features were excluded.

Data on 1,222 superficial lumps were reviewed. Overall, 269 children who had a superficial lump excised had a preoperative diagnosis of lymphadenopathy. Enlarged lymph nodes were found in 261 of these children. Thus, when a diagnosis of lymph node enlargement was based on location of the superficial lump and its physical characteristics, it was correct 97% of the time. However, when an enlarged lymph node was present in a site at which lymphadenopathy would not commonly be expected, the clinical diagnosis was often incorrect. Twenty-three enlarged midline neck lymph nodes were incorrectly diagnosed as thyroglossal duct cysts, and 6 retroauricular nodes were mistaken for "cysts"; 3 enlarged submandibular nodes were incorrectly regarded as branchiogenic cysts; an enlarged, tender, suprainguinal lymph node was operated on with a preoperative diagnosis of incarcerated inguinal hernia in 2 infants; and 4 nodes at atypical sites were misdiagnosed as miscellaneous cysts or tumors. Excluding superficial lumps that were lymph nodes, anterior midline neck masses, or

TABLE 1.—HISTOLOGIC DIAGNOSES OF 775 SUPERFICIAL LUMPS EXCISED IN CHILDREN

I. Squamous epithelial cysts		459 (59%)	V. Probably self-limited processes		47 (6%)
Presumed posttraumatic epithelial implantation	38		Pseudorheumatoid nodules and granuloma annulare	22	
Uncertain etiology, most probably of congenital origin	421		Urticaria pigmentosa	17	
			Persistent insect bite, "shot spot"	8	
II. Congenital malformations		117 (15%)	VI. Malignant tumors		11 (1.4%)
Pilomatrixoma (Malherbe's calcifying epithelioma)	79		Rhabdomyosarcoma	5	
Lymphangioma, hemolymphangioma (noninfantile)	22		Neurofibrosarcoma	1	
			Fibrosarcoma	2	
Branchial cleft cyst without sinus	10		Malignant fibrous histiocytoma	1	
Juvenile hemangioendothelioma (no overlying skin discoloration)	5		Malignant pleomorphic adenoma	1	
			Basal cell carcinoma	1	
Other hamartoma	1		VII. Miscellaneous lesions		35 (4%)
III. Benign neoplasms		56 (7%)	Pseudosarcomatous lesions— myositis ossificans and degenerating schwannoma	3	
Neurofibroma or neurolemmoma	27				
Lipoma, angiolipoma	25		Granular cell myoblastoma	8	
Sweat gland tumor	2		Traumatic neuroma	1	
Other benign tumors	2		Miscellaneous cysts without epithelial lining: sterile abscess, organizing hematoma, etc	23	
IV. Reparative or possibly neoplastic lesions, undetermined etiology		50 (6%)			
Xanthomas; xanthogranulomas	18				
Aggressive fibromatosis; recurring digital fibromas	15				
Fibroma	12				
Histiocytoma	5				

(Courtesy of Knight, P.J., and Reiner, C.B.: Pediatrics 72:147–153, August 1983. Copyright American Academy of Pediatrics 1983.)

malignant superficial lumps with a pathologic diagnosis prior to referral, there were 775 remaining superficial lumps. Of these, 11 were malignant (Table 1). Seventeen children with sarcomas diagnosed after biopsy of a superficial lump at other hospitals were referred for further therapy. Five of the total 28 malignant tumors occurred on the head and neck, 11 on the trunk, and 12 on the extremities.

Five factors were helpful in differentiating benign from malignant lumps: 3 of the 28 malignancies were in children younger than age 1 month; 8 of 25 showed rapid or progressive growth; 3 of 25 were ulcerated at presentation; 15 of 26 were deep or fixed to the fascia; and 20 of 26 were larger than 3 cm in greatest dimension (Table 2). Of the 28 children with malignancies, 22 had one or more of these five risk factors, as did 80 (10%) with benign lumps. Approximately 6% of the lumps were self-limited processes. Urticaria pigmentosa were suspected on clinical examination in 12 of the 17 affected patients whereas only 1 of the 22 patients with pseudorheumatoid nodule and granuloma annulare received a correct diagnosis prior to excisional biopsy.

The most common superficial lump excised was an epidermal inclusion cyst containing keratinaceous debris. Of these 459 cysts, 62% were correctly diagnosed preoperatively. These squamous epithelium-lined cysts were not randomly distributed, but occurred at certain typical locations, e.g., the lateral border of the eyebrow or under the scalp (Fig 10–2). The second most common lesion was pilomatrixoma, which is believed to be a hamartoma of hair follicle origin. Twenty-four of these 79 lumps were correctly diagnosed preoperatively.

Approximately 80% of malignant superficial lumps can be recognized on the basis of five risk factors. If these risk factors are absent, the child's parents can be reassured with a 99.7% accuracy as to the benign nature of the lump. About 6% of these lumps regress spontaneously and thus do not require excision. However, more than 90% of superficial lumps persist or slowly enlarge and should be electively excised.

TABLE 2.—χ^2 PROBABILITIES AND LIKELIHOOD RATIOS OF MALIGNANCY FOR FIVE RISK FACTORS

	Malignant Lumps	Benign Lumps	χ^2 Probabilities	Likelihood Ratios
Age			$\chi^2 = 18.2, P < .001$	
Neonatal age	3	5		16
> 1 mo	25	759		.90
Growth rate			$\chi^2 = 170, P < .001$	
Rapid and progressive	8	3		82
Slow or stationary	17	761		.68
Ulceration			$\chi^2 = 36, P < .001$	
Present	3	2		45
Absent	22	762		.88
Depth of lesion			$\chi^2 = 265, P < .001$	
Fixed to or deep to fascia	15	8		40
Not fixed to nor deep to fascia	11	756		.42
Size and consistency			$\chi^2 = 196, P < .001$	
>3 cm and not soft	20	34		17
<3 cm or soft	6	730		.24

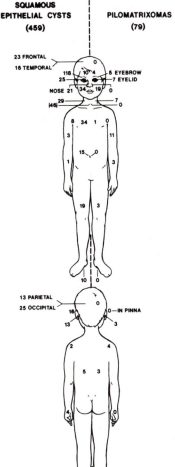

SQUAMOUS EPITHELIAL CYSTS (459)

PILOMATRIXOMAS (79)

23 FRONTAL

16 TEMPORAL

118

25

NOSE 21

146

5 EYEBROW

7 EYELID

13 PARIETAL

25 OCCIPITAL

0—IN PINNA

15 OTHER SITES

OTHER SITES 9

Fig 10–2.—Anatomical locations in which squamous epithelial cysts and pilomatrixomas were observed. (Courtesy of Knight, P.J., and Reiner, C.B.: *Pediatrics* 72:147–153, August 1983. Copyright American Academy of Pediatrics 1983.)

► Superficial lumps in children are only occasionally of serious prognostic import. They nonetheless are a source of great anxiety to parents who find an unexplained lump. When you see this sort of child in your office, there will be a potential categorization of these lumps into three possibilities: a small number requiring immediate attention, another group that can be treated expectantly, and a group of remaining masses that should be excised electively after the anxiety level of the parents has been appropriately lowered at the initial consultation. This report by Knight and Reiner, like all retrospective studies, has certain inherent and not readily quantifiable biases. This study originated out of a hospital setting, and hospitals obviously are referral centers for unusual cases. Undoubtedly, a bias for an increased number of malignant superficial bumps and a bias toward large bumps that could not be excised in physicians' offices must have existed. Despite this, the authors have provided us with valuable information concerning which child with a lump or bump is most likely to have a malignancy. As they rightfully note, very young age (less than age 1 month), rapid growth of the bump, ulceration, fixation, and odd size all tend to increase significantly the possibility of a malignancy. This is one study well worth reading in the most minute detail.

I would like to refer you to two excellent review articles that somewhat have to do with lumps and bumps in children. One of these (Marcy, S. M.: *Pediatr. Infect. Dis.* 2:397, 1983) provides a complete description of infections of lymph nodes of the head and neck. I have not seen a finer review of this anywhere. The other is an article by J. L. Sullivan (*J. Clin. Invest.* 71:1765, 1983) that gives the complete natural history of the immunodeficiency problem associated with the X-linked lymphoproliferative syndrome. Finally, no discussion of lymphadenopathy would be complete without some comment about cat-scratch disease. Researchers at the Armed Forces Institute of Pathology have found delicate pleomorphic gram-negative bacilli in lymph nodes excised from patients with cat-scratch disease (*Science* 221:1403, 1983). The organisms were intracellular and tended to increase in number as the lesions developed and decrease in number as the lesions resolved, thus fulfilling the criteria for a pathogenic organism. Unfortunately, the organisms could not be identified. It wasn't hard to see why they may have been missed previously, because they are sufficiently small as to be at the lower limit of resolution of a light microscope. Cats just don't ever seem to give up. The only thing good about a cat that I have heard recently was a joke. This was the one about a cat who ate cheese so he could sit about waiting for mice with baited breath (my apologies for this one).—J.A.S., III

LSA$_2$-L$_2$ Protocol Treatment of Stage IV Non-Hodgkin's Lymphoma in Children With Partial and Extensive Bone Marrow Involvement
Luz Duque-Hammershaimb, Norma Wollner, and Denis R. Miller (Meml. Sloan-Kettering Cancer Center)
Cancer 52:39–43, July 1, 1983   10–8

Considerable difficulty exists in distinguishing high-risk acute lymphoblastic leukemia (ALL) from stage IV non-Hodgkin's lymphoma (NHL) with bone marrow involvement. The percentage of lymphoblasts present in the bone marrow often has been used arbitrarily to distinguish between the two conditions (table). As a result, many cases of NHL are probably treated as ALL using conventional leukemic regimens, which are less aggressive than NHL regimens.

The authors used the LSA$_2$-L$_2$ protocol to treat 41 consecutive children with bulky disease and biopsy-proved NHL. The percentage of blasts in the bone marrow was 25% or less in 14 children (group IV-A) and more than 25% in the other 27 (group IV-B). The LSA$_2$-L$_2$ regimen combines cyclophosphamide, vincristine, prednisone, daunomycin, methotrexate, cytosine arabinoside, thioguanine, L-asparaginase, carmustine, and hydroxyurea in an induction, consolidation, and maintenance schedule. In-

---

CRITERIA FOR DIAGNOSIS OF ACUTE LYMPHOBLASTIC LEUKEMIA
AND STAGE IV NON-HODGKIN'S LYMPHOMA*

	Leukemia	Stage IV NHL
Blasts in marrow	>25%	<25%
Blasts in periphery	present	absent
Primary site	nodal & bone marrow extranodal rare	nodal extranodal common
All surface marker	null cell common T-cell B-cell	mostly T-cell and B-cell
Bulky disease	rare	always present
Age	generally younger	older age group
Hgb ≥ 10 g/dl	rare	common
Prognosis	50% disease-free survival 5 years if low risk 15–20% if high risk	poor prognosis

*Abbreviations: NHL, non-Hodgkin's lymphoma; Hgb, hemoglobin.
(Courtesy of Duque-Hammershaimb, L., et al.: Cancer 52:39–43, July 1, 1983.)

---

trathecal methotrexate was given throughout the three phases. Radiation therapy was given in the induction phase if only one site was to be treated and during induction and early consolidation if multiple sites needed radiation therapy.

Disease-free actuarial survival (Fig 10–3) was 64% for group IV-A (median observation time, 48+ months; range, 24–102+ months) and 65% for group IV-B (median observation time, 37+ months; range, 20–100 months).

The extent of bone marrow involvement apparently does not affect the prognosis in stage IV NHL. Improved survival is more a matter of early aggressive and multimodal therapy. Moreover, for the 24 patients in group IV-B who had unfavorable characteristics that could be considered as high-risk ALL (i.e., high initial leukocyte count, hemoglobin level above 10 gm/dl, age older than 10 years, massive adenopathy and organomegaly, and CNS disease at diagnosis), disease-free actuarial survival was 73% (median observation time, 37+ months), compared with 43% survival reported for similar patients treated with conventional leukemia therapy. Certain patients with high-risk ALL also may benefit from therapeutic regimens based on the same principles as LSA_2-L_2.

▶ Sharon Murphy, St. Jude Children's Research Hospital, Memphis, Tennessee, comments on the current status of non-Hodgkin's lymphoma:

"The authors have concluded that the extent of bone marrow involvement does not affect the prognosis in stage IV NHL, finding no significant difference in the disease-free survival between a group of 14 children with 25% or less blasts in the bone marrow and a group of 27 children with greater than 25% replacement of bone marrow elements by blasts, all being treated with the intensive 10-drug LSA_2-L_2 regimen plus radiotherapy. However, the compara-

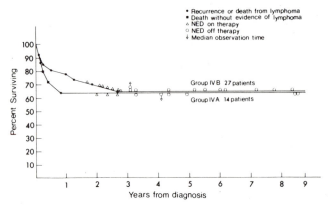

Fig 10–3.—Disease-free actuarial survival of partial and total bone marrow replacement; NED indicates no evidence of disease. (Courtesy of Duque-Hammershaimb, L., et al.: Cancer 52:39–43, July 1, 1983.)

tively small numbers of patients, along with the diversity of primary sites and histologic subtypes, diminishes levels of statistical confidence in the finding of 'no difference.' Others have noted very significant interactions between treatment and histology in childhood NHL, as reported, for instance, in the larger series of the Children's Cancer Study Group (Anderson, J. R., et al.: Childhood non-Hodgkin's lymphoma: The results of a randomized therapeutic trial comparing a 4-drug regimen (COMP) with a 10-drug regimen (LSA_2-L_2), N. Engl. J. Med. 308:559–565, 1983). For lymphoblastic disease, at least, treated with the LSA_2-L_2 therapy, one suspects that the intensity of the 10-drug regimen overrides the possible prognostic significance of partial or complete bone marrow replacement. Intuitively, the requirement to kill the last remaining tumor cell implies that the total body burden of neoplastic cells is the ultimate factor influencing prognosis. Nevertheless, the authors' conclusion that certain patients with high-risk forms of ALL might benefit from therapeutic regimens based on the same principles as the LSA_2-L_2 therapy seems unarguable from a pragmatic standpoint."

Are Cognitive and Educational Development Affected by Age at Which Prophylactic Therapy Is Given in Acute Lymphoblastic Leukemia?

L. Jannoun (Hosp. for Sick Children, London)
Arch. Dis. Child. 58:953–958, December 1983   10–9

Previous studies suggest that children treated for acute lymphoblastic leukemia (ALL) before age 5 years are likelier to have intellectual impairment than those treated similarly when older. The author used standard intelligence and achievement tests to assess development in 129 children with ALL in remission who had completed treatment. Both chemotherapy and radiation therapy had been used for treatment, which was completed at least 6 months before evaluation. Forty-three patients were treated before age 3 years, 43 when aged 3–6 years, and 43 when aged 7 or older. The patients were aged 5–17 years when evaluated. Sixty-seven healthy siblings also were assessed.

The patients in general functioned within the average range of intelligence, but had significantly lower IQs than their siblings. Only those who received cranial irradiation at age 7 or later had intelligence comparable to their siblings. Those treated before age 3 had significantly lower IQs than older patients or healthy children matched with the patients for age, sex, and parental occupation. Reading retardation was more frequent than expected in the patients. Rates of behavioral deviance did not differ significantly from those reported in general population studies. School attendance usually was reported as good to excellent.

Patients treated for ALL before age 3 years exhibit more intellectual impairment than those treated similarly at an older age. The latter also exhibit some impairment compared with healthy siblings. The possibility of delaying cranial irradiation until age 3 should be considered, and alternate methods of prophylaxis should be sought. If the risk of learning difficulties is recognized, remedial measures can be arranged for at an early stage if appropriate.

▶ It has now become apparent that standard CNS prophylaxis, as part of the management of childhood leukemia, has long-term neuropsychologic sequelae that vary in severity from minor intellectual dysfunction to severe neurologic impairment, seizures, and dementia. These clinical features represent the extremes of a spectrum of brain damage. The three chief factors implicated in causing long-term neuropsychologic dysfunction include cranial irradiation, intrathecally administered methotrexate, and moderate- to high-dose intravenously administered methotrexate. Prior YEAR BOOKS have discussed the potential hazards of CNS irradiation on intellectual functioning. Most children are not severely compromised, although they may not have IQs equivalent to those of their siblings and may have some subtle learning disorders. Enough of these problems have become recognized that alternatives to the use of radiation are being examined, although it is fair to say that any alternative therapy that is adequate prophylactically to treat the CNS may have its own set of problems. If it is found that CNS irradiation is still necessary, the dose required has been dropped from 2,400 rad to 1,800 rad (Nesbitt, M. E., et al.: *Lancet* 1:461, 1981).

I hope that we physicians who have been involved with the treatment of children with childhood leukemia will be happy with the long-term consequences of treatment. I would like to grow old and not have to worry about this. (Old age, as you know, begins at age 40 and is characterized initially by an inability to remember names and then progresses over the years to an inability to remember faces, followed by forgetfulness to pull your zipper up, and culminates at an age when you forget to pull your zipper down.)—J.A.S., III

Bone Marrow Transplantation for Acute Lymphoblastic Leukemia

Robert Peter Gale, John H. Kersey, Mortimer M. Bortin, Karel A. Dicke, Robert A. Good, Ferry E. Zwaan, and Alfred A. Rimm (International Bone Marrow Transplant Registry)

Lancet 2:663–667, Sept. 17, 1983

10–10

Although intensive chemotherapy can produce remission in more than 90% of children and more than 70% of adults with acute lymphoblastic leukemia (ALL), children with high-risk features fare less well with chemotherapy. Once relapse occurs during chemotherapy, the prognosis becomes poor, with 2-year to 4-year disease-free survival rates of less than 10% in most series. Gale et al. report the results of bone marrow transplantation from human leukocyte antigen (HLA)-identical siblings in 204 patients with various stages of ALL who were believed to be at high risk for the development of recurrent leukemia if treated with chemotherapy alone or were at high risk because of one or more relapses while receiving chemotherapy.

The actuarial probability of surviving for 4 years was 43% for the 106 patients given transplants during the first or second remission. In contrast, the probability of 4-year survival in patients with more severe disease given transplants was 15% ($P < .001$) (Fig 10–4). The actuarial probability of relapse at 4 years was 32% in patients given transplants in the first and second remissions and 67% in those with more advanced disease ($P < .001$). Of the high-risk patients, those receiving a transplant during the first remission had a higher probability of survival ($55\% \pm 22\%$) than those given transplants in their second remission ($41\% \pm 15\%$). Relapse rates in high-risk patients given transplants in their first remission were similar to those given transplants during the second remission ($28\% \pm$

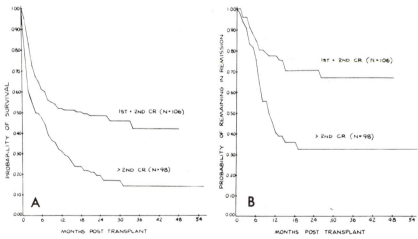

Fig 10–4.—A, probability of survival, and **B,** probability of remaining in remission in patients with acute lymphoblastic leukemia after bone marrow transplantation in the first or second remission *(upper curves)* or in more advanced disease *(lower curves);* life-table analysis. (Courtesy of Gale, R.P., et al.: Lancet 2:663–667, Sept. 17, 1983.)

24% and 31% ± 19%, respectively). Relapse rates were comparable among standard-risk and high-risk patients given transplants during the second remission, although the standard risk patients tended to have a higher probability of survival. In addition to recurrent leukemia, other major causes of treatment failure were graft-versus-host disease and interstitial pneumonia. It would appear that long-term leukemia-free survival in ALL patients can be achieved with bone-marrow transplantation.

Marrow Transplantation for Acute Nonlymphocytic Leukemia After Treatment With Busulfan and Cyclophosphamide

George W. Santos, Peter J. Tutschka, Ronald Brookmeyer, Rein Saral, William E. Beschorner, Wilma B. Bias, Hayden G. Braine, William H. Burns, Gerald J. Elfenbein, Herbert Kaizer, David Mellits, Lyle L. Sensenbrenner, Robert K. Stuart, and Andrew M. Yeager (Johns Hopkins Univ.)
N. Engl. J. Med. 309:1347–1353, Dec. 1, 1983   10–11

Fifty-one patients with acute nonlymphocytic leukemia were treated with infusion of human leukocyte antigen-identical sibling marrow after cytoreduction with high doses of busulfan and cyclophosphamide. Sixteen patients had end-stage disease (group I), 17 were in their second or third remission or in early relapse (group II), and 18 were in their first remission (group III) at the time of infusion. No patient in group I survived for more than 600 days, whereas 2-year posttransplantation survival rates in groups II and III were 29% and 44%, respectively. The difference in survival between patients in group I and group III was statistically significant (P < .01). Patients younger than age 20 years tended to have a better survival rate than older patients had; an age older than age 20 increased the risk of death by a factor of 2 (P = .06). Female patients in group II were at a higher risk than were male patients in the same group. Survival was also favorably affected by transplantation during the first remission. Twelve patients are alive and in remission 327–1,488 days after transplantation, with 10 surviving for more than 2 years. The major causes of death were acute graft-versus-host disease and viral pneumonia. In 1 patient with end-stage disease, the leukemic cells failed to clear, and another patient relapsed with meningeal leukemia. Another relapse occurred in a patient who underwent transplantation during a third remission.

Long-term remission of acute leukemia can be achieved with administration of high-dose chemotherapy with busulfan and cyclophosphamide followed by allogeneic marrow transplantation. This therapeutic approach provides an effective alternative to treatment with cyclophosphamide and total body irradiation prior to transplantation in patients with acute nonlymphocytic leukemia.

▶ Howard J. Weinstein, Assistant Professor of Pediatrics, Harvard Medical School, and Associate Clinical Director of Pediatric Oncology, the Dana-Farber Cancer Institute, comments:

"The proper application of bone marrow transplantation (BMT) for acute leukemia has not been established fully. The best results at present are in children and young adults with acute nonlymphocytic leukemia (ANLL). For patients younger than age 20 years with ANLL given transplants when in first remission, multiple studies show that long-term leukemia-free survival is greater than 50%, with leukemic relapse rates less than 20% (Thomas et al.: *Cancer Treat. Rep.* 66:1463, 1982; and Dinsmore et al.: *Blood* 63:649, 1984). In this same group, intensive chemotherapy may be equally as effective and does not expose the patient to the risks of graft-versus-host disease (GVHD) or the long-term consequences of marrow-ablative doses of busulfan and irradiation (Weinstein et al. ibid. 62:315, 1983). Bone marrow transplantation appears to be more effective than chemotherapy in ANLL with respect to preventing leukemic relapse, but overall survival is affected adversely because of GVHD and interstitial pneumonia.

"Bone marrow transplantation is currently the only treatment that offers the potential for long-term survival for the patient with ANLL who has had a relapse. The projected 5-year leukemia-free survival for patients with ANLL given transplants when in early relapse or second remission is approximately 30%.

"Santos et al. have shown that busulfan may be as effective as total body irradiation in preparing the patient with ANLL for transplantation. Unfortunately, the most serious side effect associated with irradiation, interstitial pneumonia, was observed with equal frequency after busulfan preparation.

"Bone marrow transplantation plays an important but smaller role in childhood acute lymphoblastic leukemia (ALL). With current chemotherapy, about 30% of children with ALL have a relapse. Because of this high success rate, BMT has not been generally indicated for children with ALL during first remission. However, BMT is the treatment of choice for children with ALL who relapse on chemotherapy or shortly after elective cessation of therapy (within 6 months). Multiple studies show 30% to 50% survival for patients with ALL given transplants when in second or subsequent remission (Johnson et al.: *N. Engl. J. Med.* 305:846, 1981). Gale et al., in the preceding article, report that transplants in first or second remission for patients with ALL resulted in higher survival rates than transplants in later remissions or relapse. The Seattle team has not shown a survival advantage for earlier transplantation in ALL (second versus subsequent remission). For transplant candidates with ALL who lack a histocompatible sibling, autotransplantation with in vitro monoclonal antibody treatment of bone marrow is a promising experimental procedure (Ritz et al.: *Lancet* 2:60, 1982)."

Improved Survival in Infants and Children With Primary Malignant Liver Tumors
G. Hossein Mahour, G. Udo Wogu, Stuart E. Siegel, and Hart Isaacs
Am. J. Surg. 146:236–240, August 1983   10–12

In infants and children, malignant tumors of the liver are the third most common malignant intra-abdominal neoplasm, exceeded only by neuroblastoma and nephroblastoma. The records of children with primary liver tumors seen at Childrens Hospital of Los Angeles in 1952–1981 were reviewed.

Hepatoblastoma was found in 33 patients, hepatocellular carcinoma in 9, and sarcoma in 4. In the patients with hepatoblasoma (20 boys, 13 girls) there was a preponderance of boys (14 to 5) among those younger than age 18 months, but a preponderance of girls (8 to 6) among those older than age 18 months. Most patients had abdominal enlargement and an abdominal mass. Other symptoms included irritability, weight loss, fever, and gastrointestinal complaints. Jaundice was observed in 3 patients with hepatoblastoma and in 2 with hepatocellular carcinoma; 7 had associated diseases (Table 1). Serum cholesterol levels were determined in 10 patients with hepatoblastoma and were elevated in 5.

To evaluate results of therapy, 38 patients were divided into three groups. Group 1 included 18 patients with hepatoblastoma, 1 with hepatocellular carcinoma, 1 with leiomyosarcoma, and 1 with embryonal rhabdomyosarcoma. The tumor was unresectable in these patients and biopsy was done for diagnosis only; 12 patients received chemotherapy and 5 received both chemotherapy and radiation therapy. In none was the malignancy totally eradicated, and mean survival was only 7 months. Nine patients with hepatoblastoma and 1 with hepatocellular carcinoma made up group II; all underwent hepatic lobectomy and 5 received chemotherapy and 5 received combinations of chemotherapy and radiation therapy. Mean survival was 23 months and 3 are living without disease 2, 3, and 8 years later. Five patients with hepatoblastoma and 2 with sarcoma made up group III; 6 of these patients were diagnosed and treated after 1975. They presented with unresectable tumors, and after liver biopsy they were treated with chemotherapy alone (4 patients) or in combination with radiation therapy for 3–11 months before a "second-look" celiotomy was carried out. Tumor size was reduced significantly and delayed resection of the primary lesion was possible in 5 patients. Doxorubicin was one of the chemotherapeutic agents used after operation. One patient died 2.5 years after diagnosis and 5 live without disease 2.5–7 years after diagnosis. Survival data for patients treated after 1972 are greatly improved over those of an earlier period (Table 2).

Recent publications document successful chemotherapeutic responses with improved survival in patients who initially presented with unresectable hepatoblastomas. Chemotherapy after biopsy for initial cytoreduction may allow eventual resection of initially unresectable tumors with reduced operative and postoperative mortality. Chemotherapy is useful not only

TABLE 1.—ASSOCIATED DISEASES IN SEVEN PATIENTS WITH MALIGNANT LIVER TUMOR

Patient No. and Sex	Associated Disease	Age at Diagnosis of Associated Disease	Age at Diagnosis of Liver Tumor	Type of Liver Tumor
1, F	Beckwith's syndrome	9 mo	9 mo (liver biopsy)	EHB
2, M	Sexual precocity	18 mo	18 mo (liver biopsy)	EHB
3, M	de Toni-Fanconi syndrome	6 yr	8 yr (autopsy)	HCCa
4, M	Sotos' syndrome of cerebral gigantism	1 day	14 yr (autopsy)	HCCa
5, M ⎫ Twins	Biliary cirrhosis; hydrocephalus, mental retardation	10 mo	13.5 yr (autopsy)	HCCa
6, M ⎭	Biliary cirrhosis; hydrocephalus, mental retardation	10 mo	17.5 yr (autopsy)	HCCa
7, M	Glycogen storage disease	10 mo	29 yr (autopsy)	HCCa

EHB = epithelial hepatoblastoma; HCCa = hepatocellular carcinoma.
(Courtesy of Mahour, G.H., et al.: Am. J. Surg. 146:236–240, August 1983.)

TABLE 2.—SURVIVAL DATA FOR 36
PATIENTS TREATED FOR MALIGNANT LIVER
TUMORS

	1952–1971	1972–1981
Alive	0	10*
Dead	15	7
Lost to follow-up	4	2†
Total	19	19
Time of death	1 wk–	4 mo–
(after diagnosis)	18 mo	2.5 yr
Length of survival	5.5 mo	30 mo
(mean)		
Survival rate at 2 years	0	53%

*Two patients are presently alive with disease and 8 are
without disease.
†Both patients lost to follow-up with disease.
(Courtesy of Mahour, G.H., et al.: Am. J. Surg. 146:236–
240, August 1983.)

for eradicating pulmonary metastases but also for eliminating microscopic disease at the site of liver resection if continued after operation. Improved techniques in liver resection and chemotherapy before second-look celiotomy is undertaken for an unresectable lesion have improved the prognosis in children with a malignant liver tumor.

Limb Salvage Procedures for Children With Osteosarcoma: An Alternative to Amputation
B. N. Rao, J. E. Champion, C. B. Pratt, P. Carnesale, R. Dilawari, I. Fleming, A. Green, B. Austin, E. Wrenn, and M. Kumar (St. Jude Children's Res. Hosp., Memphis, Tenn.)
J. Pediatr. Surg. 18:901–908, December 1983   10–13

Eight young patients, aged 13–21, among 32 seen consecutively with osteosarcoma who were evaluated for limb salvage surgery, underwent successful operation with endoprosthetic reconstruction to bridge the segment of resected bone. Criteria for limb salvage include age of 12 years or older, low-grade tumor or a good response to preoperative chemotherapy, or both, and lack of clinical or angiographic evidence of neurovascular involvement. Two of the 8 patients had low-grade parosteal osteosarcoma. Five patients had a Tikhoff-Linberg procedure for an upper extremity lesion, 2 had en bloc resection of a distal femoral tumor, and 1 had a segmental arthrodesis for a distal tibial lesion. Multidrug chemotherapy was administered to all patients except the 2 with parosteal osteosarcoma.

Patients have been followed for a median of 16 months. One patient died at 18 months with pulmonary involvement, but no patient has had locally recurrent disease. Two patients had minor skin necrosis requiring revision. Three had transient nerve palsy. The functional results were excellent. Patients with upper limb lesions had full hand and finger motion and more than 75% of active elbow function at follow-up. Patients with a knee endoprosthesis also had satisfactory functional results. No patient had clinical or radiologic evidence of loosening of the endoprosthesis.

Limb-sparing operations can be carried out successfully in selected patients with osteosarcoma as an alternative to amputation. Endoprosthetic joint implants are effective in restoring osseous integrity after en bloc resection. Improvements in design and materials have enhanced their safety. The chief drawback at present is a protracted postoperative course with the need to restrict activity. Newer implants that use carbon or porous prosthetic designs may reduce this problem.

▶ Prior to the 1970s, the 5-year survival of patients with osteosarcoma was in the range of 15% to 20%. Since then, reports from many institutions have indicated a threefold to fourfold increase in disease-free survival. Whether this represents the beneficial use of chemotherapy, improved staging techniques, or a biologic change in behavior of the tumor remains unknown, but we like to think it is not the last. This improved survival has been reflected in the changing concepts of the surgical management of patients with primary and metastatic osteogenic sarcoma. Initially, the concepts included resection of the entire bone or disarticulation at the joint above the primary site. This has given way in most centers to the techniques described in this article. This is an attempt to salvage the limb by removing the tumor and its soft tissue extensions en block without actually amputating the extremity. The deficit left is then corrected either with prosthetic material or bone grafts. This approach cannot be used for all osteogenic sarcomas, but when it is an option it is one that should be entertained. The investigators at St. Jude's Children's Research Hospital, from whence this article derives, arbitrarily have chosen the age of 12 or older for consideration of patients undergoing limb salvage. In the upper extremity regions, these age limitations often can be waived. In the lower extremity, and especially for lesions around the knee, the age factor is of primary importance, as most children will have a secondary growth spurt during the teens. Some leg length discrepancy can be compensated for by corrective shoes, but if the operation is performed at a very young age, the discrepancy would be expected to be extremely marked. The recommendation from St. Jude's Children's Research Hospital is that limb salvage procedures for the lower extremities are best performed when a child has reached at least 75% of his or her skeletal maturity prior to the limb salvage procedure. This seems to make sense.—J.A.S., III

Prognosis of Children With Soft Tissue Sarcoma Who Relapse After Achieving a Complete Response: a Report From the Intergroup Rhabdomyosarcoma Study I

R. Beverly Raney, Jr., William M. Crist, Harold M. Maurer, and Mary A. Foulkes (Intergroup Rhabdomyosarcoma Study Committee)
Cancer 52:44–50, July 1, 1983   10–14

Of 423 children with newly diagnosed soft tissue sarcoma who were entered into an intergroup study in 1972–1976, 80.6% achieved a complete response, but 115 of these 341 patients (33.7%) subsequently relapsed. Patients with primary tumor in the perineum-anus region, the retroperitoneum-pelvis, the gastrointestinal tract, or an extremity had the highest relapse rates. Ninety-eight patients with relapse were followed up.

About half the patients relapsed with distant metastasis at a single anatomical site. The degree of compliance with chemotherapy did not differ between patients who relapsed and the others in the overall series, and patients with local and nonlocal recurrences complied similarly. Three of 16 patients who relapsed after the completion of chemotherapy remain alive, compared with only 2 of 74 who relapsed during treatment. A second complete response was achieved in 7 of 33 patients treated by surgery, radiotherapy, or chemotherapy alone. The use of two approaches led to a complete response in 12 of 37 cases, and the use of all three approaches produced a second complete response in 14 of 20 cases. In all, 37% of retreated patients had the complete disappearance of disease.

Patients who have recurrent soft tissue tumor after completely responding to treatment have only a 5% chance of long-term survival at present, regardless of further treatment. Multimodal retrieval therapy may, however, offer a chance of prolonged survival and occasional cure to children with recurrent soft tissue sarcoma. In patients at the highest risk of recurrence, reinfusion of autologous bone marrow after high-dose chemotherapy and sequential hemibody radiation is being studied currently.

▶ Perhaps the most difficult child with malignancy to take care of is the one who relapses with a soft tissue sarcoma after having responded initially to treatment. As the authors point out, despite the best of all therapies, only about 5% of such children are likely to survive on the long haul. This is such a poor result that other alternative therapies such as autologous bone marrow transplantation seem much more attractive than conventional chemotherapy, even though the results of this approach are not all that dramatic as yet.

Two other types of soft tissue sarcomas are now well defined to be associated with poor prognosis. If rhabdomyosarcoma initially presents with any evidence of bone marrow involvement, the outlook is ominous (*Cancer* 53:368, 1984) even though initial remissions may be achieved. Likewise, patients with Hodgkin's disease in whom sarcomas of bone and soft tissue subsequently develop are not likely to do well either (ibid., p. 232).

When initially evaluating a child for a soft tissue sarcoma, one must be as certain as possible concerning the cell of origin of the disease. Very frequently, such tumors present as small cell undifferentiated tumors of soft tissue that are histologically indistinguishable among several types. Such tumors often include metastatic Wilms' tumor, neuroblastoma, lymphoma, Ewing's sarcoma, and rhabdomyosarcoma. Even electron microscopy frequently will not sort out one cell type from another. These distinctions are fairly important because the chemotherapeutic approaches to some of these disorders vary significantly. Rhabdomyosarcoma is becoming somewhat more easily distinguished by virtue of the fact that antibodies now have been developed against myoglobin. Thus, a variety of immunologic techniques can be used to help distinguish this tumor. Also, one can culture, in vitro, cells from a malignancy.

Eventually, over a period of weeks, these cells may mature from undifferentiated forms to more differentiated cells that may contain neurofibrils (suggesting that the tumor was a neuroblastoma) or myofibrils (suggesting that the tumor was a rhabdomyosarcoma).

While the overall management of the patient with newly diagnosed soft tissue sarcoma is now fairly well worked out and does not achieve reasonable response rates, we have a long way to go for the child who relapses.—J.A.S., III

Brain Metastases in Children

Francesc Graus, Russell W. Walker, and Jeffrey C. Allen (Meml. Sloan-Kettering Cancer Center, New York)

J. Pediatr. 103:558–561, October, 1983   10–15

A review of the records of the 139 children aged 21 years or younger with solid tumors in whom complete postmortem examinations were done during 1973 to 1982 revealed 18 (13%) with brain metastases. An additional 13 children with brain metastases were identified by a review of the computed tomography files over the past 4½ years.

The incidence of brain metastases was highest in children with germ cell tumor (table). Evidence of intratumoral hemorrhage was found in 50% of the autopsy cases. Pulmonary metastases were present in 28 of the 31 children (90%), and the median interval between diagnosis of lung and of brain metastases was 10 months, with a range of 0 to 60 months. No patient had evidence of brain metastases at diagnosis of the systemic cancer. In only 1 patient was the brain the only site of relapse.

Neurologic symptoms referable to brain metastases were found in 25 of the 31 patients; the other 6 had subclinical metastatic lesions discovered after death. Headache or signs of increased intracranial pressure were seen

INCIDENCE OF BRAIN METASTASIS OF SOLID MALIGNANT TUMORS EXAMINED POSTMORTEM

	Age ≤15 years			Age ≤21 years		
	Patients	*Brain metastases*		*Patients*	*Brain metastases*	
	n	*n*	*%*	*n*	*n*	*%*
Neuroblastoma	37	0	0.0	39	0	
Osteogenic sarcoma	28	4	14.3	38	5	13.5
Rhabdomyosarcoma	15	2	13.3	21	3	14.3
Ewing sarcoma	6	0	0.0	12	2	16.6
Germ cell tumor	2	1	50.0	8	4	50.0
Other	14	3	21.6	21	4*	19
Total	102	10	9.8	139	18	12.9

*Malignant schwannoma (2 patients), melanoma (1), angiosarcoma (1).
(Courtesy of Graus, F., et al.: J. Pediatr. 103:558–561, October 1983.)

in 52% of the patients, seizure in 36% (more frequently in younger children and those with germ cell tumors), and hemiparesis in 36%.

After detection of brain metastases, the median survival was 7 months in the 6 patients who underwent operation and whole brain radiation therapy (3,000 rad in 10 days) and 4 months in the 15 given radiotherapy without surgery but usually with chemotherapy. However, death was due to neurologic disease in only 4 of these 15 (27%), and of the 5 who showed a complete response to radiotherapy, none died of recurrent brain disease.

Surgery is probably indicated in patients with sarcomas who have single brain metastasis, provided they are good operative risks and have relatively long life expectancies. Higher doses of radiation therapy or the concomitant use of chemotherapy may be useful in patients with radioresistant tumors who are not candidates for surgery.

Retinoblastoma Treated in Infants in the First Six Months of Life
David H. Abramson, Robyn B. Notterman, Robert M. Ellsworth, and F. David Kitchin (New York Hosp.-Cornell Med. Center)
Arch. Ophthalmol. 101:1362–1366, September 1983   10–16

The data on 158 children in whom retinoblastoma was diagnosed and treated in the first 6 months of life, and who were then followed for a mean of 7½ years were reviewed. The mean age at diagnosis was 3½ months. About one fifth of patients had a family history of retinoblastoma. The chief complaints are shown in Figure 10–5. Fifty-one patients presented with unilateral retinoblastoma; 10 of them later developed a tumor in the fellow eye. Most unilaterally affected patients were managed by enucleation and most of the rest by irradiation. Most of those with bilateral involvement had both eyes enucleated and received irradiation. Half of the 138 treated eyes were enucleated.

Among 157 eyes that were irradiated, only 1 of the 33 requiring enucleation was lost because of complications of irradiation. In the unilateral cases that converted to bilateral retinoblastoma, disease in 6 of the second eyes was diagnosed at an earlier stage than that in the first eye. Second nonocular tumors developed in 8% of the patients. Twenty-three children died, 10 of metastatic retinoblastoma and 8 of second tumors. Nineteen of the patients who died were initially in Reese-Ellsworth stage V.

Diagnosis of retinoblastoma in the first 6 months of life does not insure that early disease is present. More than two thirds of the present infants had bilateral disease at presentation. Several patients died of metastatic retinoblastoma. The overall success of treatment was surprisingly poor, although overall patient survival was good. One fifth of infants presenting with unilateral retinoblastoma subsequently developed tumor in the fellow eye.

Homozygosity of Chromosome 13 in Retinoblastoma
Thaddeus P. Dryja, Webster Cavenee, Raymond White, Joyce M. Rapaport,

Robert Petersen, Daniel M. Albert, and Gail A. P. Bruns
N. Engl. J. Med. 310:550–553, Mar. 1, 1984   10–17

About 40% of patients with retinoblastoma can transmit the disease via a locus or loci on the long arm of chromosome 13 within band 13q14. The frequency of chromosome 13 homozygosity was determined in tumor tissue obtained from the eyes of 8 consecutive patients undergoing enucleation for retinoblastoma. The alleles determined by the enzyme esterase D, whose locus is on 13q14, and those identified by a set of cloned DNA fragments homologous to loci on chromosome 13 that reveal restriction-fragment-length polymorphisms were examined.

There was evidence for homozygosity of all or part of 13q in half the tumors examined. The homozygosity occurred in vivo, not as an event

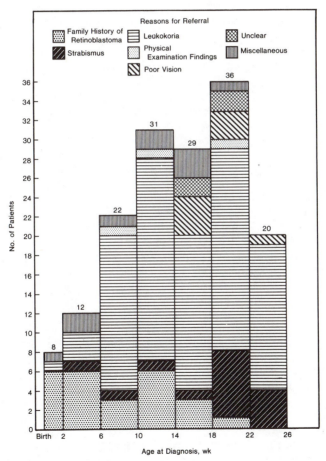

Fig 10–5.—Bar graph demonstrating age at diagnosis and reason for referral of infants with retinoblastoma in first 6 months of life. (Courtesy of Abramson, D.H., et al.: Arch. Ophthalmol. 101:1362–1366, September 1983; copyright 1983, American Medical Association.)

secondary to tumor cell culture. It did not correlate with the degree of histopathologic differentiation of the tumor. Homozygosity was associated with both sporadic and hereditary retinoblastomas. Three of the patients had unifocal and 5 had multifocal tumors; none had a family history of retinoblastoma.

The development of chromosome 13 homozygosity may represent a fundamental event in the oncogenesis of a considerable number of retinoblastomas. Homozygosity has occurred in tumors from patients with either multifocal (hereditary) or unifocal (presumably sporadic) disease. The findings may help explain variations in the penetrance of the retinoblastoma allele in different kindreds. It might be possible to predict which future family members are at risk in cases of hereditary retinoblastoma. If the tumor has lost the alleles present in one chromosome 13 homologue, it can be assumed that the chromosome 13 remaining in the tumor is the one harboring the mutant allele.

▶ Retinoblastoma is a malignant tumor arising in the eyes of newborns and young children. Approximately 10% of patients with retinoblastoma have a family history of the disease, and another 30% have multifocal disease and a negative family history. Both of these groups, or approximately 40% of patients with retinoblastoma, are capable of transmitting the disease to their offspring. This hereditary tendency is now known to be governed by a locus or loci on the long arm of chromosome 13. Although the hereditary pattern in familial retinoblastoma is that of an autosomal dominant mutation, there is evidence that the defect at the tissue level is recessive. This study seems to show this fact. All somatic cells, including the retinal cells, of a person who has the inherited form of the disease carry the tumor-predisposing allele. The malignant transformation of only a few retinal cells in such a person may be determined by some secondary event that may involve loss of the normal allele opposing the retinoblastoma locus, which would result in homozygosity for the abnormal allele, thus resulting in disease. A small percentage of patients with hereditary retinoblastoma have associated constitutional deletion of portions of chromosome 13. In such persons, a marker of this process may be found by examining the level of activity of an enzyme known as esterase D. This is an enzyme whose activity is expressed in all human tissues but whose biologic function is unknown. The gene that controls this enzyme is most likely located exactly at the site of the retinoblastoma gene or very close to it because deletion of portions of chromosome 13 that result in retinoblastoma results in a decreased level of activity of esterase D in all cells of the body, including that of red blood cells.

To make this story as simple as possible, retinoblastoma occurs in hereditary, nonhereditary, and chromosomal deletion forms. Hereditary retinoblastoma usually refers to the clinical situation in which there is a positive family history of tumor or in a case of what seems like sporadic disease but the patient has both eyes involved. No chromosomal abnormalities are present on routine karyotyping of peripheral blood. The nonhereditary form of retinoblastoma is diagnosed in persons with unilateral disease, no family history of the tumor, and no abnormality on karyotyping of peripheral blood lymphocytes (one must be cautious in this latter group, because a small percentage of these apparently sporadic cases ultimately are determined to be hereditary). The third type of retinoblastoma is the one in which peripheral blood lymphocytes can be demonstrated to have a deletion of chromosome region 13q14, and these are the cases with low esterase D activity.

After looking over this commentary, it strikes me as being a bit like a telephone book, full of facts but not containing a single, useful idea. I think it will take a little while before all the new information concerning retinoblastoma is able to be translated into practical implications that we can begin to deal with. If you would like to read a review of the diagnosis and management of retinoblastoma, see the article by D. Abramson (*CA* 32:31, 1982). Not much has changed in the past 2½ years in this regard.—J.A.S., III

Genital Clear Cell Adenocarcinoma
George A. Johnston, Jr., and Harvey A. Jones
Int. Surg. 68:257–261, July–Aug.–Sept. 1983   10–18

Genital clear cell adenocarcinoma in young women is rare and has been related to in utero exposure to diethylstilbestrol (DES). The authors analyzed data on 57 patients with genital clear cell adenocarcinoma derived from the Diethylstilbestrol Registry reported from California, the most populous state in the United States. The patients, aged 13–31 (mean, 19 years), were born between 1944 and 1965, most between 1948 and 1954. Thirty-three (57.9%) patients had a positive history of DES exposure with widely varying doses. Another 7 (12.3%) were exposed to DES and progesterone, and 1 (1.7%) was given a steroid estrogen with progesterone. In 9 patients, medications were prescribed for high-risk pregnancy, but the exact drugs could not be identified. Five patients had totally negative histories of prenatal hormone exposure. Thirty-two patients (56%) had stage I disease, 22 (38%) had stage II disease, and only 3 (6%) had stage III or stage IV disease. Although highly individualized, treatment was primarily surgical; 39 patients had radical pelvic surgery and 7 others with small, early-stage lesions had less than radical surgery. Primary exenterative surgical procedures were performed in 5 patients, and 3 underwent combined radiation and radical surgery. Radiation was used as primary or adjuvant therapy in 11 patients. Of 7 patients lost to follow-up, all but 1 was lost after 4 years of negative follow-up findings. Thirty-one patients are alive without disease since treatment. Six had recurrence, but became free of disease after further treatment. Twelve patients died of the disease, and 1 patient is living with the disease 10 years after the initial diagnosis. Of the 12 patients who died of the disease, 3 were older than age 19 years and only 1 was younger than age 15.

The upper anterior vaginal wall is the most common location for vaginal clear cell adenocarcinoma, although it may occur in other locations. A four-quadrant Papanicolaou smear is advised for those exposed to DES in utero. Patients with genital clear cell carcinoma usually have histories of bleeding after menarche. A bleeding history in a premenarchal patient exposed to DES warrants aggressive investigation. Colposcopy is useful in the evaluation of epithelial lesions of the vagina and cervix.

Teratomas in Infancy and Childhood: A 54-Year Experience at Children's Hospital Medical Center

David Tapper and Ernest E. Lack (Harvard Med. School)
Ann. Surg. 198:398–410, September 1983   10–19

The clinical and pathologic features of 254 teratomas in 245 patients younger than age 22 years treated between 1928 and 1982 were reviewed. A teratoma is a neoplasm containing at least two germ-layer derivatives typically foreign to the anatomical site of origin that, on initial resection or biopsy, contain no frankly malignant elements such as embryonal carcinoma.

Teratomas usually appear as mass lesions with signs or symptoms ascribable to a specific location and consequent impingement upon or compression of adjacent organs or tissues (Fig 10–6). Most were located in the sacrococcygeal area (40%) or ovary (37%), and 49% were detected during the newborn period. Immature teratomas were significantly larger than mature tumors in most sites.

Up-to-date follow-up data were available for 215 of the 245 patients. There were 21 tumor-related deaths (9%). Central nervous system tumors

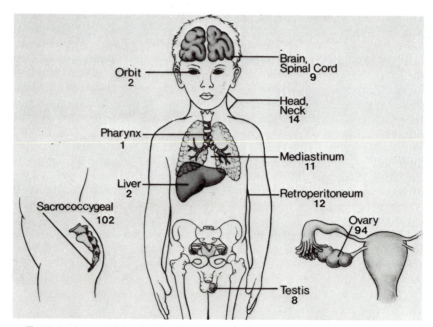

Fig 10–6.—Anatomical site of origin of the teratomas. The most common site was the sacrococcygeal area, followed by ovary, head and neck, retroperitoneum, mediastinum, testes, and central nervous system. (Courtesy of Tapper, D., and Lack, E.E.: Ann. Surg. 198:398–410, September 1983.)

involved the highest fatality rate (66%), regardless of histologic maturity or immaturity, thus reflecting the technical difficulties of complete surgical resection; patients with immature ovarian tumors had the next highest (38%). The overall mortality was significantly lower for patients with mature than for those with immature tumors. The single most important factor affecting prognosis was whether the tumor could be resected completely at initial surgery. Regardless of other treatments used, no patient survived who did not undergo surgery or in whom only partial resection was possible.

Every effort should be made to excise a teratoma completely, including possible use of cardiopulmonary bypass for large mediastinal tumors, adjunctive irradiation and chemotherapy to shrink CNS or retroperitoneal tumors and enhance resectability, and careful staging of the peritoneal surfaces of ovarian teratomas to rule out concomitant intra-abdominal disease. Assessment of tumor age and site is important in establishing a reliable prognostic profile, as are accurate determination of histologic grade, adequacy of resection, and the presence or absence of unfavorable histologic elements such as embryonal carcinoma. Tumors containing frankly malignant elements should be separated for the purpose of planning therapy and analyzing survival data. Routine adjuvant therapy may be useful for immature teratomas of the ovary. Similar teratomas in other sites must be evaluated on an individual basis, particularly in infancy. Finally, long-term follow-up is recommended for all patients, particularly those with immature teratomas.

▶ Quiz: Name the derivation of the word "teratoma."

Answer: "Teratoma" is derived from the Greek word "teratos," which literally means "monster." As such, this denotes the disturbed or malformed growth and appearance of these tumors. Throughout the earliest of times, children with such tumors seemed to be looked on as strange and fearsome individuals, as may be noted in the earliest record of a sacrococcygeal teratoma inscribed on a Babylonian cuneiform tablet dated approximately 600 BC. Teratomas are neoplasms composed of tissue elements foreign to the organ or anatomical site of origin. In children, these tumors are notable for their diversity in location and biologic behavior.

As Tapper and Lack conclude, complete surgical resection is, without question, the treatment of choice for all childhood teratomas. Furthermore, this is one of the few childhood tumors where decisions regarding adjuvant therapy must be highly individualized, particularly with regard to the site of origin and the age of the patient being treated. Surgeons tend to be extremely dogmatic in this regard and somewhat lacking in diplomacy when dealing with nonsurgeon types in discussions of this tumor. They are probably correct in this approach, even though the usual definition of surgical diplomacy means saying "nice doggy" just long enough to find a large rock.—J.A.S., III

11 Endocrinology

Method for Earlier Recognition of Abnormal Stature
A. Aynsley Green and J. A. MacFarlane (John Radcliffe Hosp., Oxford, England)
Arch. Dis. Child. 58:535–537, July 1983   11–1

The referral of children with potentially treatable abnormal growth is usually late. Because of the importance of early detection of abnormal growth, the referral age of 227 consecutive children whose height was below the third percentile or above the 97th percentile was reviewed.

More boys (126) than girls (72) were referred for short stature, whereas more girls (16) than boys (13) were referred for tall stature. Of the referrals for short stature, 45% were for children with genetic short stature. The mean age of referral for these children was 12 years (mode, 13–14 years); 36% were older than age 12 years and were experiencing psychologic difficulties related to size and the uncertainty of their final height. There was an organic reason for growth retardation in 40% of the short children, including hypothyroidism, Turner's syndrome, and growth hormone (GH) deficiency in 22%. Eighteen with hypothyroidism were referred at a mean age of 9 years (range, 3–14 years); 15 with Turner's syndrome were referred at a mean age of 12 years (range, 3–16 years); and 11 with idiopathic GH deficiency were referred at a mean age of 7 years (range, 4–11 years). Other organic causes of growth retardation included celiac disease, psychosocial deprivation, Russell Silver syndrome, dysmorphic short stature, pseudohypoparathyroidism, and hypogonadism. The mean age of patients referred because of tall stature was 13 years (range, 3–18 years). Pathologic conditions among the girls included Marfan's syndrome, unrecognized congenital adrenal hyperplasia, and thyrotoxicosis. Among the boys, all had "constitutional" tall stature, except for 3 who had XYY syndrome.

Possible reasons for delay in the referral of children with growth abnormalities include lack of appropriate measuring equipment in many practices, limited availability of appropriate percentile charts, noninclusion of routine height measurement during medical examinations at entry into school, and lack of awareness by family practitioners of recent advances in the treatment of abnormal growth. A child whose height falls between the third percentile and the − 3 SD limit, or between the 97th percentile and the + 3 SD limit, on a growth screening wall chart devised for children aged 2–9 years (Fig 11–1) should be considered for referral. This consideration should include midparental height correction using the appropriate Tanner and Whitehouse chart.

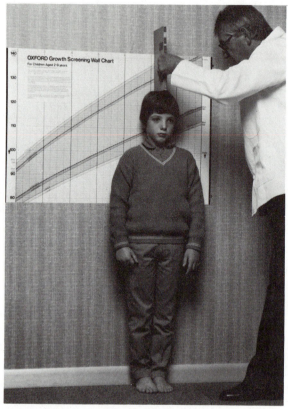

Fig 11–1.—Growth chart designed for children aged 2–9 years. The chart, printed on laminated paper, can be fixed to a wall or door at a specified height from the floor. (Courtesy of Green, A.A., and MacFarlane, J.A.: Arch. Dis. Child. 58:535–537, July 1983.)

Prospective Clinical Trial of Human Growth Hormone in Short Children Without Growth Hormone Deficiency

J. M. Gertner, M. Genel, S. P. Gianfredi, R. L. Hintz, R. G. Rosenfeld, W. V. Tamborlane, and D. M. Wilson

J. Pediatr. 104:172–176, February 1984   11–2

Rudman et al. found that some short children who are growing slowly respond well to human growth hormone (hGH) treatment, but the relation between responsiveness to hGH and the generation of insulin-like growth factor I (IGF I) is unclear. As a result, Gertner et al. examined the effects of human hGH administration over 6 months in 10 unselected, apparently healthy, prepuberal children who were more than 2.5 SD below mean height for age, but had normal growth hormone secretion on standard provocative testing. The children, aged 4½ to 11 years at the outset, had no disease or dysmorphic syndrome associated with growth failure. Intramuscular injections of 0.1 unit of hGH per kg were given three times weekly.

The mean pretreatment growth velocity was 4.3 cm per year, at the lower end of the normal range (Fig 11–2). Skeletal maturation was slightly to moderately delayed in all subjects. Treatment with hGH led to an increased growth rate in all patients, and the mean growth velocity after 6 months was 7.4 cm per year. Growth velocity subsequently slowed to 3.7 cm per year. The effect of treatment was not related to the baseline growth velocity. Concentrations of IGF I were in the low-normal range for age initially and increased twofold after four daily hormone injections. Baseline IGF II concentrations tended to be lower than in normal adults and rose significantly after short-term hGH administration. Growth velocity could not be related to either baseline IGF values or IGF responses to short-term hGH administration. Treatment was well tolerated; no adverse effects were observed. Glucose tolerance did not deteriorate, and spontaneous nocturnal growth hormone secretion was not altered by hGH therapy. The 1 child who developed antibody nevertheless had an increase in growth velocity.

The findings suggest that most unselected short children may initially respond to hGH therapy, but much longer-term studies are needed to determine the effect of such treatment on final adult stature. Measurements of IGF cannot be used to predict which children will respond to hGH administration.

▶ The prospective availability of large supplies of human growth hormone produced in bacteria by recombinant DNA techniques has rekindled interest in the

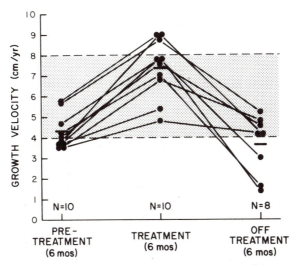

Fig 11–2.—Growth velocities before, during, and after hGH therapy. Stippled area indicates normal range for growth velocity in boys aged 8 to 10 years; from Tanner, J.M., and Whitehouse, R.H.: Longitudinal standards for height, weight, height velocity, weight velocity and stages of puberty, Arch. Dis. Child. 51:170, 1976. (Courtesy of Gertner, J.M., et al.: J. Pediatr. 104:172–176, February 1984.)

potential usefulness of this agent in short children who are not growth hormone deficient. Thus, you will be seeing more articles such as this one and the preceding one. The study of Greene et al. demonstrates that, at least in Great Britain, many short children are not recognized as being short and that our offices should be better equipped to chart the heights of the patients that we follow for routine visits. The type of chart depicted indeed is a very useful one in quickly assessing whether a child is in the normal percentile ranges.

The article of Gertner et al. followed by only a few months virtually identical data presented by Van Vliet (*N. Engl. J. Med.* 309:1016, 1983). Both studies showed that a remarkable number of short children who have normal levels of their own growth hormone would respond to exogenous growth hormone. Almost 4 years ago, Rudman et al. (ibid. 305:123, 1981) demonstrated the same finding and suggested that such patients could be selected by the presence of low plasma levels of somatomedin C concentrations. Neither the study of Gertner et al. nor Van Vliet found any good correlation with somatomedin C levels and the response to human growth hormone. All of these studies have widely opened the door now to the potential abuses of human growth hormone made available by recombinant DNA technology. If you are thinking about using growth hormone or referring a patient for its use, you may wish to read the "Ad Hoc Committee on Growth Hormone Usage, the Lawson Wilkins Pediatric Endocrine Society and Committee on Drugs" report that appeared in *Pediatrics* (72:891, 1983). This is an extremely thoughtful review that provides guidelines for what seems to be a very logical set of criteria for administration of growth hormone.

It should be said up front that growth failure due to growth hormone deficiency is the only universally accepted therapeutic indication for growth hormone treatment. However, for every short child who has growth hormone deficiency, there are scores of children who are short for other reasons. Many of these other reasons would not be expected to respond to growth hormone administration. The Ad Hoc Committee suggests that Down's syndrome, Silver-Russell syndrome, Seckel's syndrome, progeria, genetic abnormalities of cartilage and bone such as achondroplasia, or metabolic derangements associated with cardiac, renal disease, and gastrointestinal diseases would not respond to growth hormone therapy. One cannot be too definitive in this regard, however. N. Stahnke (*N. Engl. J. Med.* 310:925, 1984) did show that one patient with Silver-Russell syndrome responded to growth hormone administration. One group that clearly might benefit are children with Turner's syndrome. Some will respond and some will not respond to growth hormone therapy, but a try should at least be given if it seems indicated. The greatest number of short children in whom a study of the efficacy of growth hormone seems appropriate are those with familial short stature and constitutional growth delay. It seems probable that injections of growth hormone will promote growth in at least some of these children. There is no certainty that long-term therapy will make these children taller in the long run as adults, however. Also, there are small numbers of children who secrete normal amounts of immunoreactive growth hormone in response to provocative stimuli but who produce defective forms of growth hormone that are biologically inactive. These children, too, might profit from growth hormone administration. All these situations must be weighed against the possible effects of growth hormone therapy. The limited amounts of growth hormone that have been available for persons with true growth hormone deficiency have not resulted in any untoward side effects. One cannot predict what the increased availability of the new growth hormone products might do to the side effects that could be expected from growth hormone. Growth hormone does increase insulin resistance and can impair glucose tolerance. It also can cause hypertension, which is common in acromegalic patients.

The Ad Hoc Committee made four conclusions in their report. It is worthwhile to summarize these here:

1. Replacement of growth hormone in growth hormone-deficient children is the only established indication for growth hormone therapy. Treatment of all non-growth hormone-deficient patients must be considered experimental.

2. There is a pressing need for carefully controlled trials of effective growth hormone in patients with constitutional growth delay, intrauterine growth retardation, and Turner's syndrome.

3. Research is needed to develop reliable methods for predicting which short, non-growth hormone-deficient children will respond to growth hormone therapy.

4. Growth hormone is a potent metabolic agent and its safety when used in pharmacologic doses for the treatment of short, non-growth hormone-deficient children has not been established.

It is difficult to top the concluding sentence of the Ad Hoc Committee's report. It ends, "In selecting patients for growth hormone trials, the wise physician might adhere to the old adage, 'If it ain't broke, don't fix it.' " I would add a classier conclusion, which would be that of Voltaire, who said, "Every man must row with the oars that one has."

(If you are interested in reading about recombinant DNA and endocrine therapy in children, see the excellent review of Kappy et al. [*Am. J. Dis. Child.* 137:685, 1983].)—J.A.S., III

Evolving Hypopituitarism in Children With Central Nervous System Lesions

Cheryl E. Hanna and Stephen H. LaFranchi (Oregon Health Sciences Univ., Portland)
Pediatrics 72:65–70, July 1983   11–3

When children with suspected hypopituitarism are observed to have a subnormal growth rate, it is expected that testing will reveal human growth hormone (hGH) deficiency. Follow-up data are reported on 7 patients with organic lesions of the CNS known to be associated with hypopituitarism whose initial tests showed an adequate hGH response (greater than 7 ng/ml).

Three of the children had histiocytosis X, 1 had septo-optic dysplasia, 1 had neonatal meningitis, 1 had neurofibromatosis, and 1 had an anterior encephalocele and meningitis. When the growth rate remained subnormal or as in 1 patient became subnormal, the patients were retested for hGH deficiency. Retesting 0.5 to 4.6 years after initial evaluation showed an abnormal hGH response, as well as other pituitary hormone deficiencies. Two patients required a third test before hGH deficiency was demonstrated. Significantly delayed bone ages were observed in 6 of the 7 patients at the time hGH deficiency was documented. Five patients showed evidence of other pituitary hormone deficiencies prior to documentation of hGH deficiency, and 1 developed diabetes insipidus after hGH deficiency was demonstrated.

The mechanism for the evolving hypopituitarism in these patients is not known, but the initial subnormal growth rate may have been the result of the underlying CNS lesion or its treatment or may have involved the production of biologically inactive hGH or inadequate production of somatomedin. The findings indicate the need for careful follow-up and retesting of patients with CNS lesions and growth retardation, even if previous hGH tests have been normal.

Evaluation of Growth Hormone Release and Human Growth Hormone Treatment in Children With Cranial Irradiation-Associated Short Stature
Carolyn A. Romshe, William B. Zipf, Angela Miser, James Miser, Juan F. Sotos, and William A. Newton (Ohio State Univ.)
J. Pediatr. 104:177–181, February 1984   11–4

Subnormal growth has been described in children given cranial radiotherapy for CNS tumor or acute leukemia. Responses to growth hormone (GH) stimulation and release tests were studied in 9 children given cranial irradiation for malignancy who had decreased growth velocity subsequently, 7 children with classic GH deficiency, and 24 short but otherwise normal children whose mean height was 3.3 SD below the mean for their ages. The irradiated patients had received at least 1,500 rad to the CNS 2 years or more previously and had since grown at a rate of less than 4 cm per year. None was receiving chemotherapy at the time of the study. The most common diagnosis was acute lymphoblastic leukemia. Mean age at radiotherapy was 5½ years. All subjects were euthyroid for at least 6 months before evaluation.

Six of the 9 irradiated patients had normal GH responses to arginine and L-dopa stimulation. Only 2, however, responded normally to insulin-induced hypoglycemia, and mean peak responses were similar in the irradiated and GH-deficient groups. Pulsatile GH secretion was comparable in these groups, but differed significantly between the irradiated patients and the normal subjects. Growth velocity increased during a year of standard human growth hormone (hGH) therapy in all irradiated patients and all those in the GH-deficient group. Growth responses were comparable in these two groups.

Children with decreased growth velocity after cranial irradiation can grow more rapidly when given hGH. Present GH stimulation and release tests cannot consistently indicate which children will benefit from hGH therapy, and a 6-month trial of treatment should be considered in children who are not growing at a normal rate if they have been in prolonged remission from the primary malignancy and have no other apparent cause of growth arrest. Further follow-up will be required to determine whether the response to hGH therapy is sustained.

▶ This article and the preceding one highlight a problem of which all of us should be aware. This is the potential for growth retardation in children who either have had CNS lesions or have received cranial irradiation as part of the management of some malignant process. The data suggest that children who have received cranial irradiation resulting in subsequently decreased growth velocity and who are below normal height do achieve normalization of growth with human growth hormone therapy. These studies confirm and extend previous work in this area. Many investigators have found subnormal growth and growth hormone deficiency in children who have received cranial irradiation. These studies suggest that the loss of growth hormone secretion appears to be variably dependent on the age of the child at the time of irradiation (younger children may be more susceptible than adults), the dose of irradiation received, and other unknown individual characteristics. The site of the damage appears to be limited to the hypothalamus when doses of radiation are between 2,400 and 4,000 rad, but may involve both the pituitary gland and hypothalamus when more than 4,000 rad is delivered. The usual dose given to children with acute lymphatic leukemia is 2,400 rad. This dose may be given more than once if CNS relapse has occurred. What all this means is that because most of the children receive damage that may affect only the hypothalamus, the pituitary gland may be spared. This would result in releasable pituitary stores of growth hormone if tests for growth hormone release are used that act simply at the pituitary level. This can result in "functional" growth hormone deficiency despite the retention of the ability of the child to show a "normal" growth hormone response to stimulation. Theoretically, the use of only those tests for growth hormone release that require normal hypothalamic function should be diagnostic in these instances.

I have great difficulty in trying to remember which of the tests for growth hormone release act in which manner. In this regard, I seem always to have both feet firmly planted in the air. There are so many tests available now to detect growth hormone deficiency that you need a catalog to keep all of them in order. Most endocrinologists still seem to feel that spontaneous growth hormone release and insulin-induced hypoglycemia-associated growth hormone release may be mediated through the hypothalamic area, thus providing the · best test of the integrity of the hypothalamic-pituitary axis. Arginine-mediated growth hormone release seems to be mediated through the pituitary directly. Glucagon-mediated growth hormone release may be through effects on both the hypothalamus and the pituitary. L-Dopa infusion has inconsistent effects on growth hormone release in different animal species, and therefore its mechanism of action is less well understood. Suffice it to say, no one understands what effects irradiation of the hypothalamus has on L-dopa-induced growth hormone release. In the study by Romshe et al., an increased frequency of abnormal growth hormone responses to insulin-induced hypoglycemia, as compared with the arginine test, tends to support the concept that the damage is isolated to the hypothalamus, while the pituitary has growth hormone that is capable of being released under challenge but not under normal physiologic states that require an intact hypothalamic-pituitary axis.

Most children who have idiopathic growth hormone deficiency are thought to have defects in the hypothalamus resulting in a lack of growth hormone-releasing factor synthesis or secretion. Such a hypothesis could not be tested until recently, when there was reported the isolation and characterization of a growth hormone-releasing peptide from a pancreatic tumor in a patient with acromegaly (*Science* 218:585, 1982). This releasing hormone now allows us to classify patients with growth hormone deficiency into two subgroups according to their plasma growth hormone responses to this releasing substance. In one subgroup, there is no increase in growth hormone (type 1), and in the other (type 2) there is a subnormal but definite increase in growth hormone levels. The former represents pituitary abnormalities, whereas the other suggests hypothalamic disorder. Patients with hypothalamic disorders occasionally may show diminished responses to releasing hormone because there may have been little prior stimulation of pituitary growth hormone. Therefore, several days of administration of releasing factor may be necessary to demonstrate whether or not the pituitary is capable of producing growth hormone. We should be seeing much more written about this growth hormone-releasing factor in the near future. In the meantime, highly touted now as a better test for growth hormone deficiency than insulin or arginine is the agent clonidine. Clonidine is an α-adrenergic drug that directly stimulates growth hormone release (Fraser, N. C., et al.: *Arch. Dis. Child.* 58:355, 1983). Clonidine acts directly on central nervous system α-adrenergic receptors and appears to be a safe, reliable, and sensitive agent for testing growth hormone reserve. The drug is given by mouth, and growth hormone levels are checked 1 hour later. The real beauty of this test is that it can be done as a simple outpatient screening test. It seems to have very little side effects except for mild drowsiness and a slight decrease in systolic blood pressure. A head-to-head comparison of clonidine versus insulin-induced hypoglycemia showed it to be quite comparable and, in fact, more sensitive than L-dopa or arginine (Slover, R. H., et al.: *Am. J. Dis. Child.* 1984).

There always remains the possibility that a normal growth hormone response may not exclude treatable hormone deficiency. Immunologically reactive growth hormone may be biologically inert or the occasional patient may respond to pharmacologic stimulation but fail to release growth hormone physiologically. It has been suggested that children with psychosocial growth retardation may fall into this latter category. In any event, the ultimate proof of growth hormone deficiency is the response of the patient to replacement therapy. Children who have had prior CNS lesions or who have received irradiation and who are growing at a subnormal rate without other explanation deserve a trial of growth hormone even if the growth hormone test suggests that they are able to produce this substance. This appears to be the only definitive way of settling the issue in some circumstances. It may be a bit expensive, but in the long run it is well worth the effort.—J.A.S., III

Thyroid Abnormalities in Patients Previously Treated With Irradiation for Acne Vulgaris

Douglas B. Thomson, Charles F. Grammes, Ralph H. Starkey, Ronald P. Monsaert, and Frederick S. Sunderlin (Danville, Pa.)

South. Med. J. 77:21–23, January 1984   11–5

Despite the known association between thyroid cancer and previous head and neck radiation, cancer rarely has been reported in patients treated in adolescence for acne. An attempt was made to recall 1,203 patients irradiated for acne in 1940–1968 and 302 subjects were examined. Standard dermatologic orthovoltage therapy had been used. Generally 100 R of 100-kV therapy was delivered at each session, using lead-rubber and cones as shielding. The 203 women and 99 men examined had a mean age at initial treatment of 21 years and a mean age at follow-up of 43 years. The mean exposure was 692 R, and the range was 20–2,000 R.

The 8 patients with nodular disease included 2 with carcinoma, 2 with multinodular goiter, 2 with benign adenomas, 1 with lymphocytic thyroiditis, and 1 with a "warm" nodule that is under observation. Another patient had Graves' disease, and 1 had primary hypothyroidism. Half the cases of benign nodular disease were detected by the patients' physicians. A woman aged 38 who had received 940 R at age 16 years had papillary and follicular cancers in separate nodules. A woman aged 45 who had received 1,350 R at age 18 had papillary cancer in a single nodule. The prevalence of carcinoma was 660 per 100,000.

Reported clinical surveys suggest a linear relationship between the radiation dose to the thyroid and the risk of subsequent thyroid cancer

SUMMARY OF REPORTED SERIES: PATIENTS EXAMINED FOR
THYROID DISEASE AFTER IRRADIATION

Area Treated	Estimated Dose to Thyroid (Rads)	Prevalence Nodular Goiter	Cancer	Reference
Scalp	6.5	—	0.1	Modan et al, 1977
Thymus				
Total group	119	1.8	0.8	Hempelmann et al, 1975
Subgroup*	399	7.6	5.0	
Neck	807	27.2	5.7	Favus et al, 1976
Chest	180–1,500	26.2	6.8	Refetoff et al, 1975
Radiation	317 (Age <10 yr at exposure)	24.0	2.3	Conrad, 1977
Fallout	139 (Age >10 yr at exposure)	12.2	3.5	
^{131}I Therapy	10,000	0.17	0.08	Dobyns et al, 1974

*Patients in this subgroup were treated by one radiologist with high doses administered through large ports, including the thyroid gland in the primary x-ray beam.

(Courtesy of Thomson, D.B., et al.: South. Med. J. 77:21–23, January 1984.)

(table), as do animal studies. The present survey is the largest known recall study of acne patients given radiotherapy. The prevalence of nodular disease was within the expected range, but that of thyroid cancer was unexpectedly high, suggesting an increased risk of thyroid cancer in patients previously irradiated for acne. Such patients should be followed up to detect thyroid cancer should it develop.

▶ It has been 35 years since the first recognition of the possibility of an association between head and neck irradiation and thyroid carcinoma. Thyroid carcinoma after radiation treatment for adolescent acne vulgaris was first reported in 1967. Only a small number of cases has been reported since then, which underscores the importance of this study by Thomson et al., since it shows such a relatively significant problem. This really should have been suspected long ago. By analogy, in a study of over 70,000 Israeli children given radiation treatment for tinea capitus from 1949 to 1959, the prevalence rate for carcinoma of the thyroid was 5 times higher than expected (Mondan, B., et al.: *Radiology* 123:741, 1977). In the Israeli children the amount of radiation actually spilling over to the thyroid was only about 6 rad. The amount reaching the thyroid after radiation for acne is a bit more difficult to calculate because the way the radiation was given varied widely in different patients. The importance of all these data is that if you were taking care of children in the 1960s or earlier and know of anyone who had received this form of therapy for acne, it is imperative that some sort of follow-up be arranged even though these patients are long out of your practice.

While on the topic of thyroid disease, it may be worthwhile to digress for a few lines here to provide an update on the results of the thyroid screening programs. The results from Canada (Rovet et al.: *J. Am. Acad. Child Psychiatry* 23:110, 1984) indicate that mental retardation is being prevented by early detection and treatment of congenital hypothyroidism via the neonatal screening programs. Children in the latter study had IQs within the normal range although they were slightly below the level of their siblings. An absent thyroid gland (athyrosis) appears to be correlated with a slightly lower IQ score than was a goitrous, hypoplastic, or ectopic gland. Some children whose treatment is begun in the first month of life are showing evidence of abnormal motor coordination. This suggests that the very small amounts of thyroid hormones that cross the placenta in late pregnancy are not sufficient to allow normal development of the cerebellar cells, which are growing rapidly at that time, while parts of the brain that are developing less rapidly are not harmed so readily by intrauterine hypothyroidism. Current results fail to show any protective benefit of breast-feeding. Breast-fed and bottle-fed babies obtained almost identical scores in these studies. Indeed, using very sensitive assays, Jansson et al. (*Acta Paediatr. Scand.* 72:703, 1983) found that the concentration of thyroid hormones in breast milk when a very sophisticated assay was used was lower than that reported previously. The total daily triiodothyronine (T_3) intake of a breast-fed infant is unlikely to exceed 2.5 nmol, which is less than 10% of the recommended dose for treatment of congenital hypothyroidism. This amount of T_3 in breast milk has no influence whatsoever on the pituitary-thyroid axis in normal babies either (Mizuta et al.: *Pediatr. Res.* 17:468, 1983). A summary of all this information does confirm that screening programs for congenital hypothyroidism are likely to improve the intellectual function of affected patients considerably, although this does depend on treatment being started within 1 month of birth and being given consistently. What really is needed is some clear index of which babies may have suffered intrauterine damage early on. Currently, levels of thyrotropin and thyroxine give no clues in this regard. Some have resorted to doing skeletal x-ray studies to look for defects in skeletal maturation. This, unfortunately, involves radiation exposure. A neat idea was proposed by Larsson et al. (*Acta Paediatr. Scand.* 72:481, 1983), who suggested that serum α-fetoprotein may be useful in determining which babies are significantly affected in utero from their hypothyroidism. α-Fetoprotein decreases rapidly during the last 6 to 8 weeks of gestation in normal babies. Thus, the α-fetoprotein level at birth is a good measure of the maturity of a newborn baby. When α-fetoprotein levels in the serum of newborn infants who have been detected as having hypothyroidism were measured, the serum levels in fact did correlate with x-ray skeletal maturation indices. Therefore, it may well be that increased serum α-fetoprotein is caused by prenatal hypothyroidism and that analysis of α-fetoprotein is a valuable tool to identify those infants with congenital hypothyroidism who are at increased risk of neurologic impairment despite the fact that they are started on therapy within 1 month of life. Obviously, only time will tell if we should be adding a determination of the α-fetoprotein level to the tests that are performed once an infant is suspected of having congenital hypothyroidism. Long-term follow-up will be needed to prove this point.

If you are not yet bored by the arguments of whether to screen for congenital hypothyroidism by levels of thyroxine, thyrotropin, or combinations thereof, you will be interested in reading the summary report of the Second International Congress on Neonatal Thyroid Screening. This appeared in the *Journal of Pediatrics* almost 2 years ago (102:653, 1983). This report really is as current as any and discusses all the pros and cons and pitfalls of the screening programs that have been underway for some years. The report summarizes data on some 4,000 infants who have been detected with congenital hypothyroidism. That ain't hay and makes for the ability to make a lot of consensus out of something that ordinarily does not make a lot of sense.—J.A.S., III

Secondary Hyperparathyroidism and Bone Disease in Infants Receiving Long-Term Furosemide Therapy
Pankaja S. Venkataraman, Bokyung K. Han, Reginald C. Tsang, and Cynthia C. Daugherty
Am. J. Dis. Child. 137:1157–1161, December 1983   11–6

Four preterm infants receiving long-term furosemide therapy were examined for hypercalciuria, hyperparathyroidism, renal calcification, and bone demineralization. Gestational age ranged from 30 to 32 weeks. All 4 had developed hyperbilirubinemia and bronchopulmonary dysplasia before transfer to Children's Hospital Medical Center, Cincinnati. All were receiving long-term furosemide therapy for treatment of cor pulmonale secondary to bronchopulmonary dysplasia. The dose of furosemide had ranged from 1 to 6 mg/kg/day for 6 to 12 weeks.

Concentrations of serum calcium and serum uric acid were normal in all 4. Levels of serum alkaline phosphatase were close to the upper limit of childhood reference ranges. Levels of serum phosphorus were generally within normal range. All 4 infants had urinary calcium excretion exceeding 4.0 mg/kg/day. Levels of serum parathyroid hormone were sharply elevated above both normal adult and infant values in the 3 infants with greater amounts of urinary calcium losses. Concentrations of serum 25-hydroxy-vitamin D were slightly elevated in 2 infants. In all 4 infants bone mineral content was below the mean for preterm infants of similar gestational and postnatal age.

On abdominal roentgenograms in the prone position, all 4 infants had an abnormal calcific density in the right upper and middle parts of the abdomen. In 1 infant severe bronchopulmonary dysplasia was found at autopsy. The heart was dilated with multiple microinfarcts and extensive dystrophic calcification that involved the papillary and trabecular muscles of both ventricles. Bone findings were consistent with hyperparathyroidism.

These findings support the thesis that furosemide-induced calciuria may lead to secondary hyperparathyroidism in preterm infants. Theoretically, bone mineralization may be further compromised in such infants.

▶ Furosemide therapy is known to be associated with hypercalciuria. It therefore is not surprising that one would expect to see secondary hyperparathyroidism and bone disease if one looked for it in infants who were receiving long-term furosemide therapy. We must accept this now as a real risk with the use of this diuretic. One also must be wary of the formation of renal calcium stones.

In adults with idiopathic hypercalciuria who are stone-formers, secondary hyperparathyroidism is a frequent occurrence. This has now been described in children as well (Moore et al.: *J. Pediatr.* 103:932, 1983). Idiopathic hypercalciuria and secondary hyperparathyroidism should be considered in the differential diagnosis of children with nonobstructive, noninfectious renal calculi. This also should be considered in any child who has unexplained gross or microscopic hematuria because hypercalciuria very often causes hematuria. The reason for mentioning all this is that idiopathic hypercalciuria can be treated with the administration of thiazide diuretics. Children treated in such a way have decreases in parathyroid hormone levels and healing of their bones. Isn't it strange that one diuretic causes a problem that another diuretic can take care of?—J.A.S., III

Detection of Late-Onset 21-Hydroxylase Deficiency Congenital Adrenal Hyperplasia in Adolescents
S. J. Emans, E. Grace, E. Fleischnick, M. J. Mansfield, and J. F. Crigler, Jr. (Boston)
Pediatrics 72:690–695, November 1983   11–7

Because severe hirsutism is difficult to reverse, evaluation of the adolescent girl with progressive hirsutism should aim at the pathophysiology of androgen excess to select appropriate therapies. A prospective study was conducted to determine the occurrence of late-onset 21-hydroxylase deficiency among 22 female adolescents, mean age 17.3 years, with androgen excess. Serum 17-hydroxyprogesterone levels were measured before and after bolus intravenous infusion of 0.25 mg of synthetic adrenocorticotropin (ACTH).

Ten of the 22 patients (45%) were more than 20% overweight for height. Eight had moderate cystic acne and 4 had clitoromegaly. Seven had luteinizing hormone (LH) levels greater than 30 mIU/ml or an LH to follicle-stimulating hormone (FSH) ratio greater than 3 with a normal FSH level. Total testosterone levels were elevated in 20 patients and the free testosterone level was elevated in all 22. The serum dehydroepiandrosterone sulfate concentration was elevated in 15 patients, urinary 17-ketosteroid levels were elevated in 9, the serum dehydroepiandrosterone level was elevated in 11, and the androstenedione concentration was elevated in 8. Two patients had slightly elevated ACTH levels; the other 20, including the 2 with 21-hydroxylase blocks, had normal ACTH levels. The 2 patients with the highest baseline levels of 17-hydroxyprogesterone had a response to ACTH consistent with late-onset congenital adrenocortical hyperplasia.

Baseline androgen levels did not distinguish patients with 21-hydroxylase deficiency from other hirsute females. Infusion of synthetic ACTH did identify those needing long-term corticosteroid therapy. The use of major histocompatibility complex haplotypes could be of help in identifying affected siblings prior to the development of significant hirsutism.

▶ Alfred M. Bongiovanni, Professor of Pediatrics and Obstetrics and Gynecology, University of Pennsylvania School of Medicine and the Pennsylvania Hospital, comments:

"This paper is an important one. The so-called polycystic ovarian syndrome in women is an assortment of hyperandrogenic disorders, and certain of these appear to begin in early life. Among the causes, it is clear that adrenocortical 21-hydroxylase deficiency is one. This has been well established and the incidence in women varies from clinic to clinic and depends on the use of suitable tests. These authors rightly emphasize the usefulness of ACTH stimulation with particular attention to the rise in the level of 17-hydroxyprogesterone. In this article, the greatest concern is the prevention of severe hirsutism, which is difficult to arrest once it is well established. However, the polycystic ovarian syndrome also is characterized by a gradually increasing size of the ovary with thickening of the capsule, atretic follicular cysts, and relative infertility. In some quarters it is suggested that these difficulties, as well as the hirsutism, might be prevented by early diagnosis and treatment as described. Also, it may be that the relatively common disorder premature adrenarche which is usually considered as benign, is an early clinical manifestation. If this is so, then rather young children with this manifestation alone should be tested also. This contribution is also important because it includes studies of the HLA haplotypes, and in the 2 patients identified as having 21-hydroxylase deficiency, the genotype conformed to that previously described in the late-onset disease. The authors concede that they have not studied the possibility of deficient 3β-hydroxysteroid dehydrogenase, which turned up in a surprisingly high percentage of our studies in older females with the full syndrome (*J. Steroid. Biochem.* 18:745, 1983). One would need to include the measurement of 17-hydroxy-5-pregnenolone to detect this, and it may well be the second most common form of these disorders.''

Long-Term Treatment of Central Precocious Puberty With a Long-Acting Analogue of Luteinizing Hormone-Releasing Hormone: Effects on Somatic Growth and Skeletal Maturation
M. Joan Mansfield, Donna E. Beardsworth, Jacquelyn S. Loughlin, John D. Crawford, Hans H. Bode, Jean Rivier, Wylie Vale, David C. Kushner, John F. Crigler, Jr., and William F. Crowley, Jr. (Massachusetts Genl. Hosp., Boston)
N. Engl. J. Med. 309:1286–1290, Nov. 24, 1983   11–8

The gonadotropin-releasing hormone-like agonist D-Trp^6-Pro^6-NEt-LHRH (LHRH$_a$) has been shown to induce a reversible short-term suppression of gonadotropins and gonadal steroids in patients with central precocious puberty. Since accelerated statural growth and bone maturation are clinical features of precocity not well controlled by conventional therapies, an examination was made of the effects of prolonged LHRH$_a$ therapy for 18 consecutive months on secondary sexual development, statural growth and skeletal maturation in 9 girls with neurogenic or idiopathic precocious puberty. Sexual maturation for the 9 patients was rated at Tanner Stages II to IV of sexual development. Bone ages were advanced a mean of 4.0 ± 0.6 years beyond chronological age. Doses of LHRH$_a$ of 4–8 μg/kg body weight were given daily by subcutaneous injections; dose was adjusted until estradiol levels and maturation index were completely suppressed to prepubertal levels.

Results showed the involution of secondary sexual characteristics throughout the 18 months of treatment. Menstruation ceased in all menstruating subjects. Amount of breast tissue decreased or stabilized; pubic hair diminished in 2, but increased in another 2. Dehydroepiandrosterone sulfate levels rose in 4 of 5 patients with levels greater than 60 μg/dl before therapy. Spontaneous luteinizing hormone and follicle-stimulating hormone (FSH) pulsations were abolished throughout the treatment period in all patients. Luteinizing hormone response to LHRH fell significantly. Mean FSH levels also fell significantly during the treatment period.

During the 18 months of therapy, mean growth rate fell significantly in 6 girls previously untreated for whom data on pretreatment growth were available. Growth velocity fell from a mean rate of 9.35 ± 0.64 cm/year during the 19 months before treatment to 4.58 ± 0.60 cm/year during treatment. Bone age advanced a mean of 9.4 ± 3.3 months during treatment. These changes resulted in a mean increase of 3.3 cm in predicted height. No families discontinued treatment and no adverse psychosocial effects were noted. One patient discontinued treatment after 18 months and showed secondary sexual development progression 6 and 12 months after discontinuing the drug.

Complete suppression of the pituitary-gonadal axis can be maintained by $LHRH_a$ therapy, resulting in slowing of excessively rapid growth and skeletal maturation and in increased predicted adult height in girls with precocious puberty.

▶ Paul Saenger, Associate Professor of Pediatrics, and Head, Division of Pediatric Endocrinology, Albert Einstein College of Medicine and the Montefiore Medical Center, comments:

"Treatment of precocious puberty can be termed successful when serum gonadotropins, estrogens, or testosterone and excessive growth velocity are suppressed.

"Available therapy to date consisted of antiandrogens (e.g., cyproterone acetate or danazol) or progestogens (Depo-Provera). These drugs have well-known adverse effects (adrenal suppression, obesity) and, furthermore, none of these therapeutic modalities has been shown to improve the prognosis for adult height.

"After an initial report (Comite, F., et al.: *N. Engl. J. Med.* 305:1546, 1981) describing short-term effects of treatment of *central* idiopathic precocious puberty using a long-acting LHRH analogue, the group from the Massachusetts General Hospital now describes treatment data for 18 months' duration and provides growth data in 9 girls.

"As expected, suppression of gonadotropin pulsations and gonadal steroids was maintained in all subjects; in addition, annual growth rates fell significantly. Parallel to these desirable hormonal changes and changes in growth velocity the clinicians also noticed a decrease in behavioral problems often associated with precocious puberty.

"While these data are clearly promising, it remains unclear whether the final adult height in these youngsters will indeed be improved. The increase in predicted adult height of 3.3 cm is predicated on accuracy of (1) bone age interpretations used and (2) tables for predicting adult height from skeletal age.

"The precise mechanisms of action of LHRH agonists remains unclear, exhorting the clinician to continued vigilance. While recent evidence suggests that the effects of chronic LHRH analogues are restricted predominantly to the level of the pituitary gland, where it desensitizes the pituitary to endogenous LHRH stimulation (Evans, R. M., et al.: *J. Clin. Endocrinol. Metab.* 58:862, 1984; and Clayton, R. N.: *Endocrinology* 111:152, 1982), a direct role for LHRH in suppression of testicular or ovarian steroidogenesis cannot be ruled out completely (Warner, B., et al.: *J. Clin. Invest.* 71:1848, 1983).

"Long-term studies using LHRH agonists over several years in patients with idiopathic precocious puberty are warranted. Only then can the efficacy of this drug in improving final adult height be assessed.

"The LHRH analogues also bear considerable promise in treating precocious puberty complicating congenital adrenal hyperplasia (Pescovitz, O. H., et al.: *J. Clin. Endocrinol. Metab.* 58:857, 1984). It should be noted that LHRH analogues will not be useful in noncentral forms of precocious puberty (e.g., McCune Albright syndrome).

"The availability of intranasally administered LHRH agonists and their successful use (Luder, A. S., et al.: ibid., p. 966) will make treatment with these materials even more attractive in the future."

A Chronobiologic Abnormality in Luteinizing Hormone Secretion in Teenage Girls With the Polycystic Ovary Syndrome

Barnett Zumoff, Ruth Freeman, Susan Coupey, Paul Saenger, Morri Markowitz, and Jacob Kream (Albert Einstein College of Medicine, New York)
N. Engl. J. Med. 309:1206–1209, Nov. 17, 1983   11–9

Possible abnormalities of central nervous system regulation of luteinizing hormone (LH) were investigated over a 24-hour period in 5 girls aged 13–16 with the polycystic ovary syndrome; profiles of prolactin and cortisol were also obtained. These data were compared to those from healthy controls.

Results showed 4 of the 5 patients had plasma LH profiles that were strikingly abnormal in comparison with those of normal pubertal teenage girls. The 5 patients had a daily LH surge that was desynchronized by about 7–8 hours from their sleep period. In 3 of 4 patients the surge began at about the end of the sleep period and lasted for 6–10 hours. In normal girls, the daily LH surge is coterminous with the sleep period. Normal persons have a daily surge in prolactin that is also coterminous with the sleep period. The 5 patients with polycystic ovary syndrome had a prolactin surge that was likewise synchronous with sleep. All patients also had normal plasma cortisol profiles.

In the present study, 4 of 5 postpubertal teenage girls with the polycystic ovary syndrome had a chronobiologic abnormality of LH secretion. This finding, which appears unique to the polycystic ovary syndrome, points to the central nervous system as the probable locus of the initiating pathophysiology of the syndrome.

▶ Doctor Saenger comments on this report, which he also coauthored:

"Polycystic ovary syndrome (PCOS) may occur in teenagers soon after puberty, as documented in this report and by others (Moll, G. W., Jr., et al.: *Pediatr. Res.* 15:443, 1981).

"The chronobiologic abnormality in LH secretion resulting in a night-day reversal of LH secretion is further evidence for a hypothalamic defect among most women with PCOS. Hypothalamic modulation of prolactin and LH-FSH synthesis as well as secretion is altered whether patients have normal or increased circulating levels of these hormones (Vaitukaitis, J. L.: *N. Engl. J. Med.* 309:1245, 1983). Other clinical syndromes associated with definable causes of increased androgen secretion may share many, but not all, of the clinical and biochemical manifestations that are observed among women with PCOS. For example, the increased androgen secretion due to congenital adrenal hyperplasia or central precocious puberty will result in precocious nighttime surges in LH secretion but not in a night-day reversal of LH secretion as seen in PCOS (Boyar, R., et al.: ibid. 289:286, 1973).

"If this chronobiologic abnormality is confirmed in all or a subset of comparable patients with PCOS and also in older patients with longstanding PCOS, it may strengthen the evidence for a primary CNS defect in these patients and become a valuable diagnostic tool for PCOS."

LHRH Treatment in Unilateral Cryptorchidism: Effect on Testicular Descent and Hormonal Response
B. Karpe, P. Eneroth, and E. M. Ritzén
J. Pediatr. 103:892–897, December 1983   11–10

The effects of long-term treatment with luteinizing hormone-releasing hormone (LHRH) on unilateral cryptorchidism were evaluated in a double-blind study of 50 prepubertal boys aged 3–8 years (mean, 6.3 ± 1.4 years) seen with unilateral undescended, but palpable, testes at Karolinska Hospital, Stockholm. The boys were randomly assigned to treatment with LHRH (HOE 471, 100 μg in each nostril 6 times a day) or placebo for 28 days.

Numerical values representing changes in testicular position during treatment indicated a minor descent of the undescended testis that did not differ significantly from that in boys given placebo. This was the case for spontaneous positions assumed by the undescended testis both before and after efforts to manipulate it into the scrotum, as well as for the position obtained during moderate caudal traction. In contrast, the scrotal testis exhibited a significant descent, although its position during caudal traction did not differ significantly between the LHRH and placebo groups. Six months after treatment, a minor general ascent of the testes, compared with the immediate posttreatment position, was observed, but this was significant only for the scrotal testes during caudal traction. Of 25 boys treated with LHRH, a clinically acceptable descent of the undescended testis occurred in 5. A good response was also achieved in 4 of 23 boys in the placebo group who subsequently received LHRH therapy; 2 others had a borderline response. No serious side effects were observed. Baseline serum testosterone concentrations and testicular volume increased significantly after treatment ($P < .01$ and $P < .001$, respectively). An acute LHRH test (100 μg/sq m body surface area intravenously), before and after treatment, produced an increase in luteinizing hormone peak values and a decrease in follicle-stimulating hormone peak values in a significant number of patients ($P < .001$). A positive correlation was observed in individual patients between the increase in basal serum testosterone concentration and the extent of downward movement of the undescended testis ($P < .05$).

Although long-term intranasal treatment with LHRH in this group of boys, in whom great care was taken to exclude retractile testes, caused a significant change in posttreatment gonadotropin response, in basal serum testosterone values, and in testicular volume, any testicular descent that occurred probably resulted from decreased testicular retraction by the cremaster muscle rather than from increased length of the cord structures.

Renal Function in Relation to Metabolic Control in Children With Diabetes of Different Duration
G. Dahlquist, A. Aperia, O. Broberger, B. Persson, and P. Wilton (Stockholm)
Acta Paediatr. Scand. 72:903–909, November 1983   11–11

In a series of 157 diabetic children and adolescents, including 47 with diabetes for up to 5 years, 61 with a disease duration of 5–10 years, and 49 with known diabetes for more than 10 years, the glomerular filtration rate (GFR), measured as inulin or creatinine clearance, para-aminohippurate clearance, filtration fraction, β_2-microglobulin excretion, and albumin excretion were correlated with short-term and long-term indices of metabolic control. Reference values for GFR were obtained from 6 children having microscopic hematuria or cystitis, and urine was sampled from 21 healthy children and young adults.

As measured by inulin clearance, GFR was increased in diabetics in all disease-duration groups. In the most recently diagnosed patients, GRF correlated with the blood glucose level. Inulin clearance also correlated with the hemoglobin A_{1c} and the 24-hour urinary glucose values. In patients with diabetes for more than 10 years, the GRF and hemoglobin A_{1c} value correlated inversely. Urinary albumin excretion was significantly increased in all groups of diabetics, but excretion of β_2-microglobulin was similar to that in control subjects. Creatinine clearance correlated inversely with indices of metabolic control, but did not correlate with inulin clearance.

As measured by inulin clearance, GFR is related to metabolic control to varying degrees depending on the duration of diabetes, but the relation between increased GFR early in the course and diabetic nephropathy remains unclear. Creatinine clearance is a poor indicator of GFR in diabetics with poor metabolic control. Albuminuria, measured by a sensitive technique, might be predictive of diabetic nephropathy, but long-term prospective studies are necessary.

▶ We should be paying a lot of attention to whatever is current in the management of children with diabetes. The reason for saying this is based on the fact that we more likely than not will be seeing many more diabetic children in the future. A recent British study has found that the prevalence of diabetes in children is doubling every decade (*Br. Med. J.* 286:1855, 1983). Furthermore, this marked increase appears to be focused mostly in children of socially advantaged families. The exact relationship between the metabolic abnormalities of diabetes mellitus and the pathogenesis of its complications is still uncertain. However, the past years have brought increasing awareness of the importance of good control of blood glucose concentrations. There is no question that in diabetes the kidney is affected very early in the course of the disease. As Dahlquist et al. note, this is first manifested by an increase in the glomerular filtration rate (GFR) and slightly thereafter by an increase in protein spillage into the urine. The increase of GFR does appear to correlate with poor control. As a parameter of poor control, this is true for only the first few years of the illness; as the disease progresses, GFR ultimately decreases. No one seems to know what the mechanism of the increased GFR is early in the course of diabetes but it is a characteristic finding, especially in poor control. Clinically evident proteinuria usually is not detected for some 15 years or so after the diagnosis of insulin-dependent diabetes and prestages the development of renal failure 4 to 5 years after its detection in approximately 50% of patients whose diabetes begins in childhood. While many monitors must be used to judge the adequacy of diabetic control, each adds information and has a place in the treatment of the child with diabetes. Determinations of blood or urine glucose levels are necessary on a daily basis for insulin adjustment; 24-hour urine glucose levels or aliquots may provide information concerning the peak insulin action and glucose control for one 24-hour period. Hemoglobin A_{1c} represents biochemical control for periods of 8 to 12 weeks. Growth and development can indicate adequacy of metabolic control throughout months to years. All these measures need to be integrated into an ongoing program for monitoring of each patient.

It seems unfortunate that despite the fact that hemoglobin A_{1c} determinations have been available now for about 6 years, many practitioners do not use them to follow the degree of control of their patients. D. M. Nathan et al. (*N. Engl. J. Med.* 310:341, 1984) showed that with traditional determinations (urinary glucose levels, medical history, fasting or random glucose levels, and so forth), medical practitioners' estimates of glucose control in patients with diabetes differed markedly from the mean blood glucose level as calculated from determinations of hemoglobin A_{1c} values. Even medical practitioners who were highly experienced in the care of patients with diabetes faired only slightly better in guessing who was well controlled and who was not when hemoglobin A_{1c} was used as the gold standard. These data demonstrate the limitations of traditional clinical judgment and laboratory procedures in providing an accurate assessment of blood glucose control in such patients. This underscores the need for periodically measuring glycosylated hemoglobin levels. It is not unreasonable to expect that new technologies might require a little while to catch on. As with any new laboratory procedure, a certain amount of skepticism is to be expected. Many "important new advances" in medicine have promised more than they actually have delivered. In this respect, I have been taken for a "deride" more than once. However, hemoglobin A_{1c} determinations have been around long enough to demonstrate their validity. Sure, there are a few gaps in our knowledge. What do you do with the patient who you are convinced is in poor control and yet who has an acceptable level of hemoglobin A_{1c}? What do you do with the patient who you feel comfortable with in terms of degree of control and who has a significantly elevated hemoglobin A_{1c} level? These cases have to be handled with great care.

Two flies may have appeared in the ointment regarding strict control of diabetes. In Denmark, the effect of 1 year of very strict, near-normal blood glucose level control in insulin-dependent diabetics was actually a slightly increased degree of retinopathy in a group of adults (*Lancet* 1:200, 1983). By the same token, two girls aged 15 and 14 with poorly controlled insulin-dependent diabetes manifested the rapid development of diabetic nephropathy after the institution of an aggressive management program (*Pediatrics* 71:824, 1983). Vascular regulatory peculiarities might explain this pathogenic association between rapidly increased insulin administration and the appearance of vascular complications of diabetes. In any event, these two reports suggest that, wherever possible, rapid increases in insulin dosage should be avoided.

How to maintain better diabetic control still is an art. Self-monitoring of blood glucose levels and intensified insulin therapy have been found to be acceptable and efficacious in children with diabetes (Geffner, M. E., et al.: *JAMA* 249:2913, 1983). In patients who have poor control, continuous subcutaneous insulin infusion can be quite effective in achieving improvement in the levels of glycosylated hemoglobin (Schiffrin, A.: *J. Pediatr.* 103:522, 1983).

This commentary could not be complete without some statement regarding the introduction in the past 2 years of human insulin. A protein with an amino acid sequence identical with that of naturally occurring insulin can be manufactured either biosynthetically by DNA recombinant techniques or by chemical modification of porcine insulin. Biosynthetic human insulin (Humulin) was the first drug product developed through recombinant DNA technology approved by the Food and Drug Administration for marketing. I am not certain what the real role of this product is as yet. Biosynthetic human insulin has not been demonstrated to offer clear clinical advantages over purified animal insulins. Sure, there are isolated instances in which a patient might do better on this product, but such cases, to date, seem to be few and far between. If you do switch to biosynthetic human insulin, as with switching any insulin preparation, you may find that some patients require higher dosages, and some lower, and some others require no dosage changes at all. Because of the need for monitoring, patients should be cautioned not to switch to human insulin without notifying their physician. Nobody likes to be caught wearing last year's dress (especially those of my sex), but last year's porcine insulin is probably just as good as human insulin in all but a few cases. Perhaps my opinion in this regard will change, but I have never liked arguing or wrestling with porcines (you tend to get very dirty and, besides, the pig seems to like it).— J.A.S., III

12 Nutrition and Metabolism

Human Milk Intake and Growth in Exclusively Breast-fed Infants
Nancy F. Butte, Cutberto Garza, E. O'Brian Smith, and Buford L. Nichols (Baylor College of Medicine)
J. Pediatr. 104:187–194, February 1984   12–1

Most previous studies of human milk production have been cross-sectional and therefore unsuitable for study of the relation between milk intake and growth. Butte et al. sought to document longitudinally the voluntary milk intake and growth of exclusively breast-fed infants. Forty-five such infants were followed over the first 4 months of life. All were healthy term infants born to healthy mothers not receiving long-term medication. Mean birth weight was 3.6 kg, and mean gestational age was 39.2 weeks. There were 27 boys and 18 girls in the study. Observations were made at mean ages of 35, 64, and 119 days.

Milk intake plateaued over the 4-month observation period, with an overall mean of 733 gm daily (Table 1). Consumption declined significantly in relation to increasing body weight. Changes in milk composition over time are shown in Table 2. Energy intake did not vary significantly during the study. Overall mean intake was 476 kcal per day. Energy intake fell

TABLE 1.—HUMAN MILK AND NUTRIENT INTAKES
OF EXCLUSIVELY BREAST-FED INFANTS DURING FIRST 4
MONTHS OF LIFE*

	Age (mo)			
	1 (n = 37)	2 (n = 40)	3 (n = 37)	4 (n = 41)
Feedings (n/day)	8.3 ± 1.9	7.2 ± 1.9	6.8 ± 1.9	6.7 ± 1.8
Human milk				
Gm/day	751.0 ± 130.0	725.0 ± 131.0	723.0 ± 114.0	740.0 ± 128.0
Gm/kg/day	159.0 ± 24.0	129.0 ± 19.0	117.0 ± 20.0	111.0 ± 17.0
Protein				
Gm/day	7.6 ± 1.7	6.5 ± 1.7	6.1 ± 1.3	6.1 ± 1.4
Gm/kg/day	1.6 ± 0.3	1.1 ± 0.2	1.0 ± 0.2	0.9 ± 0.2
Lactose				
Gm/day	48.5 ± 8.9	47.8 ± 9.0	48.0 ± 8.0	49.3 ± 9.2
Gm/kg/day	10.3 ± 1.6	8.5 ± 1.3	7.8 ± 1.4	7.4 ± 1.2
Fat				
Gm/day	28.0 ± 8.5	25.2 ± 7.1	23.6 ± 7.2	25.6 ± 8.6
Gm/kg/day	5.9 ± 1.7	4.4 ± 1.2	3.8 ± 1.2	3.8 ± 1.3
Energy				
Kcal/day	520.0 ± 131.0	468.0 ± 115.0	458.0 ± 124.0	477.0 ± 111.0
Kcal/kg/day	110.0 ± 24.0	83.0 ± 19.0	74.0 ± 20.0	71.0 ± 17.0

*At onset of study, milk intake was estimated by deuterium dilution, a technique later determined to be inaccurate. Therefore, data are missing at 17 time points during first 3 months. Data are expressed as mean ± SD.
(Courtesy of Butte, N.F., et al.: J. Pediatr. 104:187–194, February 1984.)

TABLE 2.—HUMAN MILK COMPOSITION*

Age (mo)	n	Total nitrogen (mg/gm)	Protein nitrogen (mg/gm)	NPN (mg/gm)	Lactose (mg/gm)	Fat (mg/gm)	Energy (kcal/gm)
1	37	2.17 ± 0.30	1.61 ± 0.24	0.56 ± 0.28	64.7 ± 2.4	36.2 ± 7.5	0.68 ± 0.08
2	40	1.94 ± 0.24	1.42 ± 0.17	0.52 ± 0.20	65.8 ± 2.5	34.4 ± 6.8	0.64 ± 0.08
3	37	1.84 ± 0.19	1.34 ± 0.15	0.50 ± 0.13	66.5 ± 2.3	32.2 ± 7.8	0.62 ± 0.09
4	41	1.80 ± 0.21	1.31 ± 0.17	0.48 ± 0.14	66.6 ± 2.4	34.8 ± 10.8	0.64 ± 0.10

*Data are expressed as mean ± SD.
(Courtesy of Butte, N.F., et al.: J. Pediatr. 104:187–194, February 1984.)

significantly as body weight increased. Various measures of growth during the study period are shown in Table 3. Infant weight correlated with milk intake at 1 and 4 months, but it explained only 16% of the variability in intake. Growth rate tended to increase with increasing milk intake (Tables 4 and 5).

Breast-fed infants appear to achieve adequate growth on nutrient intakes substantially below current dietary recommendations. Before dietary standards are revised, however, further information is needed on the mechanisms by which infants adjust to a given plane of nutrition and adapt to suboptimal environmental conditions. Not only energy intakes, but protein intakes were considerably below recommended dietary allowances. Infants given a limited supply of dietary protein may conserve nitrogen through a decrease in protein turnover, reuse of endogenous amino acids, change in the composition of new tissues, or use of nonprotein sources of nitrogen.

▶ This is a landmark observation and highlights how little we really know about infant nutrition. The babies don't read the books and don't know that adequate growth is not believed to be possible at caloric intakes of 71 kcal/kg/day.

Kathryn Dewey and Bo Lönnerdal (J. Pediatr. Gastroenterol. Nutr. 2:497, 1983) made a similar observation. Dietary intake, milk consumption, growth, and activity were monitored monthly for 20 breast-fed infants from age 1 to age 6 months. Breast milk intake ranged from 341 to 1,096 ml/day, with mean intake increasing from 673 to 896 ml/day from age 1 to age 6 months. Energy intake averaged 113 kcal/kg/day at age 1 month, decreasing to 85 kcal/kg/day at age 5–6 months—considerably lower than the recommended 115 kcal/kg/day. All infants except 1 were above the 10th percentile of weight for age. A study from Chile (Juez, G., et al.: Am. J. Clin. Nutr. 38:462, 1983) found that 59% of 242 infants were fully nursing at age 6 months and were growing at a normal rate without receiving either supplementary milk or nondairy food. Maternal milk alone can support normal growth during the first 6 months of life. Infants do require monitoring. The milk from low-income mothers in Brazil was found to contain enough energy to sustain growth of infants at acceptable levels for the first 6 months of life (Marin, P. C., et al.: Lancet 1:232, 1984).

Remember the remarks of Oliver Wendell Holmes, who said, "A pair of substantial mammary glands has the advantage over the two hemispheres of the most learned professor's brain in the art of compounding a nutritious fluid for infants." Oliver, they don't even have to be substantial.—F.A.O.

TABLE 3.—INFANT GROWTH AND NATIONAL CENTER FOR HEALTH STATISTICS PERCENTILE RANKINGS DURING FIRST 4 MONTHS OF LIFE*

Age (mo)	n	Weight (kg)	Length (cm)	Weight gain (gm/day)	Weight gain (gm/kg/day)	Length accretion (cm/mo)	Weight-for-age Median	Weight-for-age 25th Percentile	Weight-for-age 75th Percentile	Length-for-age Median	Length-for-age 25th Percentile	Length-for-age 75th Percentile	Weight-for-length Median	Weight-for-length 25th Percentile	Weight-for-length 75th Percentile
0	45	3.58 ± 0.45	50.9 ± 2.5				72	40	86	51	18	86	45	27	64
1	45	4.76 ± 0.52	55.7 ± 2.3	37.3 ± 12.4	10.6 ± 3.8	4.6 ± 2.1	76	60	89	67	31	83	67	41	79
2	44	5.62 ± 0.67	59.0 ± 2.6	32.3 ± 13.8	6.9 ± 3.0	3.7 ± 1.6	76	57	89	63	34	88	65	37	82
3	42	6.30 ± 0.30	61.8 ± 2.4	22.4 ± 7.6	4.0 ± 1.4	2.8 ± 1.3	71	53	86	63	46	89	58	40	71
4	41	6.78 ± 0.80	63.7 ± 2.4	18.3 ± 8.1	2.9 ± 1.3	2.5 ± 1.7	69	42	86	55	37	82	49	34	72

*Data are expressed as mean ± SD.
(Courtesy of Butte, N.F., et al.: J. Pediatr. 104:187–194, February 1984.)

TABLE 4.—CORRESPONDING WEIGHT GAIN
OF INFANTS CLASSIFIED ACCORDING
TO PERCENTILE DISTRIBUTION
OF MILK INTAKE*

Percentile distribution of milk intake (gm/kg/day)

	<25th	26th to 50th	51st to 75th	76th to 100th
Age (mo)		Weight gain (gm/kg/day)		
1	11.6 ± 4.3	11.4 ± 5.2	9.5 ± 4.3	10.8 ± 1.8
2	6.0 ± 2.7	6.4 ± 3.1	6.6 ± 3.3	8.5 ± 3.4
3	4.4 ± 1.0	3.3 ± 1.2	4.3 ± 1.8	3.9 ± 1.2
4	2.6 ± 1.0	2.0 ± 1.3	3.2 ± 1.1	3.8 ± 1.1

*Data are expressed as mean ± SD.
(Courtesy of Butte, N.F., et al.: J. Pediatr. 104:187–194,
February 1984.)

TABLE 5.—CORRESPONDING MILK INTAKES
OF INFANTS CLASSIFIED ACCORDING TO
PERCENTILE DISTRIBUTION
OF WEIGHT GAIN*

Percentile distribution of weight gain (gm/kg/day)

	<25th	26th to 50th	51st to 75th	76th to 100th
Age (mo)		Milk intake (gm/kg/day)		
1	149 ± 14	169 ± 27	173 ± 31	151 ± 20
2	122 ± 19	124 ± 21	128 ± 13	142 ± 16
3	117 ± 24	119 ± 17	111 ± 19	122 ± 23
4	101 ± 16	110 ± 13	111 ± 18	121 ± 17

*Data are expressed as mean ± SD.
(Courtesy of Butte, N.F., et al.: J. Pediatr. 104:187–194,
February 1984.)

Decisions on Breast-Feeding or Formula Feeding and Trends in Infant Feeding Practices

Herbert P. Sarett, Kevin R. Bain, and John C. O'Leary (Mead Johnson Nutritional Div., Evansville, Ind.)

Am. J. Dis. Child. 137:719–725, August 1983 12–2

The development of effective programs to promote breast-feeding in the United States requires information regarding when mothers decide to breast-feed or formula feed and trends in infant-feeding practices. The results of three surveys that addressed these concerns are reported.

In the first study, 52% of 976 mothers who responded both before and after their infants were born stated that they intended to breast-feed, 43% said they planned to formula feed, and 5% were undecided (Table 1). After the infants were born, 96% of those who intended to breast-feed and 97% of those who planned to formula feed did so. Of the 51 women (5%) who had been undecided, 28 (55%) breast-fed and 23 (45%) formula fed their infants. The second study (200 expectant mothers and 200 recent mothers) showed that 85% to 92% of mothers had decided on a feeding

TABLE 1.—Comparison of Mothers' Plans for Infant Feeding Expressed During Third Trimester of Pregnancy With Practice Adopted at Birth (Study 1)

	No. (%) of Respondents (N = 976)		
	Breast-feed	**Formula Feed**	**Undecided**
Plan for infant feeding	504 (52)	421 (43)	51 (5)
Feeding practice in hospital*			
Breast-fed	482 (96)	13 (3)	28 (55)
Formula fed	22 (4)	408 (97)	23 (45)

*A total of 523 mothers (54%) breast-fed their infants; 453 mothers (46%) formula fed their infants.

(Courtesy of Sarett, H.P., et al.: Am. J. Dis. Child. 137:719–725, August 1983; copyright 1983, American Medical Association.)

TABLE 2.—Time of Choice of Breast-Feeding or Formula Feeding in Telephone Survey of Expectant Mothers During Third Trimester (Study 2)

	% of Respondents			
Time of Decision	**Total (n = 200)**	**Breast-feeding (n = 125)**	**Formula Feeding (n = 65)**	**Undecided (n = 10)**
Before pregnancy	61	64	63	...
First trimester	18	22	14	...
Second trimester	13	10	20	...
Third trimester	3	4	3	...
Undecided	5	...	...	5

(Courtesy of Sarett, H.P., et al.: Am. J. Dis. Child. 137:719–725, August 1983; copyright 1983, American Medical Association.)

TABLE 3.—Time of Choice of Breast-Feeding or Formula Feeding in Telephone Survey of Recent Mothers of Young Infants (Study 2)

	% of Respondents			
Time of Decision	**Total (n = 200)**	**Breast-feeding (n = 112)**	**Formula Feeding (n = 84)**	**Feeding Both (n = 4)**
Before pregnancy	49	55	43	...
First trimester	29	31	24	75
Second trimester	7	8	7	...
Third trimester	8	5	12	...
After delivery	7	1	14	25

(Courtesy of Sarett, H.P., et al.: Am. J. Dis. Child. 137:719–725, August 1983; copyright 1983, American Medical Association.)

method before the end of the second trimester of pregnancy and that only 5% to 7% were undecided in the third trimester; about half had decided before they became pregnant (Tables 2 and 3). The main reason given for breast-feeding was that it is healthier, whereas convenience was the most

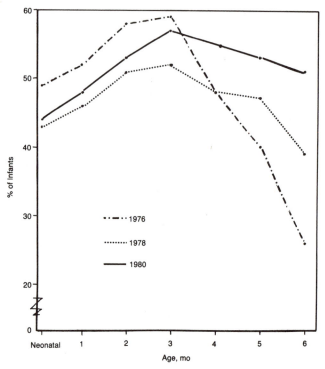

Fig 12–1.—Percentage of infants fed formula from the neonatal period to age 6 months (1976–1980). (Courtesy of Sarett, H.P., et al.: Am. J. Dis. Child. 137:719–725, August 1983; copyright 1983, American Medical Association.)

often cited reason for formula feeding. In the third study, it was found that breast-feeding during the neonatal period in the hospital increased significantly from 51% of mothers in 1976 to 57% in the period 1978 through 1980 ($P < .01$), and that breast-feeding at age 6 months increased from 20% in 1976 to 29% in 1980 ($P < .001$). The percentage of formula-fed infants during the neonatal period decreased from 49% in 1976 to 43% in 1980 ($P < .01$), whereas the percentage of formula-fed infants at age 6 months of age almost doubled, increasing from 26% in 1976 to 51% in 1980 ($P < .001$) (Fig 12–1). The use of cow's milk in infants aged 4 to 6 months decreased from 54% in 1976 to 21% in 1980 ($P < .001$) (Fig 12–2). Thus, the increase in the percentage of formula-fed infants at age 6 months may reflect to a great extent a trend toward using formula rather than cow's milk when breast-feeding is discontinued (Table 4). Supplementary baby foods were introduced later for breast-fed than for formula-fed infants, although in both groups there were similar tendencies toward the later introduction of solid foods from 1976 through 1980.

The findings indicate that many expectant mothers decide on a feeding method either before becoming pregnant or early in pregnancy and also suggest that current hospital routines do not discourage breast-feeding or

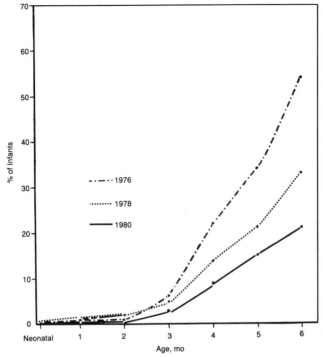

Fig 12–2.—Percentage of infants fed cow's milk from neonatal period to age 6 months (1976–1980). (Courtesy of Sarett, H.P., et al.: Am. J. Dis. Child. 137:719–725, August 1983; copyright 1983, American Medical Association.)

TABLE 4.—USE OF INFANT FORMULA AND COW'S MILK TO FEED
INFANTS WHEN BREAST-FEEDING WAS STOPPED FROM 1 WEEK TO 6
MONTHS OF AGE (STUDY 3, 1979 TO 1980 SURVEYS)

	Age at Which Breast-feeding Stopped			
	1 wk	1-2 mo	3-4 mo	5-6 mo
Exclusively Breast-fed Infants*				
No. (%) of total infants	29 (15)	87 (43)	37 (18)	49 (24)
% fed formula†	100	100	78	51
% fed cows' milk†	0	0	23	51
Breast-fed and Supplemented With Formula‡				
No. (%) of total infants	13 (2)	203 (29)	290 (40)	203 (29)
% fed formula†	100	100	94	90
% fed cows' milk†	0	0	11	27

*Total number of infants was 202.
†May add to more than 100% because of some use of both formula and cow's milk.
‡Total number of infants was 709.
(Courtesy of Sarett, H.P., et al.: Am. J. Dis. Child. 137:719–725, August 1983; copyright 1983, American Medical Association.)

cause mothers to change from their original plans for feeding. Early education concerning good infant-feeding practices is recommended.

▶ When it comes to questions related to infant nutrition, who better to ask than Lewis Barness, Professor and Chairman, Department of Pediatrics, University of South Florida? Doctor Barness comments succinctly as follows:
"Whether to breast-feed or bottle feed is a question of increasing interest. This study is important from several angles. Sarett and co-workers used an independent marketing research firm who mailed questionnaires to expectant and delivered mothers. From what appears to be a well-conceived study, if a physician is to influence the choice of feeding, he must become involved early in pregnancy, and he must give as factual information as possible to the expectant family. The increased use of formulas rather than cow's milk appears related to the recommendation that iron-containing formulas be used rather than large amounts of whole cow's milk. The authors did not specify which type of formula was used. The conclusion that current hospital routines do not discourage breast-feeding does not address two questions: (1) 'Can hospital practices affect duration of breast-feeding?' and (2) 'Would different hospital practices encourage nursing?' "

Human Milk Kills Parasitic Intestinal Protozoa
Frances D. Gillin and David S. Reiner (Univ. of California at San Diego)
Science 221:1290–1292, Sept. 23, 1983   12–3

Giardia lamblia is a common pathogenic intestinal parasite that is a major cause of waterborne enteric disease in the United States. Infection with this parasitic protozoan is prevalent in children and can cause failure to thrive. Normal human milk (NHM) contains a number of antibacterial proteins, some of which are found in other mucosal secretions. The authors assessed the ability of NHM to kill *G. lamblia* in vitro.

Low concentrations of NHM rapidly killed *G. lamblia* trophozoites: 50% were killed in less than 3 minutes by 3% NHM, in approximately 60 minutes by 1% NHM, and in 280 minutes by 0.3% NHM (Fig 12–3, A). As the *Giardia*-cidal activity of NHM was fully retained after depletion of NHM of secretory IgA (S-IgA) to undetectable levels (Fig 12–3, B), and neither IgG nor IgM was detectable in NHM, the ability of NHM to kill *G. lamblia* was not the result of antibodies. Also, NHM (1% concentration) killed more than 90% of *Entamoeba histolytica* and *Trichomonas vaginalis* trophozoites, two unrelated mucosal-dwelling pathogenic protozoa, during 3 hours of incubation.

Because of the potent antiparasitic activity of NHM in vitro, it is important to determine whether breast-fed children have a lower incidence of giardiasis or amebiasis than do children who have not been breast-fed, and to elucidate the mechanism by which these parasites are killed.

▶ I should quote Oliver Wendell Holmes once again. The anti-infective properties of milk produced by mothers giving birth to preterm infants may be even

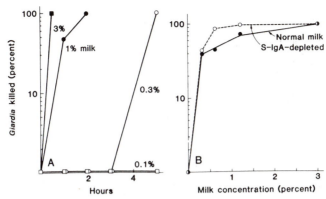

Fig 12–3.—**A,** kinetics of killing of *Giardia lamblia* trophozoites by normal human milk. The parasites (5,000/ml) were exposed to various concentration of filter-sterilized milk at about 35 C for 30–300 minutes. The percentage of parasites killed was calculated as 100 minus the percentage surviving, relative to controls lacking milk. **B,** killing of *G. lamblia* by normal human milk depleted of secretory immunoglobulin A (S-IgA). The percentage of parasites killed was determined as in **A.** No killing was observed with the control column buffer. (Courtesy of Gillin, F.D., and Reiner, D.S.: *Science* 221:1290–1292, Sept. 23, 1983. Copyright 1983 by the American Association for the Advancement of Science.)

higher than that of milk from mothers giving birth to term infants (Suzuki, S., et al.: *Acta Paediatr. Scand.* 72:671, 1983), at least with respect to antibodies to *Escherichia coli, Brucella abortus* and β-streptococci.

Another feature of breast-feeding is the observation that the infant fed human milk makes a greater antibody response to poliovirus or diptheria-pertussis-tetanus immunization than infants fed a low-protein cow's milk formula or soybean formulas (Zoppi, G., et al.: *Lancet* 2:11, 1983).

With all this evidence in favor of human milk, why would an infant receive anything else? But then again—man is the only animal that wears bow ties.—F.A.O.

Do Infant Formula Samples Shorten the Duration of Breast-Feeding?

Yves Bergevin, Cynthia Dougherty, and Michael S. Kramer
Lancet 1:1148–1151, May 21, 1983   12–4

Breast-feeding is recognized universally as resulting in lower infant morbidity and mortality due to a reduced incidence of respiratory and gastrointestinal infection, and, among higher socioeconomic groups, prevention of obesity, as well as offering important metabolic and perhaps even psychologic advantages over formula feeding. A common form of infant formula advertising consists of giving free sample packets to new mothers as they are discharged from the maternity ward.

A randomized clinical trial was designed to answer the question raised in the title. Of 696 women who gave birth at Montreal General Hospital during the study period, 448 (64.4%) breast-fed on leaving the hospital (4 were excluded from the study for various reasons). Each received a packet that contained a 120-ml bottle, a 235-ml can of ready-to-feed formula, a 120-gm can of formula powder, a reusable plastic nipple, and three information booklets with formula advertisements. Telephone interviews were conducted 3 months post partum to ascertain date of cessation of breast-feeding, defined as when the infant began taking more than one non-breast milk bottle per day and when solids were first offered.

Of the 444 eligible mothers 38 could not be reached by the interviewer. Data from the 406 who were contacted are shown in Figures 12–4 and 12–5. Of the mothers who had received a sample, 78% were still breast-feeding at 1 month versus 84% of those who had not received a sample. Among less educated mothers (no more than 14 years' schooling) the proportion was 67% versus 79%. Among primiparas the proportion was 70% versus 80%, and among mothers who had an illness in the interim the proportion was 67% versus 88%.

Eighteen percent of the 406 mothers who had received samples had introduced solid food by 2 months versus 10% of those who had received no samples. For less educated mothers the proportion was 24% versus 15%; for primiparas the proportion was 22% versus 11%; and for mothers who had been ill in the interim the proportion was 19% versus 3%.

Results suggest that receipt of infant formula samples by breast-feeding mothers may lead to a shorter duration of breast-feeding and earlier introduction of solids. This effect becomes clinically and statistically significant when the mothers are primiparous, have less education, and become ill post partum.

In North America the results shown probably would have particular

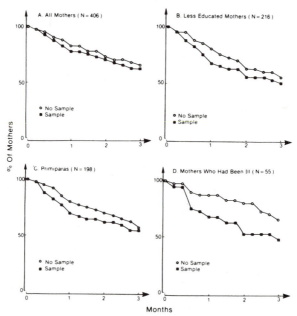

Fig 12–4.—Proportion of mothers who were breast-feeding 0 to 3 months post partum. (Courtesy of Bergevin, Y., et al.: Lancet 1:1148–1151, May 21, 1983.)

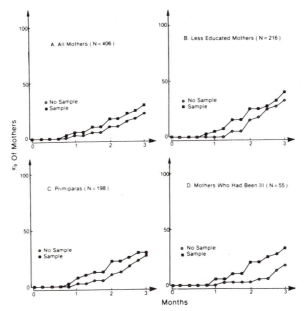

Fig 12–5.—Proportion of mothers who introduced solid food 0 to 3 months post partum. (Courtesy of Bergevin, Y., et al.: Lancet 1:1148–1151, May 21, 1983.)

relevance for primiparous women from lower socioeconomic groups. By extension, one can speculate that women and their infants in developing countries might be even more vulnerable to adverse health effects from formula samples. Other investigators with access to such populations should conduct similar studies to determine the universality of these findings. Relative risk and benefits of the "free sample" form of advertising will have to be weighed to allow health professionals to decide whether the practice should be continued in their hospitals.

▶ We turned to Calvin Woodruff for a commentary. Doctor Woodruff is Professor of Child Health, University of Missouri-Columbia School of Medicine, and a member of the American Academy of Pediatrics Committee on Nutrition. Cal writes:

"Very little is known about the sociological and cultural factors that influence the patterns of infant feeding. During the past decade we have seen a resurgence in breast-feeding, especially among the more-educated segment of our population, and it is not clear to what extent pediatricians either individually or as a group have been responsible. Nor is it clear to what extent advertising has influenced the actual practices of various groups within the population. Prospective, randomized, controlled studies in this area are difficult to design and to carry out. Consequently, this article, which attempts to deal with one very small aspect of the situation, the influence of samples of formula at the time of discharge from the hospital on the duration of nursing and the age of starting supplemental feeding, can be cited as one small step in our efforts to determine which factors in the environment have an impact on feeding practices. The distribution of formula samples in the nursery had a statistically significant influence, although it is obviously a relatively small one in the population that was studied. The influence of this form of advertising was greater among the less-educated mothers, suggesting that the more-educated group already had decided how they were going to feed their infants.

"A number of patterns of infant feeding are seen in clinical practice. The spectrum goes from exclusive breast-feeding for at least 6 months, as advocated by the La Leche League, through varying periods of feeding infant formula, to the early introduction of supplemental foods and cow's milk. These patterns are constantly changing and are probably influenced by many different trends in society, both medical and nonmedical. In order to influence the feeding of infants, pediatricians and other professionals must make greater efforts to understand and then utilize the cultural patterns that result in such diverse patterns of infant feeding at the same time that they are demonstrating which ones will promote optimal health in the infant population."

Iron, Zinc, Copper, and Manganese in Infant Formulas

Bo Lönnerdal, Carl L. Keen, Masatoshi Ohtake, and Tsunenobu Tamura
Am. J. Dis. Child. 137:433–437, May 1983   12–5

Currently, the minimum concentrations of trace elements in infant formulas recommended by the Committee on Nutrition of the American Academy of Pediatrics are 1.05 mg/L for iron (maximum, 1.75 mg/L), 3.5 mg/L for zinc, 0.42 mg/L for copper, and 0.035 mg/L for manganese. The concentrations of these trace elements in 53 regular infant formulas and

TABLE 1.—Trace Element Concentrations in Infant Formulas From Different Countries

Country	No. of Samples	Mean Concentration (Range), mg/L			
		Iron	Zinc	Copper	Manganese
United States	14	27.98 (0.17-58.50)	4.28 (0.21-13.48)	0.48 (0.31-0.65)	1.08 (0.20-7.80)
Sweden	12	3.31 (0.76-12.30)	0.82 (0.09-4.66)	0.18 (0.03-0.70)	0.57 (0.00-1.90)
West Germany	12	3.69 (0.06-12.91)	1.87 (0.18-6.20)	0.20 (0.01-1.35)	0.57 (0.00-3.68)
Japan	8	7.71 (5.58-10.35)	1.10 (0.89-1.28)	0.06 (0.02-0.15)	0.06 (0.04-0.13)
The Netherlands	2	3.50 (2.00-5.00)	0.82 (0.44-1.21)	0.28 (0.14-0.43)	0.08 (0.03-0.14)
England	2	5.90 (4.25-7.56)	1.92 (1.35-2.49)	0.14 (0.05-0.23)	0.03 (0.01-0.05)
France	2	5.69 (5.46-5.92)	1.84 (1.03-2.65)	0.12 (0.05-0.20)	0.04 (0.03-0.05)
Norway	1	9.0	2.02	0.25	0.10
Total	**53**	(0.06-58.5)	(0.09-13.5)	(0.01-1.35)	(0.00-7.80)

(Courtesy of Lönnerdal, B., et al.: Am. J. Dis. Child. 137:433–437, May 1983; copyright 1983, American Medical Association.)

TABLE 2.—TRACE ELEMENT CONCENTRATIONS IN SPECIAL
INFANT FORMULAS

Formula	No. of Samples	Mean Concentration (Range), mg/L			
		Iron	Zinc	Copper	Manganese
Soy based	6	6.15 (0.48-16.75)	2.70 (0.42-7.89)	0.69 (0.07-1.45)	1.22 (0.39-2.21)
Medium chain triglyceride	8	4.07 (0.00-9.75)	2.19 (0.48-8.74)	0.47 (0.05-1.32)	0.77 (0.00-2.91)
Low methionine	2	0.81 (5.50-8.12)	1.43 (0.36-2.51)	0.63 (0.03-1.24)	0.25 (0.07-0.43)
Corn based	1	1.51	0.39	0.13	0.17
Low histidine	1	10.87	3.80	1.32	0.74
Low leucine	1	7.50	2.70	1.04	0.21
MSUD*	2	11.41 (7.00-15.82)	2.96 (2.38-3.55)	3.41 (0.91-5.92)	3.16 (0.18-6.15)
Casein hydrolysate	2	10.95 (9.42-12.48)	2.79 (0.98-4.6)	0.47 (0.07-0.87)	0.64 (0.14-1.15)
Premature†	1	19.80	2.21	0.07	0.05
High fat	1	17.33	1.91	0.02	0.12
Low sodium	1	10.58	0.75	0.02	0.01
Low phenylalanine	8	7.53 (0.72-14.60)	3.00 (0.35-6.99)	1.03 (0.06-2.14)	1.24 (0.25-4.39)
Carbohydrate free	7	7.08 (1.59-10.67)	2.69 (0.89-9.21)	0.31 (0.02-1.52)	0.51 (0.07-2.46)
Total	**41**	(0.58-19.80)	(0.35-9.21)	(0.02-5.92)	(0.00-6.15)

*Formula used for patients with maple syrup urine disease.
†Formula used for premature infant.
(Courtesy of Lönnerdal, B., et al.: Am. J. Dis. Child. 137:433–437, May 1983; copyright 1983, American Medical Association.)

41 special infant formulas used for clinical disorders in 8 countries were analyzed.

Wide variations were found in the trace element concentrations of the 53 regular formulas (Table 1). Comparison of these concentrations with the generally accepted values for normal human milk showed that 27 of the formulas were lower in copper than human milk, 17 were lower in zinc, and 8 were lower in iron. In a high percentage of samples the concentrations were lower than the recommended minimum; however, in 6 the iron concentrations were 3 times higher than the recommended safe maximum.

Of the 41 special infant formulas, 16 were lower in copper concentration than human milk, 11 were lower in zinc, 2 were lower in iron, and 2 were lower in manganese (Table 2). None of these special formulas exceeded the recommended maximum concentrations.

In addition to variations in the absolute amounts of trace elements in formulas, ratios between the trace elements showed considerable variation. Although average ratios of zinc-copper, zinc-iron, and iron-manganese in human milk range from 3.3 to 10, 2.5 to 10, and 25 to 100, respectively, ratios in the various formulas ranged from 0.4 to 74, 0.02 to 40, and 0.04 to 425, respectively. Because a high dose of one trace element may reduce the absorption or retention, or both, of another, these differences in ratios may be important.

It is believed that greater attention should be given to the level and bioavailability of trace elements in infant formulas so that additional supplementation is not required.

▶ Quality assurance doesn't—not always, anyway.—F.A.O.

Exclusive Breast-Feeding for 9 Months: Risk of Iron Deficiency

Martti A. Siimes, Leena Salmenperä, and Jaakko Perheentupa (Univ. of Helsinki)
J. Pediatr. 104:196–199, February 1984

12–6

There is some evidence that breast-feeding can prevent or reduce the risk of iron deficiency and that iron supplementation may not be required before age 6 months. The risk of iron deficiency was assessed in healthy full-term infants given no food other than human milk up to age 9 months. A total of 198 infants of healthy mothers, the products of uncomplicated pregnancies and deliveries, were observed for 1 year. The mothers were encouraged to breast-feed their infants exclusively for as long as possible. A total of 169 were breast-fed exclusively for 3 months, 116 for 6 months, and 36 for 9 months. Infants who were weaned before age 3½ months received iron in their formula and in wheat cereal. Some of the breast-feeding mothers received 66 or 266 mg of iron daily in two doses, starting 5 days after delivery.

No breast-fed infant had evidence of anemia or iron deficiency before age 6 months, and hemoglobin concentrations were higher than in control infants at ages 4 and 6 months (Fig 12–6). Eight percent of breast-fed infants had laboratory evidence of iron deficiency at age 6 months. None of the 6 infants given iron had evidence of anemia. Iron status at age 9 months is shown in the table. The degree of maternal iron supplementation

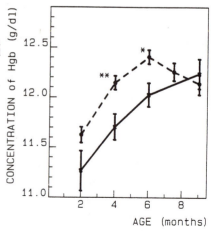

Fig 12–6.—Concentrations of hemoglobin in exclusively breast-fed infants *(broken curve)* and in control subjects *(solid curve)*. Single asterisk indicates $P < .05$; double asterisk denotes $P < .01$. (Courtesy of Siimes, M.A., et al.: J. Pediatr. 104:196–199, February 1984.)

IRON STATUS ACCORDING TO LABORATORY VALUES IN EXCLUSIVELY
BREAST-FED AND IN CONTROL INFANTS AT 9 MONTHS

	Breast-fed (n = 33)	*Controls* (n = 31)	*Breast-fed* (n = 16)	*Breast-fed* (n = 20)
Maternal iron dose (mg/day)	66 to 266		66	266
Age (mo)	9	9	7½	7½
Hemoglobin (gm/dl)	12.1 ± 0.1	12.2 ± 0.1	12.1 ± 0.2	12.1 ± 0.1
MCV	75 ± 0.6	78.0 ± 0.7*	74.0 ± 0.6	76.0 ± 1.2
MCH	26.3 ± 0.3	27.3 ± 0.2*	26.0 ± 0.4	26.8 ± 0.4
Serum iron (μg/dl)	62.0 ± 4.0	77.0 ± 4.0†	54.0 ± 5.0	67.0 ± 5.0
TIBC (μg/dl)	335.0 ± 11.0	296.0 ± 7.0	33.0 ± 15.0	325.0 ± 9.0
Iron saturation (%)	19.0 ± 1.0	26.0 ± 2.0*	16.0 ± 2.0	21.0 ± 2.0
Serum ferritin (μg/L)				
Mean	15	27*	26	27
Range	13 to 17	24 to 29	22 to 30	23 to 32

Two groups of breast-fed infants differing in dose of maternal iron supplementation are also compared, using values at age 7½ mo. These values include those of 6 infants given iron between ages 7½ and 9 mo. Data expressed as mean ± SEM (after log transformation for ferritin). MCH, mean corpuscular hemoglobin; MCV, mean corpuscular volume; TIBC, total iron-binding capacity.
*P < .01, compared with control values.
†P < .05.
(Courtesy of Siimes, M.A., et al.: J. Pediatr. 104:196–199, February 1984.)

during breast-feeding did not influence the iron status of the infants. The mothers of 4 of the 6 iron-supplemented infants had received the higher level of supplementation.

A great majority of exclusively breast-fed infants will maintain their iron status at the same level as control infants given iron supplementation. Maternal iron supplementation during breast-feeding does not prevent iron deficiency in some infants. Iron supplementation may be necessary somewhat earlier in breast-fed infants given solid foods, but exclusively breast-fed infants need not receive supplementation until age 6 months.

▶ This very nice clinical study of 36 infants who were exclusively breast-fed for a period of 9 months should settle the question of the need for iron supplementation in the term infant who is fed human milk. For the first 6 months of life, no iron supplementation is required. Some, but not all, infants who are exclusively breast-fed between 6 and 9 months of age may become iron deficient. It would be prudent to begin an iron supplement, 2 mg/kg/day, or an iron-enriched cereal for the exclusively breast-fed infant by the time the infant is age 9 months.

The ability of human milk, with an iron concentration of 0.3 to 1.0 mg/L, to provide for the iron needs of the growing infant is a direct result of the unique bioavailability of iron in human milk (McMillan, J. A., et al.: *Pediatrics* 58:686, 1976; and Saarinen, U. M., et al.: *J. Pediatr.* 91:36, 1977). At least 50% of it is absorbed. Doctor James Corrigan, of the University of Arizona, tells me that he also has completed a study that demonstrates the capacity of human milk to meet the iron needs of the infant for at least the first 6 months of life.—F.A.O.

Is Warfarin Sodium Contraindicated in the Lactating Mother?

Rajalaxmi McKenna, Edmund R. Cole, and Ushanalini Vasan (Rush-Presbyterian-St. Luke's Med. Center, Chicago)

J. Pediatr. 103:325–327, August 1983   12–7

It is recommended that lactating mothers taking warfarin sodium avoid breast-feeding their infants. However, this advice is not always followed. The findings in two mother-infant pairs studied for evidence of a reduction in Quick prothrombin activity of factor II or VII/X activities are reported. One mother had a long history of recurrent venous thromboembolic disease and began receiving warfarin sodium on the third postpartum day (mother 1). The other also was given warfarin sodium in the early postpartum period because of thromboembolic disease (mother 2). Both took heparin during pregnancy and both had a strong desire to breast-feed their infants despite having been advised against it. The duration of follow-up was 56 days for infant 1 and 131 days for infant 2. Both infants were delivered at full term.

On the three occasions that mother 1 and her infant were studied, the infant's one-stage prothrombin time activity was normal, whereas the mother's was reduced and in the therapeutic range for anticoagulation. There was no spectrophotometric evidence of warfarin sodium in this mother's milk. In mother-infant pair 2, there was no evidence of any biologic effect of warfarin sodium on the infant throughout the follow-up period, even though the infant was entirely breast-fed and gained weight (Fig 12–7). The vitamin K-dependent coagulation factors II and VII/X also remained normal in this infant.

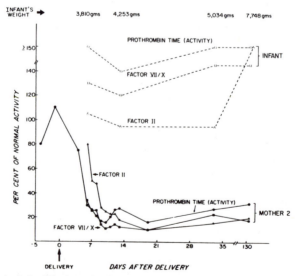

Fig 12–7.—Analysis of blood samples obtained simultaneously from a mother who was given warfarin sodium on the third postpartum day and her breast-fed infant. (Courtesy of McKenna, R., et al.: J. Pediatr. 103:325–327, August 1983.)

The findings indicate that in breast-fed infants whose mothers are given warfarin sodium, the drug has no immediate or delayed biologic effect on coagulation tests. Thus, it would appear that mothers receiving warfarin sodium should be allowed to breast-feed their normal full-term infants. However, this does not necessarily apply to other anticoagulants administered orally.

▶ Another myth is exploded. The warning to avoid warfarin still applies, however, during the later stages of pregnancy. Warfarin crosses the placenta, while heparin does not.
The more things change, the more they stay insane.—F.A.O.

Fatal Intracranial Hemorrhage in a Normal Infant Secondary to Vitamin K Deficiency

Peter A. Lane, William E. Hathaway, John H. Githens, Richard D. Krugman, and Donna A. Rosenberg (Univ. of Colorado)
Pediatrics 72:562–564, October 1983   12–8

An infant was seen with intracranial hemorrhage secondary to vitamin K deficiency.

Male infant, aged 4 weeks, was seen in a community hospital emergency room with a 1-day history of irritability, poor feeding, and decreased responsiveness without fever. Examination revealed pallor, irregular respirations, intermittent bradycardia, posturing, seizures, bulging anterior fontanelle, and excessive bleeding at puncture sites. Hematocrit value was 18%, platelet count was 125,000/μl, and arterial pH was 6.86; lumbar puncture yielded grossly bloody fluid. Initial treatment included intravenous fluids, endotracheal intubation with mechanical ventilation, and administration of Dilantin and phenobarbitol, antibiotics, cardiac drugs, dopamine, mannitol, and prednisolone. One milligram of vitamin K was given intramuscularly before transfer by air ambulance to the University of Colorado Health Sciences Center during which a transfusion of whole blood was given.

Medical history was that of a term vaginal delivery at home. No vitamin K was given. The site of circumcision oozed intermittently and required cauterization. The infant had been exclusively breast-fed and had received no vitamins or medications except amoxicillin prior to this illness.

On admission, the hemoglobin level was 7.1 gm/dl, hematocrit value was 19.3%, white blood cell count was 15,100, platelet count was 185,000/μl, and fibrinogen level was 285 mg/dl. Coagulation factor assays were performed and the abnormal prothrombin or protein induced in the absence of vitamin K was measured. Despite intensive support, the infant died the next day. At autopsy, massive, diffuse hemorrhage was revealed throughout the body without evidence of trauma.

Shortly after admission it was thought that this infant with unexplained retinal and intracranial hemorrhages had suffered nonaccidental trauma. Initial prolongation of prothrombin time (PT) and partial thromboplastin time (PTT) was consistent with disseminated intravascular coagulation secondary to head trauma, acidosis, and shock. When at 10 hours after vitamin K was administered the PT and PTT had corrected without replacement of clotting factors, vitamin K deficiency was suspected. Evaluation of the family indicated that nonaccidental trauma was unlikely.

Deficiency of vitamin K results in a functional defect of clotting factors II, VII, IX, and X with prolongation of PT and PTT. Specific action of vitamin K is the carboxylation of glutamyl residues on these clotting proteins, allowing them to bind Ca^{2+}. In the absence of this carboxylation, proteins are functionally defective. These proteins induced in the absence of vitamin K can be detected by several tests that document vitamin K deficiency and its correction over time after vitamin K is administered.

The incidence of hemorrhagic disease of the newborn was on the increase in exclusively breast-fed babies prior to routine prophylaxis with vitamin K. However, recent studies indicate that these babies are not vitamin K deficient at 1 month when they receive vitamin K at birth. It is thought that until more information becomes available defining the true incidence and risks of this deficiency in newborns, withholding vitamin K prophylaxis is ill advised. The clinician should also be alert to the possibility of vitamin K-deficient hemorrhage in older children.

▶ We mentioned James Corrigan in a comment just a while back. Now here he is, to speak for himself. Doctor Corrigan is Professor of Pediatrics and Chief, Section of Pediatric Hematology-Oncology at the University of Arizona. He writes:

"Doctor Lane and associates add another case to the growing list of infants with hemorrhage due to vitamin K deficiency outside the immediate newborn period. These patients are usually younger than age 6 months and have in common breast-feeding, intracranial hemorrhage, and either gastroenteritis or the use of antibiotics. They may or may not have received vitamin K prophylactically at birth. In the past 10 years, a vast majority of the cases (>90%) have been in exclusively breast-fed babies. Intracranial hemorrhage has been common, ranging from 25% to 65% of the cases. The case presented by Lane et al. is classic in that the infant had been noted to have bruising for about 2 weeks, then a fatal central nervous system hemorrhage; all this on a background of no vitamin K supplementation at birth, bleeding at circumcision, breast-feeding, and a 1-week course of amoxicillin therapy. In this case there was no reason to suspect a fat malabsorption disorder.

"Of the acquired coagulopathies, vitamin K deficiency easily can be diagnosed using standard, readily available, laboratory studies. These patients have a normal platelet count, normal plasma fibrinogen level, and greatly prolonged prothrombin time and partial thromboplastin time. Assays for specific coagulation factors and for PIVKA (proteins induced in vitamin K's absence or antagonists) are only needed when the diagnosis is uncertain or clouded by other possibilities (such as disseminated intravascular coagulation, liver disease, or the more rare congenital deficiency states). The techniques available to detect PIVKA are best described for prothrombin (factor II). The PIVKA II (or preprothrombin, precursor prothrombin, and others) can be measured directly or indirectly using immunologic or coagulation techniques. Both PIVKA II and factor II are antigenically similar and each can generate thrombin after activation with certain snake venoms (*Echis carinatus* and *Dipholidus typus*); only factor II will generate thrombin after the addition of physiologic activators (such as thromboplastin). The direct method employs removal of factor II by barium absorption, then measurement of the residual amount (PIVKA II) in the supernant by immunoprecipitation (using anti-factor II antibody) or by clotting activity using snake venom. The indirect method uses measurement of plasma PIVKA II and factor II by immunologic precipitation (called 'prothrombin antigen or protein level') or by venom clotting activity. Functional factor II is then measured by a standard assay using thromboplastin as the prothrombin activator. The difference between the levels obtained immunologically (or by snake venom assay) and the thromboplastin assay represents the nonfunctional factor II (i.e., PIVKA II; also called 'nonfunctional component of prothrombin protein') (*JAMA* 248:1736, 1982).

"This case also points out that what appears to be nonaccidental trauma doesn't necessarily have to be; delay in the diagnosis of vitamin K deficiency coagulopathy will only result in a disasterous outcome. Management of this condition consists of fresh-frozen plasma (15 mg/kg) infusion and intravenous, not intramuscular, administration of vitamin K. This patient had a severe coagulopathy and shock; an intramuscular injection can cause a local hematoma and the hematoma plus shock could cause delayed absorption of the vitamin. Prothrombin complex concentrates are rarely needed in this clinical setting."

"Nursing Bottle Caries" in Breast-Fed Children

Michael Brams and Joseph Maloney (Valley Pediatric Center, Apple Valley, Calif.)
J. Pediatr. 103:415–416, September 1983   12–9

The authors report the cases of 3 breast-fed infants who had rampant caries similar to those described in infants who suck on a bottle while sleeping.

CASE 1.—Boy, aged 15 months, had plaque buildup and severe pitting of all 4 maxillary incisors, primarily on the lingual surface. The mandibular incisors and molars were normal. The boy, in good general health, had been exclusively breastfed for 6 months, at which time solid foods were added to the diet. A bottle was never used, but the boy slept each night with his mother, nursing at will.

CASE 2.—Girl, aged 30 months, had extensive caries with circumferential decalcification of the upper incisors but sparing of the lower incisors and canines. She did not sleep with her mother but nursed at bedtime and usually twice during the night. Full-mouth reconstruction was scheduled.

CASE 3.—Girl, aged 9 months, had mottled mandibular incisors. She had slept with her mother since birth and nursed throughout the night, often staying at the breast for many hours. By age 16 months the maxillary incisors were severely decayed and caries were noted in the lower incisors and molars. Full-mouth reconstruction under general anesthesia was performed at age 18 months.

To prevent these early dental changes, continuous nocturnal nursing patterns should be discouraged, as should frequent, intermittent night feedings after the age of 1 year. Total weaning is probably a drastic step.

▶ We feel obliged to bring you both the good news and the bad news about breast-feeding. The good news pertained to growth rate, anti-infective properties, and iron nutrition. The bad news, this time, involved vitamin K deficiency and, in this instance, dental caries. There are two sides to breast-feeding. The authors of this piece—Brams and Maloney—should have told us what the mothers' breasts looked like with all this prolonged breast-feeding in the presence of so many teeth.—F.A.O.

Randomized Trial of Sodium Intake and Blood Pressure in Newborn Infants

Albert Hofman, Alice Hazebroek, and Hans A. Valkenburg (Erasmus Univ., Rotterdam, The Netherlands)
JAMA 250:370–373, July 15, 1983   12–10

The view that high intake of sodium contributes to high blood pressure (BP) is old, but it remains controversial. The effect of dietary sodium on BP was assessed in a double-blind trial of 245 infants randomly assigned to a normal-sodium diet and 231 infants assigned to a low-sodium diet during the first 6 months of life.

Both groups showed an increase in systolic BP with age, although the increase was smaller in the low-sodium group (Table 1). At age 25 weeks, systolic BP was 2 mm Hg lower in infants on a low-sodium diet (Table 2). The difference between the two groups over time showed a linear trend that was significantly different from zero. When the differences were adjusted for slightly different distributions of weight and length at birth, BP observers, and systolic BP in the first week, values slightly greater than the observed values were obtained, with systolic BP 2.1 mm Hg lower in the low-sodium group at age 25 weeks. Significant increases in the adjusted differences were also observed during the first 6 months of life.

The results support the view that sodium intake is causally related to

---

TABLE 1.—MEAN SYSTOLIC BP OF TWO SODIUM GROUPS

	BP, mm Hg					
	Normal-Sodium Group			Low-Sodium Group		
Week	n	Mean	SD	n	Mean	SD
1	245	87.7	19.7	231	87.0	19.5
5	243	101.9	18.6	227	102.5	19.0
9	237	108.8	14.8	227	108.3	14.9
13	243	111.9	13.4	228	111.3	13.7
17	234	113.4	13.6	224	112.4	11.9
21	241	114.9	11.0	224	113.5	12.2
25	241	116.1	11.2	225	114.1	11.9

TABLE 2.—Differences in Mean Systolic BP Between Study Groups at Various Occasions

Normal-Sodium Group Minus Low-Sodium Group, mm Hg

	Observed Difference		Adjusted Difference*	
Week	Mean	90% CI†	Mean	90% CI
1	0.7	−2.3–3.7	‡	
5	−0.6	−3.4–2.2	−0.4	−2.1–2.9
9	0.5	−1.8–2.8	0.4	−1.7–2.5
13	0.7	−1.4–2.8	0.6	−1.4–2.6
17	1.0	−1.0–3.0	1.2	−0.6–3.0
21	1.4	−0.4–3.2	1.7	0.0–3.4
25	2.0	0.2–3.8	2.1	0.5–3.7

*Adjusted for observers, weight and length at birth, and systolic BP in first week.
†Indicates 90% confidence interval.
‡Systolic BP in first week is a determinant in model.
(Courtesy of Hofman, A., et al.: JAMA 250:370–373, July 15, 1983; copyright 1983, American Medical Association.)

BP levels. Moderation of sodium intake during the very early stages of life may contribute to the prevention of high BP and of increases in BP with age.

▶ An encore for Lewis Barness. We asked for a commentary, and he sends us questions. Doctor Barness writes:

"This study is interesting and challenging. According to my calculations, the low-sodium group of infants consumed about 1 gm of salt a day and the high-sodium group, about 3 gm. Would a lesser difference in intake still cause a significant difference in blood pressure? Does this magnitude of difference cause a different imprinting of taste? The authors claim that the differences in blood pressures will persist, but what if the diets change and all children go on a low-sodium diet? This is an exciting area for further studies."

Oral Zinc Therapy for Wilson's Disease

George J. Brewer, Gretchen M. Hill, Ananda S. Prasad, Zafrallah T. Cossack, and Parviz Rabbani
Ann. Int. Med. 99:314–320, September 1983   12–11

Wilson's disease is an autosomal, recessively inherited, inborn error involving abnormal copper handling by the liver that is fatal if untreated. Present treatment involves use of penicillamine to "decopper" patients. Penicillamine is relatively toxic, causing sensitivity reactions in about 30% of patients; 10% cannot take the drug at all. Because of the low toxicity of zinc and the observation that administration of zinc for sickle cell anemia routinely induced copper deficiency, oral zinc was experimentally used for Wilson's disease in 5 patients.

The zinc regimen involved administration of 25 mg of zinc acetate every 4 hours during the day and 50 mg at bedtime; no food was allowed 1 hour before and after zinc ingestion. After initial tests with this regimen, it was decided to pretreat patients for 3 weeks before the study. This modification resulted in a negative copper balance of -0.42 mg/day over 18 days in 1 patient and of -0.44 mg/day over 8 days in another patient. The other 3 patients also showed a negative copper balance if the pretreatment period was long enough to build up zinc stores. When copper excretion and copper balance achieved on penicillamine therapy (1.0 gm/day) were compared with those achieved on zinc therapy after zinc pretreatment, the patient achieved a negative copper balance of -0.19 mg/day on penicillamine by excreting an average of 0.54 mg of copper per day in stool and 0.48 mg/day in urine. While receiving zinc therapy, the patient achieved a negative copper balance of 0.42 mg/day by excreting 1.52 mg of copper per day in stool and an insignificant amount in urine.

It is thought that the delay between the beginning of zinc therapy and the blocking of copper absorption depends on the time required for the body to induce production of metallothionein, which depends on the body's zinc status. The more zinc deficient a patient has been rendered by penicillamine therapy, the longer will be the time before zinc therapy inhibits copper absorption.

Zinc therapy is considered acceptable in patients who have been decoppered sufficiently to eliminate danger of acute copper toxicity and in whom further use of penicillamine is a major risk. Compliance should be monitored and 24-hour urinary copper levels should be measured every 3 months. Liver biopsy with copper assays, if practical, is ideal to observe patients until this therapy and patient variability in response are fully understood. Zinc therapy may also be considered for pregnant women with Wilson's disease.

It seems that zinc does more than block dietary copper uptake; it also inhibits the reabsorption of nonbiliary, endogenously secreted copper. However, until zinc has been tested as an agent for initial decoppering, the use of zinc for this purpose in acutely ill patients with Wilson's disease is not recommended.

Effects of Untreated Maternal Phenylketonuria and Hyperphenylalaninemia on the Fetus
Harvey L. Levy and Susan E. Waisbren
N. Engl. J. Med. 309:1269–1274, Nov. 24, 1983   12–12

The authors studied the effects of maternal phenylketonuria and hyperphenylalaninemia on 53 offspring from untreated pregnancies in 22 white mothers who were identified by routine screening of umbilical cord blood. Out of a total of 59 untreated pregnancies that occurred in these 22 women, 6 ended in spontaneous abortion. This rate of 10% was lower than the 15%–20% frequency expected in the general population.

Blood levels of phenylalanine in the 22 mothers ranged from 165 to 1,370 μmole/L. Complications occurred in 5 pregnancies (9%). Perinatal complications occurred in 3 births (6%) and included a nuchal cord in 2 infants and an irregular heartbeat in 1.

TABLE 1.—CORRELATION BETWEEN MATERNAL AND
OFFSPRING CHARACTERISTICS IN MATERNAL PHENYLKETONURIA
AND HYPERPHENYLALANINEMIA*

| | | MOTHERS | | |
		IQ	BLOOD PHENYLALANINE LEVEL	BLOOD TYROSINE LEVEL
OFFSPRING	IQ	r = 0.83 P<0.001 (n = 26)	r = −0.82 P<0.001 (n = 28)	r = 0.42 P = 0.013 (n = 28)
	Head circumference at birth	r = 0.24 P = NS (n = 25)	r = −0.49 P = 0.003 (n = 30)	r = 0.19 P = NS (n = 30)
	Birth weight	r = 0.002 P = NS (n = 27)	r = −0.17 P = NS (n = 33)	r = 0.30 P = 0.047 (n = 33)

*NS = not significant.
(Courtesy of Levy, H.L., and Waisbren, S.E.: N. Engl. J. Med. 309:1269–1274, Nov. 24, 1983. Reprinted by permission of the New England Journal of Medicine.)

Of the 53 offspring, 6 (11%) had either phenylketonuria or hyperphenylalaninemia. Three of the 4 children born to mothers with classic phenylketonuria had IQ scores between 64 and 69 (mild retardation) and the fourth scored 84 (borderline intelligence). Mean IQ in 13 children of mothers with atypical phenylketonuria was 95.2. One of the 13 had an IQ of 69. In children born to mothers with classic phenylketonuria, visual-motor coordination was more than 2 years below age level. Only 1 of the 53 children had congenital heart disease. Maternal characteristics were correlated with IQ, head circumference at birth, and birth weight in off-

TABLE 2.—MATERNAL BLOOD PHENYLALANINE LEVEL
AND IQ IN FAMILIES WITH MATERNAL
PHENYLKETONURIA OR HYPERPHENYLALANINEMIA IN
WHICH PATERNAL IQ SCORE WAS OBTAINED

| FAMILY | IQ | | | MATERNAL BLOOD PHENYLALANINE LEVEL |
	OFFSPRING	MOTHER	FATHER	μmol per liter
A	69	45	104	1370
B	84	94	124	1262
C	103, 92	101	125	830
D	138, 130	115	134	245
E	95	91	79	240

(Courtesy of Levy, H.L., and Waisbren, S.E.: N. Engl. J. Med. 309:1269–1274, Nov. 24, 1983. Reprinted by permission of the New England Journal of Medicine.)

spring: Table 1 indicates that IQ in offspring was significantly correlated with all three maternal characteristics. A significant correlation was found between head circumference and IQ. Three of the 4 children born to mothers with classic phenylketonuria had microcephaly at birth. In 4 of 5 families with available IQs for the father, the IQ scores of the offspring were much closer to maternal IQ than to paternal IQ (Table 2).

Classic and severe atypical forms of maternal phenylketonuria appear to have a substantial adverse effect on the fetus. Women with these disorders should be treated with a low-phenylalanine diet during pregnancy, preferably beginning before conception. The results of this study indicate that mild hyperphenylalaninemia in the mother may not damage the fetus. The data suggest there may be no effect from a less severe degree of atypical phenylketonuria on the fetus or the effect may be subtle, resulting in slight reduction in IQ and intrauterine head growth.

Dietary Management of Phenylketonuria From Birth by Using a Phenylalanine-Free Product

David B. Flannery, Elizabeth Hitchcock, and Peter Mamunes (Richmond, Va.)
J. Pediatr. 103:247–249, August 1983   12–13

Early experience with Phenylfree, a phenylalanine (PA)-free dietary product, was analyzed retrospectively in the management of 8 infants with phenylketonuria (PKU). The findings were compared with those for 8 other infants with PKU who were fed a Lofenalac-based formula that contains 0.8 mg of PA per gram of powder.

Both groups accepted and tolerated the products and both showed normal growth and mental development. At 6 months of age, the infants fed Phenylfree had significantly lower mean serum levels of PA than infants in the Lofenalac group (table). This difference was observed as late as age 24 months. In addition, infants fed Phenylfree had significantly fewer instances of serum PA values outside the desired range (68 of 276, 25%) than those fed Lofenalac (111 of 318, 35%). Calculated protein intake was within the normal range in both groups, but was about 20% higher

---

COMPARISON OF MEAN INDICES OF DIETARY CONTROL IN INFANTS*

Age (mo)	Mean daily protein intake (gm/kg body weight)		Mean serum PA (mg/dl ± 1 SD)		P
	Phenylfree	Lofenalac	Phenylfree	Lofenalac	
0 to 6	3.3	3.1	4.5 ± 2.9 (n = 145)	7.2 ± 6.4 (n = 147)	< 0.001
6 to 12	3.0	2.3	4.0 ± 2.4 (n = 29)	6.9 ± 3.8 (n = 85)	< 0.001
12 to 18	2.6	2.3	2.9 ± 1.2 (n = 36)	5.5 ± 2.7 (n = 47)	< 0.001
18 to 24	2.6	2.3	5.9 ± 4.4 (n = 16)	8.0 ± 4.0 (n = 39)	< 0.1
0 to 24	2.9	2.5	4.4 ± 2.9 (n = 276)	7.0 ± 5.1 (n = 318)	< 0.001

*n = number of individual measurements.
(Courtesy of Flannery, D.B., et al.: J. Pediatr. 103:247–249, August 1983.)

in those fed Phenylfree. Mean serum osmolality of patients fed Phenylfree was 289 mOsm/kg water, which is within the range for infants.

The results suggest that Phenylfree can be used as effectively as Lofenalac in the dietary treatment of infants with PKU. However, physicians should be aware that potentially dangerous hypophenylalaninemia can rapidly develop when Phenylfree is used without phenylalanine supplementation.

▶ Fran J. Rohr and Harvey L. Levy prepared the following commentary. Doctor Levy, of Harvard Medical School, is Director of the IEM-PKU Program.

"Less than a generation ago, it was virtually impossible to go through medical school without exposure to a mentally retarded person with phenylketonuria (PKU). At least one, if not several, pediatric rounds and perhaps even a medical grand rounds would feature PKU as the prime example of a disease that devastated the cognitive centers of the brain. A pathetically retarded child with no speech and almost uncontrollably hyperactive behavior would be shown.

"Today most medical students and even physicians 10 years out of medical school have never seen a retarded phenylketonuric individual. The reason? Newborn screening and early dietary treatment for PKU that have essentially eliminated mental retardation from this disease. This is a truly remarkable achievement in medicine.

"Thus, we now are beyond the controversies of the 1960s about whether newborn screening is justified and whether the diet prevents mental retardation. New issues are raised, such as whether the diet can be safely discontinued in childhood or must be continued even into adulthood, whether maternal PKU and its effects on the fetus can be controlled, and which of the several available diets is the best one for the treatment of PKU.

"It is the last issue with which this article is concerned. Until recently, the special formulas that are the basis of PKU therapy were hydrolysates of milk protein (casein) or albumin from which most of the free phenylalanine was removed. Since these preparations contain some phenylalanine, however, the amount of natural protein allowed in the diet is quite limited. New formulas that contain no phenylalanine are now available. These phenylalanine-free preparations are elemental, consisting of free amino acids mixed together. Their advantage lies in providing a source of protein equivalents without phenylalanine so that a larger amount of natural protein can be ingested by the child.

"Phenylfree, the phenylalanine-free product developed by Mead Johnson, has not been recommended for the treatment of PKU during the first 2 years of life because its higher osmolality and somewhat different vitamin and mineral content than low-phenylalanine formulas have been considered inappropriate for infants. Now, Flannery, Hitchcock, and Mamunes have shown that infants with PKU not only tolerate Phenylfree without difficulty but seem to maintain better blood phenylalanine level control than those receiving the low-phenylalanine formula Lofenalac. This and the fact that phenylalanine-free formulas allow the infant to receive more natural protein (e.g., breast milk, infant formula, or solid foods) in the diet indicate that these formulas (including PKU-1 of the Milupa Corporation) could become the treatment of choice for infants as well as older children with PKU."

Sialic Acid Storage Disease With Sialuria: Clinical and Biochemical Features in the Severe Infantile Type

Roger E. Stevenson, Mark Lubinsky, Harold A. Taylor, David A. Wenger, Richard J. Schroer, and P. M. Olmstead
Pediatrics 72:441–449, October 1983
12–14

Two infants were seen with a new disorder characterized biochemically by elevated levels of free sialic acid in urine, serum, and cell lysates. Three other biochemically diagnosed cases and 2 possible cases have appeared in the literature (table).

Clinical findings present at birth or soon after include facial coarsening, hypopigmentation and sparseness of the hair (Fig 12–8), hepatosplenomegaly, diarrhea, anemia, profound inactivity, slow growth, and severe mental and physical impairment. Osseous stippling may be present, and clear vacuoles may be demonstrated in lymphocytes and cultured fibroblasts. The course is one of relentless deterioration, with death in early childhood.

In both new cases, urinary excretion of free sialic acid was increased

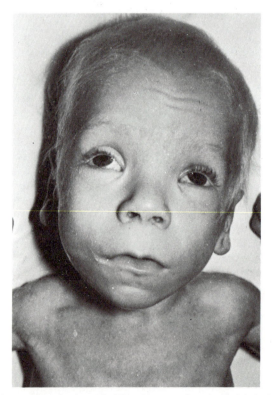

Fig 12–8.—Infant, aged 16 months, with sialic acid storage disease with sialuria. Note coarse facies with prominent philtrum, divergent strabismus, and sparse, fine hair. (Courtesy of Stevenson, R.E., et al.: Pediatrics 72:441–449, October 1983. Copyright American Academy of Pediatrics 1983.)

CLINICAL FEATURES IN FIVE INFANTS WITH SIALIC ACID STORAGE DISEASE WITH SIALURIA AND TWO POSSIBLE CASES FROM LITERATURE

	This Report		Hancock et al	Tondeur et al		Crocker and Farber*	Lachman et al*
	Case 1	Case 2		Case 1	Case 2		
Sex	M	F	M	M	F	M	M
Ancestry	Unknown	German	German-Swedish	Yugoslavian	Yugoslavian	Unknown	Unknown
Birth weight	3.1 kg	3.1 kg	...	2.2 kg	1.8 kg	2.7 kg	...
Growth retardation	Yes	Yes	Unknown	Yes	Yes	Yes	Unknown
Mental retardation	Severe	Severe	Probable	Severe	Severe	Probable	Unknown
Hepatosplenomegaly	Yes	Yes	Yes	Yes	Yes	Yes	Unknown
Hypopigmentation	Yes	Yes	Unknown	Yes	Yes	Yes	Unknown
Coarse facies	Yes	Yes	Unknown	Yes	Yes	Yes	Unknown
Radiologic abnormality	Yes	Yes	No	No	No	Yes	Yes
Punctate calcification	No	Yes	No	No	No	Yes	Yes
Diarrhea	Yes	No	Unknown	Unknown	Unknown	Yes	Yes
Anemia	Yes	Yes	Unknown	Yes	Yes	Yes	Unknown
Circulating storage cells (light microscopy)	Yes	Yes	Unknown	Yes	No	Yes	Unknown
Other problems	Recurrent pneumonias	Pneumonia	Neonatal ascites	Inguinal hernia, pneumonias	Rickets, pneumonias	...	...
Course	Died 3.3 yr	Profound delay 8 mo	Died 5 mo	"Terminal" 4.5 yr	Bedridden 2 yr	Died 4 mo	Died 8 mo

*These cases are from older literature and have no biochemical data included; they were described as cases of atypical Niemann-Pick disease.
(Courtesy of Stevenson, R.E., et al.: Pediatrics 72:441–449, October 1983. Copyright American Academy of Pediatrics 1983.)

20- to 60-fold. Free sialic acid levels also were elevated in serum leukocytes, cultured fibroblasts, and liver. No lysosomal hydrolase deficiencies were found. On the contrary, increased activities were found for sialidase, α-mannosidase, β-N-acetylglucosaminidase, α-fucosidase, and β-glucuronidase.

The infantile form of sialic acid storage disease with sialuria may be suspected on the basis of clinical findings present at or soon after birth. The diagnosis depends on demonstration of elevated urinary and tissue levels of free sialic acid. The condition should be included in the differential diagnosis of any patient with undiagnosed clinical features of the lysosomal storage disorders. It is not detected by routine urine metabolic screening tests; a specific assay for free sialic acid is necessary. Prenatal diagnosis may be possible by measuring sialic acid in amniocytes and amniotic fluid.

▶ A powerful clue in these patients is the presence of vacuolated lymphocytes in the peripheral blood. This is by no means a specific diagnostic finding, but it should serve to arouse your suspicions. Speaking of having your suspicions aroused, always be suspicious when a man dressed in Arab robes comes into your office carrying a suitcase full of money and offers you a million dollars in cash for a prescription for Robitussin with codeine. There may be a scam in the making.—F.A.O.

13 The Musculoskeletal System

Cardiac Involvement in Juvenile Rheumatoid Arthritis: A Follow-up Study
Helena Svantesson, Gudrun Björkhem, and Renate Elborgh (Univ. Hosp., Lund, Sweden)
Acta Pediatr. Scand. 72:345–350, May 1983   13–1

The authors attempted to determine if residual cardiac abnormalities can be detected by echocardiography in children during remission. A series of 320 patients with juvenile rheumatoid arthritis (JRA) were observed over 10 years; 33(10.3%) had systemic-onset disease and 15 (4.7%) had cardiac involvement. Age of these 15 patients ranged from 4 to 22 years, follow-up period from first signs of cardiac involvement was 1–16 years, and from last attack of pericarditis or myocarditis 1–12 years.

Primary diagnosis of cardiac involvement was based on clinical symptoms, ECG chest x-ray study, and (in 9 patients) echocardiography. The 10 patients with pericarditis had remittent fever, constant tachycardia, dyspnea, and a friction rub. The 2 patients with myocarditis had moderate fever, ECG showed inverted T waves and a chest x-ray study indicated moderate cardiac enlargement. There were 2 patients with perimyocarditis. One with valvulitis had no clinical symptoms but an impressive murmur of aortic regurgitation; chest x-ray study showed enlargement of the left ventricle.

In 9 patients (60%) recurrent episodes of clinically evident pericarditis or myocarditis occurred (Fig 13–1). Usually such attacks lasted 1–12 weeks, but in 1 girl the pericardial effusion remained for 3 years with only short remissions.

All patients were treated with corticosteroids (between 0.5 and 2 mg/kg/day) and 2 patients, additionally with cytostatic drugs. Response to treatment was rapid in most cases, but weaning from steroids was often associated with flare-up of the disease.

At the final follow-up, echocardiographic findings of the 10 patients with pericarditis showed 1 with a hypertrophic left ventricular wall and 1 with dilated aortic root. Of the 2 patients with myocarditis 1 had evidence of impaired left ventricular function. Of the 2 patients with perimyocarditis, 1 each showed impaired ventricular function and a dilated left ventricle.

Cardiac involvement can begin concomitantly with or even precede arthritis; the highest risk of carditis was during the first 3 years. Risk of relapsing episodes was greatest during the first 5 years. Prognosis of pericarditis seems to be good because no patient developed cardiac tamponade or constrictive pericarditis. Prognosis in myocarditis and perimyocarditis

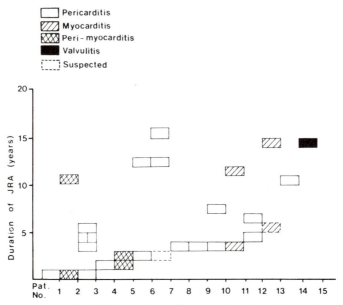

Fig 13–1.—Duration of JRA before cardiac involvement and number of relapses for the different patients. (Courtesy of Svantesson, H., et al.: Acta Pediatr. Scand. 72:345–350, May 1983.)

seems to be less favorable, because only 1 of 4 patients in these groups had a normal echocardiogram. In valvulitis, the prognosis must depend on which valve is involved and to what extent.

Early use of corticosteroids in systemic cases can be important in preventing occurrence of manifest cardiac symptoms if asymptomatic carditis is suppressed.

▶ Cardiac complications can be among the most disastrous problems that children with juvenile rheumatoid arthritis (JRA) face. Pericarditis is not the major difficulty, although it is the most common cardiac complication, with a reported occurrence as frequent as 7% to 10% in children with JRA. This should not be expected to cause cardiac tamponade or constrictive pericarditis. The major problem is with myocarditis, which can lead to congestive heart failure and death during flareups of cardiac involvement with JRA. The treatment of choice is steroids. The problem with cardiac involvement in JRA is that it can be the initial presentation of the systemic, more generalized, disorder. When this type of presentation occurs, one rarely thinks of JRA as being the culprit. Usually various viruses, etc., are implicated and there may be a reluctance to use steroids. We clinicians constantly must be aware of this potential happenstance. Recently, 3 cases were reported in which cardiac problems were the initial manifestation of JRA (*Pediatrics* 73:394, 1984). Indeed, included among these cases is the first clearly documented presentation of JRA as myocarditis. These patients presented with very typical signs of chest pain and shortness of breath along with tachypnea, gallop, and a friction rub.

As suggested in this study by Svantesson et al., the outlook for cardiac involvement in JRA is quite good if it is limited to pericarditis. The prognosis may be guarded if the myocardium is involved.

We gradually are learning more and more about some of the basic facts of JRA. Indeed, for the first time we actually may have a handle on exactly how often this problem presents itself. In a very detailed prevalence study in New York, it has been estimated that one should expect to see 0.5 case of JRA per 1,000 children. Thus, in the average solo practice of pediatrics, it is even money that you should be taking care of a child with JRA. Based on the 1980 census data, these numbers translate into approximately 32,000 children in the United States with JRA (Gewanter, H. L., et al.: *Arthritis Rheum.* 26:599, 1983). We also are getting some information about the long-term prognosis in children with JRA who have systemic onset of disease. In a study reported from Sweden (*Scand. J. Rheumatol.* 12:139, 1983), 33 patients with systemic-onset JRA were followed for up to 24 years. None of these patients ever developed positive rheumatoid factors or antinuclear antibodies. Most ultimately developed polyarthritis. Cardiac involvement eventually occurred in 42% of the patients. As was noted in the reports previously mentioned, cardiac prognosis was good for pericarditis but seemed to be worse for myocarditis. About 10% of patients ultimately developed renal amyloidosis. Severe growth retardation was observed in 40% of the patients. The average time to complete remission of the disease was 6 years from the time of diagnosis in those who did achieve a remission. Two thirds of the patients were in a good functional state and the best prognosis was seen when the progression of disease was fairly limited in the first 5 years of diagnosis and when the disease was diagnosed after age 5. These are very important observations because of the long-term follow-up.

While on the subject of pericarditis and arthritis, I would call to your attention a new syndrome of familial pericarditis, arthritis, and camptodactyly. This appeared as an autosomal recessive disorder in 5 siblings in one family (*N. Engl. J. Med.* 309:224, 1983). This disorder appears to be distinctly unique from JRA, but we should think of it any time we see a patient with flexion contractures of the fingers. While on the topic of camptodactyly, it should be mentioned that *Campylobacter* infection can cause an arthritic pattern virtually identical clinically in some cases to JRA (please pardon the flight of free association between camptodactyly and *Campylobacter*). In many patients with arthritis secondary to *Campylobacter* infection the joints themselves are sterile and the arthritis is thought to be an immune complex reactive phenomenon. Although it has been suggested that HLA-B27-positive persons might be more prone to this sort of reactive arthritis after infection with Campylobacter, this HLA type is not uniformly present (Johnsen, K., et al.: *Acta Med. Scand.* 214:165, 1983). It was nice to think that being prone to arthritis in general might be a consequence of having HLA-B27, but this association was based on scattered and anecdotal reports with respect to *Campylobacter*. "For example," in such cases, as the saying goes, is not proof.—J.A.S., III

Children With Juvenile Chronic Arthritis: Their Beliefs About Their Illness and Therapy

J. Gerald Beales, P. J. Lennox Holt, John H. Keen, and Valerie P. Mellor (Manchester, England)
Ann. Rheum. Dis. 42:481–486, October 1983   13–2

Seventy-five patients, aged 7–17 years, with juvenile chronic arthritis were interviewed to identify their beliefs about the physical nature of their illness and the relevance and modes of action of their clinical treatment. Forty-eight patients were girls. Thirty-nine children were aged 7–11 and 36 were aged 12–17.

A broad difference was discerned between the beliefs and concepts of children aged 7–11 years and those aged 12–17 years. A large majority of those in the 7–11 age group perceived arthritis in terms of its immediate, concrete manifestations. Only 5 children in this age group perceived the subjective feelings, surface appearance, and restricted motor capacity as consequences of some internal pathologic condition. The children in the younger age group generally judged the relevance and likely effectiveness of therapy according to its directly recognizable effect on what they perceived the disease to be. The table shows some of these beliefs. In the group aged 7–11, injections were more frequently seen to constitute physical assault on the body, adding to total discomfort. Younger children assumed that recovery of a damaged limb was contingent on the affected part being rested and left undisturbed. No one in this younger group had any conception why having blood taken was necessary.

Children in the older age group generally understood that treatment that was unpleasant could have a long-term benefit on their condition. About two thirds of the children in this group perceived arthritis as a state of internal pathologic change and recognized the signs and symptoms as consequences of damage existing out of sight. The pathologic condition that was imagined was frequently more extreme than was in fact the case.

This study indicates that children aged 7–11 and those aged 12–17 require explanations of their arthritis for different reasons and that they also require qualitatively different types of explanations. Although a significant difference was found between the two age groups, there was an appreciable overlap, so that it cannot be assumed that any 12-year-old patient can cope with a "textbook" description or that any 10-year-old requires the use of analogies. If clinicians are to tackle the problem of explaining juvenile chronic arthritis to their young patients with any degree of confidence, simple and reliable means of identifying the child's level of cognitive development in relation to the disease must be found.

▶ Although a child's belief about the physical nature of his or her illness greatly influences the amount of emotional stress experienced and even perhaps the willingness to comply with therapy, there has been hardly any systematic investigation of how patients of different ages with juvenile rheumatoid arthritis (JRA) (in this study called by the now modern term "juvenile chronic arthritis") perceive the condition. Such studies as this are important because secondary

BELIEFS ABOUT VALUE OF TREATMENTS*

If you have arthritis:	Is more likely to: make you better		make you worse		p
	7–11	*12–17*	*7–11*	*12–17*	
Taking nice-tasting medicine	39 (100%)	30 (83%)	0 (0%)	6 (17%)	0·024
Taking nasty-tasting medicine	19 (49%)	31 (86%)	20 (51%)	5 (14%)	0·002
Swallowing tablets	23 (59%)	28 (78%)	16 (41%)	8 (22%)	NS
Having injections	11 (28%)	20 (56%)	28 (72%)	16 (44%)	0·028
Doing exercises	24 (62%)	29 (81%)	15 (38%)	7 (19%)	NS
Wearing splints	22 (56%)	24 (67%)	17 (44%)	12 (33%)	NS
	Yes		*No*		p
	7–11	*12–17*	*7–11*	*12–17*	
Having blood taken helps the doctor to make you better	19 (49%)	29 (81%)	20 (51%)	7 (19%)	0·009

*(Courtesy of Beales, J.G., et al.: Ann. Rheum. Dis. 42:481–486, October 1983.)

emotional problems can make this disorder much more difficult to treat, and some investigators have felt that part of the cure of this disorder is a "self-cure" with final eradication of the underlying immunologic problem. It is only honest to say that not much is known in this regard. For example, an unrelated observation is the fact that a paralyzed extremity in a child with JRA is not likely to be affected with joint disease. The same is true of osteoarthritis and of gout. Recently, an 8-year-old girl with paraplegia resulting from a high lumbar meningomyelocele was described who had severe JRA with practically every joint involved except for the paralyzed lower extremities (Hepworth, R. C.: *Pediatrics* 73:400, 1984). There is no easy explanation to these series of observations, although the immobility of a paralyzed joint is suspected to be the protector of these joints. It should not be concluded from these cases that children with JRA should have immobilization as part of the therapeutic management. Generally, this significantly worsens the preservation of joint function, as pointed out by a commentary in *Pediatrics* (73:402, 1984).—J.A.S., III

Significance of a Positive Antinuclear Antibody Test in a Pediatric Population

David S. Chudwin, Arthur J. Ammann, Morton J. Cowan, and Diane W. Wara
Am. J. Dis. Child. 137:1103–1106, November 1983   13-3

Data on 1,442 patients seen at the Pediatric Immunology/Rheumatology Clinic, Univ. of California, San Francisco, was reviewed retrospectively. Of 138 patients younger than age 18 years who had a positive antinuclear antibody (ANA) test, 91 had specific autoimmune or rheumatic diseases (table).

DIAGNOSIS OF PEDIATRIC PATIENTS WITH POSITIVE ANTINUCLEAR
ANTIBODY TESTS

Diagnosis	No. of Patients	F	M	ANA Pattern		
				Diffuse	Speckled	Other
Systemic lupus erythematosus	37	30	7	25	9	3
Discoid lupus	2	2	0	1	1	0
Juvenile rheumatoid arthritis **Subtotal**	**33**	**26**	**7**	**18**	**12**	**3**
Pauciarticular, early onset (type 1)	19	17	2	11	7	1
Pauciarticular, late onset (type 2)	3	0	3	1	1	1
Polyarticular, positive rheumatoid factor	3	3	0	2	1	0
Polyarticular, negative rheumatoid factor	6	4	2	2	3	1
Systemic	2	2	0	2	0	0
Sjögren's syndrome	9	7	2	0	8	1
Mixed connective tissue disease	7	4	3	0	7	0
Dermatomyositis	3	3	0	1	1	1
Suspected autoimmune disease	27	22	5	12	14	1
IgA deficiency	9	8	1	2	7	0
Postinfectious (presumed)	10	6	4	5	3	2
Leukemia	1	1	0	1	0	0
Total	**138**	**109**	**29**	**65**	**62**	**11**

The ANA test was performed by indirect immunofluorescence; it was considered positive if significant fluorescence was observed when serum was applied at a 1 : 20 dilution. Diagnosis of mixed connective tissue disease was made in patients with a titer of antibody to extractable nuclear antigen (ENA) of 1 : 100,000 and typical clinical features such as Raynaud's phenomenon and arthritis.

The most common diagnosis in children with a positive ANA test was systemic lupus erythematosus (SLE), and it is recommended that these patients undergo clinical and laboratory studies for SLE, including anti-DNA and anti-ENA tests, determination of the total hemolytic complement (or C3 and C4) level, urinalysis, and complete blood cell count. Other diagnoses need to be considered because less than one third of pediatric patients with a positive ANA test had SLE. A positive ANA test in a child with arthritis should alert the examiner to the possibility of associated iridocyclitis and the need for ophthalmologic follow-up.

Speckled ANA patterns were most frequent among children with mixed connective tissue disease and Sjögren's syndrome. Children with SLE, mixed connective tissue disease, Sjögren's syndrome, or suspected autoimmune disease tended to have higher ANA titers (mean, >1:240) than those with other diagnoses.

In 92% of patients, a positive ANA test was associated with an autoimmune or rheumatic disorder; only 11 patients had other causes for the positive ANA test, including presumed infection (usually viral) and malignancy (leukemia).

Pediatric patients with a positive ANA test should have the test repeated; if the results are again positive, complete clinical and laboratory studies for autoimmune disorders should be undertaken. The patients should be followed up regularly for future development of disease.

Childhood Dermatomyositis: Factors Predicting Functional Outcome and Development of Dystrophic Calcification
Suzanne L. Bowyer, Caroline E. Blane, Donita B. Sullivan, and James T. Cassidy (Univ. of Michigan)
J. Pediatr. 103:882–888, December 1983   13–4

The medical records of 33 girls and 14 boys with dermatomyositis who were seen in the pediatric rheumatology clinic at the University of Michigan between 1964 and 1982 were reviewed in an attempt to identify variables in mode of presentation or treatment that might predict which children were at risk for the more severe sequelae of the disease. Age at onset of illness ranged from 3 months to 15 years. Disease course was classified as (1) monophasic without permanent functional impairment; (2) polyphasic with an outcome of minimal or no disability; (3) persistent disease with significant impairment; (4) inactive muscle disease with moderate impairment; and (5) death. Treatment included prednisone in divided doses of 2 mg/kg/day for the first month of illness, with subsequent reductions predicted on a favorable clinical and laboratory response.

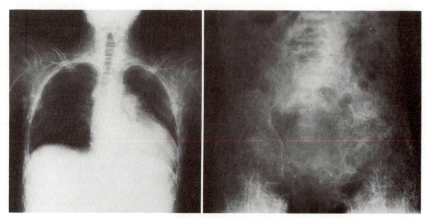

Fig 13–2.—Extensive linear superficial calcification almost creating exoskeleton in girl aged 16. (Courtesy of Bowyer, S.L., et al.: J. Pediatr. 103:882–888, December 1983.)

In 28 of 47 patients (60%), the disease followed course 1 or 2. The remaining 17 had at least one relapse during the treatment course. In 18 (40%), disease followed course 3 or 4. In only 1 case was death attributed to the primary disease: a girl aged 12 died of widespread gastrointestinal vasculitis and bleeding 2 months after diagnosis. Of the 18 given treatment with corticosteroid within 4 months of onset of symptoms, 14 (78%) had good results (disease course 1 or 2). If treatment was delayed until 4–12 months after onset but optimal corticosteroid doses were used, the outlook for functional recovery was still favorable. If treatment was delayed for longer than 4 months after symptoms began and included low steroid doses, outcome was worse. In the group as a whole, sex of the patient had no effect on outcome and neither did age of onset. Seventeen girls and seven boys (51%) developed dystrophic calcification. Calcium deposition was first noted from 1–7 years after disease onset. Figure 13–2 demonstrates an example of a lacy, reticular pattern of calcification extending throughout the body at the level of the subcutaneous tissue, which was considered the severe form of dystrophic calcification. Fourteen of 18 patients (78%) given treatment within 4 months of onset with high doses of corticosteroids had no calcium deposits or only type 1 calcification.

A subgroup of children with dermatomyositis who appear to do poorly despite optimal therapeutic regimens has been identified. These patients are distinguished by a severe disease course responding minimally to corticosteroid therapy and manifested by persistent muscle weakness, elevations of muscle enzyme activity, and severe generalized cutaneous vasculitis. These children are at high risk for development of exoskeleton-like calcification.

The Hypermobility Syndrome

Frank Biro, Harry L. Gewanter, and John Baum (Univ. of Rochester)

Pediatrics 72:701–706, November 1983

The hypermobility syndrome has been recognized as a definitive diagnostic entity among children referred to a Pediatric Arthritis Clinic with musculoskeletal complaints. Diagnosis of hypermobility was made by the ability of the patients to perform at least three of the following maneuvers: (1) extension of the wrists and metacarpal phalanges so that the fingers are parallel to the dorsum of the forearm (Fig 13–3); (2) passive apposition of thumbs to the flexor aspect of the forearm; (3) hyperextension of elbows (≥10 degrees); (4) hyperextension of the knees (≥10 degrees); (5) flexion of trunk with knees extended so palms rest on the floor (Fig 13–4).

From January 1979 to July 1981, 262 patients attended the clinic; 15 (5.7%) were identified as hypermobile and 109 (41.6%) had juvenile arthritis. Three of the 15 hypermobile children also had juvenile arthritis. The remainder of the clinic population had various other rheumatic and nonrheumatic conditions. The usual presenting complaints of the hypermobile patients were pain or swelling, or both, of various joints, with the most common complaints about the knees; the fingers and hands were the second most frequent sites. Except for the 3 patients with concomitant juvenile arthritis and the patient with trisomy 21 and viral illness, the Westergren sedimentation rate was less than 20 mm per hour. Of the 12 patients without juvenile arthritis, 6 responded to treatment with salicylates, 2 to tolmetin sodium, and 1 to sulindac, in addition to rest and physical therapy. Hypermobility was not diagnosed at the time of initial evaluation in any of the 3 patients with juvenile arthritis. Most cases of hypermobility were noted to occur between ages 10 and 15 years (7 patients), but there were 3 in this group younger than age 5 years.

The authors note that most hypermobile children with minor or recurrent musculoskeletal complaints do not seek attention from the health care system. Early recognition of this syndrome and appropriate reassurance and therapy will help reduce patient and parental anxiety.

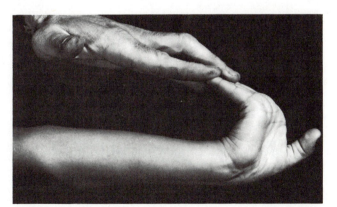

Fig 13–3.—Hyperextension of wrist and metacarpal phalangeal joint with fingers parallel to forearm. (Courtesy of Biro, F., et al.: Pediatrics 72:701–706, November 1983. Copyright American Academy of Pediatrics 1983.)

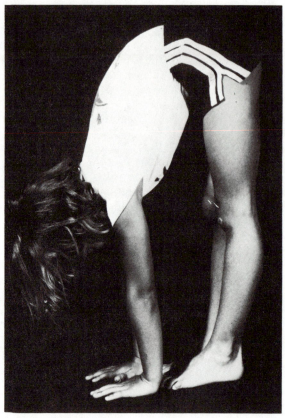

Fig 13–4.—Flexion of trunk with knees extended and with palms resting on floor. (Courtesy of Biro, F., et al.: Pediatrics 72:701–706, November 1983. Copyright American Academy of Pediatrics 1983.)

Treatment of Congenital Osteopetrosis With High-Dose Calcitriol

Lyndon Key, David Carnes, Sessions Cole, Marijke Holtrop, Zvi Bar-Shavit, Fred Shapiro, Robert Arceci, James Steinberg, Caren Gundberg, Arnold Kahn, Steven Teitelbaum, and Constantine Anast

N. Engl. J. Med. 310:409–415, Feb. 16, 1984   13–6

Osteopetrosis is a group of disorders caused by defective osteoclast function. Some patients are not candidates for bone marrow transplantation, and the procedure carries much risk in any event because of the need for profound immunosuppression and the chance of a graft-versus-host reaction. The authors used the bone-resorbing agent calcitriol in an attempt to stimulate osteoclastic activity in a child with osteopetrosis.

Girl, aged 8 weeks, had a diagnosis of osteopetrosis, which was confirmed by bone biopsy at age 11 months. No marrow donor was available. The infant was blind. The liver extended 3 cm below the costal margin and 2 cm beyond the midline, and the spleen extended to the pelvic brim. A leukoerythroblastic reaction was evident. The long bones were diffusely osteosclerotic and had no medullary spaces (Fig 13–5). Computed tomography of the skull showed narrowed optic and internal auditory foramina. Visual stimulation evoked no brain stem response, and delayed auditory nerve conduction was documented. Transfusion requirements were reduced after 6 weeks of high-dosage calcitriol therapy, and the spleen was much smaller. Treatment was stopped after 3 months, however, at the parents' request, because of the patient's poor neurologic prognosis.

Calcitriol was given in dosages up to 32 μg daily in conjunction with a low-calcium diet. Measures of bone turnover increased during treatment. Hydroxyproline excretion increased in parallel with the urinary calcium-creatinine ratio, the urinary γ-carboxyglutamic acid concentration, and the serum osteocalcin concentration and alkaline phosphatase activity. Bone biopsies showed numerous osteoclasts with ruffled borders and associated bony disruption after 3 months of treatment. The capacity of the patient's monocytes for in vitro bone resorption rose substantially during treatment.

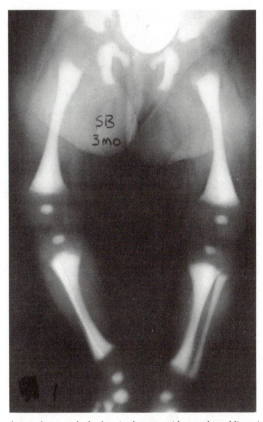

Fig 13–5.—Long bones show marked sclerotic changes, with complete obliteration of bone marrow cavity, at age 3 months. (Courtesy of Key, L., et al.: N. Engl. J. Med. 310:409–415, Feb. 16, 1984. Reprinted by permission of the New England Journal of Medicine.)

High-dosage calcitriol therapy led to bone resorption in this child with osteopetrosis. There were no apparent complications. Such treatment may be useful as an adjunct to bone marrow transplantation or as primary therapy when transplantation has to be delayed or is not feasible. Optimal treatment will require a better understanding of the basic defect in osteopetrosis.

▶ Calcitriol is the most potent stimulator of osteoclastic bone resorption known. In case you forgot, calcitriol is 1,25-dihydroxy vitamin D_3. 1-Hydroxylation occurs in the kidney after 25-hydroxylation in the liver, to produce the vitamin D hormone that is the most physiologically active form of vitamin D metabolite. Osteopetrosis represents a disequilibrium between the normally balanced process of bone formation and bone resorption. The net result is deposition of excessive mineral osteoid, skeletal radiopacity, and encroachment on bone marrow spaces and cranial nerve foramina. This results in marked extramedullary hematopoiesis, massive splenomegaly, and transfusion dependency because of bone marrow failure. The osteoclast, residing in bone, is the cell that normally is responsible for taking bone apart when it isn't needed. It now has been shown that peripheral-blood monocytes and tissue macrophages also can do the same thing. Hence, one can expect bone marrow transplantation, which provides normally active cells that can break down bone, to be effective in helping to reverse this process. One theory is that patients' own cells are insensitive to signals to resorb bone whereas exogenous cells would do a proper job. Peter Coccia has reviewed all this recently (N. Engl. J. Med. 310:456, 1984). He notes that a total of 14 bone marrow transplantations have been done for infantile osteopetrosis, of which 6 have been successful. Deaths in the other patients were a result of transplantation complications. To date, transplantation of bone marrow is the only known true cure for this condition. The child described in this study had no bone marrow donor and had to be treated with calcitriol. Although there was evidence of improvement on x-ray studies and biochemical evidence of improvement in the laboratory, the overall clinical response of this child was disappointing. The use of calcitriol was obviously worth a try, and I am sure that we will be reading much more about its use. If nothing else, it will give us a great deal of further insight into the mechanism by which cells resorb bone. It is the only hope for children who do not have a bone marrow donor.—J.A.S., III

Osteofibrous Dysplasia (Ossifying Fibroma of Long Bones): A Study of 12 Cases

Yasuaki Nakashima, Takao Yamamuro, Yuzo Fujiwara, Yoshihiko Kotoura, Eigo Mori, and Yoshihiro Hamashima
Cancer 52:909–914, Sept. 1, 1983   13–7

The findings in 9 girls and 3 boys with osteofibrous dysplasia seen at one of four hospitals in Japan and followed for an average of 5.3 years are reviewed. Average age at diagnosis was 5.1 years. Average duration of symptoms was 1 month. The most common features were tibial swelling and local pain. Two patients presented with fracture. No patient had associated extraskeletal anomalies. The tibia was involved in all cases, and in 1 patient the ipsilateral fibula was also involved. Radiograms of all patients showed diaphyseal involvement, with either solitary or multiple lytic lesions, thinning and expansion of the cortex, and in many cases, bowing deformity. The lesion usually became multifocal with recurrences (Fig 13–6).

Ten patients were treated by curettage, with or without bone grafting, but all had recurrences in an average of 7 months. Two patients with lesions of the distal third of the tibia had recurrences with pathologic fractures, followed by pseudarthrosis. Two recent patients had biopsy only and have had no evidence of progression of the disease during follow-up for 23 and 13 months, respectively. No spontaneous regression has been observed. Cartilaginous foci were seen in two lesions. Primary and recurrent lesions had similar histologic features. None of the lesions were malignant.

The cause of osteofibrous dysplasia is not known, and it is not clear whether it is a primary neoplasm of bone or a congenital anomaly of the tibia. The lesion has a marked tendency to recur, even after wide resection

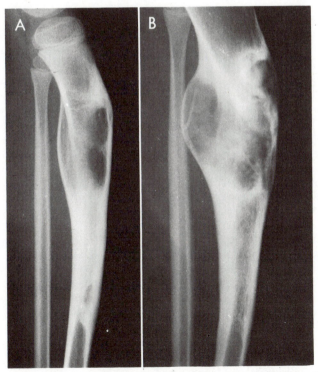

Fig 13–6.—A, third recurrence of osteofibrous dysplasia. Patient was aged 7 years and underwent segmental resection of tibia, including periosteum. **B,** film of same patient at age 12 years. (Courtesy of Nakashima, Y., et al.: Cancer 52:909–914, Sept. 1, 1983.)

that includes the periosteum. Ablative surgery would appear to be contraindicated in patients younger than age 10 years. Bracing is indicated to prevent fracture. Patients with pseudarthrosis may require conservative surgical treatment. There is no apparent indication for radiation therapy, and postradiation sarcoma has been reported in cases of fibrous dysplasia. Long-term prognosis of osteofibrous dysplasia remains unclear, but malignant change has not been described.

▶ Ossifying fibromas of long bones are usually not difficult to distinguish radiologically from nonossifying fibromas. The distinction is important because the latter condition may be associated with neurofibromatosis. Any time you see lesions like this, of the bone, however, you should do a careful examination to look for the telltale signs of neurofibromatosis.—J.A.S., III

Bone Scintigraphy of Hip Joint Effusions in Children

Reinhard Kloiber, William Pavlosky, Oliver Portner, and Kathleen Gartke (Children's Hosp. of Eastern Ontario, Ottawa)
AJR 140:995–999, May 1983   13–8

Twenty-two boys and 16 girls, aged 12 months to 14 years, with hip pain of acute onset were studied by bone scintigraphy. Twelve patients had aspiration of the affected hip within 24 hours of radionuclide imaging. Each patient received ^{99m}Tc-methylene diphosphonate intravenously in a dose of 250 μCi/kg.

Of the 38 patients, 4 had septic arthritis, 1 with associated osteomyelitis. Nineteen were diagnosed as having transient synovitis. Three patients had total absence of femoral head activity, and aspiration yielded large quantities of purulent material in all. Follow-up studies showed normal head uptake in 2 cases, after 7–10 days. Femoral head uptake reverted to normal in 2 patients who had follow-up scintigraphy 1 and 2 days after aspiration (Fig 13–7). Eight of 10 cases with photon deficiency on blood pool images had joint aspiration confirming the presence of fluid. Of the 9 cases of impaired femoral head uptake, the 3 without identifiable activity proved to be septic. Of the 19 cases of transient synovitis, 6 had entirely normal scintigraphic studies.

The authors conclude bone scintigraphy is useful in the diagnosis of joint effusions and can give information as to the state of perfusion of the femoral head. Follow-up studies after aspiration can differentiate infarction from reversible ischemia. Joint aspiration in cases with decreased uptake may prove to be not only diagnostic but also therapeutic for the prevention of Legg-Perthes disease.

▶ Data from this report should not be interpreted to mean that bone scans obviate the need for aspiration of the hip joint in patients who have symptoms referable to that joint. Septic arthritis of the hip joint may be sufficiently mild that there is not enough elevation of joint pressure to decrease the perfusion of the femoral head. Conversely, abnormal scans can be seen in Legg-Calvé-

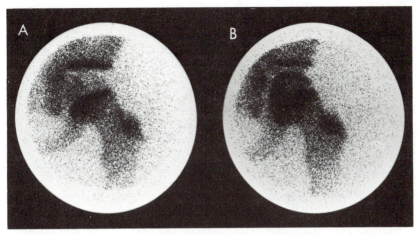

Fig 13–7.—Boy, aged 7, with joint effusion due to transient synovitis of left hip. **A,** marked reduction of radiotracer uptake in femoral head (grade 1). Involvement of head is uniform, and apparent greater activity medially is due to overlap by ischium. **B,** repeat study 1 day after aspiration. Normal uptake. (Courtesy of Kloiber, R., et al.: AJR 140:995–999, May 1983.)

Perth's disease with ischemic infarction of the femoral head. With the latter disorder, aspiration of the hip joint is also diagnostic in that it shows little or no abnormalities consistent with septic arthritis. Bone scan and joint aspiration should be considered complementary in all but the most obvious of cases. Another point made by this study also should be well digested, that is that joints affected by septic arthritis can have elevations of joint pressure that will result in necrosis of the femoral head as a result of ischemia. This can occur in less than 24 hours, and the only way of knowing if permanent damage has occurred is by repeat follow-up bone scan within 1 or 2 days after aspiration and the start of treatment for septic arthritis.

On an unrelated topic, well worth your reading time, is an article by Cunningham et al. (*Lancet* 1:668, 1984). This article was entitled "A Clicking Hip in a Newborn Infant Should Never Be Ignored." During a newborn screening program to detect congenital dislocated hips, examination of 8,000 infants showed 46 with obvious evidence of hip problems. About 8% of the overall group in addition to these 46 patients had minor signs such as clicking or a grating of the hip. Among these infants, on follow-up examination 63 turned out to have definitive hip abnormalities at age 4 months. Thus, dislocated or dislocatable hips were 30 times more common in infants who had such minor signs as a click on physical examination in the immediate newborn period. Another interesting observation of this study was the fact that another 7 patients who were absolutely normal in the newborn period turned up later to have dislocated hips. This has been observed in two other letters to the editor of *The Lancet* (2:340, 1983). Quite frankly, previously it had been felt that all cases of dislocated hips that showed up later were, in fact, cases that had been missed in the newborn period. This probably simply isn't so, because in one of these two reports an infant actually had hip films performed in the first few months of life (for other reasons) which were normal and then showed up with dislocated hips by age 16 months. This makes life simple and complex for us at the same time. It clearly means that lawsuits will be much more difficult to come by for late-diagnosed congenital dislocations of the hip. It also means, however, that hip examinations should be extended well beyond our first one or two contacts with infants.—J.A.S., III

Localized Immune Complexes and Slipped Upper Femoral Epiphysis
Raymond T. Morrissy, Russell W. Steele, and Michael H. Gerdes (Little Rock, Ark.)
J. Bone Joint Surg. [Br.] 65–B:574–579, November 1983   13–9

The cause of slipped upper femoral epiphysis remains unknown. It probably is not caused by an accident, because the magnitude of trauma experienced is not great, familial occurrence has been demonstrated, and there is a constant association with synovitis even before slippage is demonstrated.

The local occurrence of immune complexes was determined by the authors in a series of 12 consecutive patients treated for slipped capital femoral epiphysis. Except for 1 with hypothyroidism who was under treatment, no patient had an apparent cause for slipped epiphysis. Five cases were rated as mild and 7 as moderate. Only 1 case was acute. Twenty-one control patients with synovitis requiring surgery or arthroscopy also were assessed. All but 1 patient were followed up for at least a year without developing chondrolysis or avascular necrosis.

Immune complexes were detected in 10 of 11 synovial fluid samples from patients with slipped epiphysis. Both the C1q-binding assay and the Raji-cell assay were positive in a majority of cases. No patient had circulating immune complexes. None of the positive synovial fluid specimens contained rheumatoid factor or hepatitis B antigen. No significant changes in serum or synovial fluid immunoglobulin or complement levels were noted. Only 2 control patients had synovial fluid immune complexes; 1 had known juvenile rheumatoid arthritis and 1, marked synovitis associated with lumbar myelomeningocele and subluxation of the hip. No patient in either group exhibited positive synovial immunofluorescence. Synovial biopsy specimens from study patients showed edema, synovial cell proliferation, increased vascularity, and infiltration by lymphocytes and plasma cells. Large groups of plasma cells often were observed.

The synovitis of slipped capital femoral epiphysis can be distinguished from that seen in most other orthopedic disorders by the presence of immune complexes in the synovial fluid. In contrast to rheumatoid arthritis, circulating immune complexes are not present.

▶ Slipped upper femoral epiphysis remains a disease of unknown etiology despite much investigation. Its most unusual feature is its occurrence in a narrow age range of puberty. This has led to the speculation that this disease is secondary to some type of hormonal imbalance. In fact, very occasionally a patient can be defined to have some endocrine disorder such as hypothyroidism, but this is rare. Most orthopedists tend to favor trauma as the etiology of slipped epiphysis, including the femoral head. As attractive as this concept might be, it has several problems. Firstly, these children do not give you a history of trauma invariably. Secondly, familial occurrence has been described. Thirdly, and most importantly, many, if not most, children with slipping give a long history of synovitis of the hip. It is the last point that led these investigators to examine evidence for an immune cause for slipped femoral epiphysis.

Immune complexes have now been demonstrated in a number of diseases. Except for rheumatoid diseases, disordered immune function has not been implicated as an etiologic factor in orthopedic diseases. Immune complexes are formed by the reaction of antibody with antigens generated from microorganisms, autologous cells, or any exogenous substance. In most instances, such complexes do not cause any problem. If antigen does persist, complexes may trigger a variety of biologic processes, such as the fixation of complement, the release of chemotactic factors and vasoactive amines, an increased vascular permeability, and infiltration with neutrophils and mononuclear leukocytes. This all results in tissue destruction.

Two problems with the present study (which are common to any similar study that seeks the presence of immune complexes) are whether the material identified truly is an immune complex and what, if any, role it plays in the disease process. The authors of this study were very careful to use the best assays for immune complexes. There does not appear to be any question that they have correctly identified such complexes in the synovial fluid of patients with slipped femoral epiphysis. Less conclusive is any direct evidence that the immune complexes are participating in the pathologic process. The fact that complexes can be isolated from joints affected by disease does not prove that the immune complexes are the cause of the disease. This is incriminating if not conclusive evidence, however. That immune complexes are not found at other sites in a variety of other orthopedic disorders is also incriminating. Indeed, this finding of immune complexes at the site of a particular disease and their absence from a variety of other diseases that may affect the same tissues and organs is strongly suggestive that they play a part in the pathologic process. I personally would have never bet that slipped femoral epiphysis was an immune-mediated phenomenon. In fact, I would have argued strongly in the opposite direction. Data from this study, however, are suggestive to me that I should buy a clothes hamper and throw in the towel.—J.A.S., III

Lateral Electric Surface Stimulation for the Treatment of Progressive Idiopathic Scoliosis
Jens Axelgaard and John Carlisle Brown (Ranchos Los Amigos Hosp., Downey, Calif.)
Spine 8:242–260, April 1983   13–10

Transcutaneous lateral electric muscle stimulation was evaluated as an alternative to bracing in the management of patients with progressive scoliosis. The goal was to produce rib movement by electrically induced muscle contractions on the lateral thorax or trunk to reduce the spinal curvature and counteract the exaggerated compressive biomechanical forces on the concave side of the vertebral epiphyseal growth plates, hopefully preventing further disk and bony deformity.

For this study a portable electronic stimulator was connected to removable skin electrodes. Monophasic 200-µsec pulses of 60 to 80 mamp were delivered at a rate of 25 pulses per second to produce muscle contractions that closely resemble voluntary contractions. Electrode placement was guided by the apical vertebra of the curve (Fig 13–8). The target muscles lie in a band that stretches laterally from the edge of the paraspinal muscles to the anterior axillary line.

Between April 1977 and March 1982, 80 female and 10 male patients have been treated with this technique. Sixty-one had single primary curves and 29 had double primary curves. Only one of the curves was treated in 17 of the latter cases. Stimulation was applied nightly for an average of 15 months. Arrest of progression or curve correction was observed in 84% of patients with single primary curves and in 83% of those with double primary curves. The respective rates for patients who complied fully with the program were 97% and 93%. Follow-up for up to 2 years of 13 patients with skeletally mature curves showed no increase in curvature. The most common cause of discontinuation of treatment was inadequate stimulation time.

Transcutaneous nighttime lateral electric stimulation can arrest the progression of juvenile and adolescent idiopathic scoliosis. The outcome has not been related to the severity or location of the curve. No adverse effects on rotation or wedging have been noted. Curve stabilization was evident

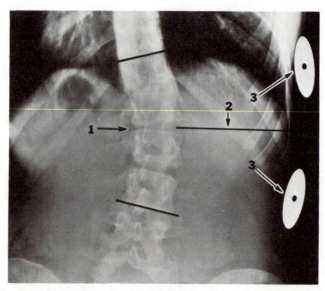

Fig 13–8.—Electrode placement technique for lumbar curves. (Courtesy of Axelgaard, J., and Brown, J.C.: Spine 8:242–260, April 1983.)

on posttreatment follow-up at 2 years. Inclusion only of cooperative patients with adequate family support would improve the success rate.

▶ William P. Bunnell, Director of Orthopaedics and Assistant Medical Director, Alfred I. DuPont Institute, comments:

"Two multicenter studies with the goal of evaluating the results of electric stimulation for the treatment of idiopathic scoliosis are currently under way. Axelgaard and Brown have reported their early experience with this treatment modality; in their series, arrest of progression occurred in 84% of patients.

"Given that the report of Axelgaard and Brown is a preliminary one, there remain several problems with the study. To begin, 70% of the patients actually did not meet all of the criteria for inclusion in this study, thus raising the distinct possibility that many of them would have had a 'good' result, even without treatment. In addition, the average length of follow-up was only 15 months. This is much too short a time to evaluate the results of scoliosis treatment, which ideally should begin at least 1 year prior to the end of growth and continue for 1 year following cessation of growth. Further, one fourth of the patients in the authors' series discontinued this method of treatment prior to reaching skeletal maturity; this indicates that a rather high percentage of patients did not complete the treatment protocol. Less than half of these patients had further curve progression.

"Surface electric stimulation offers many advantages over conventional brace treatment. It eliminates the necessity of wearing a brace during the daytime, is more readily accepted by most patients, and represents less of an intrusion into the patient's life. The studies reported to date, however, do not adequately demonstrate that this method will yield results as good as those achieved with conventional bracing; therefore, the technique can only be recommended with 'guarded optimism.' "

High School Football Injuries in Birmingham, Alabama

Michael I. Culpepper and Kurt M. W. Niemann (Univ. of Alabama)
South. Med. J. 76:873–875, July 1983   13–11

The authors analyzed 1,877 injuries treated in 1976–1979 at the Sports Medicine Clinic.

Approximately 600,000 football injuries occur annually. Comprehensive understanding of the mechanisms of injury may lead to prompt diagnosis and treatment. The most common injuries are listed and their incidence is compared to the North Carolina study (Table 1). The reduced incidence of lacerations and concussions may be due to the improvement of such equipment as helmets and shoes and the institution of rules against "spear" tackling. Contact injuries, fractures and contusions, account for 35% of all injuries. Injuries to head and neck, shoulder, hand and fingers, knee, and ankle account for 65.8% of all injuries. Instead of the old seven-post cleated shoes, most players in the Birmingham area wear now soccer-type shoes, which may account for the reduction in ankle injuries.

TABLE 1.—COMPARISON OF NORTH CAROLINA STUDY
WITH BIRMINGHAM STUDY AS TO INJURY TYPE

Injury Type	North Carolina Study (%)	Birmingham Study (%)
Sprain	20.4	32.2
Contusion	24.1	24.8
Fracture	10.6	11.0
Strain	16.2	12.4
Laceration	5.8	0.4
Concussion	5.4	1.0
Dislocation	2.1	2.1
Separation	1.1	0.4
Neuropathy	1.5	0.6
Tear	7.2	3.8
Other/not specified	5.6	11.5
Total	100.0	100.2

(Courtesy of Culpepper, M.I., and Niemann, K.M.W.: South. Med. J. 76:873–875, July 1983.)

In offensive play, players who handle the ball most often sustain the greatest number of injuries; the quarterback position is inherently the most hazardous. In defensive play, linebackers and defensive backs sustain the greatest number of injuries (Table 2).

Of the 1,877 injuries recorded, 661 (35.2%) were sustained during games. Considering the time involved, the number of game injuries is higher than practice injuries because the intensity of playing is greater during

TABLE 2.—DISTRIBUTION OF INJURIES BY PLAYER
POSITION

Player Position	No.	%
Quarterback	163	8.7
Runningback	367	19.6
Wide receiver	136	7.2
Tight end	97	5.2
Tackle	218	11.6
Guard	146	7.8
Center	80	4.3
Defensive back	172	9.2
Defensive end	89	4.7
Defensive tackle	54	2.9
Defensive guard	48	2.6
Linebacker	168	9.0
Other/not specified	139	7.4
Total	1,877	100.2

(Courtesy of Culpepper, M.I., and Niemann, K.M.W.: South. Med. J. 76:873–875, July 1983.)

games than during practice. It appears that a substantial number of players younger than 15 are prone to injury and in need of medical attention.

Changes in rules, equipment, and style of play change the patterns of injury. Further study of the characteristics associated with such changes could reduce the number and severity of football injuries.

▶ The authors of this study that evaluated football injuries in Alabama conclude the report by saying that further knowledge of the reasons for certain types of football injuries could reduce the number and severity of these problems. A very interesting article that reviewed the sports injuries in 1 academic year among about 7,000 Irish schoolchildren does provide some insights in this regard (Watson, A.: *Am. J. Sports Med.* 12:65, 1984). In the study from Ireland, the incidence of injuries overall was anywhere from one half to one tenth of the reported incidence in a similar age group of children in the United States. When I first read this detailed report, I thought this was just "luck of the Irish," but the real difference appears to be based on the fact that Irish teachers and coaches are reluctant to classify an incident as an injury unless the level of incapacity is high, and they tend to ignore conditions that would be referred for medical treatment in the United States, where, the Irish authors say, "The level of involvement of medical and paramedical personnel in sports is considerably greater." This report from Ireland does highlight one very important characteristic of school athletic injuries. It was noted that illegal play was the major cause of injury in school matches and if this problem could be corrected, much of the trauma associated with athletics would disappear. In the United States we tend to focus on newer technologies in protective equipment rather than on playing by the rules. This is a bit of an overstatement, but it has some truth to it. One must be honest about the fact that improvements in equipment have produced significant declines in injury. For example, a switch from the old seven-post cleated shoes to soccer-type shoes for football players has dramatically decreased the incidence of ankle injuries. In my opinion, soccer shoes should be worn only on the football field if you want to prevent ankle injuries. The reason for saying this may be found in the following article, which demonstrates that among soccer players, trauma to the ankle is the most frequent injury. We have been seeing a great deal more European soccer matches on cable television. I am firmly convinced that the way some soccer is played, it is like nuclear warfare—there are no winners, only survivors.—J.A.S., III

Profile of Youth Soccer Injuries
John R. McCarroll, Craig Meaney, and Jon M. Sieber
Physician Sportsmed. 12:113–117, February 1984   13–12

Soccer is the most popular sport worldwide and is increasing in popularity in the United States. The occurrence of soccer injuries in 4,018 children and adolescents on 253 teams in Indiana was reviewed. A total of 176 injuries occurred, for a rate of 4.4%. Rates were less in the younger teams. Competitive teams had higher injury rates than recreational teams

TYPES OF INJURY BY LOCATION IN YOUTH SOCCER

	No.	%
ANKLE	35	19.9
Sprain	32	
Fracture	1	
Tendinitis	2	
KNEE	25	14.2
Medial collateral ligament	7	
Anterior cruciate ligament	3	
Patella	9	
Osgood-Schlatter disease	5	
Meniscus	1	
SHIN	23	13.1
Contusion	21	
Laceration	2	
MUSCLE CONTUSION	20	11.4
Quadriceps	16	
Gastrocnemius	4	
FRACTURES	17	9.7
Arm	3	
Tibia	4	
Rib	2	
Thumb	2	
Wrist	4	
Finger	2	
ACHILLES TENDON	17	9.7
MUSCLE STRAIN	12	6.8
Groin	5	
Hamstring	2	
Quadriceps	5	
FOOT INJURIES	9	5.1
Sprain	5	
Fracture	4	
CONCUSSION	5	2.8
FACE	5	2.8
BACK	4	2.2
Neck	1	
Lower	3	
SHOULDER (contusion)	2	1.1
KIDNEY (contusion)	1	0.6
AORTA (rupture)	1	0.6

(Courtesy of McCarroll, J.R., et al.: Physician Sportsmed. 12:113–117, February 1984. Reprinted by permission of The Physicians and Sports Medicine, a McGraw-Hill publication.)

at all ages. All but 2 of the injuries that necessitated operation occurred on competitive teams. Ankle injuries were most frequent, followed by knee injuries (table). Sprains and contusions were the most common types of injury. Six operations on the knee were necessary, as were 1 ankle operation and 1 operation to repair an aortic rupture resulting from a blow to the abdomen.

Soccer appears to be a comparatively safe sport for young athletes. Knee injuries are the most serious concern. Prevention of soccer injuries requires a well-trained coaching staff, sound conditioning and training procedures, and knowledgeable medical personnel.

Medical History Associated With Adolescent Powerlifting
Eugene W. Brown and Richard G. Kimball (Michigan State Univ.)
Pediatrics 72:636–644, November 1983   13–13

A questionnaire was administered to obtain data about the training, experience, and medical history of adolescent powerlifters from 71 contestants in the 1981 Michigan Teenage Powerlifting Championship.

The average powerlifting experience of the 71 subjects was 17.1 months. The subjects began participation in powerlifting at an average 15.3 years of age and had previously participated in an average of 3.4 contests. Seventy percent of the subjects had participated in three contests or less. The subjects trained an average of 4.1 times per week, 99.2 minutes per training session. On the average, training was performed alone or with friends, without the supervision of a "trained coach," 51.6% of the time. There was a tendency toward a direct relationship between increased age and percent of knowledge obtained by trial and error. The percent of knowledge obtained from "trained coaches and instructors" tended to be inversely related to age. About 44% of the subjects engaged in intentional weight loss to compete in a lower weight class in the Michigan Teenage Powerlifting Championship. The greatest percentage of subjects indicated higher incidence and levels of pain in the knee than in other areas of the lower body. Evaluation of all regions of the body showed that the highest percent of subjects indicated an increased occurrence and level of pain in the axial regions of the upper and lower back. Figure 13–9 shows the types and sites of injuries severe enough to discontinue training for at least one day. Of 71 subjects, 28 recorded at least one such injury. The injury type with the highest incidence was muscle pull at 61.2%.

The authors caution that these findings are specific to the teenage populations studied, and prognosis about the long-term effects of powerlifting is not warranted.

▶ Powerlifting is a form of competitive weightlifting. It consists of three events, "a squat lift, a dead lift, and the bench press." The goal of competition obviously is to lift the maximum weight for each event. Competition in this sport is sanctioned by the International Powerlifting Federation for various age groups, including boys as young as age 14. In teenage powerlifting, it is com-

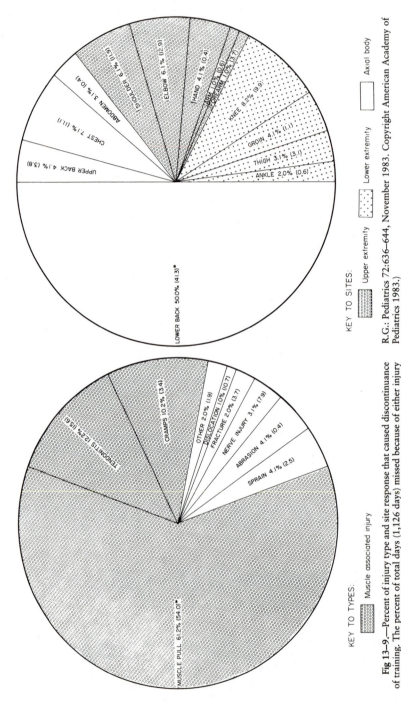

Fig 13–9.—Percent of injury type and site response that caused discontinuance of training. The percent of total days (1,126 days) missed because of either injury type or site is shown in parentheses. (Courtesy of Brown, E.W., and Kimball, R.G.: Pediatrics 72:636–644, November 1983. Copyright American Academy of Pediatrics 1983.)

mon for the musculoskeletal system to be exposed to loads that exceed body weight by as much as two to three times. It is not hard to see why the body can be injured by this, because in order for the body to support these kinds of loads, opposing muscular torques must be exerted that are at least equal to the resistive torques resulting from the load to be lifted.

The long-term effects of the injuries associated with powerlifting are not known. Fortunately, the young age of the patients in this study by Brown and Kimball was inconsistent with life-threatening complications of powerlifting. In an interesting letter to the editor (*Lancet* 1:393, 1984), A. W. Fowler speculated that much of the sudden death during certain sport activities was related to breath holding during isometric exercise accompanying tonic muscular contraction. Obviously, powerlifting is about as close to this description as you can come. Fowler's letter actually dealt with sudden death in squash players. This has reached almost epidemic proportions, apparently, in Great Britain. In a series of 30 sudden deaths associated with squash playing, the mean age was only 46 years. Most of the deaths were from coronary heart disease (Northcote, R. J., et al.: ibid., p. 148). As far as this sport is concerned, it seems obvious "to get fit to play squash, don't play squash to get fit."

In prior YEAR BOOKS you may have sensed that this commentator hates most exercise as rabidly as a person who loves exercise hates common sense. That is correct. The following are philosophies that I adhere to in this regard.

1. Exercise is a waste of calories. Science has shown that 1 hour of intense productive mental effort consumes only the calories equivalent to one oyster cracker or one-half a salted peanut.

2. Never exercise before breakfast; if you have to exercise before breakfast, eat your breakfast first.

3. Golf is nothing but a good walk spoiled.

4. Jogging is very beneficial—it makes the ground feel needed.

5. Just in case you are too confident, remember that behind every good tennis player there is another good tennis player.

6. Sitting is better than standing. Show me a man with both feet on the ground and I'll show you a man who can't put his pants on.—J.A.S., III

Performance Measurement and Percent Body Fat in the High School Athlete

William D. McLeod, Stephen C. Hunter, and Bill Etchison
Am. J. Sports Med. 11:390–397, Nov.–Dec. 1983   13–14

The authors derived standards for performance from preseason assessments of high school athletes. Strength, endurance, and power measurements were obtained from 3,174 athletes in a 2-year period, 2,342 boys aged 14–17 years and 832 girls of the same age. The assessment included the number of sit-ups done in 1 minute, the total number of dips, total pull-ups for boys and the flexed arm hang time for girls, right and left-hand grip strength, and vertical jump height. Body fat measurements were made at the subscapular site and anterior thigh in boys and at the triceps and iliac crest in girls. Measurements were converted to the amount of work done or force developed, and nondimensional ratios were calculated.

The average performance decreased dramatically as body fat increased above 10% in boys and above 19% in girls. Tests of endurance showed significantly poorer performance when these limits were exceeded. Single effort performance showed some improvement with increasing body fat, but average performance was impeded by excess body fat. Performance measurements could help coaches and trainers determine whether an athlete who performs inadequately should lose body fat or condition himself to increase his strength.

▶ Evaluation of body composition can provide valuable information on the status of competitive preparation for many athletes. I asked someone well versed in studies of body composition to comment on this particular article. He found many difficulties with the report. One concern was that the age span of 14 to 17 years was too wide. This is just the time when boys are experiencing a considerable increase in lean weight and some fall in body weight, and one would expect on the basis of age alone that performance would increase. Thus, attempting to relate a higher body fat to poor performance could be an "epi" phenomenon. Also, no attention was paid to height as a variable. It is well known that some aspects of athletic performance are related to stature. As an example, professional athletes are generally taller than nonathletes. Despite these flaws, I assume the reviewers who accepted this article for publication in the *American Journal of Sports Medicine* did find some merit in it, especially since the study was the Winner of the Sports Science and Performance Award. That's better than I often do. Sometimes the only thing I can get accepted by a journal is my check for the subscription.—J.A.S., III

14 Ophthalmology

Ophthalmia Neonatorum Caused by β-Lactamase-Producing *Neisseria gonorrhoeae*

Brinda Doraiswamy, Margaret R. Hammerschlag, George F. Pringle, and Lorraine du Bouchet (SUNY Downstate Med. Center)

JAMA 250:790–791, Aug. 12, 1983   14–1

Data are reported on what appears to be the second case of ophthalmia neonatorum caused by penicillinase-producing strains of *Neisseria gonorrhoeae* in the United States.

Infant girl, weighing 1,940 gm, was born by normal spontaneous vaginal delivery at an estimated gestational age of 36 to 37 weeks. Apgar scores were 9 at 1 minute and 10 at 5 minutes. Routine ocular prophylaxis with 1% silver nitrate was given in the delivery room. A copious, bilateral conjunctival discharge was noted on the third day of life. Cultures were obtained and therapy with penicillin G potassium, 50,000 units/kg/day intravenously, in 3 divided doses was instituted. Cultures from the eyes yielded β-lactamase-producing *N. gonorrhoeae* on the third day after starting therapy. Antibiotic therapy was changed to cefotaxime sodium, 100 mg/kg/day, in 3 divided doses for 7 days. Remainder of the course was unremarkable and follow-up cultures of the eyes were negative. There was no evidence of corneal damage.

The mother's cervical cultures were also positive for penicillinase-producing strains of *N. gonorrhoeae*. A single dose of 2 gm of spectinomycin hydrochloride was given intramuscularly. Minimum inhibitory concentration (MIC) of penicillin and cefotaxime against the organisms isolated from the neonate was 16 and 0.125 mg/L, respectively.

Penicillinase-producing strains of *N. gonorrhoeae* have become highly endemic in some countries of East and Southeast Asia. The initial cases may have been brought to the United States by members of the Armed Forces. Between 1979 and 1980 the number of reported cases in the United States rose 235%.

The risk of acquiring gonococcal ophthalmia with or without silver nitrate prophylaxis is approximately 0.04% of all live births. This result is probably secondary to the present policy of maternal detection and treatment. The Centers for Disease Control (CDC) recommend ointments or drops containing tetracycline hydrochloride or erythromycin for neonatal ocular prophylaxis. Penicillinase-producing strains of *N. gonorrhoeae* frequently demonstrate low-level resistance to tetracycline with MIC of 2 mg/L or more, compared with MIC of 1 mg/L or less for β-lactamase-negative strains. Similarly, 90% of β-lactamase-negative strains and penicillinase-producing strains of *N. gonorrhoeae* are inhibited with 1 mg and 2 mg of erythromycin per liter, respectively.

The CDC currently recommend either parenteral cefotaxime or gentamicin sulfate for ophthalmia neonatorum caused by penicillinase-producing strains of *N. gonorrhoeae*. However, no clinical experience with these regimens has been reported.

To prevent corneal damage and subsequent blindness, appropriate therapy for gonococcal ophthalmia should be initiated promptly. It may be prudent to begin initial therapy for suspected gonococcal ophthalmia with a drug that is β-lactamase resistent, e.g., cefotaxime.

► By now, most of us are wishing that gonorrhea had been eradicated from the face of the earth just like smallpox. The permutations and complications of what this infection can cause in neonates are becoming so increasingly complex it is difficult to keep up with the changes and recommendations regarding treatment. At the time this article was published, only 2 cases of ophthalmia neonatorum caused by β-lactamase-producing *N. gonorrhoeae* had been reported in the United States. Although these 2 cases have peaked our interest, it is really the potential as to where this may lead that is of most concern. The first case of gonococcal ophthalmia neonatorum caused by penicillinase-producing strains of *N. gonorrhoeae* was reported from Singapore in 1978. Within 2 years, over one third of all cases of gonococcal ophthalmia neonatorum in Singapore were due to resistant strains (Thirumoorthy, T., et al.: *Br. J. Vener. Dis.* 58:308, 1982). The 2 cases from New York City represented between 10% and 20% of all cases of gonococcal ophthalmia in 1982. If we are seeing anything like what is going on in Asian countries, this whole problem will reach epidemic proportions quite shortly.

The practitioner obviously has a potpourri of choices to pick from when attempting prophylaxis of the newborn eyes against gonococci. These include the use of silver nitrate, topical use of tetracycline or erythromycin, and intramuscular administration of penicillin. The story that goes with each of these has been discussed in some length in previous YEAR BOOKS and will not be dealt with here. You may recall that the 1984 YEAR BOOK (p. 355) included the very first case report of ophthalmia neonatorum caused by penicillinase-producing *Neisseria gonorrhoeae*. No conclusions could be reached at that time as to the best mode of prevention. Penicillin-resistant organisms can produce low levels of resistance against tetracycline and erythromycin in vitro. The very high topical concentrations achieved in the eye might be expected to handle these resistant organisms, although the cases are so few and far between that this has never had to be tested. Clearly, intramuscular use of penicillin as a routine prophylaxis in the newborn period would not be expected to be effective. That, of course, leaves us with silver nitrate. There is no a priori reason to assume that silver nitrate would not work against resistant strains because the way the drug works is by depositing silver in the membrane of the bacteria. Curiously, however, one of the 2 described cases from New York City was in a patient who did receive silver nitrate prophylaxis in the immediate newborn period and then went on to develop resistant ophthalmia neonatorum. This should not be meant to imply that silver nitrate failed, since some other manner in which the bug could have reentered the eye is always conceivably possible. It simply leaves one a little unsettled, at best. What is more straightforward (relatively) is the manner of treatment once resistant organisms have been defined as a cause of ophthalmia neonatorum. The Centers for Disease Control have recommended (*Morbidity Mortality Weekly Rep.* 31:33S, 1982) the use of either parenterally administered cefotaxime or gentamicin sulfate as therapy for established disease. These infants should be hospitalized and so treated unless other recommendations are forthcoming. What is so unpleasant about this entire situation is that it may lead some to conclude that silver nitrate is still the best way to go. I still have problems with this drug. Once the chemical conjunctivitis comes along, you may not be able to differentiate it clearly from an infectious conjunctivitis and off you go on a complex and somewhat expensive evaluation precipitated by all this nonsense regarding resistant organisms. There just doesn't seem to be any perfect solution.

While on the topic of *Neisseria gonorrhoeae* conjunctivitis, it is well worth reminding ourselves that we should think of this organism anytime a patient has what appears to be an uncomplicated viral conjunctivitis that progresses to a purulent discharge. Alfonso et al. (*JAMA* 250:794, 1983) called this to our attention among a group of infants and adults who presented with fairly typical epidemic hemorrhagic conjunctivitis. The most common cause for acute hemorrhagic conjunctivitis is viral. This usually goes away by itself, but in the 10 cases described, a purulent discharge developed. In each instance, the 10 patients had applied urine to their eyes as a folk remedy for treatment of pink eye. Obviously, the urine was contaminated with *Neisseria gonorrhoeae* and thus a viral process soon became an important bacterial one. The use of urine and other biologic products of the body for treatment of eye ailments is historically well known. The clay tablets of Niefeh, Assyria, reported that saliva and breast milk from prostitutes were frequently prescribed for sore eyes. *Eber's Papyrus,* the most comprehensive Egyptian medical text dating from about the 15th century B.C., contains a reference in which urine mixed with flies' dirt and ochre was reported to prevent and cure eye ailments, while urine from prepuberal children would dissolve sores on the cornea and cure diseases of the eyelids (Gifford: *The Evil Eye: Studies in the Folklore of Vision,* New York, McMillan Company, 1958). Stranger things in life must happen, but I can't think of many.

We obviously have not heard the end of the story of resistant organisms and ophthalmia neonatorum. Please stay tuned. For what it's worth, the disease in the United States is a by-product of our involvement in the Viet Nam War and a reflection of our continued military presence in Southeast Asia, because this is where the problem began; it was transmitted here via infected servicemen. Enough said.—J.A.S., III

Gnat Sore Eyes: Seasonal, Acute Conjunctivitis in a Southern State
James W. Buehler, John T. Holloway, Richard A. Goodman, and R. Keith Sikes (Georgia Dept. of Human Resources, Atlanta)
South. Med. J. 76:587–589, May 1983   14–2

A widespread outbreak of acute bacterial conjunctivitis occurred in September 1981 in southeast Georgia, primarily in grade-school children. The condition was similar to seasonal conjunctivitis described periodically since

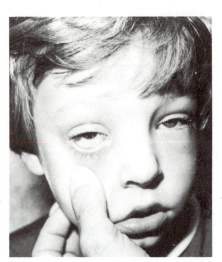

Fig 14–1.—Acute, seasonal conjunctivitis in child aged 6. (Courtesy of Buehler, J.W., et al.: South Med. J. 76:587–589, May 1983.)

1929 in Southern states and attributed to the eye gnat, *Hippelates pusio,* which transmits the suspected causative agent, the Koch-Weeks bacillus (known formerly as *Hemophilus aegyptius* and currently as *Hemophilus influenzae* biotype III).

Clinical features ranged from a dramatic presentation accompanied by severe lid edema, conjunctival hyperemia, and purulent drainage (Fig 14–1) to mild illness with only minimal conjunctival infection and lid swelling. Fever and gastrointestinal and respiratory symptoms were seldom present. Most cases occurred in children younger than age 10 years and lasted 2 to 18 days (median, 6.5 days). Various ophthalmic medications were used in treatment, but their relative effectiveness is unknown.

This outbreak, which involved more than 2,000 persons from 20 counties in southeast Georgia, shows that "gnat sore eyes," or seasonal acute conjunctivitis, remains a potential problem in the Southern United States during warm months and especially during periods when the gnats are unusually prevalent.

► If the title of this article doesn't grab you, you just aren't grabbable. I am sure there is not one of us who has not been bothered by the little critter called the gnat. They are well known among insectologists as being the tiny bug that flies around your head when you walk outside on warm moist summer and early fall evenings. For some reason, I never realized that if one of those pesty things got into your eye it could cause such trouble. This outbreak of conjunctivitis that occurred in south Georgia in 1981 is strikingly similar to outbreaks described in southern California and in the southern states more than 20 to 50 years ago. Unfortunately, most of the reports appeared in the public health literature and never appeared in the journals that most of us commonly read. For example, in 1949 and 1950 in Thomas county, Georgia, absenteeism during the months of September and October was so high that the entire matter had to be investigated by the Public Health Service. In these southern states, the problem begins in the summer but peaks in the early fall and has attack rates that are as high as 50% in children younger than age 4 years. In children aged 5 to 9 this declines to 32%, while in adults the attack rates are only about 5%. That's a lot of red eyes. In all fairness to the little gnats *(Hippelates pusio)*, this vector has been suspected, although never proved, as the mode of transmission. It is a highly likely suspect, however, because a number of children with the syndrome have gnats in their eyes when they are examined. The presumption is that *Hippelates pusio* carries a variety of *Hemophilus aegyptius,* also known as the "Koch-Weeks bacillus." My presumption is that this would be treatable with the usual topical sulfa preparations that most use for common run-of-the-mill conjunctivitis. Credit for making us all aware of the problem of gnat sore eyes goes to the Office of Public Health in the Georgia Department of Human Resources. However, I would like to quote for you a reference from a somewhat older article. It reads as follows, "Fifteen hundred children in the Coachella Valley Unit High School, at Thermal, California, are suffering with serious conjunctivitis or pink eye, due to the ravages of the California eye gnat. . . . The gnat, known specifically as *Hippelates pusio, . . .* hovers and swarms about the eyes, noses, and mouths of persons and stock. Small children are especially helpless against it. Over one hundred of the schoolchildren in this region now have serious eye trouble caused by the gnat. . . ."—anonymous—*Science,* 1929. It is axiomatic that it is unfortunate that credit goes to the man who convinces the world, not the man to whom the idea first occurs. Perhaps we should call this "anonymous sore eyes."—J.A.S., III

Congenital Aniridia: Histopathologic Study of the Anterior Segment in Children
Curtis E. Margo (Armed Forces Inst. of Pathology)
J. Pediatr. Ophthalmol. Strabismus 20:192–198, Sept.–Oct. 1983   14–3

Children with congenital aniridia frequently exhibit abnormal development of the macula and optic nerve as well, and most have progressive changes during life that involve the cornea, anterior chamber angle, and lens. Seven eyes from 7 children with congenital aniridia were examined to elucidate the relation between congenital and acquired abnormalities. The children were aged 6 days to 14 years at enucleation or autopsy. None had had an intraocular operation. The clinical findings are summarized in the table.

Apart from iris and ciliary body hypoplasia, the eyes exhibited anomalous development of the anterior chamber angle, incomplete cleavage of the chamber angle, and attenuation of Bowman's membrane. The 2 cases of anomalous development of the anterior chamber angle were in children with partial deletion of the short arm of chromosome 11. These children were among the 3 with urogenital tumors and the 4 with sporadic rather than familial aniridia. Major portions of Bowman's membrane were focally attenuated or absent in 2 eyes. The acquired abnormalities of the anterior segment included corneal pannus, peripheral anterior synechiae, and len-

CLINICAL DATA ON 7 CASES OF CONGENITAL ANIRIDIA

Case	Age*/Sex/Race	Family History of Aniridia	Additional Diagnosis	Clinical Diagnosis of glaucoma	Reason for enucleation, or cause of death
1	6 da/?/?	Yes	None	No	Autopsy-intracranial hemorrhage
2	6 mo/F/?	No	Mental retardation; Wilms' tumor	No	Autopsy-Wilms' tumor
3	19 mo/M/?	No	None	No	Autopsy-sudden death
4	21 mo/F/W	No	Partial deletion 11 p; mental retardation; gonadoblastoma	Yes	Autopsy-pneumonia
5	6 yr/F/?	No	Partial deletion 11 p; mental retardation; Wilms' tumor; congenital heart disease	Yes	Enucleation-rule out metastatic Wilms' tumor
6	11 yr/M/W	Yes	None	Yes	Enucleation-blindness and pain
7	14 yr/M/W	Yes	Blunt ocular trauma 2 wks prior to enucleation	Yes	Enucleation-blindess and pain

*Age at enucleation or autopsy.
(Courtesy of Margo, C.E.: J. Pediatr. Ophthalmol. Strabismus 20:192–198, Sept.–Oct. 1983.)

ticular degeneration. The lens was cataractous in all cases but 1. Various degrees of nuclear and cortical degeneration were frequent findings. Retinal detachments were present in 2 eyes; 1 was secondary to a choroidal granuloma due to *Histoplasma capsulatum,* and the other was in a child with a history of blunt ocular trauma.

Iris hypoplasia is rarely an isolated abnormality and usually is not the chief determinant of visual function. Glaucoma is thought to result from angle closure due to synechia formation in most aniridic eyes. Whether the corneal abnormalities are primary or secondary is uncertain.

The Development of Binocular Summation in Human Infants
Eileen E. Birch (Univ. of Texas) and Richard Held (Masachusetts Inst. of Technology)
Ophthalmol. Vis. Sci. 24:1103–1107, August 1983   14–4

Studies of binocular vision in infancy using the psychophysical and electrophysiologic approaches have suggested that the visual paths through which signals from the eyes converge for disparity processing require a period of maturation after birth. The authors used the difference in pupil diameter under monocular and binocular viewing conditions as a measure of binocular luminance summation in assessing 97 infants in the first year of life. This is an objective approach that requires minimal time and cooperation and can be used even in the presence of large angle tropias. Stereopsis also was evaluated. Studies were done in 10 normal adults aged 20–50 years as well.

No significant difference in pupil diameters under monocular and binocular viewing conditions was found until the end of the fourth month of life, and the age at onset correlated with that for stereopsis, as assessed by preferential looking. An adult-like difference in pupil diameters was present by the end of the sixth month of life. The coefficient of correlation between the ages of onset obtained by the two procedures in 12 infants who were tested twice a month over ages 2–6 months was 0.775.

Binocular summation is measurable by age 4 months in normal infants and is comparable in magnitude to that in adults by age 6 months. The age at onset of binocular summation correlates closely with that of stereopsis. The findings are consistent with the absence of binocular summation in the pupillary response of strabismic adults. The development of bifoveal fixation is not the only factor determining the onset of stereopsis. Rather, the visual paths by which signals from the eyes converge must undergo maturation over the first few months of postnatal life. The binocular summation procedure may prove especially useful in evaluating strabismic infants.

▶ This article and the preceding one deal with various aspects of either normal or abnormal development of the eyes. The association of congenital aniridia with urogenital malformations and mental retardation (now quickly becoming known as the "AGR triad") is found mostly in sporadically occurring cases. This may be the result of a partial deletion of the short arm of chromosome 11. It appears likely that the well-established aniridia-Wilms' tumor association is also a result of this chromosome deletion. Hittner et al. have described an inherited form of aniridia in association with chromosome 11 deletion (*Ophthalmology* 86:1173, 1979). Obviously, anytime a congenital aniridia is detected, serial follow-up for the development of Wilms' tumor (perhaps best done by frequent sonography) is in order. Chromosomal studies looking for partial deletion of the short arm of chromosome 11 likewise should be done.

Regarding the development of normal vision in infants as partly discussed in the article by Birch and Held, we are seeing a great deal more information concerning exactly what goes on in the first few months of life, particularly in infants who may have some difficulties with the development of normal vision. As is discussed in the following article, the term "delayed visual development" has been applied to full-term infants who, at age 6 weeks or older, show no visual awareness of their surroundings and have an inability to fixate or follow a bright object. The delay in visual maturation is often part of a general neurologic disorder or delay, but the severity of the visual impairment tends to be greater than that of the other disabilities if they are present at all. A high percentage of these infants are either premature or small for gestational age. This association suggests that a neurologic insult in the neonatal period may be a causative factor. A delayed visual development can manifest itself throughout the first year of life and then gradually resolve. As we will see in the following article, the theory that cortical dysfunction is the cause of delayed visual maturation receives further support from the fact that in most of the reported cases the infants were of low birth weight and were thus prone to hypoxic ischemic brain damage. Partial ischemia tends to cause selective neuronal necrosis in the cortex, diencephalon, and midbrain. The visual cortex is particularly vulnerable. Despite reports of neurologic normality in some infants with delayed visual maturation, existing data favor the view that this condition is a marker of neurologic damage. In most instances, an early positive diagnosis can be made by clinical examination and electrodiagnostic tests, and the parents can be reassured of a good prognosis for visual outcome. However, these infants still run a high risk of late neurologic troubles and learning disabilities, so they should be closely and expertly monitored throughout the rest of childhood.—J.A.S., III

Cortical Blindness in Infancy: A Follow-up Study
S. Ronen, I. Nawratzki, and L. Yanko (Hadassah Univ., Jerusalem)
Ophthalmologica 187:217–221, 1983   14–5

Cortical blindness is a cause of loss of vision in childhood. It is diagnosed on the basis of blindness, presence of the pupillary reflex, normal ophthalmoscopic findings, and the absence of optokinetic nystagmus and spontaneous nystagmus. The authors report the long-term follow-up of 6 children with cortical blindness in the prenatal and perinatal periods or shortly after birth. The diagnosis should be confirmed electrophysiologically. The electroretinogram is intact, while the visual evoked potentials are generally abnormal. Older children have been reported usually to have at least partial recovery of vision.

Some visual recovery was observed in the present cases, but recognition capacity remained impaired. The children had difficulty in recognizing or identifying objects and, especially, symbols. Older children who were mobile were seen to move about without bumping into obstacles even though they did not recognize them, and they sometimes reached out to touch them. Three patients were taught to move about by a combination of touching and seeing. The children learned to recognize persons and objects at home, but failed to identify them when presented in pictures. A lack of educational effort may produce the picture of a mentally retarded child, and some children have been confined in institutions. Associated severe brain damage can, however, lead to mental deficiency, as in 1 of the present cases.

It is difficult to predict whether and to what extent visual functions will return, but recovery tends to occur slowly and to be incomplete when cortical blindness develops perinatally or in early infancy.

▶ Missing cortical blindness in an infant is relatively easy. That is not to say that parents will not be quite dismayed by not being told their child is blind earlier. Indeed, the suspicion that a baby with otherwise normal-looking eyes does not see is usually raised by the parents. These infants usually do not present with squint or "roving" eyes as do many babies with other forms or combined forms of blindness. The detection occurs usually at the time at which a parent feels that the child is not following objects appropriately or has a somewhat blank expression. The presence of the typical symptomatology triad of blindness, the presence of the pupillary reflex, and a normal ophthalmoscopic picture, as well as absence of the optokinetic nystagmus and the spontaneous nystagmus, which occurs in all other cases of organic blindness occurring in the first month of life, lead to the diagnosis of cortical blindness. Various causes leading to cortical blindness in children have been reported in the literature. Except for cases of cortical blindness caused by infections, as in meningitis, or head injuries, the etiology is mostly a vascular event leading to hypoxia or anoxia with possible necrosis of tissues. Although an unusual event, it certainly is possible that anoxia in the perinatal period can affect only the occipital lobes without producing more diffuse signs that one typically associates cerebral palsy. Among the 6 patients described in this series, at least 1 had no other evidence of diffuse anoxic damage by later infancy or early childhood. Thus, we must be constantly aware of the potential for blindness in the absence of any other neurologic deficits in babies coming out of our intensive care nurseries. Some have felt strongly enough about this that recommendations for routine visual evoked potentials have been suggested for babies who have complicated perinatal courses.

Cortical blindness is different from all other cases of congenital blindness due to damage to the afferent visual pathways. Children with cortical blindness actually may learn to see partially but will have difficulty in recognizing or identifying objects, especially symbols. For example, these children very frequently are mobile, crawling or walking, but are never seen to bump into objects even though they do not recognize what is in front of them. It is somewhat of an anachronism that the healthy among us generally see only what the mind is prepared to comprehend while these unfortunate children, despite their anoxic damage, are capable of comprehending, but do not see.—J.A.S., III

Ocular Presentation of Sarcoidosis in Children

Sudesh Kataria, G. Earl Trevathan, James E. Holland, and Yash P. Kataria (East Carolina Univ., Greenville, N.C.)
Clin. Pediatr. (Phila.) 12:793–797, December 1983   14–6

In sarcoidosis in children, ocular involvement is the second most common manifestation, exceeded only by hilar adenopathy and pulmonary abnormalities. The authors describe a black boy who presented with redness of the left eye, blurred vision, and decreased visual acuity. He was subsequently diagnosed as having sarcoidosis.

Boy, 14, had a 3-month history of irritation, redness, and discomfort of the left eye in bright light. Four days prior to admission he noted decreased visual acuity and blurred vision in this eye. He also had intermittent cough productive of scanty white sputum and had been fatigued and sleepy. The right pupil was round and reactive; the left pupil was irregular, middilated and fixed (Fig 14–2) by posterior synechiae. Slit-lamp examination of the left eye revealed diffuse haziness of the cornea with the endothelial surface showing diffuse mutton-fat keratitic precipitates. The anterior chamber showed flare with occasional cells. The iris contained multiple superficial vascularized nodular lesions. The lens had multiple posterior synechiae. Fundoscopic examination of the right eye showed multiple discrete, slightly elevated yellowish-white lesions of the periphery of the retina. Fundoscopic examination of the left eye revealed multiple vitreous veils.

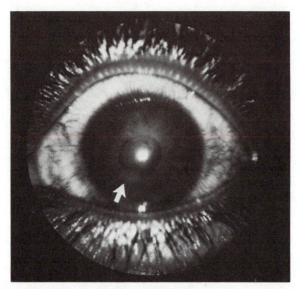

Fig 14–2.—Left eye showing marked congestion of conjunctiva, especially around limbus, and irregular pupil (anterior uveitis). Koeppe's nodule is seen at inferior margin of pupil. (Courtesy of Kataria, S., et al.: Clin. Pediatr. (Phila.) 12:793–797, December 1983.)

Total leukocyte count was 4,700/µl with 13% eosinophils. A biopsy specimen from a right cervical lymph node showed noncaseating granulomatous inflammation compatible with the diagnosis of sarcoidosis.

The patient was started on orally administered prednisone, 40 mg daily, and prednisolone acetate 1% eyedrops, one drop three times a day in the left eye. At 2-week follow-up there was subjective improvement in visual acuity of the left eye. At 6-month follow-up there was marked reduction of vision in the left eye, with best corrected visual acuities of 20/200 in the left and 20/20 in the right eye.

The prognosis of sarcoidosis in symptomatic children is not easy to determine because there has been no long-term follow-up of a large number of patients. All patients with suspected sarcoidosis should have complete ophthalmologic examinations and patients with ocular findings suggestive of sarcoidosis should have thorough medical examinations that include chest films. In the study patient the chest film showed bilateral diffuse reticulonodular infiltrates.

▶ We don't tend to think a great deal about sarcoidosis in children. It generally is considered a "rarity" among the patients that we treat and it is often not recognized for what it is despite the presence of absolutely classic signs and symptoms. It is true that the prevalence and incidence in the United States are not known, because mass screening chest radiographs have not been as popular in the United States as in other parts of the world. In Hungary and Japan, where routine chest x-ray studies are much more prevalent, the incidence of sarcoidosis in asymptomatic children is at least equal to that of adults in the same population. This destroys the myth that sarcoidosis is principally a disease of adults. Most reported cases of sarcoidosis in the United States have been symptomatic and have occurred predominantly in blacks. Preadolescents and adolescents account for the highest frequency. Because of the multisystem presentation of sarcoidosis in children, the disease is diagnosed at a considerably later stage than the disease in adults. What is particularly unique to children, however, is the fact that the incidence of ocular involvement, which is perhaps as high as 20% in older people, is virtually 100% in the very young patient. This is the importance of this study from *Clinical Pediatrics.* In contrast to older children and adults, the child younger than age 5 with sarcoidosis rarely has pulmonary disease and typically has involvement of joints, skin, and eyes. Uveitis may be the first and only clinical manifestation of sarcoidosis in such young children. If unrecognized and not treated for what it is, cataracts can develop, leading to blindness as well as other serious ocular complications. Steroids are the drugs of choice in the management of sarcoidosis. If the only significant clinical problem is that of uveitis, topical treatment might suffice although systemic therapy or management with steroids or other immunosuppressive therapies may ultimately be necessary. The goal of treatment is not to eliminate the signs and symptoms, which is not always possible, but to prevent visual loss and other sequelae such as posterior synechiae, secondary glaucoma, cataract formation, and optic nerve involvement. The prognosis in all of these children is difficult to determine because of the relatively small sizes of the individual series that have been reported. The purpose of having this article in the YEAR BOOK is obvious. It is to remind us that sarcoidosis is a problem of childhood and can have significant effects on vision if not managed properly. It is a bad disease in some instances and we wish that someone had a better idea about its true prognosis. For right now, I would view the prognosis through rose-colored glasses but with a jaundiced eye.— J.A.S., III

Conjunctival Scarring in Kawasaki Disease: A New Finding?

Edwin H. Ryan and David S. Walton (Harvard Med. School)
J. Pediatr. Ophthalmol. Strabismus 20:106–108, May–June 1983   14–7

Characteristically, in Kawasaki disease there is bilateral injection of the bulbar conjunctiva. Chemosis and purulent discharge are generally absent. An instance of Kawasaki disease with resultant bilateral palpebral conjunctival scarring is presented here.

Male infant was first seen at age 4 months and was diagnosed as having a residual pupillary membrane structure in the left eye; his twin brother had a similar plaque. At 10 months he had a rash covering the entire body that was associated with a temperature up to 104.8 F. This condition persisted and on the sixth day the lips became red and cracked. When the infant refused to eat, he was admitted to the hospital. A tentative diagnosis of Kawasaki disease was given. Laboratory data included a white blood cell count of 28,300; platelet count of 508,000; cerebrospinal fluid with 5 white blood cells, all lymphocytes; and urine with 1 to 3 white blood cells per high-powered field. Multiple small, firm posterior cervical and supraclavicular nodes were palpated. Cardiovascular examination was normal;

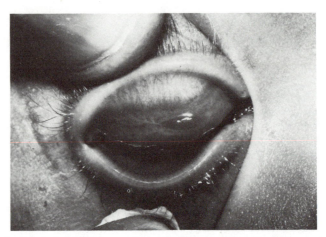

Fig 14–3.—Scarring is visible in 3-mm–wide band 2 mm removed from tarsus along superior forniceal conjunctiva. Normal conjunctiva can be seen prolapsing through defect in scar. (Courtesy of Ryan, E.H., and Walton, D.S.: J. Pediatr. Ophthalmol. Strabismus 20:106–108, May–June 1983.)

mild conjunctival injection without exudate was revealed on eye examination.

After day 11, the patient was afebrile. A conjunctival exudate was noted that grew *Staphylococcus aureus* on culture and he was started on erythromycin ointment. Ocular examination on day 17 was normal, except for the cataract and the conjunctivae that were injected. Hands and feet began to desquamate and he was discharged on day 20 of illness. When seen 3 weeks later he was found to have bilateral scarring of the superior and inferior forniceal conjunctivae to within 2 mm of the tarsal plate (Fig 14–3). (His HLA-identical twin was never sick.)

This patient showed all six major symptoms of Kawasaki disease: fever unresponsive to antibiotics, bilateral congestion of ocular conjunctivae, changes of lips and oral cavity, changes of peripheral extremities, polymorphous exanthema of body trunk without vesicles or crusts and acute nonpurulent swelling of cervical nodes. He also had most of the minor symptoms, including elevated sedimentation rate and thrombocytosis.

Bilateral scarring of the superior and inferior forniceal conjunctivae in this patient seemed to have developed within 3 weeks of discharge from the hospital. Although these abnormalities were not seen during the course of Kawasaki disease, it is assumed that they were a complication of the disease. Although Kawasaki disease appears to be a separate clinical entity, it is clearly closely related to other mucocutaneous syndromes, such as erythema multiforme and Stevens-Johnson syndrome that also has scarring as a sequel.

Careful examination of the palpebral and forniceal conjunctivae of patients who have Kawasaki disease is needed to establish the incidence of conjunctival scarring in this disease.

▶ Eye findings are not at all uncommon in cases of Kawasaki disease. In fact, bilateral injection of the bulbar conjuctivae in the presence of fever, erythema of the oropharynx, generalized rash, edema of the hands and feet, and non-suppurative lymphadenopathy, all together, form the diagnostic complex of Kawasaki disease. What this study is telling us, however, is that one should not take too lightly the "conjunctivitis" of Kawasaki disease, because it may leave residual scarring that is capable of impairing vision. R. L. Font et al. (*Ophthalmology* 90:569, 1983) summarize for us the eye findings of Kawasaki disease. Specifically, 89% of cases will have conjunctivitis, 78% will have iridiocyclitis, 22% will have superficial punctate keratitis, 11% will have vitreous opacities, 11% will have papilledema, and 6% will have subconjunctival hemorrhages. Most important was the observation by the latter investigators of bilateral severe retinal ischemia in a child aged 4 months who died of cardiovascular complications of Kawasaki disease. At autopsy, this baby showed aneurysmal dilatation and thromboses in the coronary blood vessels, the abdominal aorta, and in both carotid arteries. Vasculitis and thrombosis of the ophthalmic artery also were present. Curiously, the mitochondrial ultrastructure of cells from the retina showed marked abnormalities similar to those found in other tissue, including blood vessel walls. Without question, this is a multisystem disorder in which one must pay careful attention to the ophthalmologic complications as well as the cardiac ones.—J.A.S., III

Uveitis Complicating Autoimmune Chronic Active Hepatitis
Jeffrey N. Bloom, I. Matthew Rabinowicz, and Stanford T. Shulman (Univ. of Florida)
Am. J. Dis. Child. 137:1175–1176, December 1983   14–8

A patient with autoimmune hepatitis B surface antigen-negative chronic active hepatitis (CAH) developed uveitis during the course of the disease.

Girl, 8, had insidious onset of icterus. General physical examination showed an otherwise healthy girl with obvious scleral and mucosal icterus. Ophthalmologic examination showed a visual acuity of 20/25 in the right and left eyes. Scleral icterus was noted bilaterally. Multiple keratic precipitates of medium size were seen in the right eye and were associated with moderate inflammatory reaction in the anterior chamber and vitreous cavity. No autoimmune hepatitis B surface antigen (HBsAG) was detected. Antinuclear antibodies were present at low serum titer. Antibody to smooth muscle was present. Histologic examination of a percutaneous needle biopsy specimen of the liver demonstrated cirrhosis, reticular collapse, and portal and periportal mononuclear inflammation with piecemeal necrosis, consistent with the diagnosis of CAH. Initial treatment consisted of orally administered prednisone (40 mg/day), scopolamine hydrobromide ophthalmic solution (0.25%) twice daily, and fluorometholone three times daily. Within 2 weeks, the icterus had greatly improved, the uveitis had cleared, and the serous retinal detachment was minimal. Persistent elevation of serum transaminase levels was noted. After 4 doses of transfer factor during 10 weeks only modest improvement in serum transaminase levels was seen. Subsequent administration of prednisone with azathioprine (50 mg/day) resulted in normalization of liver chemistry. This therapy was continued for 2 years. Three months later, uveitis was again noted in the right eye but resolved after a short course of prednisone.

Clinicians should be alert to the association of uveitis with CAH so that patients at risk may be examined for this potentially serious ocular disease.

▶ Chronic active hepatitis which is hepatitis B surface antigen negative most likely represents an autoimmune process and often is associated with extra-hepatic manifestations such as arthritis, glomerulitis, hemolytic anemia, and pericarditis. Occasionally all this is associated with specific HLA types (A–1 and B–8). Some patients also show a form of Hashimoto's thyroiditis, Sjögren's syndrome, ulcerative colitis, pleuritis, and myasthenia gravis. Presumably what is going on with the liver disease in these patients is that an antibody with specificity for liver membrane antigens is being attached to hepatocytes. From this report we must have a heightened awareness of the extension of this panautoimmune phenomenon to the eye. Now that the association be-tween uveitis and chronic hepatitis has been well described, it is incumbent on us to recognize these cases when they cross our path. This is one of those unusual associations that we must file away in our Betz cell computers to recall when the information is needed. Good intentions won't diagnose this, only brute memory. As the old southern saying goes, " 'Mean to' don't pick no cotton."—J.A.S., III

Hypertensive Retinopathy in the Newborn Infant
Mary Ellen Leder Skalina, William L. Annable, Robert M. Kliegman, and Avroy A. Fanaroff (Case Western Reserve Univ., Cleveland)
J. Pediatr. 103:781–786, November 1983   14–9

Hypertension (blood pressure greater than 70 mm Hg on 3 days) was noted in 23 of 1,941 infants, or 1.2% of all neonatal admissions to the intensive and intermediate care nurseries at Rainbow Babies and Childrens Hospital, Cleveland, from December 1978 to November 1980. Indirect ophthalmoscopy was performed in hypertensive infants only after their acute medical condition had stabilized or improved.

Of the 23 patients with symptomatic systemic arterial hypertension, 2 died. The other 21 infants had a mean birth weight of 2,566 gm and mean gestational age of 35.6 weeks. The infants were found to be hypertensive by routine monitoring of vital signs. In 11, a spectrum of retinal abnor-malities was detected during the initial ophthalmologic examination. A consistent observation in all 11 was an increased ratio of venous to arterial calibers. Hemorrhages and exudates, frequent findings in adults, were less common in these infants. Two infants had retinal exudates (Fig 14–4). To date, 7 patients with definite retinal abnormalities have had follow-up examinations. As a group, these 7 had all of the disorders described (arterial spasm, venous dilation, hemorrhage, and exudate). Five of the 7 had com-plete clearing of all hypertensive changes when reexamined 1–6 months later.

The retinal abnormalities observed in these infants may be related to the primary medical diagnoses. Certain elements of the retinopathy ob-served resemble the retinopathy of prematurity. It is not known yet whether

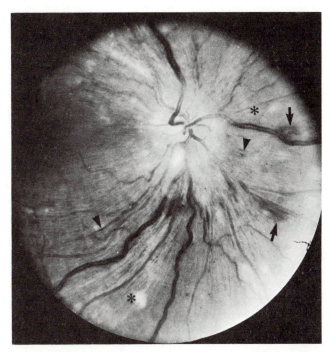

Fig 14–4.—Severe hypertensive retinopathy, with arterial spasm, vascular tortuosity, cotton wool exudates *(asterisks)*, and both streak *(arrowheads)* and blot *(arrows)* hemorrhages. (Courtesy of Skalina, M.E.L., et al.: J. Pediatr. 103:781–786, November 1983.)

hypertensive retinopathy has the same implications for the newborn as for the adult patient. The presence of signs of cardiac or renal dysfunction in many of these hypertensive neonatal patients indicates there may be an association between vascular disease in other organs and retinal changes in this age group as well.

Corneal Scarring Associated With Daily Soft Contact Lens Wear
Stephen T. Conway (Rhode Island Hosp., Providence) and Safa F. Wagdi (Massachusetts Eye & Ear Infirm., Boston)
Ann. Ophthalmol. 15:868–871, September 1983   14–10

Three adolescent and young adult subjects were recently encountered who developed scarring of both corneas with loss of visual acuity while wearing cosmetic soft contact lenses daily. All 3 had bilateral involvement. The scarring began superiorly and spread inferiorly and was associated with conjunctival injection and corneal staining at the time of presentation. Conjunctival injection resolved rapidly when lens wear was discontinued, but the corneal staining and scarring resolved much more slowly, and 1 patient was left with a permanent reduction in visual acuity associated with induced astigmatism secondary to corneal change. The best corrected acuity in this subject was 20/40 in the right eye and 20/50 in the left. Keratometry showed the corneal mires to be irregular.

This condition definitely appears related to contact lens wear. All patients had bilateral involvement starting 6–12 months after the onset of lens use, and all improved when lens wear was discontinued. The patient with a residual decrease in acuity had resumed lens wear after initially improving. Possible specific causes include a reaction to a chemical in the solution used to care for the lenses or in proprietary eyedrops, an allergic reaction to surface deposits on the lenses, and the "tight lens" or "overwear" syndrome. The last state appears to be due to epithelial hypoxia. The disorder may be more frequent than the ophthalmologic literature indicates.

▶ E. Lee Stock, Director of the Cornea and External Eye Disease Laboratory, Department of Ophthalmology, Northwestern University, comments:

"Soft contact lenses have become increasingly popular over the past 10 years. They are more comfortable than hard lenses and are easier to fit. However, these lenses are thought to cause diseases that only recently have been recognized. Giant papillary conjunctivitis is the most common of these disorders. The tarsal conjunctiva becomes inflamed and the inflammatory cells collect around blood vessels, resulting in the irregular elevations known as giant papillae. Small white dots may be seen at the edge of the cornea (Trantas' dots). This condition is associated with redness of the eyes as well as discomfort and itching. The more serious complications involve the cornea, because inflammation can lead to vascularization and scarring that may lead to loss of vision. These patterns include inflammation of the superior part of the cornea and peripheral corneal inflammation.

"Inflammation may be based on an allergy to the preservatives in the contact lens solutions, but also may be caused by allergic reactions to the contact lens material itself or some antigenic material that is concentrated on the surface of the lens.

"Criteria for a good contact lens fit include good vision and absence of redness, irritation, discomfort, or decreased vision. Any of these symptoms is unacceptable and may indicate poor lens fit or a reaction to the lens.

"Any symptom should be investigated by complete ophthalmologic examination, including slit-lamp examination, in order to diagnose corneal and conjunctival complications that may lead to visual loss."

15 Neurology and Psychiatry

Long-term Outcome of Children With Severe Head Trauma and Prolonged Coma
William J. Mahoney, Bernard J. D'Souza, J. Alex Haller, Mark C. Rogers, Melvin H. Epstein, and John M. Freeman
Pediatrics 71:756–762, May 1983   15–1

Trauma is the leading cause of death in children older than age 1 year, with head trauma being the major contributing factor. Recent advances in the management of head trauma have decreased mortality; however, it was predicted that this decline in mortality would be accompanied by a concomitant increase in morbidity in survivors.

The long-term outcome is reported in the 46 children with significant head trauma admitted to the Pediatric Intensive Care Unit (PICU) of Johns Hopkins Childrens Center between January 1976 and December 1979 who remained in coma for more than 24 hours. Twelve (38%) of the 46 children died. They were either dead on arrival (group A), died of causes not related to the central nervous system (CNS) (group B), died as a result of increased cranial pressure (ICP) (group C), or died of other causes (group D) (table). The 4 children in group A were believed to be brain dead at the time of arrival; cerebral function did not return despite extensive resuscitative efforts and maintenance of vital functions for more than 24 hours. The 1 patient in group D appeared to have died of hypotension. Eleven of the 12 children were declared brain dead. The mean duration of coma in the survivors was 15.5 days. Intracranial pressure was monitored in 12 of the 46 children and all underwent computed tomography scanning. The children were classified according to outcome: return to normal after trauma (class I); learning or behavioral problems (class II), further subdivided into those with similar problems prior to trauma (class IIA) and those reportedly normal before trauma (IIB); handicapping motor residua but normal intellect (class III); and significant mental retardation or motor problems that could preclude independent functioning (class IV). Of the 3 class IV survivors, 2 were younger than age 2 years and were the only children in this age group who survived. Ten of 12 children younger than age 4 years survived. Of the 34 survivors, 10 were in class I, 11 in class IIA, 7 in class IIB, 3 in class III, and 3 in class IV. Although children who were in a prolonged coma tended to have a poor outcome, 9 of 14 children in coma for more than 2 weeks had little or no handicapping neurologic residua (Fig 15–1). Despite major complications, the degree of recovery in the surviving children was impressive.

DATA CONCERNING 12 CHILDREN WHO DIED OF SEVERE HEAD TRAUMA

Patient No.	Age (yr)	Sex	Condition on Admission	Course	Length of Coma (d)	Criteria for Death	Comment
A. Dead on arrival							
1	10	M	Cardiac arrest prior to arrival; cyanotic; clinical criteria BD	Cardiac arrest in emergency room	2	BD*	Nonpreventable
2	12	F	Brain dead	No recovery	3	BD	Nonpreventable
3	6	F	Apneic	Pupils fixed at 10 mm; CT, edema; hypotension	3	BD	Nonpreventable; no response to treatment
4	1	F	Respiratory arrest prior to transfer; clinical criteria BD	No response to therapy	2	BD	Nonpreventable
B. Death due to factors outside CNS							
5	7	F	Combative, stuporous	BD at 4 h; CT, edema; cardiac arrest; operating room (OR), splenectomy postoperative cardiac arrest	3	BD	Possibly preventable
6	5	M	Conscious on arrival; decreased consciousness; shock	Response with resuscitation; OR, liver laceration; vena caval tear; multiple cardiac arrests	3	BD	Possibly preventable
7	1½	M	Crying prior to transfer; pupils react; hypotension	OR, liver and spleen laceration; postoperative responsive, hypotension	2	BD	Possibly preventable
8	5	M	Shock; pupils fixed	OR, liver and spleen laceration; postoperative responsive, disseminated intravascular coagulopathy; return to OR, kidney laceration; postoperative, arrest	4	BD	Possibly preventable
C. Death due to increased intracranial pressure (ICP)							
9	12	M	Decerebrate; pupils react	ICP; nonaggressive therapy; therapy abandoned	10	BD	Possibly preventable
10	13	F	Cardiac arrest at scene; decorticate; pupils sluggish	Impossible to control ICP	3	BD	Nonpreventable
11	4	M	Decorticate; pupils sluggish	Progressive ICP despite vigorous treatment	3	BD	Nonpreventable
D. Other							
12	15	M	Open skull fracture; decorticate; pupils nonreactive	OR, immediate frontal lobectomy; postoperative hypotension twice	2	BD	Possibly preventable

*BD, brain death.

(Courtesy of Mahoney, W.J., et al.: Pediatrics 71:756–762, May 1983. Copyright American Academy of Pediatrics 1983.)

The findings indicate that intensive medical and surgical care in patients with serious head trauma does not result in a large number of severely disabled survivors.

▶ Robert Kanter, Assistant Professor of Pediatrics and Director, Intensive Care Unit, State University of New York Upstate Medical Center, comments:
"This study confirms the impression of Brink and associates (*J. Pediatr.* 97:721–727, 1980) that most pediatric survivors of coma due to head trauma

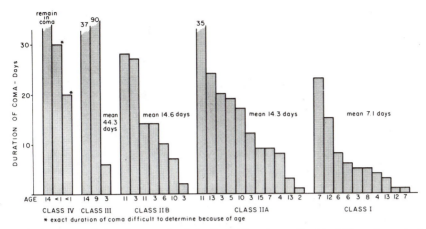

Fig 15–1.—Correlation of outcome by class with duration of coma (days) in children who survived severe head trauma. Age of each child is shown along the ordinate. (Courtesy of Mahoney, W.J., et al.: *Pediatrics* 71:756–762, May 1983. Copyright American Academy of Pediatrics 1983.)

recover without serious disability. Why are the survival and recovery in these patients improving so dramatically? Most importantly, advances in organizing prehospital care and resuscitation have provided early control of circulatory and respiratory derangements. When systematic management by experienced personnel is lacking, avoidable complications are common. Studies in Glasgow, Scotland, revealed preventable airway obstruction in 27%, respiratory arrest in 12%, and inadequately treated hypotension in 11% of head-injured patients during transfer between hospitals (Gentleman, D., et al.: *Lancet* 2:853–855, 1981). Earlier observations had identified head trauma victims whose avoidable deaths appeared to be due to airway obstruction in 35% and inadequately treated shock in 29% (Rose, J., et al.: *Br. Med. J.* 2:615–618, 1977). Beyond prevention, the most productive areas for efforts to improve trauma morbidity and mortality are development of regional trauma care centers and objective assessment of methods of prehospital care (West, J. G., et al.: *Arch. Surg.* 114:455–460, 1979; and Trunkey, D. D.: *J. Trauma* 24:86–87, 1984), for example: What techniques should be applied in the prehospital resuscitation? What is the relative value of time spent on stabilization in the field versus rapid transportation to a hospital? What are the most effective mechanisms for physician supervision of prehospital care?

"Rapid CT scan detection of surgically treatable lesions and control of intracranial hypertension also contribute to improved outcome. Survival with traumatic acute subdural hematoma falls from 70% to 10% when surgery is delayed longer than 4 hours after the injury (Seelig, J. M., et al.: *N. Engl. J. Med.* 304:1511–1518, 1981). Aggressive efforts to control intracranial pressure resulted in reduced severity of intracranial hypertension as well as lower mortality even when episodes of intracranial hypertension did occur, compared to mortality in patients treated in a more conservative fashion (Saul, T. G., et al.: *J. Neurosurg.* 56:498–503, 1982).

"Because of the multiplicity of variables, Mahoney and associates emphasize that their findings do not represent the prognosis for all comatose victims of head trauma. Their results should not be extrapolated to patients with prolonged coma due to other causes, such as anoxia, for whom outcome is likely to be far less favorable (Margolis, L. H., et al.: *Pediatrics* 65:477–483, 1980).

"Future efforts to refine techniques of intensive care and rehabilitation of head-injured patients require identification of the many risk factors predisposing to poor outcome, allowing matching of treatment and control groups in therapeutic trials. Adopting a consistent classification of outcome will facilitate comparisons among studies (Jennett, B., et al.: *Lancet* 1:480–484, 1975)."

Neonatal Convulsions: A 10-Year Review
H. J. Goldberg (Melbourne)
Arch. Dis. Child. 58:976–978, December 1983   15–2

The incidence and causes of neonatal convulsions in a hospital population are reviewed. There were 12,904 live births in 1971–1974, 13,304 in 1975–1977, and 14,849 in 1978–1980. The incidence of neonatal convulsions increased from 2–6 to 8.6 per 1,000 live births. The major causes are given in Table 1. Prematurity was strongly associated with cerebral hypoxia and meningitis, especially in the later years of the review period (Table 2). Other, less frequent causes of seizures are listed in Table 3. Hypoxia was the chief cause of seizures in the first 2 days of life. Another peak was associated with fifth-day fits. Neonatal mortality is related to the cause of seizures in Table 4. Overall mortality fell from 33% to 18% during the review period, but mortality in infants with cerebral hypoxia remained at about 50%.

These findings are compared with those in other reported series in Table 5. An increasing number of infants have received an etiologic diagnosis, and this has been of therapeutic and prognostic benefit.

▶ This survey article and the article to follow provide the reader with a picture of the chief causes over the past decade for seizures in early infancy. It can be

TABLE 1.—Neonatal Convulsions

Aetiology	1971–4 No (%)		1975–7 No (%)		1978–80 No (%)	
Fifth day fits	8	(29)	30	(37)	48	(38)
Cerebral hypoxia	11	(41)	23	(30)	38	(30)
Unknown	2	(7)	14	(17)	14	(11)
Hypocalcaemia	1	(4)	4	(5)	8	(6)
Hyponatraemia	—	—	1	(1)	5	(4)
Meningitis	1	(4)	3	(4)	7	(5)
Hypoglycaemia	3	(11)	1	(1)	1	(1)
Others	1	(4)	4	(5)	7	(5)
Total	27	(100)	80	(100)	128	(100)

(Courtesy of Goldberg, H.J.: Arch. Dis. Child. 58:976–978, December 1983.)

TABLE 2.—NEONATAL CONVULSIONS RELATED TO
NUMBERS OF INFANTS BORN BEFORE 37 WEEKS
OF GESTATION

Aetiology	1971–4		1975–7		1978–80	
	No	(%)	No	(%)	No	(%)
Fifth day fits	0/8	(0)	0/30	(0)	0/48	(0)
Cerebral hypoxia	4/11	(36)	14/23	(60)	27/38	(71)
Unknown	1/2	(50)	2/14	(14)	0/14	(0)
Hypocalcaemia	1/1	(100)	2/4	(50)	2/8	(25)
Hyponatraemia	—	—	1/1	(100)	5/5	(100)
Meningitis	0/1	(0)	1/3	(33)	5/7	(71)
Hypoglycaemia	1/3	(33)	0/1	(0)	1/1	(100)
Others	0/1	(0)	1/4	(25)	3/7	(43)
Total	7/27	(26)	21/80	(26)	43/128	(34)

(Courtesy of Goldberg, H.J.: Arch. Dis. Child. 58:976–978, December 1983.)

TABLE 3.—OTHER CAUSES OF CONVULSIONS
(1971–1980)

Aetiology	No
Cerebral haemorrhage after birth trauma	4
Cerebral haemorrhage after parental abuse	1
Cerebral haemorrhage after antenatal motor car accident	1
Zellweger's syndrome	1
Intrauterine CMV	1
Uraemia	1
Congenital hydrocephalus	1
Overdose of intralipid	1
Hypernatraemia	1

*CMV = cytomegalovirus.
(Courtesy of Goldberg, H.J.: Arch. Dis. Child. 58:976–978, December 1983.)

TABLE 4.—NEONATALITY MORTALITY ACCORDING
TO ETIOLOGY OF FITS

Aetiology	1971–4		1975–7		1978–80	
	No	(%)	No	(%)	No	(%)
Cerebral hypoxia	5/11	(45)	14/23	(61)	20/38	(53)
Hypoglycaemia	1/3	(33)	0/1	(0)	0/1	(0)
Meningitis	1/1	(100)	0/3	(0)	2/7	(29)
Zellweger's syndrome	1/1	(100)	—	—	—	—
Congenital hydrocephalus	—	—	—	—	1/1	(100)
Unknown	1/2	(50)	0/14	(0)	0/14	(0)
Birth trauma	—	—	0/3	(0)	1/1	(100)
Total	9		14		24	
As % of total number with fits	33·5%		17·5%		18·5%	

(Courtesy of Goldberg, H.J.: Arch. Dis. Child. 58:976–978, December 1983.)

TABLE 5.—COMPARATIVE SERIES

Year	Source	Incidence per 1000 live births	Aetiology unknown (%)	Mortality (%)
1959	Leeds	—	47	42
1969	Gothenburg	3·7	31	13·5
1970	Boston	—	27	—
1972	Edinburgh	14	56	10
1979	Stockholm	1·5	29	13
1974	Melbourne	2·0	7	33·5
1977	Melbourne	6·0	17	17·5
1980	Melbourne	8·6	11	18·5

(Courtesy of Goldberg, H.J.: Arch. Dis. Child. 58:976–978, December 1983.)

observed that hypocalcemia and hypoglycemia are rarely a cause for neonatal seizures today. In nurseries currently, particularly those with many low birth weight infants, seizures as a consequence of hypoxia and ischemia top the list.

The outcome of neonates with convulsions who were seen in a neonatal intensive care unit was examined by Ira Bergman and associates (*Ann. Neurol.* 14:642, 1983). A total of 131 survivors of neonatal seizures, now aged 1 to 5 years, were evaluated. Half of the children had been born before 37 weeks' gestation and one fourth, before 31 weeks. From this group of 131 infants, 50 (38%) were normal while 30 (23%) had severe disabilities and 6 (4.6%) had died because of profound neurologic handicaps. Recurrent nonfebrile seizures had developed in about one fifth of the group. Most of the children with motor handicaps or visual loss were intellectually retarded, but 10 of 15 children with bilateral hearing loss were intellectually normal. Of the 77 children whose neonatal seizures were caused by a hypoxic-ischemic insult, 41 had developed moderate or severe disabilities. When predictors of poor outcome were examined, it was found that infants with seizures who ultimately did the worst were those who had late-onset fits, tonic seizures, and seizures lasting many days. Although seizure frequency and neonatal mortality associated with seizures were greatest in the premature infants, the outcome in premature infants who survived was as good as that of the term infant.

"Fifth-day fits," by the way, is a term invented in France. The diagnosis is commonly made in Australia (see 1983 YEAR BOOK, pp. 36–37); the cause is unknown. It has not been imported to the United States as yet. We already have enough diseases without an explanation.

For a comprehensive discussion of the management of neonatal seizures, particularly those secondary to a hypoxic-ischemic insult, please see the commentary by Joseph Volpe in the 1984 YEAR BOOK (pp. 363–365).—F.A.O.

Etiologic Factors and Long-term Prognosis of Convulsive Disorders in the First Year of Life

A. Matsumoto, K. Watanabe, M. Sugiura, T. Negoro, E. Takaesu, and K. Iwase (Nagoya Univ.)

Neuropediatrics 14:231–234, November 1983

Data on 562 patients with convulsive disorders in the first year of life were reviewed to identify etiologic factors and determine the long-term outcome. Fifty-seven of the infants had febrile convulsions, excluding cases of CNS infection. Mean patient age at last follow-up was 7¼ years.

The classification of the cases is given in Table 1. Over 60% of the prenatal group had cerebral anomalies. Most infants with perinatal cases had asphyxia and an abnormal delivery. A positive family history was most frequent in cryptogenic cases (Table 2). The type of seizures is related to the age at onset of seizures in Figure 15–2. Infantile spasms were the most common initial seizure type in the prenatal and doubtful groups and partial seizures in the postnatal group (Table 3). The prognosis for seizures

TABLE 1.—ETIOLOGIC CLASSIFICATION OF 562 CASES

	No. of cases	%
Prenatal	114	20.3
Perinatal	114	20.3
Postnatal	24	4.3
Doubtful	53	9.4
Cryptogenic	257	45.7
Total	562	100.0

(Courtesy of Matsumoto, A., et al.: Neuropediatrics 14:231–234, November 1983.)

TABLE 2.—CLINICAL FEATURES

	Prenatal N* (%**)	Perinatal N* (%**)	Postnatal N* (%**)	Doubtful N* (%**)	Cryptogenic N* (%**)
1. Boys	114 (47.0)	114 (62.3)	24 (39.1)	53 (67.9)	257 (49.8)
2. Positive family history	67 (10.4)	70 (15.7)	19 (26.3)	28 (10.7)	119 (23.5)
3. Head circumference < −2SD	113 (42.7)	101 (12.9)	19 (10.5)	46 (4.3)	228 (2.2)
4. Low birthweight < 2500g	108 (27.8)	109 (4.6)	19 (5.3)	50 (0)	249 (2.0)
5. SFD	110 (26.4)	109 (1.8)	21 (4.8)	50 (0)	251 (1.6)
6. Neurological abnormality	114 (74.8)	114 (46.4)	24 (65.2)	53 (18.9)	257 (0)
7. Delayed development before the onset	113 (80.5)	110 (63.6)	23 (17.4)	53 (100)	257 (0)
8. Age at 1st seizure < 6 months	114 (61.7)	114 (67.9)	24 (21.7)	53 (47.2)	257 (36.2)

*Total no. cases for which information on each item was sufficiently detailed.
**Percent of affected patients in total no. of cases.
(Courtesy of Matsumoto, A., et al.: Neuropediatrics 14:231–234, November 1983.)

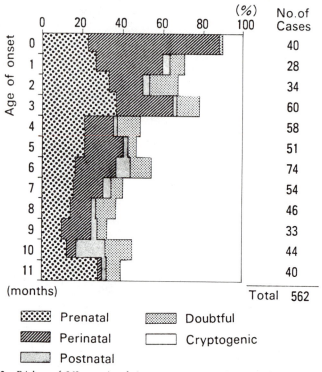

Fig 15–2.—Etiology of 562 cases in relation to age at onset. (Courtesy of Matsumoto, A., et al.: Neuropediatrics 14:231–234, November 1983.)

was best in cryptogenic cases (Table 4). The prognosis for mental and physical development is shown in Table 5. Over 80% of patients with cryptogenic cases and only 10% of those with prenatal and postnatal seizures had normal physical and mental development at follow-up. Nearly

TABLE 3.—TYPE OF SEIZURES

	Prenatal N %	Perinatal N %	Postnatal N %	Doubtful N %	Cryptogenic N %
1. Generalized motor seizures	24 (21.1)	46 (41.8)	6 (26.2)	16 (30.2)	167 (78.8)
2. Infantile spasms	71 (62.3)	38 (34.5)	5 (21.7)	27 (50.9)	20 (9.4)
3. SGE *	15 (13.1)	17 (15.5)	3 (13.0)	6 (11.3)	7 (3.3)
4. Partial seizures	3 (2.6)	6 (5.5)	5 (21.7)	2 (3.8)	13 (6.1)
5. Hemiconvulsive seizures	1 (0.9)	3 (2.7)	4 (17.4)	2 (3.8)	5 (2.4)
Total	114 (100)	110 (100)	23 (100)	53 (100)	212 (100)

*SGE: seizures belonging to secondary generalized epilepsy, other than infantile spasms.
(Courtesy of Matsumoto, A., et al.: Neuropediatrics 14:231–234, November 1983.)

TABLE 4.—Prognosis: Persistence of Seizures

	Prenatal N* %**	Perinatal N* %**	Postnatal N* %**	Doubtful N* %**	Cryptogenic N* %**
Seizure free ≥ 3 yrs.	60 (35.0)	62 (54.8)	19 (42.1)	26 (26.9)	117 (80.3)
Seizure stopped ≤ 3 yrs. of age	65 (20.0)	65 (23.1)	19 (15.8)	27 (14.8)	118 (50.8)

*Total no. cases for which information on each item was sufficiently detailed.
**Percent of affected patients in total no. of cases.
(Courtesy of Matsumoto, A., et al.: Neuropediatrics 14:231–234, November 1983.)

TABLE 5.—Prognosis: Mental and Physical Development*

	Prenatal N %	Perinatal N %	Postnatal N %	Doubtful N %	Cryptogenic N %
I	9 (13.2)	20 (28.6)	2 (10.5)	1 (3.6)	100 (84.0)
II	2 (2.9)	0 (0)	0 (0)	0 (0)	0 (0)
III	12 (17.6)	14 (20.0)	4 (21.1)	19 (67.9)	14 (11.8)
IV	12 (17.6)	10 (14.3)	10 (52.6)	5 (17.9)	3 (2.5)
V	21 (30.9)	15 (21.4)	1 (5.3)	1 (3.6)	0 (0)
Dead	12 (17.6)	11 (15.7)	2 (10.5)	2 (7.1)	2 (1.7)
Total	68 (100)	70 (100)	19 (100)	28 (100)	119 (100)

*I, mentally and physically normal; II, mentally normal but physically handicapped; III, mentally subnormal and physically normal; IV, mildly to moderately handicapped mentally and physically; V, mentally and physically severely handicapped; Dead, died before age 6 years.
(Courtesy of Matsumoto, A., et al.: Neuropediatrics 14:231–234, November 1983.)

half the patients with prenatal seizures were severely handicapped or died before age 6 years. Mortality was highest in the prenatal and perinatal groups.

The cause of convulsive disorder in the first year was known in 45% of this series. Primary generalized epilepsy may be rare. Some so-called generalized motor seizures in the first year may represent partial seizures evolving to secondarily generalized seizures. The prognosis for both seizures and mental and physical development has been best in cryptogenic cases.

ACTH and Prednisone in Childhood Seizure Disorders
O. Carter Snead III, John W. Benton, and Gary J. Myers (Univ. of Alabama, Birmingham)
Neurology (Cleve.) 33:966–970, August 1983   15–4

The data from most previous studies of steroids and ACTH in the treatment of seizure disorders are conflicting and difficult to interpret because of the variability of dosage regimens. Snead et al. used standardized regimens of either prednisone or ACTH to treat 52 children with infantile spasms and hypsarhythmia and 64 with other types of intractable seizures (Table 1). Treatment was standardized (Table 2) but not blind or randomized (1 author used prednisone exclusively, 1 used ACTH, and 1 used both). No attempt was made to control for use of other anticonvulsant drugs.

Seizure control, defined as existing when no seizures were noted by the parents, was better ($P < .005$) with ACTH than with prednisone in all groups (Table 3). There was no instance of improved EEG findings without seizure control, or vice versa. Acceptable cosmetic side effects were seen in all patients (Table 4); more troublesome side effects were seen only with ACTH, but no child experienced the serious side effects of ACTH reported by others. Seizures recurred in 40%–50% of patients within 4–14 months after completion of therapy (Table 5). No child who was neurologically normal at the onset of seizures and whose seizures were controlled with either drug relapsed after cessation of therapy.

▶ Richard Hrachovy and associates (*J. Pediatr.* 103:641, 1983) conducted a

TABLE 1.—CHARACTERISTICS OF PATIENT POPULATION*

	ACTH-treated			Prednisone-treated		
Seizure type	No. patients	Mean age (mos)	Mean follow-up (mos)	No. patients	Mean age (mos)	Mean follow-up (mos)
Infantile spasms with hypsarhythmia	30	6.8	24.6	22	6.2	47.1
Infantile spasms— myoclonic jerks without hypsarhythmia	16	13.4	25.3	14	10.7	46.7
Other intractable seizures	18	47.8	21.4	16	42.5	29.5
Preexisting neurologic disease	41 (63%)			30 (60%)		

*(Courtesy of Snead, O.C., III, et al.: Neurology (Cleve.) 33:966–970, August 1983.)

TABLE 2.—TREATMENT REGIMEN*

Prednisone
First 4 weeks: 3 mg per kg per day
Second 8 weeks: 3 mg per kg every other day
Final 4 weeks: Taper

ACTH
First week: 150 units per M² per day of ACTH gel
                                   IM in two divided doses
Second week: 75 units per M² per day of ACTH gel
                                   IM once daily
Third and fourth   75 units per M² per day of ACTH gel
week: IM every other day
Final 8 weeks: Taper

*(Courtesy of Snead, O.C., III, et al.: Neurology (Cleve.) 33:966–970, August 1983.)

TABLE 3.—RESULTS OF TREATMENT*

	ACTH	Prednisone
Seizure control achieved		
Infantile spasms with hypsarhythmia	30/30	13/22
Infantile spasms—myoclonic seizures w/o hypsarhythmia	13/16	0/14
Other intractable seizures	12/18	0/16
Mean time to seizure control (days)		
Improvement	2	7
Seizure-free	5	14
Improvement of EEG abnormalities hypsarhythmia		
Normal	29/30	11/22
Improved	1/30	2/22
No change	—	9/22
Improvement of other EEG abnormalities		
Normal	14/34	0/30
Improved	11/34	0/30
No change	9/34	30/30

*(Courtesy of Snead, O.C., III, et al.: Neurology (Cleve.) 33:966–970, August 1983.)

TABLE 4.—SIDE EFFECTS OF THERAPY*

	ACTH	Prednisone
Cushingoid appearance	62/64	48/52
Extreme irritability	6/64	0/52
Hypertension	4/64	0/52
Transient glucosuria	4/64	0/52

*(Courtesy of Snead, O.C., III, et al.: Neurology (Cleve.) 33:966–970, August 1983.)

TABLE 5.—RECURRENT SEIZURES

	ACTH			Prednisone		
	No. patients	No. with preexisting neurol disease	Mean time to recurrence from cessation of ACTH (mos)	No. patients	No. with preexisting neurol disease	Mean time to recurrence from cessation of prednisone (mos)
Infantile spasms with hypsarhythmia	14/30	14	6.3	8/13	8	4.2
Recurrent spasms	6*			2		
Other seizures	8			6		
Infantile spasms— myoclonic seizures without hypsarhythmia	4/13	4	7.1	—	—	—
Other intractable seizures	6/12	6	14	—	—	—

*All recontrolled with second course of ACTH.
(Courtesy of Snead, O.C. III, et al.: Neurology (Cleve.) 33:966–970, August 1983.)

double-blind, placebo-controlled study to compare the therapeutic effectiveness of ACTH with that of prednisone in 24 patients with infantile spasms and a hypsarhythmic EEG pattern. Response to therapy was defined as a complete cessation of seizures and the disappearance of the hypsarhythmic EEG pattern.

The two drugs were very similar in their therapeutic response. Nine patients responded to ACTH and 7 responded to prednisone. Responses were rapid; 12 patients responded within 2 weeks and 4 others within 6 weeks. Therapy was tapered and discontinued immediately after a response was obtained. Five patients relapsed; 4 responded to a second course of therapy. Of the 8 patients who failed to respond to hormonal therapy, 7 were treated with clonazepam without improvement.

Adenocorticotropin or prednisone should not be used for the treatment of seizures without some good evidence that the patient does, in fact, have infantile spasms. Other anticonvulsants should be used. Computed axial tomography examinations should be performed in the evaluation of such patients because they are extremely helpful in establishing prognosis with infantile spasms (Singer, W. D., et al.: ibid. 100:47, 1982; and 1983 YEAR BOOK, pp. 401–403) and ruling out tuberous sclerosis as a cause for the problem (Haglund, M., et al.: *Acta Paediatr. Scand.* 70:751, 1981).

Adenocorticotropin produces a variety of undesirable side effects, including cerebral atrophy, increased incidence of infection, hypertension, osteoporosis, and electrolyte problems (Riikonen, R., et al.: *Arch. Dis. Child.* 55:664, 1980). The optimal dose and duration of ACTH therapy have yet to be established. The larger doses (120–160 units) do not appear to produce a better result than 20- to 40-unit doses. Side effects are more common with the larger doses (Riikonen, R.: *Acta Paediatr. Scand.* 73:1, 1984).—F.A.O.

Pyridoxine-Dependent Seizures: A Wider Clinical Spectrum
A. Bankier, M. Turner, and I. J. Hopkins (Melbourne)
Arch. Dis. Child. 58:415–418, June 1983   15–5

Four cases of pyridoxine-dependent seizures were seen in which the clinical features and subsequent course were atypical. One case is described below.

Girl, a full-term neonate with a normal neonatal course, developed multifocal motor seizures at age 8 days, which were treated with phenytoin. After a 5-day absence the seizures recurred and she was admitted at age 19 days. Phenytoin plus phenobarbitone briefly controlled the seizures. Anticonvulsant drugs and steroids failed to control subsequent recurrences, and at age 2 months she was treated with thiopentone, assisted ventilation, and intravenous megavitamin therapy. Seizures did not recur after withdrawal of thiopentone. All vitamins were withdrawn at age 3 months, and prednisolone was withdrawn over 1 week, but phenobarbitone, phenytoin, and sodium valproate were continued. On this regimen, she had no seizures and became more alert and responsive to visual and auditory stimuli. Her head control improved. Multifocal motor seizures recurred at age 9½ months. Anticonvulsants had no effect, but the seizures stopped approximately 3 minutes after intravenous administration of 100 mg of pyridoxine. A recurrence 10 days later was stopped within 1 minute after intravenous administration of 50 mg of pyridoxine. A maintenance dose of 75 mg of oral pyridoxine daily was initiated and other anticonvulsants were discontinued.

An EEG at age 9½ months showed frank epileptiform discharges. Within 48 hours after the intravenous dose of 100 mg of pyridoxine there was marked improvement with no epileptiform discharges, but some slow components and sharp wave forms persisted. When last seen at age 1 year, she was sitting without support but was unable to crawl or pull herself to a standing position.

The unusual features in these 4 infants that led to diagnostic uncertainty included late onset of seizures, which occurred as late as age 6 weeks in 1 case; prolonged seizure-free period with anticonvulsant drugs before administration of pyridoxine; prolonged remission after discontinuation of pyridoxine; presentation with seizure types commonly associated with structural brain pathology; and a history of fetal distress in labor (2 cases) that incorrectly suggested intrauterine hypoxia as a cause of the seizures.

Pyridoxine-dependent seizures should be considered in any infant with intractable epilepsy, regardless of the pattern of seizures and the response to anticonvulsant medications. In such infants, 100 mg of pyridoxine should be given intravenously and the child should be observed for 30 minutes before anticonvulsant drugs are administered. If there is a clinical response to pyridoxine, it should be given orally indefinitely. An increase in dose may be required as the child grows and when there is an intercurrent illness.

Childhood Migraine and Motion Sickness

Gabor Barabas, Wendy Schempp Matthews, and Michael Ferrari (New Jersey-Rutgers Med. School, Piscataway)
Pediatrics 72:188–190, August 1983   15–6

The incidence of motion sickness was compared in four groups of children aged 4.8 to 19.9 years, including those with migraine headaches (60 patients); those with nonmigraine headaches (42 patients); those with seizure disorders (60 patients); and those with learning disability or perceptual or neurologic impairment, with no complaint of headache (60 patients).

Of the 60 children with migraine headache, 27 (45%) had had at least

FREQUENCY OF MOTION SICKNESS IN FOUR GROUPS
OF CHILDREN

	No. of Patients	Incidents of Motion Sickness	
		No.	%
Migraine headaches	60	27	45.0
Nonmigraine headaches	42	3	7.1
Seizure disorders	60	4	6.6
Learning disability/neurologic or perceptual impairment	60	3	5.0
Total	222	37	

(Courtesy of Barabas, G., et al.: Pediatrics 72:188–190, August 1983. Copyright American Academy of Pediatrics 1983.)

three episodes of motion sickness (table), a much higher incidence than in each of the other categories. Overall, 73% of the 37 children suffering from motion sickness were migraine sufferers.

This association of motion sickness with migraine headache may be regarded as a minor diagnostic criterion for arriving at the diagnosis of migraine. A common underlying neurotransmitter abnormality is suggested and discussed in relation to the relative predominance of brain stem cholinergic systems over serotonergic systems. Hypersensitivity of peripheral receptors (semicircular canals) to motion in migraine sufferers is also postulated. This may be the result of intermittent vasoconstriction in the distribution of the basilar artery and ischemia in the region of its labyrinthine branches.

▶ The clinical criteria used in making a diagnosis of migraine in children include the presence of at least three of the following: paroxysmal headaches with pain-free intervals; unilateral, throbbing headaches; nausea, vomiting, or abdominal pain associated with the headache; a visual aura preceding the headache; and a close family history of migraine. Physicians using these criteria are very unlikely to misdiagnose serious underlying problems such as brain tumors or vascular malformations (Tal, Y., et al.: *Acta Paediatr. Scand.* 73:55, 1984).

The presence of motion sickness or, as seen in the following article, sleepwalking, are helpful clues to the presence of migraine in a child. The role of food in triggering migraine headaches is discussed in Chapter 3, "Allergy and Dermatology."

The poor child with migraine! The family takes him for a ride—he gets sick. They stop at McDonald's—he gets sick again. He comes home to go to bed and ends up walking around all night. Meanwhile, one of his parents is very grumpy because of a "splitting headache."—F.A.O.

Childhood Migraine and Somnambulism

Gabor Barabas, Michael Ferrari, and Wendy Schempp Matthews (New Jersey-Rutgers Med. School, Piscataway)
Neurology (Cleve.) 33:948–949, July 1983   15–7

The possibility of an association between migraine and somnambulism in children was studied by sending questionnaires to the parents of 222 children, aged 4.8 to 19.9 years, who had migraine headache; nonmigraine headache; seizure disorders; or learning, perception, or neurologic problems without headaches or seizures. All four groups were matched for mean age (11.1 years). No child was mentally retarded or incapable of walking due to a physical handicap.

Two or more episodes of sleepwalking had occurred in 30% of the children with migraine headaches but in only 4.8% to 6.6% of children in the other three groups ($P < .0001$) (table). The estimated incidence of somnambulism in the general population is 1% to 6%.

The major diagnostic criterion of migraine is that of paroxysmal headache with symptom-free intervals. Minor criteria include a prodrome (gen-

FREQUENCY OF SOMNAMBULISM IN FOUR GROUPS OF CHILDREN

Children with:	Number of patients	Percentage who sleepwalk	Percentage of total sleepwalkers (n = 18)
Migraine headaches	60	30.0%	66.6%
Nonmigraine headaches	42	4.8%	7.4%
Seizure disorders	60	6.6%	14.8%
Learning disability/perceptual or neurologic impairment	60	5.0%	11.1%

(Courtesy of Barabas, G., et al.: Neurology (Cleve.) 33:948–949, July 1983.)

erally visual, 10% to 50%), gastrointestinal symptoms (70% to 100%), a throbbing quality to the pain, lateralization to one side, positive family history (72%), and relief after sleep. The high frequency with which somnambulism apparently occurs in childhood migraine may warrant its inclusion as a minor diagnostic criterion. Its presence could obviate the need for extensive laboratory testing. Because it differentiated migraine from nonmigraine headache so markedly, it could expedite appropriate treatment for children with headache symptoms.

Migraine and somnambulism are both thought to be related to abnormalities in serotonin metabolism; this could explain their coexistence.

▶ Even benign paroxysmal vertigo of childhood may be a migraine equivalent or a migraine precursor (Mira, E., et al.: *ORL* 46:97, 1984). In a study of 13 children with benign paroxysmal vertigo, 9 were found to have positive headache provocation tests with nitroglycerin, histamine, and fenfluramine. Several children had a positive family history for migraine, and headache was frequently associated with motion sickness, cyclic vomiting, or abdominal pain. Some children with vertigo responded to migraine treatment.

How common is migraine or other headaches in young adolescents? A survey was conducted in Finland of 1,954 boys and 1,909 girls who were aged 14 (Sillanpaa, M., et al.: *Scand. J. Primary Health Care* 2:27, 1984). In the 12 months prior to the survey, 68% of the children had experienced some form of headache. In 10.2% of the schoolchildren migraine attacks appeared to have occurred. They were more common in girls (13.8%) than in boys (6.7%). With 2 out of 3 young teenagers having headaches, is it any wonder that our airways are filled with analgesic commercials?—F.A.O.

A Progressive Syndrome of Autism, Dementia, Ataxia, and Loss of Purposeful Hand Use in Girls: Rett's Syndrome—Report of 35 Cases
Bengt Hagberg, Jean Aicardi, Karin Dias, and Ovidio Ramos (Ostra Hosp., Göteborg, Sweden)
Ann. Neurol. 14:471–479, October 1983   15–8

In 1966, Rett described a syndrome of "cerebral atrophy and hyperammonemia" observed only in girls and characterized by autistic behavior and dementia, apraxia of gait, loss of facial expression, and stereotyped use of the hands. The authors report on a pooled series of 14 French, 4 Portuguese, and 17 Swedish female patients with Rett's syndrome. All 35 patients fulfilled the following criteria: (1) normal neurologic and mental development during the first 7–18 months of life; (2) stagnation of developmental acquisitions after this period, followed by rapid deterioration of behavior and mental status; (3) loss of purposeful use of the hands; (4) jerky ataxia of the trunk and extremities, ataxic gait, and acquired microcephaly; (5) a protracted period with a relatively stable mental status.

At examination the patients demonstrated no sustained interest in persons or objects, although they were able to see and visually to follow them. Spontaneous motor activity was stereotypic and monotonous. Thirty had learned to walk when supported by one or both hands. Only 13 of the ambulant girls became able to walk independently. Signs of corticospinal tract dysfunction usually appeared late, at a median age of 60 months. Vasomotor disturbances predominating in the legs and feet were common at school age. Epileptic seizures were a late symptom, recorded in 25 patients. Four patients had an unusually rapid and severe course. In these girls the disease started soon after age 6 months, and they had completely lost the ability to maintain a sitting position by age 4 years. Family histories revealed no instance of known consanguinity or any abnormal clustering of cases of mental retardation. Laboratory investigations were generally unhelpful. In 2 early cases, serum copper levels were intermittently raised and in 1 of these patients urinary copper excretion was also high. The EEG was abnormal in all patients older than age 3 years. Neuroradiologic examinations in 21 of the 35 girls were either normal or showed slight cortical atrophy.

The clinical symptom complex displayed by these patients suggests a progressive degenerative disorder of the brain predominantly involving the gray matter. The nature and cause of this progressive disorder remain unknown. The exclusive involvement of girls, correlated with findings in family data analyses, suggests a dominant mutation on one X chromosome that results in affected girls and nonviable male hemizygous conceptuses.

▶ It is surprising that Rett's syndrome has not been reported, as yet, from the United States. As a matter of fact, it seems that we usually import most of our interesting diseases from the East rather than from Western Europe, e.g., Kawasaki's disease, Reye's syndrome, Asian flu, and sushi bars.— F.A.O.

A Study of the Neurological Disorder Associated With Acute Hemorrhagic Conjunctivitis due to Enterovirus 70

N. H. Wadia, P. N. Wadia, S. M. Katrak, and V. P. Misra (Bombay)
J. Neurol. Neurosurg. Psychiatry 46:599–610, July 1983 15–9

Ninety cases of neurologic manifestations associated with acute hemorrhagic conjunctivitis occurred during the 1971 and 1981 epidemics; 84 patients had acute hemorrhagic conjunctivitis whereas 6 were only close contacts but had the same neurologic symptoms. Male adults predominated in the study population.

Electromyography and blink reflex studies were done. Samples of sera and cerebrospinal fluid (CSF) were collected during the 1981 epidemic and analyzed for antibody titers to enterovirus (EV 70), poliovirus, and coxsackie A24 variant virus.

Over half of the patients had fever and malaise, usually preceding, but at times continuing with, the neurologic symptoms; the constitutional symptoms either accompanied the acute hemorrhagic conjunctivitis (8.6%), or the neurologic illness (43.4%) alone, or were present with both (17.6%), or were absent (30.4%).

Illness often began with backache and muscular or root pains mostly in the legs, lasting sometimes up to 3 weeks. Pains were accompanied or followed within 4 days by acute essentially asymmetric, proximal, hypotonic, areflexic paralysis of the lower extremities. Acute, isolated, unilateral lower motor neuron facial paralysis, often misdiagnosed as "Bell's palsy," was another form of the disease. These and less frequent signs of varying duration are listed in the table. It is noteworthy that 20 of 46 patients with limb paralysis had recently received intramuscular injections in the more paralyzed leg and that 4 of 14 women were pregnant when the paralysis developed. Neurologic symptoms followed acute hemorrhagic conjunctivitis in 83 of 90 patients. Cerebrospinal fluid was abnormal in 47 of 61 patients during the acute stage of spinal disease.

The principal lesion is believed to be in the anterior horn cells of the spinal cord and the cranial motor neurons. Serial neurophysiologic ex-

CLINICAL FEATURES (90 PATIENTS)			
	No of patients		Total
	1971	1981	
Acute haemorrhagic conjunctivitis	18	66	84
Prodromal Symptoms			
Constitutional	7	43	50
Limb pains (muscular or root)	13	41	54
Lower motor neuron paralysis			
Lower limbs	17	44	61
Diminished deep reflexes	18	44	62
Facial	1	28	29
Upper limb with lower limb	1	23	24
Upper limb alone	0	2	2
Trigeminal	0	4	4
Abucens	0	2	2
Vagus	0	2	2
Mild, infrequent, transient features			
Brisk reflexes; Extensor Plantars	6	2	8
Cutaneous sensory loss	0	8	8
Retention of Urine	0	7	7
Vertigo	0	4	4
Impaired vibration	1	2	3

(Courtesy of Wadia, N.H., et al.: J. Neurol. Neurosurg. Psychiatry 46:599–610, July 1983.)

amination was very helpful in localization and diagnosis of lesions. The abnormal F wave response along with persistently normal motor conduction also pointed to acute anterior horn cell or anterior root disease, or both. Two persistent abnormalities in the blink reflex examination were an absent or prolonged R_1 and increased intereye difference of R_1 and R_2 responses.

Antibody titers against EV 70 were demonstrated in the serum and CSF. While other viruses can cause epidemic conjunctivitis, the combination of hemorrhagic conjunctivitis and neurologic disease mostly simulating poliomyelitis is caused by EV 70 alone. The virus grows in the epithelial cells of the conjunctiva and spreads mainly by the eye-hand-fomite route. Its spread from the conjunctiva to the CNS is believed to be similar to that of poliomyelitis.

Based on the two components of the disease, it is suggested that it be called "enterovirus 70 disease." This would insure more urgent health measures and prevent its acceptance as a benign self-limiting local eye disease rather than as one that can cause permanent disabling paralysis.

▶ It would be hard not to recognize this disease in your midst—hemorrhagic conjunctivitis and paralysis of the extremities or cranial nerves. "Enterovirus 70 disease" seems to be an appropriate name. Most of the patients in this report were aged 20 to 40 years, so the viral syndrome is more likely to attack you than your patients, but, presumably, the younger individual is not immune from the virus-related syndrome.

Enterovirus infections may produce long-term neurologic consequences for the very young. At the 1984 meetings of the Society for Pediatric Research (*Pediatr. Res.* 18:230A, 1984), J. A. Jenista and co-workers in Rochester described their experience with a summer enterovirus epidemic. In a prospective study of 688 normal newborns, 12.8% had a culture-proved enterovirus infection during the first month of life. Of the infected infants, 1 in 5 were hospitalized. At approximately 18 months of age, 71 of the 75 neonatally infected infants and their matched controls underwent neurologic evaluation. Infected infants were found to display delays in development, receptive language, and expressive language. Respect, and fear, the enteroviruses.—F.A.O.

Management and Outcome in Anorexia Nervosa: Standardized Prognostic Study

H. G. Morgan, Joan Purgold, and Jill Welbourne (Univ. of Bristol)
Br. J. Psychiatry 143:282–287, September 1983   15–10

Outcome was examined in 78 patients with anorexia nervosa treated in a special clinic in Bristol between 1973 and 1978. The diagnostic criteria included purposeful weight loss, amenorrhea or impotence and loss of libido, typical psychopathology including a distorted concept of body size, and nonspecific depressive, phobic, obsessional, or hysterical symptoms. Treatment was based on a psychosomatic approach and ranged from prolonged personal treatment to firm authoritarian management. The general approach was pragmatic. Treatment was generally on an outpatient basis, unless weight loss was severe or other problems were present. Most patients received antidepressants, and nearly half received tranquilizers.

Direct contact was made with many patients for follow-up evaluation (Table 1). A good outcome was more frequent in the Bristol series than in the others. An increased duration of illness and disordered relations between patient and family correlated with a poor prognosis (Table 2). Family hostility toward the patient and personality difficulties were also poor prognostic features. The outcome could not be related to age at onset, degree of weight loss, social class, neurotic-behavioral disorder at school, mental illness in the nuclear family, or anomalous family situation.

Early intervention may be important in the effective management of patients with anorexia nervosa. Long-term, ongoing outpatient care may be useful. Further studies are needed to assess chronic morbidity from anorexia nervosa and to evaluate treatment programs prospectively.

▶ Despite the spate of articles about eating disorders in adolescence, the pediatric literature is almost as thin as some of the patients when it comes to meaningful follow-up studies.

For example, there were no articles on anorexia cited in the *Combined Cumulative Index to Pediatrics* for 1983. This index lists all articles that have appeared in *American Journal of Diseases of Children, Clinical Pediatrics, Journal of Pediatrics, Pediatric Annals, Pediatric Clinics of North America,* and *Pediatrics.*

Patients with anorexia nervosa are characterized as being "resistant" to

TABLE 1.—Duration and Method of Evaluation at Follow-up

	Maudsley Hospital %	Bristol Royal Infirmary %	St George's Hospital %
Duration of follow-up (range of years and mean)	4–10 (5.0)	4–8.5 (5.8)	4–8 (5.9)
Direct interview with patient	83	69	75
Direct interview with relative	7	8	13
Postal questionnaire from patient	5	9	12
Other informants (direct or indirect)	5	14	—
	100	100	100

(Courtesy of Morgan, H.G., et al.: Br. J. Psychiatry 143:282–287, 1983.)

TABLE 2.—Prognostic Indicators

	General outcome categories (χ^2)	Average outcome scores (χ^2)
Duration of illness		
Food difficulties	$(P < 0.05)$	$(P < 0.01)$
Amenorrhoea	$(P = 0.029)$	$(P < 0.0042)$
Family hostile to patient	N.S	$(P < 0.05)$
Disturbed relationship between patient and family	$(P\ 0.02)$	$(P\ 0.018)$
Personality difficulties	N.S	$(P\ 0.05)$

(Courtesy of Morgan, H.G., et al.: Br. J. Psychiatry 143:282–287, 1983.)

treatment. A clinical study of 133 inpatients described a dropout rate of 50% (Vandereycken, W., et al.: *Br. J. Med. Psychol.* 56:145, 1983). H.-C. Steinhausen and K. Glanville (*Psychol. Med.* 13:239, 1983) reviewed all of the follow-up studies of anorexia nervosa and found that the published rates of improvement ranged from 10% to 86%, most falling between 30% and 50%. This study by Morgan and associates agrees with those previous estimates. The most important prognostic features still remain unclear. Even if all the facts were known with respect to prognosis, they would be of limited help to the physician confronted with a new anorectic patient in his office. As Tom Weller states in his book entitled *Minims,* "A knowledge of Sanskrit is of little use to a man trapped in a sewer."—F.A.O.

16 Child Development

Diet and Sleep Patterns in Newborn Infants
Michael W. Yogman and Steven H. Zeisel
N. Engl. J. Med. 309:1147–1149, Nov. 10, 1983   16–1

Sleep behavior is modulated by serotonergic neurons within the brain; the synthesis and release of serotonin by such neurons are thought to be influenced by the availability of tryptophan, the amino acid precursor of serotonin. The effects on sleep patterns of diet variations designed to affect tryptophan availability were investigated in 20 healthy newborns aged 2–3 days. The infants randomly were assigned to receive a feeding consisting of tryptophan in 10% glucose or valine in 5% glucose; valine competes with tryptophan for entry into the brain. Sleep patterns during the 3 hours after this feeding were compared with those after a feeding of routine formula (Similac).

The two groups did not differ significantly in birth weight or gestational age. The infants in the tryptophan group ingested a mean of 19.8 mg of tryptophan (60 ml), and those in the valine group ingested a mean of 27 mg of valine (53 ml). The significant results for mean difference scores are summarized in Figure 16–1. After ingesting tryptophan, infants entered quiet sleep a mean of 20 minutes earlier, and active sleep 14.1 minutes earlier, than after ingesting Similac. Infants given valine entered quiet sleep a mean of 39 minutes later, and active sleep 15.8 minutes later, than after ingesting Similac ($P < .005$ for quiet sleep, $P < .01$ for active sleep; tryptophan vs. valine). In contrast to results in the tryptophan group, infants fed valine spent a mean of 21.8 minutes less in active sleep, 36.2 minutes less in total sleep, and 31.8 minutes more in a wakeful, alert state than after ingesting Similac. All infants displayed the normal newborn pattern of entering sleep through the active, rapid-eye-movement stage.

These data demonstrate that modification of the preparations fed to newborns can influence the length of time it takes them to fall asleep after a feeding. These results reflect only short-term effects. The changes observed in sleep behavior could have been caused by changes in serotonin synthesis and neurotransmission within the newborns' brains.

▶ Rudolph Leibel, of Rockefeller University, a man who is never caught napping, provided us with the following:

"This study is based on the intriguing concept, developed over the past 15 years by Wurtman, Fernstrom, and others, that the tissue concentrations and bioactivities of certain brain neurotransmitters (e.g., serotonin, norepinephrine, and acetylcholine) reflect, to some extent, ambient levels of relevant precursor molecules (e.g., tryptophan, tyrosine, and choline). Because tryptophan hydroxylase, which catalyzes the rate-limiting step in the synthesis of

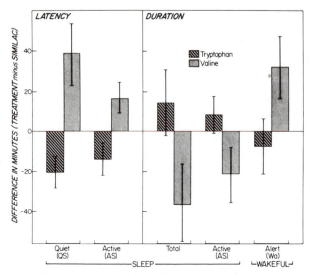

Fig 16–1.—Sleep behavior changes associated with feedings. Data are presented as mean differences (between behavior after treatment with tryptophan or valine and after Similac) in minutes ± SEM. "Latency" refers to the time taken to enter quiet or active sleep. In the tryptophan vs. valine groups, the results were as follows: latency to quiet sleep (QS), $F_{(1,16\ df)}$ = 10.39, $P < .005$; latency to active sleep (AS), $F_{(1,16\ df)}$ = 8.49, $P < .01$; duration of total sleep, $F_{(1,16\ df)}$ = 3.55, $P = .077.$; duration of active sleep, $F_{(1,16\ df)}$ = 3.18, $P = 0.93$; and duration of wakefulness (WA), $F_{(1,16\ df)}$ = 3.67, $P = .073$. (Courtesy of Yogman, M.W., and Zeisel, S.H.: N. Engl. J. Med. 309:1147–1149, Nov. 10, 1983. Reprinted by permission of the New England Journal of Medicine.)

serotonin, is not saturated with substrate at normal concentrations of brain tryptophan, and because there is no end product inhibition of this pathway, the rate of neuronal serotonin synthesis is largely controlled by the availability of tryptophan. Thus, altering of brain levels of tryptophan (e.g., with diet) can presumably change the rate of serotonin synthesis.

"Given the structural stability of the central nervous system, and its intricate mechanism—the 'blood-brain barrier'—for excluding a wide variety of substances, it is hard to accept the notion that this organ would subject its most critical biochemical processes to the short-term vicissitudes of diet quality and quantity. That liver, kidney, and pancreas may dance at the end of metabolic strings held by diet seems altogether reasonable and physiologic; that the brain should be in the same hands does not. Although the biologic 'wisdom' of such an arrangement can be readily argued, the evidence continues to accumulate that brain chemistry can be affected by short-term manipulations of diet. In a sense, this is the ultimate pavlovian phenomenon—in which the stimulus (i.e., diet) directly alters the chemistry and function of the brain. We should, I suppose, have been prepared for all of this by the observation of the efficacy of L-dopa in the treatment of Parkinson's disease. After all, this drug is, in fact, a neurotransmitter precursor that is metabolized to dopamine in the substantia nigra.

"Serotonergic neurons in the brain stem send axons to regions of the brain implicated in the control of sleep, appetite, and mood. In animals, the administration of tryptophan has been associated with changes in a wide range of behaviors: increased sleep, diminished locomoter activity, pain response to electroshock, male homosexual behavior, muricidal behavior and protein intake (Fernstrom, J. D.: *Annu. Rev. Med.* 32:413–425, 1981). In man, diminished brain serotonin levels have been reported in people who committed suicide. Administration of tryptophan has been reported to decrease posthypoxic intention myoclonus, sleep latency, and carbohydrate craving (Wurtman, R. J., et al.: *Pharmacol. Rev.* 32:315–335, 1981).

"One of the problems facing clinical investigators in this field is the selection of relevant, quantifiable, dependent behavioral variables that can be related to actual or putative brain neurochemical status. An additional problem is the control of composition and quantity of overall diet when discrete nutritional manipulations are being performed. Yogman and Zeisel chose a clever way around both of these issues by using readily quantified aspects of sleep in infants on an otherwise constant formula diet. Strictly speaking, the experiment is not perfectly controlled because the concentration of glucose used as the vehicle for the two amino acids was not identical, and no glucose control was included. Additionally, plasma levels of the relevant amino acids were not measured, and so no dose (amino acid)-response (sleep) relationship has been demonstrated. Nonetheless, the data are impressive and probably physiologically meaningful.

"The effects described in this paper are subtle and of more interest from a biologic than a clinical perspective. They are important for the support they lend to the hypothesis relating neurotransmitter synthesis and function to diet. Pediatricians have long been sensitized to the critical role of nutrition in organ (including brain) growth. A new level of subtlety must now be introduced into our thinking about the diet-brain axis. This is not, of course, to imply that all hyperactivity is due to food additives, refined sugar, or zinc deficiency; that Al Capone ate too much tyrosine; or that tryptophan should be added to the drinking water.

"It seems unlikely that tryptophan will enter the therapeutic armamentarium as a somnifacient for infants. In the study by Yogman and Zeisel, the total amount of sleep time was not affected by this agent, and its efficient administration is a nuisance in that it must be given in a vehicle (glucose) that maximizes its potential to enter the central nervous system. Perhaps most importantly, nothing is known about the ultimate effects of exposing the developing brain to supraphysiologic surges of neurotransmitter precursors. Thus, for the time being, infants should be left to their own devices. Weary parents may, however, want to avail themselves of a slug of tryptophan from time to time."

Night Waking in 4- to 8-Month-Old Infants
Marc Weissbluth, A. Todd Davis, and John Poncher (Northwestern Univ.)
J. Pediatr. 104:477–480, March 1984   16–2

Night waking is frequent in infancy but is not well understood. The sleep patterns of 141 normal infants aged 4–8 months from middle-class families were investigated. The infants were seen in 5 independent pediatricians' offices; 43% were boys, and 46% were predominantly breast-fed. The mean birth weight was 3.5 kg.

Infants who had colic had briefer total sleep and more frequent night wakings than observed in those without colic (Table 1). Infants whose parents reported current night waking had briefer total sleep and an increased frequency of night wakings. Threshold ratings were not related to the frequency of night wakings, and the number and duration of night wakings did not correlate with night sleep duration. A past history of colic covaried significantly with current night waking (Table 2). Signs suggesting partial airway obstruction during sleep, including snoring and mouth breathing, were not significantly associated with a past history of colic or with current night waking.

TABLE 1.—SLEEP DURATION AND NIGHT AWAKENING

	Total sleep duration (hr)	Number of night awakenings
Colic		
Yes	13.5 ± 0.3*	2.3 ± 0.3†
No	14.3 ± 0.2	0.9 ± 0.1
Night waking as a problem		
Yes	13.3 ± 0.3*	2.3 ± 0.3†
No	14.2 ± 0.2	0.9 ± 0.1
Snoring		
Yes	12.9 ± 0.4‡	2.1 ± 0.5‡
No	14.4 ± 0.2	1.0 ± 0.1
Mouth breathing when asleep		
Yes	14.3 ± 0.7§	2.4 ± 0.6*
No	14.1 ± 0.2	1.0 ± 0.1

Data expressed as mean ± SEM.
*$P < .05$.
†$P < .001$.
‡$P < .005$.
§Not significant.
(Courtesy of Weissbluth, M., et al.: J. Pediatr. 104:477–480, March 1984.)

TABLE 2.—COMPARISONS BETWEEN 2 GROUPS OF INFANTS

	Colicky infants who developed night waking as a problem		Infants who snore
	Past history of colic	Night waking a current problem	Snoring or mouth breathing when asleep
Past history of colic	—	Yes*	No
Night waking a current problem	Yes	—	No
Snoring or mouth breathing when asleep	No	No	—
Difficult or labored breathing when asleep	No	No	Yes
Sex difference	No	Boys predominate	No
Increased frequency of night waking	Yes	Yes	Yes
Brief sleep duration	Yes	Yes	Yes (snoring only)

*Correlation coefficient or Student's t test, $P < .05$.
(Courtesy of Weissbluth, M., et al.: J. Pediatr. 104:477–480, March 1984.)

Several reports support the present observation that colic early in infancy is associated with the later occurrence of frequent night awakenings with brief sleep duration. It is possible that certain constitutional CNS characteristics lead directly to both colic and sleep disturbance. It also is possible that parental behaviors cause these infant behaviors or that an interaction between constitutional infant factors and resultant parental behaviors is operative. Other studies suggest that infants with colic, brief sleep duration, and frequent night wakings may be at an increased risk of developing a "difficult" temperament.

▶ Weissbluth and his associates put forth an attractive, and testable, hypothesis—infants who previously had colic are at greater risk for developing sleep disturbances such as brief sleep duration or frequent night awakening. In a prospective study, Weissbluth and co-workers (*J. Pediatr.* 104:951, 1984) reduced the incidence of colic with dicyclomine hydrochloride but failed to produce easier temperament or longer sleep durations at age 4 months in infants whose colic stopped during therapy. Nice try, Weissbluth, but apparently once a crab, always a crab.—F.A.O.

Clinicians' Assessments of Children's Understanding of Illness
Ellen C. Perrin and James M. Perrin (Vanderbilt Univ.)
Am. J. Dis. Child. 137:874–878, September 1983   16–3

The accuracy of professionals in estimating the age at which children give developmentally characteristic answers to a series of questions about illness was studied.

A total of 127 children (age range, 5 to 13 years; average IQ, 118) were randomly selected from suburban schools and asked five questions: "How do children know they're sick?" "How do children get sick?" "How can children keep from getting sick?" "How do children get better?" "How does medicine work?"

Illness-related concepts were found to progress through a systematic and predictable sequence from prelogical and magical notions of causality in the preoperational child to coherent descriptions of complex physiologic mechanisms in the operational child (Table 1). Health professionals (residents and full-time staff of the pediatrics department, nurse clinicians, nurses, and members of the local pediatricians' association) were asked (by questionnaire) (Table 2) to estimate the age at which they would expect a child to make typical responses to the five questions.

Overall, there was a tremendous variability in professionals' estimates of children's ages, in both direction and degree of accuracy. Mean difference scores ranged from 5 years above true age to 5 years below it. Most accurate estimates were made regarding the question, "When children get sick, how do they get better?" Here, the mean difference score was only 1.7 years. Respondents varied widely in underestimating or overestimating the level of children's understanding of concepts on which the questions were based (Fig 16–2). The proportion of correct estimates varied from

TABLE 1.—Examples of Children's Responses to Illness-Related Questions at Different Ages

Age, yr	Responses

If a child does get sick, how can he or she get better again?
5-7	Stay warm . . . get lots of rest
	Eat foods that are good for you
	Take medicine
9-11	Take the right medicines that can fight off the germs
	Do what the doctor says; you do different things for different sicknesses
13-15	Medicines help the body repair itself
	Eating good foods gives your body extra energy to fight off germs

How do children get sick?
5-7	By going out in the rain without boots
	From other people
	Eating bad foods or poisons
9-11	From breathing in sick people's germs
	From germs getting inside your chest
13-15	By eating something that is a poison to your body so your heart doesn't work right
	Certain germs might get in your blood stream and mess up the muscles and things

How can children keep from getting sick?
5-7	Eat good foods . . . get lots of rest
	Take the medicines you're supposed to
	Stay away from sick people
9-11	Get shots to build up your tolerance to germs
	Eat vitamins so you can fight off germs
13-15	Take good care of yourself so your body will be strong enough to fight off the sickness
	Good foods nourish the fighting cells so they'll kill germs if they get inside you

(Courtesy of Perrin, E.C., and Perrin, J.M.: Am. J. Dis. Child. 137:874–878, September 1983; copyright 1983, American Medical Association.)

TABLE 2.—Sample Format of Questionnaire

	Age

At what age would you expect a child to make each of these responses in answer to the question indicated?

1. Everyone gets sick once in a while. How do children know when they're sick?

You don't have any energy	_____
You can't go to school	_____
It just depends what's the matter with you	_____
You might have a headache or a stomachache	_____

2. How do children get sick?

If germs get into your system when your resistance is down	_____
By sitting near someone who's sick	_____
By going out in the rain without boots on	_____

(Courtesy of Perrin, E.C., and Perrin, J.M.: Am. J. Dis. Child. 137:874–878, September 1983; copyright 1983, American Medical Association.)

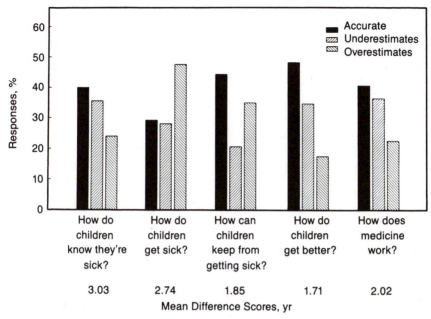

Fig 16–2.—Accurate and inaccurate estimates of children's age according to question asked. (Courtesy of Perrin, E.C., and Perrin, J.M.: Am. J. Dis. Child. 137:874–878, September 1983; copyright 1983, American Medical Association.)

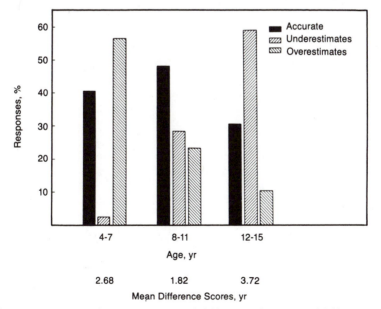

Fig 16–3.—Accurate and inaccurate estimates of children's age, by true age of child. (Courtesy of Perrin, E.C., and Perrin, J.M.: Am. J. Dis. Child. 137:874–878, September 1983; copyright 1983, American Medical Association.)

48% for the question, "How do children get better?" to 29% for the question, "How do children get sick?"

When arranged according to the true ages at which children made the 34 statements, mean difference scores ranged from 2.7 years for the youngest children's responses to 3.7 years for the oldest children's responses (Fig 16–3). Within each age group, physicians were more likely to overestimate children's ages than were nonphysicians and were less likely to underestimate them. This may indicate that professionals do not expect children to understand, for instance, the notion of prevention even at a relatively unsophisticated level at which most children do conceptualize it. Children's understanding of the mechanisms of medicine and healing seems to be better anticipated by professionals, and children's age is usually underestimated rather than overestimated.

Data from this study suggest that adults may expect more of young children than they can understand and that adults expect too little and perhaps talk down to children older than age 10 years. Frustration and miscommunication may result in either case.

▶ Barbara Korsch, Professor of Pediatrics, University of Southern California, and Head, Division of General Pediatrics, Children's Hospital of Los Angeles, provided the following commentary:

"The latest contribution of the Perrin team, in their studies on chronic illness in childhood, focuses on children's perceptions of their bodily functioning in health and disease and the extent to which health care providers, pediatricians, and others are aware (or, more often, not aware) of these levels of understanding. The Perrins demonstrate, not surprisingly, that children's thinking about illness and causation generally reflects developmental progress and is not dissimilar to the Piaget kind of schema for children's ability to reason in general. The fact that pediatricians and others caring for sick children are not aware of children's own concepts concerning illness and treatment is also not surprising. However, it definitely needed to be pointed out and documented in the workmanship-like manner that the Perrins' careful study demonstrates.

"The significance of this work cannot be overestimated. All serious studies of the health behavior of patients in general, and of parents and children in pediatric practice specifically, underscore that health behavior is going to reflect the patient's perception of treatment and illness rather than the scientific explanations or the perceptions on the part of the physician.

"Thus, in order to reduce anxiety, to motivate children to appropriate health behavior, and to make for optimal adaptation, it is crucial that explanations to children be given in awareness of the limitations and understanding that prevail. Obviously, from a general scheme the pediatrician is not going to be able to assess the nature of a particular child's understanding. However, it at least gives him a frame of reference in which to operate and, most of all, alerts him to the need for assessing the individual patient's readiness for certain kinds of explanations and advice.

"Besides emphasizing specific problems relating to children's perceptions and comprehension of health-related concepts, this work once again highlights another very significant aspect of pediatric practice, namely, the importance of communication directly with the child patient as opposed to communication with parents and other caretakers. The work of Pantell and others has shown that there is a tendency for significant communications about the child's illness and treatment to be addressed to the parents or caretakers without inclusion of the patient, even at moments when the patient's cognitive level and general developmental needs would clearly indicate the need for inclusion in the interaction. The Perrins' work focuses on the need for specific awareness and sensitivity to children's readiness to understand and accept certain concepts of causality and of the nature of disease in order to be able to benefit from this type of communication.

"Especially because there is also a great deal of evidence to suggest that a child's sense of competence and self-esteem is an important determinant of his adaptation and functional level in the presence of chronic illness, the presence of such communication appears to be an essential and often neglected feature in the process of offering health care to children."

A Near-Death Experience in a 7-Year-Old Child
Melvin Morse (Univ. of Washington)
Am. J. Dis. Child. 137:959–961, October 1983   16–4

An unwitnessed incident of near-drowning in a girl aged 7 occurred in a community swimming pool.

Girl, 7, was comatose with fixed and dilated pupils when seen by a physician at the poolside. She was intubated at the scene, cardiopulmonary resuscitation was started, and sodium bicarbonate was given. At the emergency room of the nearby hospital, she initially had spontaneous respirations, pupils midpoint and reactive to light, and intact brain stem reflexes. There were no spontaneous movements, no response to commands, and decerebrated posturing in response to pain. Massive pulmonary edema and respiratory distress syndrome rapidly developed. The Po_2 was never greater than 40 mm Hg during the first 4 hours. The patient was transported to Primary Children's Hospital in Salt Lake City where she required mechanical ventilation for 3 days. She regained consciousness on the third day and was discharged after 1 week. Two weeks after the initial event she returned to school, apparently fully recovered. Short-term memory deficit was present for about 4 weeks.

The patient was the second of 6 children; the parents were active Mormons and the patient attended church and Bible school. Her home environment was stable and loving.

When asked what she remembered of the experience, she said, "talking to the Heavenly Father," and did not want to discuss it further. Later she stated, "It feels good to talk about it." Her affect was that of a person who had had an intensely personal experience. Her first memory of the near-drowning was that of being in the water. "I was dead. Then I was in a tunnel. It was dark and I was scared. I couldn't walk." She said that a woman named Elizabeth appeared, and the tunnel became bright, and they walked together to heaven. "Heaven was fun, it was bright and there were lots of flowers."

She said that there was a border around heaven that she could not see past and that she met her dead grandparents, her dead maternal aunt, and Heather and Melissa, who were waiting to be reborn. She then met the "Heavenly Father and Jesus," who asked her whether she wanted to return to earth; she replied, "No." Elizabeth asked whether she wanted to see her mother; she said, "Yes," and woke up in the hospital. She could not supply any details of the 3 days during which she was comatose, although she claimed to remember the author. To her mother she said, "I'd like to go back there (heaven); it was nice."

This child had a near-death experience consistent with that reported among adults: feelings of peace, entering a dark tunnel, being out of the body, encountering a being of light, meeting others (relatives), and reaching a border. It is thought that these near-death experiences represent a defense mechanism against the fear of dying, although children's anxiety about death usually is focused on concrete concerns, not on an abstract perception of death.

The pediatrician should be aware that children who experience near-death events may benefit from counseling concerning such experiences.

▶ It is amazing to me how closely this child's near-death experience resembles those reported by adults. I think these stories go a long way in establishing that there is life after death. Now it remains to be established if there is life after birth.—F.A.O.

American Children Who Claim to Remember Previous Lives
Ian Stevenson (Univ. of Virginia, Charlottesville)
J. Nerv. Ment. Dis. 171:742–748, December 1983   16–5

Children who report they recall previous lives are rather readily found in many Asian countries. This is the first report of cases of the reincarnation type from the United States. Data from 79 American cases were compared with those of 266 cases of the same general type seen in India. The American series includes 43 boys and 36 girls.

A recent survey indicated that only about one fourth of Americans believe in reincarnation. Many cases in this study have occurred in families in which the parents do not believe in reincarnation and perhaps are not even familiar with the idea. Many informants have indicated that the idea is a strange or uncongenial one, and parental statements often have conflicted seriously with those made by the children.

Features of the American and Indian cases are contrasted in the table. American children have made fewer specific statements. The child's statements correctly corresponded to a deceased person in 77% of Indian cases but in only 20% of American cases. The mode of death in the previous life was mentioned less often by American children, and it was more often violent than in Indian cases. When violent death was reported, both groups of children tended to be phobic about the instrument or mode of death.

COMPARISON OF PRINCIPAL FEATURES OF
AMERICAN AND INDIAN CASES[a]

Item	U. S. A.	India	p
1. Percentage of solved cases among all cases of country	20%	77%	.001
2. Percentage of "same family" cases among solved cases	94%	16%	—[b]
3. Age (in months) of subject's first speaking about the previous life (mean)	37	38	NS[c]
4. Age (in months) of subject's stopping speaking about the previous life (mean)	64	79	.05[c]
5. Number of different statements made by subject			
Mean	23.3	18.2	NS[c]
Median	14	14	NS[d]
6. Subject mentioned previous personality's name	34%	75%	.001
7. Subject mentioned previous personality's mode of death	43%	78%	.001
8. Cases with violent mode of death	80%	56%	.01
9. Phobias in subject when previous personality died violently	48%	39%	NS
10. Phobias in subject when previous personality died naturally	11%	3%	—[b]
11. "Sex change" cases	15%	3%	.005

[a]Unless otherwise stated, all statistical analyses were done with chi-square tests of 1 df. Number of cases for which information was available was not the same for all variables.
[b]Analysis not done due to low-frequency cells.
[c]Independent means t test, two-tailed.
[d]Mann-Whitney U test.
(Courtesy of Stevenson, I.: J. Nerv. Ment. Dis. 171:742–748, December 1983.)

The occupation and socioeconomic status of the deceased persons mentioned by the American children varied greatly.

American and Indian children who report they recall previous lives are similar in many respects but different in others. The episodes differ markedly from cases of imaginary playmates in important respects. It is not easy to discern a wish-fulfilling motive in most instances. Hopefully, the study of more cases will permit conclusions to be drawn regarding the origin of this phenomenon.

▶ Out of the mouths of babes—but, then again—no one achieves immortality in his own lifetime.—F.A.O.

Behavioral Assessment in Youth Sports: Coaching Behaviors and Children's Attitudes

Ronald E. Smith, Nolan W. S. Zane, Frank L. Smoll, and David B. Coppel (Univ. of Washington, Seattle)
Med. Sci. Sports Exerc. 15:208–214, 1983   16–6

The authors coded 15,449 behaviors of 31 youth basketball coaches in terms of a 10-category system to define the characteristics and dimensional patterning of coaching behaviors. Postseason attitude and self-esteem data were obtained from players on 23 teams and were related to the behavioral measures. All 31 coaches were male volunteers in a parks department program and were aged 22–46 years. The children included 182 boys on 23 teams, aged 9–12 years. An adaptation of the Coaching Behavior Assessment System (CBAS) was used to collect behavioral data. Observers were 7 male and 10 female undergraduates who successfully completed a 4-week training program in the use of the CBAS. Observers positioned themselves unobtrusively to observe and hear the coach.

Data were collected on the 31 coaches during a total of 110 complete games, each averaging 57.4 minutes. Coaches most frequently engaged in reinforcement, general encouragement, and general technical instruction. Nearly 75% of the coaches' behaviors during games fell into these three categories. Punitive responses occurred in only 6% of the behaviors. Three factors accounted for 72.5% of total behavioral variance exhibited by all coaches: general, mistake-contingent, and punitive technical instruction; reinforcement, mistake-contingent encouragement, and general encouragement; and a tendency to engage in conversation unrelated to the game and to respond to misbehavior with verbal attempts to maintain order. As a group, the children had extremely positive attitudes toward the sport and evaluated their coaches positively. Coaching behaviors accounted for 53% of the variance in mean player attitude toward the sport and 42% of the variance in evaluation of the coach. The strongest predictor of players' liking for basketball was the coach's rate of technical instruction in response to mistakes. General technical instruction had a significant negative relationship to both team solidarity and player self-esteem.

The authors conclude that coaching behaviors are most highly related to player attitudes toward the sport. This finding suggests a coach can indeed affect a child's enjoyment of sport participation.

▶ Technical instruction and a willingness to teach—even after mistakes on the part of the player—were most valued by the group. The same attributes probably apply to other forms of teaching as well. I tried to get a commentary from Bobby Knight.—F.A.O.

Developmental Assessment at Four Years: Are There Any Differences Between Children Who Do, or Do Not, Cooperate?

M. Ounsted, J. Cockburn, and V. A. Moar (John Radcliffe Hosp., Oxford, England)
Arch. Dis. Child. 58:286–289, April 1983   16–7

The significance of the failure of preschool-aged children to cooperate in developmental assessment was investigated. The study group included 203 children whose motor and intellectual abilities were assessed at age 4 years and at age 7½ years.

At age 4 years, 37 (18%) of the children did not cooperate fully or at all in the tests; thus, an overall developmental score could not be calculated. When scores could be determined for the uncooperative children, those who cooperated completely had higher development scores that were significant with regard to visuomotor skills, language, and comprehension. At age 7½ years, boys and girls had similar scores for the five British Ability Scales processes, but girls generally were more advanced in reading. The mean reading quotients for boys, including the noncooperators, did not differ, but significant differences were found among the girls, with cooperators scoring significantly higher than noncooperators. Children in the lower social classes who were not cooperative at age 4 years had lower scores in all six areas of ability tested at age 7½ years than those found in children who were fully cooperative (table). There were no significant differences between cooperative and uncooperative children from an upper-class background.

The results suggest that the refusal of young children to cooperate in developmental assessment tests may indicate an inability to perform and that such children should not be ignored or excluded from follow-up analyses.

▶ Betsy Lozoff, of the Departments of Pediatrics and Geographic Medicine, Case Western Reserve University, kindly provided the following comments:

"This article is especially valuable because it stimulates us to pay attention to a frequently observed but often dismissed phenomenon—a young child's refusal to try some or all of developmental tests. In this study, excessive shyness was the most common apparent reason for lack of cooperation. Although Ounsted and colleagues emphasize the importance of 'noncooperators' in relation to follow-up studies of high-risk neonates, their observations also seem highly pertinent to general pediatricians who are screening children for mental and motor delay and often encounter a child who refuses to try parts of a test like the Denver, a screening test quite similar to that used by Ounsted et al. Perhaps such refusal should alert pediatricians to the possibility of limitations in the child's cognitive functioning. The data of Ounsted et al. suggest that this is particularly true in lower-class children. Because children who were uncooperative at age 4 had deficits in receptive and expressive language, it is not altogether surprising that they had lower scores at age 7½ years, because IQ tests are so heavily involved with verbal capacities.

"Affective response to developmental testing may be an important indicator of developmental dysfunction even earlier, in infancy. In our study of iron de-

REFUSALS AT 4 YEARS AND INTELLECTUAL ABILITY AT 7½ YEARS

	Cooperative at 4 years			Uncooperative at 4 years				
	Mean	SD	n	Mean	SD	n	F	P
Reading quotient								
Non-manual	110·8	19·7	71	105·8	15·5	12	0·69	NS
Manual	100·8	16·0	92	93·1	20·2	25	4·09	<0·05
Reasoning								
Non-manual	109·8	14·9	71	109·3	14·3	12	0·01	NS
Manual	103·5	12·9	92	96·5	13·6	25	5·67	<0·05
Spatial imagery								
Non-manual	116·4	17·3	71*	124·3	14·1	12	2·28	NS
Manual	110·6	16·8	91*	101·3	16·1	25	6·13	<0·05
Perceptual matching								
Non-manual	114·7	12·6	71*	115·1	11·8	12	0·01	NS
Manual	114·6	13·4	91*	104·7	14·8	25	10·2	<0·01
Memory								
Non-manual	109·4	15·1	71	111·7	17·9	12	0·22	NS
Manual	104·6	14·5	92	96·9	19·8	25	4·69	<0·05
Retrieval and application of knowledge								
Non-manual	111·2	13·0	71	106·8	13·1	12	1·20	NS
Manual	106·0	13·5	92	100·0	9·9	25	4·32	<0·05

*Test equipment not available for 1 child.
NS = not significant.
(Courtesy of Ounsted, M., et al.: Arch. Dis. Child. 58:286–289, April 1983.)

ficiency anemia in Guatemala, developmental delays were not found in all ane-mic infants. Instead, delays were noted almost exclusively in those who showed disturbed affect during Bayley testing. These infants, characterized as tense, fearful, and withdrawn, had mental scores worrisome for mental re-tardation, albeit mild (Lozoff, B., et al.: Abnormal behavior and low develop-mental test scores in iron-deficient anemic infants. Submitted for publication.)

"Such observations, both in infants and preschool-aged children, suggest that a child's refusal to try developmental test items or extreme shyness should be taken seriously and pursued by retesting the child on another occasion, including a more thorough evaluation if the disruptive affect persists."

Child Snatching: New Epidemic of an Ancient Malady
Lenore C. Terr (Univ. of California, San Francisco)
J. Pediatr. 103:151–156, July 1983   16–8

The number of reports of children being kidnapped by parents has increased alarmingly in recent years. The findings on psychiatric evaluation of 18 children who were kidnapped successfully or abortively by a parent are presented.

Sixteen of the 18 children showed one or more emotional effects of being successfully or abortively snatched by a parent. Eleven showed posttraumatic stress response syndrome or the aftereffects of severe fright, 7 showed the effects of mental indoctrination, 7 expressed grief or rage about an absent parent, 9 rejected the offending parent, and 2 had an exaggerated identification with a parent or wish fulfillment about a parent (table).

These functional emotional disturbances occurred whether or not the kidnapping was successful, the law sanctioned the snatching, it was a first or second snatching, or the parents or court regarded the experience as a "vacation." The 2 girls who showed no direct psychiatric effects had been told the truth from the beginning, maintained phone contact and visitations with their mother while staying with their father, and lived in so many different settings afterward that the kidnapping seemed little more than another episode in an otherwise disorganized young life.

Serious problems exist at the law-psychiatry interface regarding stolen children. In both areas, efforts must be directed toward prevention of these family tragedies. Every child who returns from a child-stealing experience should undergo psychiatric evaluation. Pediatricians and child psychiatrists may assist the court in understanding the child's point of view by testifying to the medical findings and by interpreting the child's testimony and behavior to the court.

Growth of Intelligence: Failure and Catch-up Associated Respectively With Abuse and Rescue in the Syndrome of Abuse Dwarfism
John Money, Charles Annecillo, and John F. Kelley (Johns Hopkins Univ.)
Psychoneuroendocrinology 8:309–319, 1983   16–9

A relationship between child abuse, neglect, or both, and impaired intellectual growth is now recognized. The IQ changes over time were examined in 19 male and 15 female patients with a diagnosis of abuse-related dwarfism, confirmed by endocrinologic and follow-up studies. All patients but 4 were below the third percentile in stature, and these were at about the fourth percentile. Initial IQ values were obtained during the stage of abuse or when the patient was equivocally rescued. Repeat measurements

PSYCHIATRIC FINDINGS IN SNATCHED OR ABORTIVELY SNATCHED CHILDREN

Patient	Age when taken (yr)	Age when returned (yr)	Parent who snatched	Psychic trauma or fright	Mental indoctrition	Long-term grief or rage	Rejection of parent by child	Exaggerated identification or wish fulfillment
"Successfully" snatched children								
1	3	5	Mother / Father (+ detective)	Psychic trauma	Mother	Father / Mother		
2	4	5	Father / Mother	Psychic trauma	Father / Mother	Mother / Father	Mother	
3	4	8	Father		Father			Oedipal wishes
4	7	11	Father	Fright	Father	Mother		
5	5–6?	6	Father?	Fright			Father	
6	6	7	Mother / Father (+ detective)					
7	8	9	Father (+ detective)					
8	8	8	Mother		Mother	Mother		Identification with mother

Abortive snatches						
9	5	Father (+ detective)	Psychic trauma			Father
10	7	Mother	Psychic trauma			Mother
11	7	Father	Fright			Father
Threatened snatches						
12	8	Father	Fright			Father
13	10	Father	Fright			Father
"Vacation" snatches						
14	5	Father	Psychic trauma	Mother		Father
15	2	Father			Mother	
16	3	Father	Psychic trauma		Mother	
17	3	Mother		Mother	Father	
18	8	Mother				Mother

(Courtesy of Terr, L.C.: J. Pediatr. 103:151–156, July 1983.)

were made in an environment of rescue in 23 cases, when abuse persisted in 2, and in an equivocal state in 9.

The findings in subjects who were consistently rescued are shown in the table, and the IQ changes at various intervals after rescue are shown in Figure 16–4. A mean rise in IQ of 24 was found in this group of subjects. Greater gains in IQ were apparent in subjects who were younger when rescued. A progressive rise in IQ was evident in the 16 patients with more than one postrescue IQ determination. A similar trend was seen in 8 patients who were assessed as juveniles, again around puberty, and later.

Strong evidence against IQ constancy was obtained in this study. Intelligence grows just as the body does, and its growth can be slowed and stunted or advanced and elevated. A proper environment is needed for the normal development of intelligence, just as normal body growth requires proper nutrition. Permanent intellectual impairment can occur in children who spend most of their juvenile years without rescue from abusive living conditions. The duration of rescue was the main factor associated with IQ elevation in this study. Elevation of IQ was gradual and progressive over the years of follow-up when rescue was maintained. The most marked change was from an IQ of 36 to 120 in a girl assessed at ages 3½ and 14 years, respectively.

▶ The last lines of the original manuscript deserve constant repetition. They state, "The truth about intelligence is that it grows, just as the body grows—

BASELINE OF ABUSE TO FINAL FOLLOW-UP AFTER CONSISTENT RESCUE ($n = 23$)

	Baseline abuse IQ	Age at rescue (yr, month)	Final IQ in rescue	Age (yr, month)	Time in rescue (yr, month)	IQ change
B68D	50	4, 3	48	4, 7	0, 4	– 2
C67D	62	7, 7	77	7, 11	0, 4	+ 15
M71R	83	3, 2	105	3, 6	0, 4	+ 22
S58R	57	7, 4	77	9, 9	2, 5	+ 20
W58V	42	6, 11	56	9, 8	2, 9	+ 14
M69S	83	4, 0	118	7, 3	3, 3	+ 35
H63R	101	4, 3	89	7, 8	3, 5	– 12
T72Tb	80	2, 4	107	5, 9	3, 5	+ 27
T72Ta	80	2, 4	104	5, 9	3, 5	+ 24
S67P	43	8, 10	63	13, 3	4, 5	+ 20
N61S	74	12, 3	91	17, 1	4, 10	+ 17
R60M	56	12, 8	73	17, 7	4, 11	+ 17
R62V	55	10, 0	73	14, 11	4, 11	+ 18
H54G	80	7, 10	80	12, 10	5, 0	0
S67T	62	7, 0	93	12, 3	5, 3	+ 31
H54Rb	80	17, 5	90	23, 7	6, 2	+ 10
H55Rn	68	15, 1	96	22, 9	7, 8	+ 28
B64S	81	5, 8	99	13, 8	8, 0	+ 18
T63S	57	5, 5	112	13, 8	8, 3	+ 55
I63T	79	6, 8	93	15, 2	8, 6	+ 14
K53J	51	15, 7	87	24, 1	8, 6	+ 36
D64M	61	4, 1	133	12, 11	8, 10	+ 72
B63S	36	3, 10	115	16, 4	12, 6	+ 79
Mean	66	7, 7	90	12, 8	5, 1	24
S.D.	16	4, 4	21	5, 11	3, 1	21

(Courtesy of Money, J., et al.: Psychoneuroendocrinology 8:309–319, 1983.)

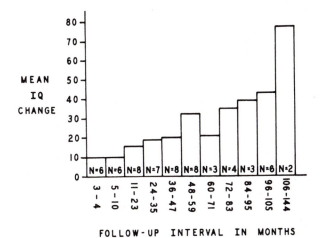

80 –
70 –
60 –
MEAN 50 –
IQ 40 –
CHANGE 30 –
20 –
10 –
0

N=6 | N=6 | N=8 | N=7 | N=8 | N=8 | N=3 | N=4 | N=3 | N=6 | N=2

3 – 4 | 5 – 10 | 11 – 23 | 24 – 35 | 36 – 47 | 48 – 59 | 60 – 71 | 72 – 83 | 84 – 95 | 96 – 105 | 106 – 144

FOLLOW-UP INTERVAL IN MONTHS

Fig 16–4.—Change in IQ at different intervals of follow-up after rescue (*n* = 23, with 16 tested more than once during follow-up). (Courtesy of Money, J., et al.: Psychoneuroendocrinology 8:309–319, 1983.)

and its growth can be slowed and stunted, just as the growth of the body can be slowed and stunted or, conversely, advanced and elevated. For healthy, optimal growth, the body needs proper nutrition. So also does the intelligence, though its diet is, of course, food for the mind." All the children in our society require mind food.—F.A.O.

Failure To Thrive: Controlled Study of Familial Characteristics

Milton Kotelchuck and Eli H. Newberger
J. Am. Acad. Child. Psychiatry 22:322–328, July 1983   16–10

The significance of ecologic stress factors in the etiology of failure to thrive (FTT) was explored through structured interviews with mothers of

TABLE 1.—Demographic Characteristics
of the Children With Failure to Thrive:
Control and Pediatric Social
Illness Diagnoses

Variable	Failure to Thrive	Controls	Pediatric Social Illnesses
Number of subjects	42	42	165
Age (% 18 months or younger)	81	81	50
Sex (% male)	69	69	56
Race (% white)	83	83	61
SES (% of families receiving welfare or medical assistance)	33	33	54

(Courtesy of Kotelchuck, M., and Newberger, E.H.: J. Am. Acad. Child. Psychiatry 22:322–328, July 1983.)

TABLE 2.—Familial Characteristics of Failure to Thrive (FTT) and Control Families: Mean Values and Statistical Comparisons

Variables	FTT Means	Control Means	p Value
DEMOGRAPHIC CHARACTERISTICS			
Months residing in present home	31.80	33.90	—
Number of housing moves in last year	0.45	0.42	—
Number of family members	4.29	4.76	—
Birth order of index	2.48	2.64	—
Father's age	26.98	28.10	—
Presently married (no/yes)	0.71	0.67	—
Number of years married	5.91	5.77	—
English not spoken at home (no/yes)	0.07	0.05	—
SOCIAL CLASS			
Family lives in apartment (no/yes)	.52	0.48	—
Number of rooms in home	4.74	5.62	0.089
Mother's years of education	11.50	12.60	0.084
Father's years of education	13.20	12.80	—
Father's job status (Hollingshead)	4.64	4.81	—
Mother employed full-time (no/yes)	0.80	0.85	—
Father employed full-time (no/yes)	4.61	6.10	—
Mother's job status (Hollingshead)	0.17	0.19	—
Family has private physician (no/yes)	0.81	0.76	—
Discrepancy in years of parent's education	1.70	0.20	0.010
MOTHER-CHILD SEPARATION			
Separated for more that one week (no/yes)	0.50	0.31	0.077
Age in months of initial separation	12.60	11.30	—
Child initiated the separations (no/yes)	0.86	0.67	—
PREGNANCY			
Index premature (no/yes)	0.05	0.12	—
Physically felt during pregnancy (bad/ambivalent/good)	1.31	1.45	—
Wanted child (no/ambivalent/yes)	1.33	1.57	—
CHILD-CENTERED PROBLEMS			
Health of index (okay/minor/major problems)	1.24	0.43	0.001
Problem with feeding (no/yes)	0.48	0.14	0.005
Problem with sleeping (no/yes)	0.19	0.12	—
Problem with discipline (no/yes)	0.07	0.10	—
Number of childrearing problems	0.72	0.36	0.022
FAMILY AND NEIGHBORHOOD SUPPORT			
Number of people accompanying child to hospital	1.55	1.69	—
Has own phone (no/yes)	0.88	1.00	0.021
Child care help available (no/yes)	0.93	0.81	—
Visits neighbors (no/yes)	0.70	0.83	—
Neighborhood friendly (no/yes)	0.60	0.91	0.002
Mother likes neighborhood (no/yes)	0.59	0.86	0.007
Nearby family exists (no/yes)	0.69	0.77	—
Sees family often (no/yes)	0.67	0.88	0.019
MATERNAL STRESSES			
Mental problems (no/yes)	0.19	0.22	—
Mother's childhood family intact (no/yes)	0.51	0.46	—
Mother's childhood family movile (no/yes)	0.69	0.65	—
Mother's childhood family healthy (no/yes)	0.19	0.17	—
Number of mother's childhood family troubles	1.39	1.18	0.091
Structural housing problems (no/yes)	0.50	0.60	—
Mother's health (okay/minor/major problems)	0.33	0.21	—

(Courtesy of Kotelchuck, M., and Newberger, E.H.: J. Am. Acad. Child. Psychiatry 22:322–328, July 1983.)

42 affected infants and 42 matched controls. Table 1 shows the characteristics of the FTT infants. None was older than age 36 months and 83% were white. Table 2 shows that demographic measures of family structure do not distinguish FTT infants from controls. Because the FTT group and the controls were matched initially on a crude index of socioeconomic status (SES), no differences emerged on the more comprehensive Holl-

ingshead SES index. No significant differences between cases and controls were noted with regard to pregnancy. Slightly more separations from the mother were experienced by the children with FTT than by controls. The FTT infants were perceived by their mothers as substantially more sickly than controls ($P < .001$), as 38% of FTT children were perceived as in poor health compared to 7% of controls. Although no single historical stress variable distinguished between mothers of FTT infants and controls, a composite measure of stress in childhood, including frequent family mobility, a broken home, and family illness, did moderately distinguish the two groups. There was less perceived positive support for mothers of FTT children from family and neighbors than for control mothers. Three variables significantly accounted for all of the variances explained in discriminant analysis: the families of infants with FTT have children with ill health, they live in an unfriendly neighborhood, and they have a larger discrepancy in parents' education.

The findings suggest that the widely held assumption that maternal behavior is the primary cause of FTT needs reexamination. More attention should be paid to the contribution of the sickly child to the diagnosis of FTT. Such a child could contribute to maternal psychologic distress and to the disrupted mother-child interaction patterns seen in the clinic. Maternal behavior may be the consequence, not the cause, of FTT.

▶ Speaking of mind food, this study should provoke a reexamination of certain assumptions. It is a good way to end the chapter. Now just close the book and think.—F.A.O.

17 Adolescent Medicine

Birth Weights Among Infants Born to Adolescent and Young Adult Women
Isabelle L. Horon, Donna M. Strobino, and Hugh M. MacDonald (Johns Hopkins Univ.)
Am. J. Obstet. Gynecol. 146:444–449, June 15, 1983   17–1

National figures indicate that a greater proportion of infants weighing 2,500 gm or less are born to mothers younger than age 15 than to any other maternal age group. Birth weights of infants born to 422 primigravid patients younger than age 16 were compared with the birth weights of infants born to a control group of 422 primigravid patients aged 20–24 years who matched the adolescent group in race and year of delivery; control patients were selected from an eligible population of 5,894 women.

The adolescent group consisted of a higher proportion of clinic patients who lived in less affluent neighborhoods, were more likely to be unmarried, had lower prepregnancy weights, were shorter in stature, initiated antepartum care later, and had a shorter length of gestation than the group aged 20–24 years. However, there was no significant difference in birth weights: infants born to adolescents had a mean birth weight of 3,051 gm compared to 3,093 gm for the group aged 20–24 years. Low birth weight ratios were 13.3% for the younger and 11.8% for the older group. Mean birth weight for 5,894 women eligible for the study was 3,274 gm. The percentage of nonwhite women in this group was 13.6%, compared to 68.2% among the adolescents.

Gestational age was the most important variable in predicting birth weight. Race, prepregnancy weight, change in weight during pregnancy, and number of antepartum visits were significantly associated with birth weight. Infants born to white women age 20–24 years were an average of 251 gm heavier than those born to black women for this age group; for adolescents, the difference was 99 gm. Average birth weight among adolescents who delivered prior to 33 weeks' gestation was 1,471 gm lower than that of adolescents who delivered at term. For the group aged 20–24 years, this difference was 1,867 gm.

Adolescents are at greater risk of being delivered of premature infants, but these infants have higher birth weights than premature infants delivered to older women. Adolescents had lower prepregnancy weights and shorter lengths of gestation; they appeared to compensate for these deficits by gaining more weight relative to body size during pregnancy and by more rapid intrauterine growth. Maternal gain in weight during pregnancy was a more important predictor of birth weight among adolescents than among adults. Sex of the infant was a significant indicator only among the older group. Male infants born to 20- to 24-year-olds weighed an average of

90 gm more than female infants; among adolescents the difference was only 11 gm.

Adolescent mothers contend with a greater number of risks and may require more careful management than young adult women. However, much of this risk is due to the sociodemographic characteristics of women of this age who carry pregnancies to term.

Are Pregnant Teenagers Still in Rapid Growth?
Stanley M. Garn, Marquisa LaVelle, Shelly D. Pesick, and Stephen A. Ridella (Univ. of Michigan)
Am. J. Dis. Child. 138:32–34, January 1984   17–2

The cause of the greater pregnancy weight gain observed in the youngest mothers has not been clarified. A longitudinal analysis was made of data on 1,601 teenage girls participating in the National Collaborative Perinatal Project. They were followed through at least 2 pregnancies in order to determine whether younger teenage mothers are in a period of rapid growth during pregnancy, thus accounting for a relatively large pregnancy weight gain. A total of 216 subjects have been followed through 3 successive pregnancies.

Weight gains during pregnancy are given in Table 1, and weight gains relative to the time since menarche are shown in Table 2. There was no evidence that a larger weight gain in younger teenagers could be attributed to rapid growth. Comparable conclusions were drawn from analyzing data on girls followed through 3 pregnancies.

These findings fail to support the view that rapid body growth is re-

TABLE 1.—Weight Before Pregnancy and Weight and Stature Gains in Teenage Pregnancy*

Race Group	n	Menarcheal age, yr†	Age at Pregnancy, yr† 1	2	Weight Gain, kg‡ Before Pregnancy 1	2	D	During Pregnancy 1	2	D	Stature, cm‡ 1	2	D
Black	8	11.6	13.5	15.3	51.1	54.4	3.3	11.6	11.4	−0.2	156.0	157.4	1.4
	35	12.5	14.5	17.1	53.0	56.7	3.7	12.5	11.3	−1.2	158.7	159.4	0.7
	96	12.6	15.5	17.5	53.8	55.5	1.7	10.3	10.3	0.0	159.5	160.1	0.6
	174	12.8	16.5	18.6	54.1	56.1	2.0	10.1	9.9	−0.2	160.1	160.1	0.0
	182	12.9	17.5	19.4	53.5	54.9	1.4	9.4	9.5	0.1	159.4	159.8	0.4
	237	13.2	18.5	20.4	56.0	57.6	1.6	9.8	9.2	−0.6	160.5	160.9	0.4
	198	13.2	19.5	21.4	55.7	57.3	1.6	9.6	9.7	−0.3	160.9	160.9	0.0
White	2	11.5	13.5	17.0	48.5	50.5	2.0	15.5	10.0	−5.5	159.5	162.0	2.5
	5	11.7	14.5	17.3	50.6	60.0	9.4	14.8	11.0	−3.8	157.8	158.8	1.2
	23	12.1	15.5	17.2	52.9	54.2	1.3	10.8	9.8	−1.0	158.4	158.8	0.4
	51	12.5	16.5	18.3	53.1	55.4	2.3	11.1	9.0	−2.1	159.7	160.3	0.6
	129	12.8	17.5	19.2	53.4	54.5	1.1	11.1	10.4	−0.7	160.6	160.6	0.0
	204	12.9	18.5	20.3	54.0	55.5	1.5	10.4	9.5	−0.9	160.2	160.2	0.0
	257	12.9	19.5	21.3	56.2	57.5	1.3	10.3	9.2	−0.9	161.2	160.9	−0.3

*Data for first and second pregnancies are given.
†Corrected to midpoint of class interval.
‡D = difference.
(Courtesy of Garn, S.M., et al.: Am. J. Dis. Child. 138:32–34, January 1984; copyright 1984, American Medical Association.)

TABLE 2.—STATURE AND WEIGHT GAINS RELATIVE
TO YEARS SINCE MENARCHE*

Table 2.—Stature and Weight Gains Relative to Years Since Menarche*

Years Since Menarche	Interval Between Pregnancies, yr	Long-term Change					
		Stature Gain, cm			Weight Gain, kg		
		n	Observed	Expected	n	Observed	Expected
			White Subjects				
2	2.2	17	1.3	1.4	19	2.9	3.7
3	1.9	41	−0.2	0.8	48	1.8	2.0
4	1.8	100	0.2	0.2	120	1.1	1.1
			Black Subjects				
2	2.1	103	0.6	1.4	101	1.3	3.8
3	2.0	162	0.3	0.8	161	1.5	2.0
4	1.9	191	0.4	0.1	193	1.2	1.0

Based on size at first pregnancy, interval between pregnancies, and values reported by Moerman. Observed and expected stature and weight gains for interval between pregnancies are given.
(Courtesy of Garn, S.M., et al.: Am. J. Dis. Child. 138:32–34, January 1984; copyright 1984, American Medical Association.)

sponsible for the greater pregnancy weight gains seen in younger teenage mothers. Fluid retention and an increased fluid volume are more likely factors in the relatively great pregnancy gain of these subjects.

▶ Richard H. Aubry, Professor, Department of Obstetrics and Gynecology, State University of New York Upstate Medical Center, comments:

"The article by Garn et al. is very timely, informative, and thought provoking. Teenage pregnancy, particularly early teenage pregnancy (younger than age 16), is considered to be riskier chiefly because of an increased rate of anemia, toxemia, preterm birth and low birth weight. All of these problems seem to have their roots in insufficient nutrition, especially regarding calories, protein, iron, and certain vitamins. Two potential mechanisms to explain this seeming nutritional inadequacy in the early teenage pregnancy have been proposed. First is the possibility that these patients still are experiencing significant growth in their own body that thus competes with the nutritional needs of the rapidly growing products of conception. The study of Garn et al. documents what many obstetricians have suspected: that by the time the ovaries have functioned long enough to allow for establishment of a pregnancy, further significant growth is largely over. Such evidence is extremely valuable in directing our attention to the second potential mechanism whereby early teenage pregnancy is associated with complications that have their roots in poor nutrition— that these young women simply do not eat well enough for the needs of the pregnancy. This perspective is easy for the obstetrician to accept given the frequent history of poor dietary intake in such patients. How, then, do we explain the seemingly contradictory observation that the younger the patient is, the larger the weight gain? There is not enough breadth of data to answer from the study itself. However, because the weight gain of pregnancy includes a significant expansion in interstitial fluid and the amount of such fluid is greatly increased in toxemia of pregnancy, a condition that occurs in as many as one third of early teenage pregnancy, it may be that the greater weight gain in the very young gravida is due to the higher rate of toxemia. This also fits with the unusually poor nutrition in these patients because toxemia is known to be more frequent in the poorly nourished, especially protein-malnourished, gravida. Thus, we can thank Garn et al. for helping us focus on the real problem— insufficient dietary intake for the needs of the pregnancy in these early teenage pregnant women.''

Teenage Fathers: Stresses During Gestation and Early Parenthood

Arthur B. Elster and Susan Panzarine (Univ. of Utah)
Clin. Pediatr. (Phila.) 22:700–703, October 1983   17–3

Twenty boys, aged 17 to 18 years, were interviewed from one to four times during the pregnancy and early postpartum period of their girlfriends. All conceptions occurred out of wedlock but 15 of the couples married before delivery. Four interviews were conducted during the first trimester, 12 during the second, 17 during the third, and 11 at 4 to 6 weeks postpartum.

The boys reported concerns in four major areas (table), and the intensity of these concerns changed during the prenatal and postnatal periods. Vocational and educational stresses were greatest during the first trimester and remained at a relatively high level throughout the study period. Concern for the health of the mother and child peaked during the third trimester and dropped off substantially after delivery. Concerns about parenting arose during the second trimester, dropped slightly during the third trimester, and increased again after the birth of the baby. Problems with relationships were greatest during the first trimester and dropped off at each

STRESSORS REPORTED BY TEENAGE FATHERS (N = 20)	
Group	Concern(s)
I	Vocational-educational
	Financial concerns
	Job concerns
	School disruption
II	Health
	Mother's health
	Baby's health
	Labor and delivery concerns
III	Parenthood
IV	Relationships
	Problems with mate
	Problems with parents
	Problems with friends
	Feelings about church

(Courtesy of Elster, A.B., and Panzarine, S.: Clin. Pediatr. (Phila.) 22:700–703, October 1983.)

subsequent interval. Relatively few boys reported any concern about parenthood; at the third-trimester interview, only 35% noted parenthood as a stressor, whereas 100% had vocational and educational concerns, 94% had health concerns, and 76% had problems with relationships.

The pregnancy had been expected in 58% of the cases and unexpected in 42%. Boys who had expected it tended to report less stress during the third trimester than did those who had not anticipated conception.

The stresses found in these young, unmarried, 90% white, middle-class prospective fathers were similar to those reported in black, lower-class boys in a similar situation. Young fathers can be helped by involving them in the clinical services provided to the pregnant teenager. Health care counseling provided to the couple may improve the paternal knowledge and feeling of involvement in the pregnancy.

▶ Elizabeth R. McAnarney, Professor of Pediatrics, and Director, Division of Biosocial Pediatrics and Adolescent Medicine, comments:

"We know relatively little about the experience of adolescent fathers compared to adolescent mothers. One of the major problems of studying adolescent fathers is that, as a group, they may not be readily accessible to investigators and clinicians. They often see no reason to go to traditional health facilities where studies usually are performed.

"Elster and Panzarine have studied two very different groups of adolescent fathers during the past several years. They first studied a group of predominantly black, unmarried, lower-socioeconomic-status adolescent fathers who were unlikely to marry after the pregnancy was diagnosed (*J. Adolesc. Health Care* 1:116–120, 1980). More recently, they have studied a group of predominantly white, married (after the pregnancy), middle-socioeconomic-status adolescent fathers. Their findings are similar in these two groups.

"Their findings have implications for clinical care of adolescent fathers; vocational and educational stresses were common throughout the pregnancy. There were specific changes in the intensity of concerns for the health of the mother and child, concerns about parenting, and problems with relationships during different times in the prenatal and postnatal periods. Adolescent fathers who had expected pregnancy reported less stress during the third trimester.

"Clinical experience indicates that many prospective adolescent fathers would like to become involved in contacts with professionals during their partners' pregnancies. Prospective adolescent fathers often do not know how to become involved, and the professionals have not been very creative in either reaching these young men or developing effective services for them.

"The authors of this article suggest a blueprint for addressing issues with prospective fathers. Several additional ideas come to mind: (1) placement of services for prospective adolescent fathers in non-health-related facilities that are more accessible to them and that do not imply they have to be "sick" to go there; (2) use of groups as a vehicle to address vocational-educational stresses, concerns for the health of the mother and child, concerns about parenting, and relationships; (3) invitation to prospective adolescent fathers to meet their partners' prenatal caretakers and to join any sessions to which they and their partners agree; (4) training of both adolescent boys and adolescent girls about the 24-hour responsibilities of child care through participation in day-care facilities.

"The authors have been working in a very difficult area, but have contributed substantially to our knowledge about adolescent fathers."

Risks Associated With Teenage Abortion
Willard Cates, Jr., Kenneth F. Schulz, and David A. Grimes (Centers for Disease Control, Atlanta)
N. Engl. J. Med. 309:621–624, Sept. 15, 1983   17–4

Data from the Joint Program for the Study of Abortion, a multicenter prospective study of nearly 165,000 legal abortions (including more than 50,000 in teens), and data from a national surveillance of abortion-related deaths were used to study the risks associated with teenage abortion.

For suction-curettage procedures at or before 12 weeks' gestation, teenagers had a risk of short-term major complications similar to that for older women (Table 1). Regardless of age, the rate of major complications was approximately 3 per 1,000 procedures between 1971 and 1975, and 1–2 per 1,000 between 1975 and 1978. Compared with older women, teenagers

TABLE 1.—Rates of Complication or Treatment Associated With Suction-Curettage Abortion at 12 Weeks' Gestation or Earlier

Type of Complication or Treatment	Rate of Complication or Treatment *					
	Woman's Age (yr)					
	≤17	18–19	20–24	25–29	≥30	P †
1971–1975						
All major complications	2.7	2.9	2.6	3.6	3.0	NS
Fever ≥3 days	1.4	1.8	0.9	1.6	0.3	NS
Transfusion	0.2	0.0	0.6	1.1	0.9	<0.01
Major surgery	0.0	0.1	0.6	0.7	1.5	<0.001
Fever ≥1 day	8.6	6.3	7.1	8.0	5.5	NS
Hemorrhage	2.1	4.2	3.4	3.0	4.6	NS
Cervical injury	16.8	9.4	10.9	8.0	8.4	<0.001
Uterine perforation	0.9	1.1	2.0	2.7	2.3	<0.05
1975–1978						
All serious complications	0.8	1.5	2.0	2.1	1.5	NS
Fever ≥3 days	0.4	0.7	0.9	1.0	0.9	NS
Transfusion	0.1	0.2	0.3	0.4	0.2	NS
Major surgery	0.3	0.5	0.9	0.7	0.5	NS
Fever ≥1 day	10.0	11.0	10.4	11.2	7.3	NS
Hemorrhage	2.8	2.1	3.4	3.2	3.5	NS
Cervical injury	5.5	3.3	3.1	2.6	1.7	<0.001
Uterine perforation	0.5	1.3	1.5	1.6	1.3	NS

*Number of complications or treatments per 1,000 procedures.
†Based on Mantel-extension method for testing linear trends; NS denotes not significant ($P > .05$).
(Courtesy of Cates, W., Jr., et al.: N. Engl. J. Med. 309:621–624, Sept. 15, 1983. Reprinted by permission of the New England Journal of Medicine.)

had lower rates of unintended major surgery, including hysterectomy, but higher rates of cervical injury.

Age was an important factor influencing the risks of abortion procedures used after 12 weeks' gestation (Table 2), with teens having the lowest rate of major complications of any age group for dilation and evacuation and for saline administration. Age also affected the specific complications of both of these procedures.

Between 1972 and 1978, teens were at a lower risk of dying after legal abortions than older women (Table 3). The crude death-to-case rate was 1.3 per 100,000 procedures for teenagers and nearly twice as high for older women. Teenagers had a slightly higher risk of dying of infectious complications and a slightly lower risk of dying of embolic events or reactions to anesthesia than older women, but they were only one ninth as likely to die of hemorrhage (Table 4).

A teenager contemplating abortion is at no higher risk than an older woman of having a serious complication, and she is at lower risk of death. Efforts to reduce the risk of cervical injury in teenage mothers should

TABLE 2.—RATES OF COMPLICATION OR TREATMENT ASSOCIATED WITH ABORTIONS AT 13–24 WEEKS' GESTATION

ABORTION METHOD AND TYPE OF COMPLICATION OR TREATMENT	RATE OF COMPLICATION OR TREATMENT *					
	WOMAN'S AGE (YR)					
	≤17	18–19	20–24	25–29	≥30	P †
1971–1975						
Dilation and evacuation						
All major complications	3.5	6.7	4.8	7.2	9.0	NS
Fever ≥3 days	0.0	2.2	1.6	4.3	4.5	<0.05
Transfusion	0.0	1.5	1.1	1.4	4.5	NS
Major surgery	1.7	2.2	0.0	4.3	4.5	NS
Saline administration						
All major complications	10.5	13.5	18.0	18.4	34.6	<0.001
Fever ≥3 days	2.3	6.5	4.7	6.4	6.9	NS
Transfusion	5.5	5.4	7.9	11.0	25.4	<0.001
Major surgery	0.5	0.0	1.1	2.8	3.5	<0.01
1975–1978						
Dilation and evacuation						
All serious complications	4.7	2.6	6.3	6.7	4.6	NS
Fever ≥3 days	2.5	1.3	0.7	2.5	0.0	NS
Transfusion	0.8	0.0	5.3	3.4	4.6	<0.005
Major surgery	1.3	1.3	3.3	2.5	2.3	NS
Saline administration						
All serious complications	11.0	15.4	25.5	42.7	32.4	<0.001
Fever ≥3 days	2.2	3.1	6.7	7.4	10.0	<0.02
Transfusion	8.1	13.3	19.4	33.4	27.4	<0.001
Major surgery	0.7	1.0	0.0	1.9	2.5	NS

*Number of complications or treatments per 1,000 procedures.
†Based on the Mantel-extension method for testing linear trends; NS denotes not significant (P > .05).
(Courtesy of Cates, W., Jr., et al.: N. Engl. J. Med. 309:621–624, Sept. 15, 1983. Reprinted by permission of the New England Journal of Medicine.)

TABLE 3.—Death-to-Case Rates for Legal
Abortion in 1972–1978, According to Woman's
Age and Gestational Age

WOMAN'S AGE (YR)	DEATH-TO-CASE RATE *				
	GESTATIONAL AGE (WEEKS)				
	≤8	9–12	13–16	≥17	TOTAL
≤19	0.2	0.6	3.4	7.8	1.3
20–24	0.3	1.5	7.4	21.0	2.1
25–29	0.3	1.9	7.5	22.4	2.0
≥30	0.9	2.6	13.9	23.1	2.9
Total	0.4	1.4	6.5	14.8	1.9

*Number of deaths per 100,000 abortions.
(Courtesy of Cates, W., Jr., et al.: N. Engl. J. Med. 309:621–624, Sept.
15, 1983. Reprinted by permission of the New England Journal of Medicine.)

TABLE 4.—Death-to-Case Rates for Legal
Abortion in 1972–1978, According to Age and
Cause of Death

WOMAN'S AGE (YR) AND CAUSE OF DEATH	NO. OF ABORTIONS	NO. OF DEATHS	DEATH-TO-CASE RATE *
≤19			
Infection		12	0.52
Embolic events		7	0.31
Anesthesia reactions		4	0.17
Hemorrhage		1	0.04
Other		5	0.22
Total	2,292,000	29	1.27
≥20			
Infection		22	0.45
Embolic events		26	0.53
Anesthesia reactions		17	0.35
Hemorrhage		19	0.39
Other		25	0.51
Total	4,878,000	109	2.23

*Number of deaths per 100,000 abortions.
(Courtesy of Cates, W., Jr., et al.: N. Engl. J. Med. 309:621–624, Sept. 15,
1983. Reprinted by permission of the New England Journal of Medicine.)

include more gradual preoperative cervical dilation with *Laminaria* or the
use of osmotic dilators or prostaglandins to soften and widen the cervix
before evacuation in teenagers with small, immature cervices.

Reexamining the Concept of Adolescence: Differences Between Adolescent Boys and Girls in the Context of Their Families

John F. McDermott, Jr., Albert B. Robillard, Walter F. Char, Jing Hsu, Wen-Shing Tseng, and Geoffrey C. Ashton (Univ. of Hawaii)
Am. J. Psychiatry 140:1318–1322, October 1983
17–5

A questionnaire on individual attitudes toward family values was administered to 74 Japanese-American and 84 white families as part of a larger study on family functioning in an attempt to determine how ethnicity, generation, and sex affected responses of family members. Participants had at least 2 unmarried children between the ages of 13 and 20. There were 121 Japanese-American and 126 white teenagers falling within the age constraints. All families were intact with 158 fathers and 158 mothers.

Results showed that general differences between parents and their adolescent offspring were as one might expect. Differences between white and Japanese-American adolescents about family values were fewer than one might expect, while differences between boys and girls, regardless of ethnic or cultural backgrounds, were most striking. Mothers and fathers showed stronger agreement than their adolescent offspring that there should be a clear line of authority within the family. Adolescents agreed significantly more strongly than their parents that every member of the family had a right to privacy. Only two items generated significant differences between the two ethnic groups of adolescents. White adolescents believed older children should have more privileges than younger, while Japanese-American adolescents felt youngsters older than age 7 or 8 should be able to watch whatever television they wanted. For sex differences, compared to boys, girls stand firmly for strong interrelationships and obligations within the family, affectional ties, and open expression of emotion.

The findings suggest that adolescent boys and girls differ significantly both in the rate and degree of separation from the nuclear family and in the way they handle it. Daughters in this study appeared to be struggling for their individuality within the family, while sons appeared to try to break away from the family. The findings also appear to challenge the notion that adolescent boys and girls have the same family experience. The variations may mean they have different routes in achieving the common goal of maturity.

▶ Stanford Friedman, Professor of Pediatrics and Psychiatry, University of Maryland, comments:

"I have chosen to comment on only two aspects of this study. First, the finding of fewer differences than one might expect between white and Japanese-American adolescents about family values adds further support that there has been a major mixing of cultural values in Hawaii. Such a convergence of attitudes and values, including those related to the family, is probably most pronounced in the 'younger generation.' Further, the lack of differences might well have been enhanced by selecting for study only those families consisting of two parents. These findings suggest that perhaps Hawaii is not the ideal location for doing cross-cultural studies.

"Second, it is of general interest that the adolescents in the study placed more emphasis than their parents on each member of the family having a right to 'privacy.' This is a critical issue relevant to all health professionals involved in counseling of adolescents and their families. It has been my experience that many parents do not acknowledge that a desire for privacy is a reflection of healthy adolescent development and therefore should be encouraged. Rather, they frequently interpret the wish for privacy and confidentiality by their teenager as a sign of rejection. When the pediatrician hears from parents that they have read the diary of or letters addressed to their teenager, he should be alert to the possibility that the parent-adolescent relationship may not be optimal. Likewise, going through the desk or bureau of a teenager is not respectful of his or her need to develop a life increasingly independent from parents. The developing adolescent should share many of his most personal thoughts and feelings with selected peers and not necessarily with his parents."

Adolescent Chest Pain: A Prospective Study
Robert H. Pantell and Benjamin W. Goodman, Jr.
Pediatrics 71:881–887, June 1983   17–6

One hundred adolescents with chest pain (mean age, 16.4 years) seen at the Medical University of South Carolina were studied prospectively to determine the etiology, functional implications, and illness attributions of such patients at an adolescent clinic.

TABLE 1.—CLINICAL CHARACTERISTICS
OF CHEST PAIN

	No. of Patients
Time course: <1 mo	29
1–6 mo	35
6–12	12
>1 yr	24
Episodes: 1	9
2–6	20
>6	71
Frequency: Daily or more often	27
2–6/wk	36
1–7/mo	29
<1/mo	8
Location: Left precordium	28
Central/substernal	40
Right precordium	8
Combination of these	24
Duration: <1 min	13
1–5 min	36
6–60 min	32
>60 min	19
Quality: Sharp	68
Dull	19
"Pinprick"	6
Other (includes both)	7
Radiation: None	75
Arms	5
Back	7
Other	13

(Courtesy of Pantell, R.H., and Goodman, B.W., Jr.: Pediatrics 71:881–887, June 1983. Copyright American Academy of Pediatrics 1983.)

Ninety-one percent of the patients were black and 63% were female. Typical patients reported frequent episodes of sharp pain (63% had two or more episodes weekly) of moderate duration (51% of episodes lasted longer than 6 minutes) that had been occurring for many months (36% of patients had had pain for more than 6 months) (Table 1). Sixty-nine percent of adolescents had restricted their physical activity because of the pain and 41% were absent from school.

Except for chest wall tenderness, physical examination was normal in most patients. A single specific cause of pain was determined in 46 patients, a pattern not suggestive of a specific organic problem was observed in 43, and 11 patients were believed to have multiple etiologies. Of those with a definite diagnosis, 23 had hyperventilation and 10 of the 11 patients with multiple etiologies had hyperventilation as one of the causes (Table

TABLE 2.—ETIOLOGY OF CHEST PAIN

	Patients	Diagnoses	
		No.	%
Idiopathic	43 (3)*	46	39
Musculoskeletal			
Chest wall syndrome	13 (2)	15	13
Traumatic	1 (2)	3	2
Costochondritis	9 (7)	16	14
Ribcage anomaly	1 (1)	2	2
Hyperventilation	13 (10)	23	20
Mixed	11		
Others			
Breast-related	5 (1)	6	5
Respiratory	2	2	2
Gastrointestinal	2 (1)	3	2
Mitral valve prolapse	0 (1)	1	1
Total	100 (28)	117	100

*Values in parentheses indicate diagnoses included under mixed category.
(Courtesy of Pantell, R.H., and Goodman, B.W., Jr.: Pediatrics 71:881–887, June 1983. Copyright American Academy of Pediatrics, 1983.)

TABLE 3.—RESPONSES TO QUESTIONS ABOUT CAUSES OF CHEST PAIN*

	"What do you think caused your pain?"	"What were you afraid caused your pain?"
Heart attack	4	44
Heart disease	6	12
Cancer	2	12
Gas	7	0
Don't know	61	23
Miscellaneous	20	9

*Data indicate importance of how a question is phrased.
(Courtesy of Pantell, R.H., and Goodman, B.W., Jr.: Pediatrics 71:881–887, June 1983. Copyright American Academy of Pediatrics, 1983.)

2). The most commonly diagnosed cause was musculoskeletal problems (31%), including costochondritis (14%), chest wall syndrome (13%), skeletal trauma (2%), and rib cage anomaly (2%). Breast-related problems were diagnosed in 5% of patients, including 4 male patients with gynecomastia.

When questioned about their understanding of their illness, 56 patients feared that they had a cardiac problem, including 44 who were afraid they were experiencing a heart attack (Table 3). Twelve feared cancer. Occurrence of significant, stressful, negative events within 6 months of the onset of pain was reported by 31% of patients; 26% reported such events had occurred within 3 months of the onset.

Chest pain is a common problem that usually is caused by a benign process, but it often is misunderstood and can be the source of considerable dysfunction and anxiety in adolescents.

▶ In my experience, the most common cause of chest pain in adolescents as well as young adults is the entity that has been termed "precordial catch" (Miller, A., and Texidor, T.: *JAMA* 159:1364, 1955). It has three major aspects.

1. Patients are light or of medium build; they are younger than age 35, and there is no sex prevalence.

2. The pain is severe, sudden in onset, does not radiate, and regularly is located near or above the cardiac apex.

3. The pain occurs at rest or during mild activity and frequently is related to a "slouched posture."

Taking a deep breath, or moving, makes the pain go away. It is frightening the first few times it is felt. Frightening—until you learn that you are not about to die. The cause of this pain is unknown, although it has been suggested that the pain is caused by some pinching of the pleura or the pericardium. It has been estimated that "Texidor's twinge" occurs in about one half of all persons sometime between ages 15 and 35 years. Did you ever have it?—F.A.O.

18 Therapeutics and Toxicology

Chloramphenicol Toxicity in Neonates: Its Incidence and Prevention
Anne Mulhall, John de Louvois, and Rosalinde Hurley
Br. Med. J. 287:1424–1427, Nov. 12, 1983   18–1

Despite its potential toxicity, chloramphenicol is used widely in the treatment of neonatal meningitis. The incidence of dose-related chloramphenicol toxicity was assessed in 64 neonates treated at 12 hospitals with chloramphenicol for life-threatening meningeal infections.

Ten infants had symptoms clinically attributable to chloramphenicol treatment. Nine were given the prescribed dose, but in 6 this was greater than the recommended dose (Table 1). Four of the 9 infants collapsed suddenly and became gray; cardiac arrest developed within 48 hours after the first dose of the drug was given. Four infants had reversible hematologic reactions. Four accidents occurred with regard to the use of chloramphenicol, 3 of which involved a tenfold overdose. One infant received 40 mg of chloramphenicol intraventricularly rather than intravenously. High serum concentrations, possibly the result of an unrecognized overdose, were observed in 4 infants, but only 2 had toxic reactions. Peak serum concentrations greater than 25 mg/L or trough concentrations greater than 15 mg/L were detected in 23 of 45 infants, 16 of whom received more than the recommended dose of chloramphenicol (Table 2). Of the 64 infants, 32 of 54 receiving the prescribed dose had peak serum chloramphenicol concentrations greater than 25 mg/L or trough concentrations greater than 15 mg/L; 9 of these 32 had clinical signs or symptoms of toxicity (Table 3).

In this series, serious toxic reactions were associated with prescription of doses exceeding the recommended dose or overdosage. This can be avoided by prescription and administration of the recommended dose, followed by careful monitoring. Serum concentrations of chloramphenicol should be maintained between 15 mg/L and 25 mg/L.

▶ It wouldn't be a YEAR BOOK without a contribution from George McCracken, Jr. Sorry to keep you in suspense so long. Doctor McCracken, Professor of Pediatrics, The University of Texas, Southwestern Medical School, comments:

"The paper by Mulhall and associates chronicles the issue of chloramphenicol dosage and toxicity in neonates. Despite the fact that cardiovascular instability or collapse (gray baby syndrome) was described more than 20 years ago, it is still encountered in neonates, principally as a result of failure of physicians to monitor serum concentrations as the only reliable guide to proper dosage.

TABLE 1.—SIGNS OF TOXICITY IN 9 NEONATES RECEIVING CHLORAMPHENICOL

Case No	Evidence of toxicity	Dose (mg/kg/day)	Recommended dose (mg/kg/day)	Serum concentration (mg/l)	Time after dose (hours)
1	Sudden collapse, grey coloration, cardiac and respiratory difficulties	34	25	>38 >80 4	4·5 25 92
2	Sudden collapse, grey coloration, cardiac and respiratory difficulties	53	25	35	2
3	Sudden collapse, grey coloration, cardiac and respiratory difficulties	77 77	25	>60 140* 124* 90	7·5 5* 7·5* 7
4	Sudden collapse, grey coloration, cardiac and respiratory difficulties	50 36 36	25	31 46 35 >43	12 0·5 12 6
5	Haematological	22	25	45 36 40	1 12 1
6	Haematological	50	25	38 47 47	12 1 12
7	Haematological	25	25	19 34 30 56	12 1 12 1
8	Haematological	37·5	37·5-50	72 100	1 3
9	Very grey	29	25	21 28 10	12 0·5 24

*Values before and after exchange transfusion.
(Courtesy of Mulhall, A., et al.: Br. Med. J. 287:1424–1427, Nov. 12, 1983.)

TABLE 2.—Dosage Schedules and Serum Chloramphenicol
Concentrations in 45 Neonates Without Signs of Toxicity

Serum chloramphenicol concentrations

Dosage given	Peak <15 mg/l	Peak 15-25 mg/l trough <15 mg/l	Peak >25 mg/l trough >15 mg/l	Total
Recommended	4	4	3	11
> Recommended	1	3	16	20
< Recommended	9	1	4	14
Total	14	8	23	45

(Courtesy of Mulhall, A., et al.: Br. Med. J. 287:1424–1427, Nov. 12, 1983.)

TABLE 3.—Relationship Between Dosage, High Serum
Concentrations, and Toxicity

	No	Peak concentration >25 mg/l or trough >15 mg/l or both	Clinical signs or symptoms of toxicity
Prescribed dose	54	32	9*
Known overdose	4	3 + 1 (CSF)	1
?Overdose	2	2	
Not evaluated	4		
Total	64	37 + 1 (CSF)	10

CSF = cerebrospinal fluid.
*All 9 infants had peak concentrations of more than 25 mg/L or trough concentrations of more than 15 mg/L, or both. In 2 infants an overdose was suspected.
(Courtesy of Mulhall, A., et al.: Br. Med. J. 287:1424–1427, Nov. 12, 1983.)

Although guidelines have been suggested, there is no standard dosage of chloramphenicol for newborn infants. It should be emphasized that chloramphenicol is *not* a first-line therapeutic agent for newborn infants for the following reasons: In vitro studies demonstrate that chloramphenicol is only bacteriostatic against many gram-negative enteric bacilli and it can antagonize the bactericidal activity of ampicillin on *Listeria* and on group B streptococci and of the new broad-spectrum β-lactams on *Klebsiella pneumoniae.* In experimental meningitis due to *Proteus mirabilis,* the bactericidal action of gentamicin against the infecting strain was abolished by the simultaneous intravenous administration of chloramphenicol. Additionally, pharmacologic antagonism has been demonstrated between phenobarbital or phenytoin and chloramphenicol. Phenobarbital induces hepatic microsomal enzyme activity resulting in subtherapeutic serum concentrations of chloramphenicol in many infants. By contrast, phenytoin has been shown to elevate chloramphenicol levels into the potentially toxic range. Finally, and most importantly, there are no data from properly controlled, prospective studies that demonstrate therapeutic superiority of chloramphenicol over conventional regimens of ampicillin and an aminoglycoside or over the new β-lactam compounds cefotaxime or moxalactam. Thus, I urge pediatricians to refrain from using chloramphenicol during the neonatal period unless there are compelling reasons to do so. In such uncommon situations, serum concentrations of chloramphenicol *must* be monitored and the dosage adjusted accordingly in order to insure therapeutic and safe levels."

A System for Individualized Dosing of Intravenous Aminophylline Using a Programmable Calculator

J. Chris Mitsuoka and Richard J. Fleck
Pediatrics 73:64–67, January 1984   18–2

Individualization of aminophylline dosing is indicated because of wide variability in drug clearance among patients. A dosing program that calculates a clearance value before reaching steady state in the early stage of treatment was evaluated. The program follows the basic approach of giving a loading dose over a short period, followed by a continuous infusion of the drug. The initial dose is based on weight, age, and other relevant parameters. The program is written for the Texas Instruments TI-59 programmable calculator. A typical run is shown in the table. The loading dose is reduced appropriately if the patient has taken theophylline before admission. If the preloading dose value is much lower than expected, an additional loading dose is given before the maintenance infusion is continued, and serum is drawn after at least 4 hours of continuous infusion.

This program can provide clinically useful information on projected plasma concentrations before steady state is reached, on the basis of the serum concentration and an accurate history of dosing. The iterative technique utilized would be impractical without the assistance of a calculator. Only a single serum sample is needed if no xanthene has been administered previously. The closer to steady state the sample is obtained, the more accurate the prediction will be. Programmable calculators are an economical and portable means of rapidly performing complicated mathematical

Typical Program Run

Printed Output	Symbol	Explanation
375.	D^*	Loading dose
60.	MD	Maintenance dose
0.	CO	Initial serum concentration
18.	CT	Observed serum concentration at time (t)
10.	TP	Time after loading dose
63.	KG	Weight in kg
30.24	V	Volume of distribution
1.645019531	CL	Clearance
0.054398794	Ke	Elimination rate constant
29.15321062	CSS	Projected state concentration
30.84411621	MD	New maintenance dose to maintain desired concentration
12.	$T3$	Time of dose adjustment in hours after loading dose
19.15321062	$C3$	Concentration at T3
4.493117193	TE	Time to hold infusion to reach desired serum concentration

(Courtesy of Mitsuoka, J.C., and Fleck, R.J.: Pediatrics 73:64–67, January 1984. Copyright American Academy of Pediatrics 1984.)

manipulations, and their routine clinical use can improve the quality of patient care and reduce the number of serum samples required for determining the correct dose of aminophylline in a given patient.

Childhood Lead Poisoning: Controlled Trial of the Effect of Dust-Control Measures on Blood Lead Levels
Evan Charney, Barry Kessler, Mark Farfel, and David Jackson
N. Engl. J. Med. 309:1089–1093, Nov. 3, 1983   18–3

Lead-contaminated house dust is a factor in childhood lead poisoning. However, most lead-reduction programs do not emphasize the control of house dust. They studied whether lead-reduction plus dust-control measures would lower blood lead levels in children with class II or III poisoning (blood lead levels of 30–49 μg/dl) more effectively than lead-reduction measures alone. An experimental group of 14 children and a control group of 35 children whose homes already had been treated were studied. In experimental homes, sites with elevated lead levels (greater than 100 μg/ 930 sq cm) were wet-mopped twice monthly, and families were encouraged to clean and to wash the child's hands frequently.

All subjects were black, and all lived within the city of Baltimore. There was a significant fall in mean blood lead level in the experimental group after 6 months (from 38.6 to 33.3 μg/dl); there was a further drop after 1 year (to 31.7 μg/dl) (Table 1). Four of the 14 experimental subjects had values that fell below 30 μg/dl by the end of the study, and none had values that exceeded 50 μg/dl. In contrast, the mean value for control subjects did not change significantly over the course of the study (Table 2). In 13 of the 14 experimental cases, sites within the home had sample values that exceeded 100 μg, which is the level of lead commonly seen in new homes (Table 3). Interior windowsills and floor areas adjacent to those windows were the sites with the highest values. Only 5 of the 14 homes had continuing values below 100 μg of lead per site before cleaning. There was no significant relation between the reduction in lead-contaminated dust in a given home over time and a reduction in a child's blood lead level. The reduction in blood lead value was most marked in children who had initial levels in the upper range for class II lead poisoning and were therefore most at risk of requiring chelation therapy if they had a further increase. Four (11.4%) of the 35 control subjects were hospitalized for such therapy during the course of the study.

House-dust sampling and dust-control efforts, including dust analyses after home treatment, should be incorporated as a regular part of the strategy for controlling childhood lead poisoning.

▶ Herbert Needleman, Director, Behavioral Science Division, Children's Hospital of Pittsburgh, and one of the first clearly to demonstrate the intellectual damage produced by an increased body lead burden, comments:

"With justification, lead continues to receive considerable attention by both scientists and regulators here and in Europe. A strong movement has been set

BLOOD LEAD AND FREE ERYTHROCYTE PROTOPORPHYRIN LEVELS

Blood lead (μg/dl) [†]	At Start		At 6 Months		At 12 Months	
	EXPER GROUP (N = 14)	CONTROL GROUP (N = 35)	EXPER GROUP (N = 14)	CONTROL GROUP [*] (N = 33)	EXPER GROUP (N = 14)	CONTROL GROUP (N = 35)
			no. of subjects			
≥50	0	0	0	3	0	4
45.5–49.5	2	5	0	1	0	2
40.5–45	4	7	1	9	0	3
35.5–40	3	12	3	8	1	11
30–35	5	11	9	11	9	12
<30	0	0	1	1	4	3
Mean ±S.D. [‡]	38.6±5.2	38.5±5.2	33.3±3.6 [‡]	38.7±7.6 [‡]	31.7±2.6 [‡]	37.8±7.9 [‡]
Free erythrocyte protoporphyrin (μg/dl of red cells) [§]	203±99	231±103	158±76	216±125	144±82	208±130

[*]Two observations not obtained at 6 months.
[†]Values are rounded to nearest 0.5 μg.
[‡]Difference between groups at 6 and 12 months is significant ($P < .001$).
[§]Mean ± SD. $P < .05$ for difference between groups at 12 months.
(Courtesy of Charney, E., et al.: N. Engl. J. Med. 309:1089–1093, Nov. 3, 1983. Reprinted by permission of the New England Journal of Medicine.)

in motion on both continents to remove all lead from gasoline, and the Centers for Disease Control have lowered the defined threshold for elevated lead levels in children to 25 μg/dl. These efforts spring from two forces: (1) concern in Europe over the deterioration of the Black Forest due to acid rain and (2) the steadily growing body of evidence that lower and lower doses of lead have

CHANGES IN INDIVIDUAL BLOOD LEAD LEVELS*

CHANGE IN LEAD LEVEL (μg/dl)	FROM 6 MO BEFORE TO START		FROM START TO 6 MO		FROM START TO 12 MO	
	EXPER GROUP	CONTROL GROUP	EXPER GROUP	CONTROL GROUP	EXPER GROUP	CONTROL GROUP
	no. of subjects					
Increase ≥6	2	2	0	3	0	6
Increase 3.5–5.5	1	3	0	1	0	0
±3	8	15	5	22	2	18
Decrease 3.5–5.5	2	2	2	3	3	5
Decrease ≥6	0	2	7	3	9	6
Mean change	+1.0	+1.0	−5.3	+0.2	−6.9	−0.7

*Observations were not obtained in all subjects 6 months before study and 6 months after start. Experimental group lacks 1 observation 6 months before study; control group lacks 11 observations 6 months before study and 3 observations 6 months after start.
(Courtesy of Charney, E., et al.: N. Engl. J. Med. 309:1089–1093, Nov. 3, 1983. Reprinted by permission of the New England Journal of Medicine.)

LEAD LEVELS IN HOUSE DUST OF 14 EXPERIMENTAL HOMES*

SITES WITH LEAD IN DUST	LEAD LEVEL	AT START	AT 12 MO
	μg	*no. of homes*	
None	>100	1	5
≥ One	100–200	1	4
≥ One	200–400	1	1
≥ One	400–800	3	4
≥ One	800–1600	4	0
≥ One	≥1600	4	0

*(Courtesy of Charney, E., et al.: N. Engl. J. Med. 309:1089–1093, Nov. 3, 1983. Reprinted by permission of the New England Journal of Medicine.)

adverse health effects in children. Recent studies have shown that 1,25-dihydroxyvitamin D levels are reduced at very low doses of lead (Mahaffey, K. R., et al.: *Am. J. Clin. Nutr.* 35:1237–1331, 1982) and that lead cleaves the phosphate-ribose backbone of transfer RNA in catalytic fashion, suggesting that there is no threshold for this effect (Brown, R. S., et al.: *Nature* 303:543–546, 1983). Lead levels in umbilical cord blood are related to minor malformations and Bayley scores at ages 6 and 12 months, controlling for other covariates (Needleman, H. L., et al.: *JAMA* 251:2956, 1984; and Needleman, H. L., et al.: *Pediatr. Res.* 17:179A, 1983).

"High technology generally gets the lion's share of public attention in matters of health, but a strong case can be made that the most effective means for changing the state of affairs for most people are often ordinary procedures, readily available, of low cost. These are usually devoid of drama. This article by Charney and colleagues is a neat example of this principle. Here, mops and buckets, combined with teaching and supervision, are rigorously shown to lower children's blood lead levels. This is an important contribution, but a cautionary note is in order. Studies of compliance to long-term medical regimens yield pessimistic prognoses. While mothers may be willing and able to participate in this program for a finite period, one confidently could predict that the curve of compliance will be a declining one.

"It is reasonable, at the same time, to ask whether the responsibility for the control of a generally distributed threat to health should be imposed on individual consumers for more than a brief time. Lead should be recognized and treated for what it is, a public health problem, and the responsibility for its control bestowed on those institutions that are responsible for public health. If the disease were cholera, would we ask mothers to boil their water forever?"

Assessment of Lead Stores in Children: Validation of 8-Hour CaNa2EDTA Provocative Test

Morri E. Markowitz and John F. Rosen (Albert Einstein College of Medicine, New York)

J. Pediatr. 104:337–341, March 1984   18–4

The standard 24-hour edetate disodium calcium (CaNa2EDTA) provocative test is a sensitive means of estimating the mobile and potentially toxic fraction of body lead stores and assessing the response to chelation therapy; however, it requires hospitalization, two intramuscular injections, and a 24-hour quantitative urine collection. A simplified 8-hour provocative test was evaluated in 36 asymptomatic children with blood lead levels of no more than 69 µg/dl and erythrocyte protoporphyrin levels of at least 50 µg/dl. Lead excretion during the first 8 hours of a 24-hour CaNa2EDTA test was compared with excretion during the entire test period. One child was tested 3 times. The test doses of CaNa2EDTA consisted of 500 mg/sq m. Twenty-five children had not received a chelating agent in the past 6 months. The mean age was 46 months. Most children were from families living in substandard housing.

The test results are given in Table 1. On the basis of a 24-hour urinary lead limit of 500 µg, an 8-hour value of 200 µg or more was most successful in correctly predicting the test outcome (Table 2). The coefficient of correlation between the 8-hour and 24-hour urinary lead-EDTA ratios was 0.79. An 8-hour ratio of 0.70 or more best predicted the test outcome. Correlations between blood lead and erythrocyte protoporphyrin values and the urinary excretion of lead after administration of CaNa2EDTA are shown in Table 3. All of the children who had positive results by the ratio criterion also had lead excretion of at least 500 µg/24 hours.

The excretion of at least 200 µg of lead in 8 hours after administration of a test dose of CaNa2EDTA or a urinary lead-EDTA ratio of 0.70 or more can identify children who will respond to chelation therapy by lead diuresis. Some children may receive unnecessary chelation therapy, but

TABLE 1.—Results of Edetate Disodium Calcium (CaNa$_2$ EDTA) Provocative Test

	n	Age (mo)	PbB (µg/dl)	EP (µg/dl)	UPb (µg)		UPb/EDTA		Total 24-hr dose CaNa$_2$EDTA
					8 Hr	24 Hr	8 Hr	24 Hr	
Total population	36	46 ± 23	41 ± 11	169 ± 105	210 ± 169	497 ± 301	0.60 ± 0.43	0.70 ± 0.41	686 ± 158
Negative test*	22	42 ± 18	36 ± 9	166 ± 121	128 ± 50	301 ± 110	0.39 ± 0.15	0.46 ± 0.16	644 ± 105
PbU ≥500 µg/24 hr	14	54 ± 29	48 ± 10	201 ± 99	339 ± 209	804 ± 452	0.92 ± 0.53	1.07 ± 0.42	752 ± 205
PbU · EDTA ≥ 1.0/24 hr	7	47 ± 23	53 ± 10	228 ± 73	434 ± 255	1043 ± 556	1.21 ± 0.59	1.40 ± 0.37	713 ± 226

Data expressed as mean ± SD.
*Negative CaNa$_2$ EDTA provocative test result by both criteria of absolute lead excretion and lead-drug ratio.
(Courtesy of Markowitz, M.E., and Rosen, J.F.: J. Pediatr. 104:337–341, March 1984.)

only a few who require treatment will be missed by the 8-hour test. If the ratio criterion is used, none will be missed.

▶ Markowitz and Rosen have made a valuable contribution by documenting the utility of the 8-hour EDTA provocative test in identifying the child with an increased body lead burden. No more hospital admissions for the collection of 24-hour urine specimens! It still remains to be demonstrated what the "safe" lead-EDTA ratio really is. With 4% of all children between ages 6 months and 5 years having blood lead values in excess of 30 µg/dl and 18.6% of poor central-city black children in this category (Mahaffey, K. R., et al.: *N. Engl. J.*

TABLE 2.—PREDICTIVE VALUE OF 8-HOUR PROVOCATIVE TEST

	Criterion 1 24-hr PbU ≥500 µg 8-hr PbU ≥200 µg		Criterion 2 24-hr PbU/EDTA ≥1.00 8-hr PbU/EDTA ≥0.70	
	n	%	n	%
Sensitivity*	12/14	86	7/7	100
Specificity†	20/22	91	27/29	93
False negative‡	2/14	14	0/7	0
False positive§	2/22	9	2/29	7

Standard test outcome
(24-hr provocative test)

		+	−
Screening test outcome (8-hr provocative test)	+	True+	False+
	−	False−	True−

*Sensitivity = True+/(True+) + (False−).
†Specificity = True−/(True−) + (False+).
‡False− = False−/(True+) + (False−).
§False+ = False+/(False+) + (True+).
(Courtesy of Markowitz, M.E., and Rosen, J.F.: J. Pediatr. 104:337–341, March 1984.)

TABLE 3.—COMPARISON OF BLOOD AND
URINE INDICATORS OF LEAD BURDEN*

			UPb		UPb/EDTA
	PbB	EP	8 Hr	24 Hr	8 Hr
PbB	—				
EP	0.21	—			
UPb 8 hr	0.50†	0.09	—		
UPb 24 hr	0.62‡	0.12	0.86‡	—	
UPb/EDTA 8 hr	0.49†	0.27	0.90‡	0.68‡	—
UPb/EDTA 24 hr	0.68‡	0.33§	0.82‡	0.91‡	0.79‡

*Linear correlation coefficients (n = 36).
†$P < .01$.
‡$P < .001$.
§$P < .05$.
(Courtesy of Markowitz, M.E., and Rosen, J.F.: J. Pediatr. 104:337–341, March 1984.)

Med. 302:573, 1982), it is time we had an answer to the question, "Is any lead safe?"

Jeanne Maracek and others (*Arch. Environ. Health.* 38:355, 1983) reported that lead, even at concentrations generally regarded as asymptomatic, was associated with deficits in visual-motor functioning and perceptual integration, right-left orientation, and verbal abstraction.

Perhaps the worse lead story of 1984 was a political one and reflects the power of the lead industry. A story in *Science* (223:672, 1984) reported that Vernon Houk, director of the environmental health center within the Centers for Disease Control (CDC), received a note demanding that he call off a scientific meeting that planned to go over a document entitled "Preventing Lead Poisoning in Young Children." The letter came from a law firm representing the Lead Industries Association and warned of "further legal proceedings" if the meeting was not cancelled. The meeting was called off. The lead manufacturers were concerned that the meeting would produce a document suggesting that the "safe" blood level was to be reduced from 30 to 25 µg/dl. The lead people think that this is "alarmist." The fox is now guarding the henhouse.—F.A.O.

Button Battery Ingestions: A Review of 56 Cases
Toby L. Litovitz (Georgetown Univ. Hosp.)
JAMA 249:2495–2500, May 13, 1983   18–5

Fifty-six cases of button battery ingestions were reviewed to identify features of serious cases and to determine whether miniature button batteries can pass spontaneously without adverse consequences. Ingestions were studied with respect to size, components, locations, and passage of the battery and the ingestor's age, symptoms, and therapy.

In 5 symptomatic children the button cell lodged in the esophagus and the only 2 deaths reported in this series occurred in this group; in the 3 most severe cases the ingestion initially was unsuspected and medical evaluation was delayed. Large button cells with diameters of 21 to 23 mm were involved in these 5 cases and the identical manganese dioxide battery was implicated in 4.

In the remaining 51 cases the button cell passed spontaneously beyond the esophagus and only 4 were symptomatic. Of 14 asymptomatic patients who underwent endoscopy or surgery, 7 were found to have unanticipated mucosal lesions of the gastrointestinal tract. Transit time through the gut, documented in 25 patients, ranged from 14 hours to 7 days. In 36% of cases it was delayed beyond 48 hours. In 62.5% of cases in which endoscopic retrieval was attempted, the button cell could not be removed because the instrument lost hold of the slippery foreign body.

Twelve of 17 corroded, pitted, or split batteries passed through the gastrointestinal tract spontaneously and 5 were surgically removed. Corrosion or evidence of leakage did not correlate with the magnitude of the patient's symptoms. There was a statistically significant association of mercuric oxide cells with symptoms or mucosal lesions.

It is believed imperative that every button battery ingestor should have an emergent chest roentgenogram to exclude the possibility of an esophageal location, as esophageal injury has been observed only 4 hours after ingestion. Symptoms may include dysphagia, vomiting, anorexia, and fever. Although batteries located in the esophagus must be removed immediately, a less invasive approach is indicated if the battery has passed beyond the esophagus. Administration of ipecac is not advised because of the risk of airway obstruction when the foreign body is regurgitated.

Only 1 of the 51 cases in which the battery passed beyond the esophagus was associated with a severe complication, a perforated Meckel's diverticulum. No correlation was found between length of transit time and presence of even minor symptoms. Although daily roentgenograms to monitor battery progression are often espoused, careful observation (at home) for symptoms would seem to be sufficient. Cathartics routinely are advocated to hasten transit. In theory, cimetidine, antacids, or metoclopramide hydrochloride to minimize gastric acid-induced corrosion may be of some additional value, but these recommendations require confirmation in animal studies. All instances of button battery ingestion should be reported to the National Capital Poison Center 24-hour emergency line: 202–625–3333.

▶ The ingestion of these small, disk-shaped batteries used to power watches, cameras, calculators, small games, and hearing aids is increasing at an alarming rate (Kulig, K., et al.: *JAMA* 249:2502, 1983; and Votteler, T. P., et al.: ibid., p. 2504). Physicians must become familiar with the current rules of management. H. Barry and Carol M Rumack (ibid., p. 2509) suggest:

1. If there has been an ingestion of a battery, an x-ray study must be obtained as soon as possible. Initial radiologic examination must include the area from the nasopharynx to the anus.

2. Once an x-ray study demonstrates the presence of an object in the esophagus, the object must be removed immediately.

3. If the battery has passed through the esophagus and is in the stomach or beyond, the patient need only be followed up and observed for symptoms. If the battery is not passed by rectum in 7 days, then an enema should be administered, depending on the location. If this fails or the patient is symptomatic, then surgery should be used.

4. If the battery has come apart in the lower bowel, enema removal is safer and more effective than surgery to remove all of the dispersed particles.

5. If the battery comes apart, heavy metal levels should be obtained in blood and urine to determine if chelation therapy is necessary.

Ingestion of a battery is not like ingestion of a roll of film, where you can tell a parent, "Don't worry, nothing will develop."—F.A.O.

Burn Injury Related to Improper Use of Microwave Oven

Mark Puczynski, Dennis Rademaker, and Robert L. Gatson (Loyola Univ., Maywood, Ill.)
Pediatrics 72:714–715, November 1983   18–6

An infant aged 1 week sustained a microwave oven-related burn injury.

Male infant, aged 1 week, was hospitalized with second-degree scald burns over 6% of the body surface. The mother reported that the burns resulted from overheated formula that was poured into a bottle having a rubber nipple tightly stretched over the top. The formula was heated for about 1 minute under the highest microwave oven setting. While holding the infant in one arm, the mother removed the bottle of formula from the oven; the plastic liner exploded and hot formula spilled over the infant. Vital signs and results of physical examination were normal except for second-degree burns over the abdomen and right thigh. The infant was hospitalized for 2 weeks and discharged in good condition.

Physicians caring for children should be aware of the dangers of microwave ovens and warn parents of the potential hazards. Parents should be cautioned about the dangers of incorrect heating and should be advised to follow manufacturer's instructions for preparing foods.

▶ Here is another disease of "progress." In 1982 it was estimated that microwave ovens were present in 25% of all homes (*Business Week,* p. 28 Mar. 8, 1982). By now, the figure is probably much higher. More burns will come.— F.A.O.

19 Miscellaneous

Profile of Pediatric Practice in the United States

Robert A. Hoekelman, Barbara Starfield, Marie McCormick, Hallie DeChant, Christy Moynihan, Stephen Radecki, and Robert C. Mendenhall
Am. J. Dis. Child. 137:1057–1060, November 1983
19–1

Under the auspices of the Division of Research and Medical Education, University of Southern California School of Medicine, Los Angeles, a random sample of 429 office-based pediatricians was drawn from 20,999 pediatricians listed in American Medical Association files. Data gathered from each respondent included: summary of daily encounters for 1 week, a detailed account of activities during 3 consecutive days, and personal,

TABLE 1.—CHARACTERISTICS OF PEDIATRICIANS STUDIED

Certification Status and Practice Arrangement (%)*	Age, yr (Mean ± SD)	Urban Practice Location, %	% Female (N = 53)
Certified (73.4)	49.1 ± 10.6	86.3	56.6
Solo (28.9)	53.0 ± 11.1	87.5	32.1
Partnership (21.2)	48.0 ± 9.6	88.0	9.4
Group (23.3)	45.2 ± 9.4	83.0	15.1
Noncertified (26.6)	49.0 ± 12.4	74.1	43.4
Solo (14.5)	54.3 ± 10.9	68.8	26.4
Partnership (6.1)	44.4 ± 11.1	80.8	7.5
Group (6.1)	41.0 ± 10.9	80.0	9.4
Total	49.1 ± 11.1	83.0	12.4

*Percentage of total sample.
(Courtesy of Hoekelman, R.A., et al.: Am. J. Dis. Child. 137:1057–1060, November 1983; copyright 1983, American Medical Association.)

TABLE 2.—TIME SPENT BY PEDIATRICIANS CONDUCTING OFFICE VISITS

All Visits		Visits by Age of Patient		
Duration, min*	% of Visits	Patient Age, yr	No. of Visits Sampled	Duration, min (Mean ± SEM)
1-5	15	<1	4,693	11.2 ± 0.09
6-10	40	1-4	7,564	10.3 ± 0.07
11-15	24	5-9	4,999	10.5 ± 0.10
16-20	17	10-14	2,757	11.0 ± 0.13
≥21	4	15-19	1,153	11.6 ± 0.27

*Mean duration of all office visits was 10.7 minutes.
(Courtesy of Hoekelman, R.A., et al.: Am. J. Dis. Child. 137:1057–1060, November 1983; copyright 1983, American Medical Association.)

TABLE 3.—ANNUAL NUMBER OF VISITS TO OFFICE-BASED
PEDIATRICIANS

Patient Age, yr	Children in US, ×1,000*	No. of Visits, ×1,000	Av No. of Visits/yr	% of All Visits	% Male
<1	3,279	11,310	3.45	25.3	54.0
1-4	12,784	16,657	1.36	37.3	54.4
5-9	17,530	9,710	0.55	21.7	52.4
10-14	19,504	5,045	0.26	11.3	52.2
15-19	21,477	1,937	0.09	4.3	48.2
Total	**74,574**	**44,659**	0.60	**99.9**	53.3

*Data from *Preliminary Estimates of the Population of the United States, by Age, Sex, and Race, 1970 to 1981*, U.S. Department of Commerce publication 917, 1982.
(Courtesy of Hoekelman, R.A., et al.: Am. J. Dis. Child. 137:1057–1060, November 1983; copyright 1983, American Medical Association.)

TABLE 4.—DIAGNOSIS FOR PATIENTS OF ALL AGES

Diagnosis	All Diagnoses		Principal Diagnosis Only	
	No., ×1,000 (%)	Cumulative %	No., ×1,000 (%)	Cumulative %
Well-child care (health supervision)	15,615 (30.3)	30.3	15,442 (34.6)	34.6
Otitis media	7,560 (14.7)	45.0	6,225 (13.9)	48.5
Acute pharyngitis	5,105 (9.9)	54.9	4,228 (9.5)	58.0
Pneumonia	4,357 (8.5)	63.4	3,592 (8.0)	66.0
Upper respiratory tract infection	3,181 (6.2)	69.6	2,741 (6.1)	72.1
Bronchitis	2,198 (4.2)	73.8	2,037 (4.6)	76.7
Acute tonsillitis	2,089 (4.0)	77.8	1,794 (4.0)	80.7
Gastroenteritis	1,954 (3.8)	81.6	1,662 (3.7)	84.4
Dermatitis	1,372 (2.7)	84.3	855 (1.9)	86.3
Laryngitis and tracheitis	1,089 (2.1)	86.4	969 (2.2)	88.5
Complication of medical care	973 (1.9)	88.4	673 (1.5)	90.0
Asthma	885 (1.7)	90.0	723 (1.6)	91.6
Urinary tract symptoms	704 (1.4)	91.4	323 (0.7)	92.3
Viral infection, unspecified site	669 (1.3)	92.7	606 (1.4)	93.7
All other diagnoses	3,762 (7.3)	100.0	2,790 (6.3)	100.0
Total	**51,513 (100.0)**	. . .	**44,660 (100.0)**	. . .

(Courtesy of Hoekelman, R.A., et al.: Am. J. Dis. Child. 137:1057–1060, November 1983; copyright 1983, American Medical Association.)

professional, and practice characteristics. Each practitioner completed a series of questionnaires, log-diaries, and patient encounter forms.

Characteristics of pediatricians studied as to certification, practice arrangement, location, and sex are detailed in Table 1. Practice of pediatrics is heavily weighted toward ambulatory care, which accounts for 88% of the time spent in professional activities. Patients' access to pediatricians is primarily by appointment, with 97.9% of visits scheduled beforehand.

TABLE 5.—Distribution of Primary Problem Focus

Primary Problem Focus	All Ages (21,784)	<1 (4,799)	1-4 (7,784)	5-9 (5,179)	10-14 (2,841)	15-19 (1,181)
			Age, yr, % of Visits*			
Well patient	28.0	54.6	24.8	14.7	18.3	22.2
Upper respiratory tract†	15.0	11.3	19.0	15.2	12.2	10.0
Ears	12.2	9.4	16.7	13.1	6.3	3.4
Mouth/throat	10.6	3.4	10.9	17.1	7.6	16.1
Lower respiratory tract	8.5	3.9	8.8	10.8	15.2	7.4
Skin	5.5	4.4	5.4	8.2	10.5	9.8
Gastrointestinal	5.1	6.7	4.9	4.4	5.1	3.7
Nose	1.9	1.3	1.9	2.4	1.8	1.7
Skeletal	1.7	0.2	0.7	1.8	5.1	5.2
Head/neck	1.2	0.9	1.1	1.5	1.7	1.8
Emotional/behavioral	1.0	0.3	0.2	1.9	2.1	3.3
Eyes	1.0	0.9	0.9	1.3	1.2	0.7
Neurologic	0.7	0.4	0.5	0.9	1.7	0.8
Muscular	0.7	0.2	0.2	0.6	2.2	2.7
Blood/lymphatics	0.6	0.3	0.5	0.8	0.7	1.2
Renal	0.6	0.0	0.1	0.9	0.5	0.0
Circulatory (heart)	0.3	0.3	0.2	0.3	0.3	0.6
Genital (M)	0.2	0.1	0.2	0.3	0.3	0.7
Gynecologic	0.2	0.0	0.1	0.2	0.4	2.0
Endocrine	0.2	0.0	0.0	0.3	0.8	0.8
Liver/gallbladder	0.1	0.3	0.0	0.1	0.1	0.2
Breasts	0.1	0.1	0.0	0.0	0.3	0.2
Circulatory (other)	0.1	0.0	0.1	0.1	0.2	0.1
Arthritis/rheumatism	0.1	0.0	0.1	0.2	0.2	0.3
Other and multisystem	2.0	1.4	1.5	1.5	4.3	4.1

*Number of visits to sample of pediatricians studied are indicated in parentheses.
†Not localized to ears, nose, mouth, or throat.
(Courtesy of Hoekelman, R.A., et al.: Am. J. Dis. Child. 137:1057–1060, November 1983; copyright 1983, American Medical Association.)

However, 82% of pediatricians said they saw patients who "walked in." Mean duration of all office visits was 10.7 minutes, with 55% of visits lasting 1–10 minutes (Table 2). Visits by patients younger than age 1 year constituted the largest percentage (25%) of all visits (Table 3). Male patients accounted for most visits, except for the group aged 15–19 years.

Respondents were asked to record the principal diagnosis made for each visit and to list two other diagnoses, if indicated. Of all diagnoses, 81.6%— and of principal diagnoses, 84.5%—were accounted for by health supervision and diseases of the upper and lower respiratory tract (Table 4). The primary problem for each office visit and the age groups of patients are identified in Table 5. Health supervision, respiratory, gastrointestinal, dermatologic, and musculoskeletal illnesses accounted for two thirds to seven eighths of patient visits, depending on age of patient (Table 6).

The numbers in Tables 3 and 4 have been extrapolated from the study sample of pediatricians to all pediatricians in the United States. The diagnoses listed in Tables 5 and 6 are skewed heavily to respiratory tract

TABLE 6.—FIVE MOST FREQUENT PRIMARY PROBLEM FOCI BY
PATIENT AGE

	Age, yr, % of Visits*				
Primary Problem Focus	<1 (4,799)	1-4 (7,784)	5-9 (5,179)	10-14 (2,841)	15-19 (1,181)
Well patient	54.6	24.8	14.7	18.3	22.2
Upper respiratory tract†	11.3	19.0	15.2	12.2	10.0
Ears	9.4	16.7	13.1	. . .	. . .
Gastrointestinal	6.7	. . .	. . .	. . .	. . .
Skin	4.4	. . .	. . .	10.5	9.8
Mouth/throat	. . .	10.9	17.1	15.2	16.1
Lower respiratory tract	. . .	8.8	10.8	7.6	. . .
Musculoskeletal	. . .	. . .	. . .	. . .	7.9
Total for 5 Most Frequent Foci	86.4	80.2	70.9	63.8	66.0

*Number of visits to sample of pediatricians studied are indicated in parentheses.
†Not localized to ears, nose, mouth, or throat.
(Courtesy of Hoekelman, R.A., et al.: Am. J. Dis. Child. 137:1057–1060, November 1983; copyright 1983, American Medical Association.)

illnesses because the sampling of this study was conducted during November and December and is not characteristic of patient visits made throughout the year.

The data of this study should be useful to pediatric educators in planning pediatric residency programs and to health planners and legislators and will enable individual pediatricians to compare the content of their practice with those of their colleagues.

▶ Robert J. Haggerty, President, American Academy of Pediatrics, and President, William T. Grant Foundation, comments:

"These data on pediatric practice are the most representative and up-to-date of what the office-based pediatrician in the United States does today. As the authors state in their paper, they were collected in the months of November and December and, therefore, are more heavily weighted to respiratory tract infections than would be the case throughout the entire year. In addition, they represent what pediatricians now diagnose, not necessarily what problems children have. It seems clear from other studies that these diagnoses underrepresent the frequency of behavioral, social, and learning problems and also underrepresent both the number of and problems related to adolescents. Work by these and other authors have shown how variable are the rate of diagnoses in these areas between different pediatricians seeing approximately the same type of patient. Therefore, provider variation appears to be a major reason for different and often low rates of diagnosis of these problems. These social and behavioral problems are also undoubtedly present in some children seen in well-child supervision visits, since it has been shown that many children presenting for well-child visits actually have a considerable number of problems and are not 'well.' These data, therefore, represent what is, not what should be, the content of pediatric practice as such. They are vey important openings into that 'black box' of pediatric practice."

Behavioral, Health, and Cost Outcomes of an HMO-Based Prenatal Health Education Program

Daniel H. Ershoff, Neil K. Aaronson, Brian G. Danaher, and Fred W. Wasserman

Public Health Rep. 98:536–547, Nov.–Dec. 1983   19–2

A prenatal health education program conducted within a health maintenance organization (HMO) setting was evaluated by comparing the behavioral, birth, and treatment cost outcomes for 57 women given personal nutrition counseling and participating in an 8-week, home-correspondence stop-smoking program and 72 control women given standard prenatal care. The HMO enrollees were a heterogeneous group ethnically and socioeconomically. Two personal nutrition counseling sessions were offered the experimental subjects, and a follow-up session was held about 3 months later.

More experimental than control women stopped smoking during pregnancy (49% vs. 37.5%). Among women who continued to smoke, those in the experimental group reduced their smoking more during pregnancy. Significantly more women in the experimental group adjusted their diets ante partum (91% vs. 68%). Particular success was achieved in consumption of more dairy products and vegetables and less coffee and in achievement of adequate weight gain during pregnancy. Mean infant birth weight was higher in the study group, and there were fewer low birth weight infants in this group (7.0% vs. 9.7%). The cost savings associated with less hospital care for low birth weight infants in the study group yielded an overall benefit-cost ratio for the study program of about 2:1. Costs are compared in the table.

This experience supports the feasibility of conducting small-scale evaluations of various health education and promotion programs within HMOs. Programs that encourage and facilitate healthful life-style changes are an alternative, or at least a complementary, strategy to traditional methods of limiting health care expenditures. This approach can be expected to yield savings in both human and economic terms.

INCIDENCE RATE AND TREATMENT COSTS ASSOCIATED WITH PRETERM, SMALL FOR DATE, AND OTHER DELIVERIES AMONG EXPERIMENTAL AND CONTROL GROUP SUBJECTS

Variables	Experimental group		Control group		Both groups	
	Incidence (percent)	Cost per delivery	Incidence (percent)	Cost per delivery	Incidence (percent)	Cost per delivery
Deliveries:						
Low birth weight	7.0	$1,771	9.7	$2,914	8.6	$2,498
Preterm	1.7	4,138	6.9	3,959	4.7	3,989
Small-for-date	5.3	982	2.8	301	3.9	709
Other	93.0	315	90.3	452	91.4	391
Average cost per delivery		417		692		570
Adjusted cost per delivery		466		649		

(Courtesy of Ershoff, D.H., et al.: Public Health Rep. 98:536–547, Nov.–Dec. 1983.)

Parental Response to Repeat Testing of Infants With "False Positive" Results in a Newborn Screening Program

James R. Sorenson, Harvey L. Levy, Thomas W. Mangione, and Stephen J. Sepe (Boston Univ.)
Pediatrics 73:183–187, February 1984
19-3

Most infants who are rescreened for initial abnormal findings will have normal results, and there is concern that the parents will be subjected to unwarranted anxiety or depression. Parental concern over repeat screening and responses as a function of parental understanding of the reason for retesting were assessed among the parents of 60 infants requiring retesting in a newborn screening program for metabolic disorders, 55 mothers and 5 fathers. In 63% of cases some special action, such as a call from the clinic or physician, was taken to notify the parents of the need for a specimen.

Reasons given the parents for repeat testing are listed in Table 1. Forty-five percent of the parents understood why retesting was necessary, but most believed that retesting was routine or that a mistake had been made on initial testing or reported having been told nothing specific about the testing. Few parents reported having discussed the results of repeat testing with the spouse or friends or relatives. Those who understood that the initial result was abnormal were no more anxious or depressed than the others (Table 2). Both groups were less distressed at a second interview when told of the normal results of the repeat test. Over a third of the parents of normal infants, however, reported concern over their infant's health because of the repeat testing. Such concern was greater among parents who reported that they had not received adequate information on the screening-testing process and its import for the health of the infant.

The findings support the disclosure of aberrant initial test results to parents before the infant is retested. Some concern about the infant's health may result, however, and a more complete understanding of the screening-testing process might be helpful.

TABLE 1.—REASONS PROVIDERS GAVE
PARENTS FOR REPEAT TEST (N = 59)

Parent Told	%
Initial test result abnormal	45
1st sample elevated 25%	
1st sample ambiguous 12%	
May be a "problem" 8%	
Other reason	55
Told nothing specific 23%	
Repeat testing routine 19%	
Mistake made on 1st test 10%	
1st test lost 3%	

TABLE 2.—MEAN MULTIPLE AFFECT ADJECTIVE CHECKLIST ANXIETY AND DEPRESSION SCORES BY INTERVIEW AND PARENTAL KNOWLEDGE OF INITIAL TEST RESULTS

Psychological Dimension	1st Interview			2nd Interview			Mean Difference Scores 1st to 2nd Interviews Total Population	
	1st Test Abnormal (1)	Other Reason for Repeat Test (2)	P†	1st Test Abnormal (3)	Other Reason for Repeat Test (4)	P†	(5)	P‡
Anxiety	10.7* (3.6)	9.9 (4.4)	NS	6.2 (3.3)	5.3 (3.1)	NS	4.5 (4.8)	.000
Depression	18.7 (4.5)	16.8 (5.5)	NS	15.6 (4.9)	14.0 (5.8)	NS	2.8 (6.4)	.001
N	27	32		25	32		58	

*Values shown in columns 1 to 5 are means; SD is shown in parentheses.
†Determined by t test, independent samples.
‡Determined by t test, dependent samples.
(Courtesy of Sorenson, J.R., et al.: Pediatrics 73:183–187, February 1984. Copyright American Academy of Pediatrics 1984.)

▶ Honesty is usually the best policy. I once heard a cynic remark, ''You can fool all of the people some of the time; you can fool some of the people all of the time; and that should be sufficient for most purposes.''—F.A.O.

Concerns of Mothers Seeking Care in Private Pediatric Offices: Opportunities for Expanding Services

Gerald B. Hickson, William A. Altemeier, and Susan O'Connor

Pediatrics 72:619–624, November 1983

19–4

A surplus of general pediatricians is predicted for 1990. This surplus could provide both the opportunity and need for practitioners to identify areas of maternal concern that might guide expansion of marketable physician services. Maternal concerns were assessed in interviews of 207 mothers seeking care in private pediatric offices. Several weeks later, the 10 pediatricians participating were given a copy of the interview and asked to predict the results.

The total number of specific concerns per mother averaged 6.4; those mentioned most frequently are shown in Table 1. When only the most important specific concern was considered by category, 30% of the women selected some aspect of physical health as their greatest concern. Pediatricians provided relatively little help with psychosocial needs; only 28% of mothers indicated they discussed or planned to present their most important psychosocial concern to the pediatrician. The 149 mothers who had not communicated their greatest psychosocial concern did not do so for the following reasons: unawareness that the pediatrician could be a source of assistance (39%); belief that the pediatrician was too busy (16%); denial of needing help (15%); belief that the pediatrician was not qualified (12%); belief that the pediatrician was unwilling to help (10%); and embarrassment in discussing the problem (8%). When the 10 pediatricians were asked to predict these responses, they responded as follows: parents' perception of pediatricians as too busy (8/10), maternal embarrassment (5/10), not being aware pediatricians can help (3/10), and feeling that pediatricians are unsympathetic or unqualified (1/10). Rates of commu-

TABLE 1.—MOST FREQUENTLY MENTIONED
SPECIFIC CONCERNS OF 207 MOTHERS WAITING IN
PRIVATE PEDIATRIC OFFICES

	% of Mothers Expressing Concern
Working takes too much time away from my child	35
Best method for discipline	24
Effects of divorce on child	17
Assessment of personality development	13
Effects of family member's death on child	10
Fear of developing a serious childhood disease	10
Excessive shyness	9
Inadequate discipline from father	9
Child rearing is confining	8
Child may be misled by peer pressure	8
Child's social skills need improvement	8
Inconsistent discipline	7
Assessment of mental development	7
Learning problems	7
Husband loses control when disciplining	7

(Courtesy of Hickson, G.B., et al.: Pediatrics 72:619–624, November 1983. Copyright American Academy of Pediatrics 1983.)

TABLE 2.—Effects of Type of Concern,
Sociodemographics, and Physician Attitudes
on Communication of Psychosocial Needs

	Correlation with Communication
Category of concern	
Mental development	.169*
Quantity or quality of time with child	−.154*
Adjustment to adolescent transition	−.141*
Sociodemographic characteristics	
Father's occupation score	.213†
White race	.211†
Maternal age	.162*
Maternal education	.151*
Intensity of concern	.126
Reason for visit (well *v* sick)	.113
Married	.101
No. of children	.101
Mother's occupation score	.016
Physician attitudes	
Interest score	.336†
Self-perceived capability score	.268†

*$P < .05$.
†$P < .01$.
(Courtesy of Hickson, G.B., et al.: Pediatrics 72:619–624, November 1983. Copyright American Academy of Pediatrics 1983.)

TABLE 3.—Regression Analysis
Examining Relative Importance of
Physician Attitude and Family
Socioeconomic Characteristics on
Communication of Psychosocial Needs

	β Weight
Physician interest score	0.313
Race	0.149
Mother's age	0.106
Father's occupation	0.062
Physician capability score	0.046
Mother's education	0.038

(Courtesy of Hickson, G.B., et al.: Pediatrics 72:619–624, November 1983. Copyright American Academy of Pediatrics 1983.)

nication of greatest psychosocial concerns to the 10 individual pediatricians ranged from 0% to 57%. Effects of various factors on communication of psychosocial needs are listed in Table 2. Table 3 shows the results of regression analysis, which suggested that physician interest was the most important determinant of communication.

Mothers waiting in private pediatric offices perceive a variety of needs for their children. Physician interest is a more important predictor of communication than are family socioeconomic characteristics. The major question is how counseling for psychosocial needs can be delivered in a way that is acceptable and economically feasible for both parents and pediatricians.

▶ Barbara Starfield, Professor of Pediatrics and Public Health, Johns Hopkins University, comments:

"Not everyone (but perhaps most pediatricians) would agree that psychosocial problems should be in the purview of medical care. There is relatively little time devoted to psychologic phenomena in the curricula of medical school and virtually none devoted to social phenomena. What makes us think that pediatricians have anything to offer their patients?

"Effective medical care, as provided by practitioners, consists of four parts: (1) recognition of the problems that have an impact on health status and on ability to function to maximum potential, (2) reaching an appropriate diagnosis, (3) ability to recommend appropriate management, and (4) reassessment to assure that the problem actually has been addressed adequately. The literature shows that the most imporant determinant of the quality of care is the setting in which it is conducted; group practices, in particular, seem to provide the incentives that lead to optimum results. Settings in which the care is prepaid seem better able to deal with psychosocial problems in children, perhaps because of the absence of fee-for-service reimbursement for these services under current conditions. Another major determinant is the nature of the practitioner's training; physicians do best what they have been most trained to do. Unfortunately, neither training nor most work settings provide the basis for doing what should be done. Fortunately, this study shows that practitioners appear to realize their deficiencies and seem to feel that they could do better. There is little evidence that medical academia, concentrating as it does primarily on organic problems, will be of much help. Primary-care pediatricians should increase their insistence that the agencies mainly responsible for child health research and that the academies responsible for setting and monitoring educational standards take psychosocial problems as seriously as they take organic child health problems. Practitioners also might consider engaging in collaborative research on the recognition and management of psychosocial concerns so that more information would be available on the distribution and nature of the problems and experiences in handling them where they usually are found. But real change may have to await major reform in health care financing. Psychosocial problems in children do not exist in isolation; serious attention to them could well improve the results of care for the more traditional conditions."

The Zeta Sedimentation Ratio in Children

Michael Bennish, James Vardiman, and Marc O. Beem (Univ. of Chicago)
J. Pediatr. 104:249–251, February 1984   19–5

The erythrocyte sedimentation rate (ESR) has several disadvantages for use in pediatric patients, including the need for 2 ml of blood, the time

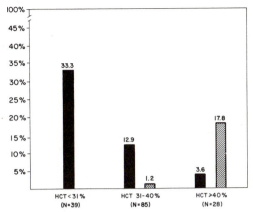

Fig 19–1.—Frequency and nature of discrepant (one test normal and other test elevated) ESR and ZSR measurements according to HCT range. Solid bars indicate ESR elevated, ZSR normal; and hatched bars denote ZSR elevated, ESR normal. Normal ZSR is less than 57% in females and less than 55% in males. Normal ESR is less than 21 mm per hour in females and less than 16 mm per hour in males. (Courtesy of Bennish, M., et al.: J. Pediatr. 104:249–251, February 1984.)

required for the determination, and artifactual elevations by anemia. The zeta sedimentation ratio (ZSR) is a modification that uses slow-speed centrifugation to speed sedimentation. Only 0.1 ml of blood is needed, and the determination takes only 3 minutes rather than an hour. Correction is made for anemia.

The usefulness of the ZSR was examined in studies of 120 normal children and comparative studies of the ESR and ZSR in 120 acutely and chronically ill children. A total of 152 patient samples were evaluated.

The mean ZSR in normal boys was 44%, with an SD of 5%, and the mean for girls was 46%, with an SD of 5%. The respective upper limits of normal were 54% and 56%. No significant sex differences in age or mean hematocrit (HCT) were found. Reported normal ranges for men and women have been less than 55%. The ESR and ZSR were in agreement in 80% of patient samples. Discrepant values were most frequent in specimens with either a low or a high HCT (Fig 19–1). Only 8% of pairs were markedly discrepant. Nine of these 12 pairs were in samples with an HCT of less than 31%. Eleven of the samples had an elevated ESR and a normal ZSR.

The ZSR correlates closely with the ESR in most pediatric patients, and it is probably superior in anemic patients. It now is used routinely at the authors' center. The expanded scale of the ESR may be of use in assessing disease progression in patients with markedly elevated values, such as those with severe inflammation.

▶ This is a test that, because of its speed and simplicity, should replace the classic erythrocyte sedimentation rate. Both are nonspecific. It is unclear at present if one is any more or less nonspecific than the other. Both tests are indirect measures of the plasma concentration of the acute-phase reactants fibrinogen and γ-globulin. Both these macromolecules act to decrease the negative charge, or zeta potential, on the surface of the red blood cell.—F.A.O.

Major Dog Attack Injuries in Children

Nathan E. Wiseman, Harvey Chochinov, and Virginia Fraser
J. Pediatr. Surg. 18:533–536, October 1983   19–6

Data on the 57 patients sustaining injuries resulting from dog attacks over a 5-year period (1977–1981) who have been treated at the Children's Hospital of Winnipeg, in Manitoba, Canada, were reviewed. Half of the victims were aged 5 years or younger. Injuries occurred more often in boys (55%). Soft tissue injuries occurred alone in 51 patients and were associated with fractures in 3 patients. There were a total of 78 sites of soft tissue injury, with 60 being in the head and face region and 18 in the extremities. Fracture sites in 3 patients were to the skull, nasal bone, and zygoma. Treatment was successful in all cases. In 3 patients, a life-threatening visceral injury resulted from the dog attack, and a fourth patient died prior to arrival at the hospital.

CASE 1.—Girl, aged 28 months, sustained a bite wound to the abdomen while playing with her pet St. Bernard dog. She was febrile, had tachycardia, and had signs of generalized peritonitis. An upright abdominal radiogram showed free air within the peritoneal cavity and confirmed a perforated viscus. At laparotomy, lacerations to the left lobe of the liver and a puncture wound to the anterior wall of the stomach were repaired. The animal was not destroyed.

CASE 2.—Boy, aged 5 years, had gone into the bush to have a bowel movement when he was assaulted sexually by a neighbor's large dog. Operation disclosed a discrete anterior rectal wall perforation located just above the peritoneal reflection. He also had fecal pelvic peritonitis. Colostomy was performed and later closed. The dog was destroyed.

CASE 3.—Boy, aged 22 months, was at play when he was attacked and mauled by a large chained mongrel dog. Surgical treatment consisted of debridement and closure of the gastric wounds, suture of the duodenal laceration, and creation of an ileostomy and a left lower-quadrant mucous fistula. There were also fractures of the right 9th, 10th, and 11th ribs. The chest was reconstructed primarily. The patient was discharged from the hospital after 2 months.

CASE 4.—Boy, aged 3½ years, crawled unwitnessed into a closure occupied by four 10-month-old Husky sled dogs and was savaged to death. Postmortem examination revealed a total of twelve deep anterior and posterior cervical lacerations. Death was attributed to acute exsanguination. The dogs were destroyed.

The authors conclude such incidents are preventable if large dogs and small children are kept apart. They present 10 rules for human beings: Do not (1) hold your face close to a dog, (2) allow dogs to roam unleashed, (3) pet a strange dog, (4) tease a dog, (5)startle a dog, (6) touch a sleeping dog, (7) leave a small child and dog alone, (8) omit vaccination of a dog, (9) leave a dog alone with strangers, and (10) ignore warning signals of aggressive behavior.

▶ I thought everyone was familiar with Rule 6—"Let sleeping dogs lie." It has been estimated that 1 in every 275 persons will be bitten by a dog each year (Klein, D.: *N. Y. State J. Med.* 66:2306, 1966) and that 1 in every 200 visits to a pediatric emergency room is occasioned by a dog bite (see 1983 YEAR BOOK, pp. 461–462). We gave it to the cats in Chapter 2, "Infectious Disease and Immunity", so it is now time to turn our attack on dogs.

Equal time for the pet owners: A survey of 13,000 owners published in the August, 1984, issue of *Psychology Today* revealed the following:

1. Nine of 10 pet owners said that their pet was "extremely" or "very" important to them. Owners ranked their pets right behind their friends and relatives and ahead of their work in importance.

2. Almost 8 of 10 owners said that sometimes their pet was their closest companion.

3. About one half of the owners keep pictures of their pet in their wallet, at home, or in the office. One-half allow the pet to sleep with a member of the family and one-fourth celebrate their pet's birthday.

With all those advantages, what is so bad about 100,000 dog bites more or less?—F.A.O.

Circumcision: Study of Current Practices

Thomas J. Metcalf, Lucy M. Osborn, and E. Mark Mariani (Univ. of Utah)
Clin. Pediatr. (Phila.) 22:575–579, August 1983   19–7

In 1975 the American Academy of Pediatrics Ad Hoc Task Force on Circumcision stated, "There is no absolute medical indication for routine circumcision of the newborn." Nevertheless, there has been little change in the incidence of circumcision in the United States. A survey of hospital and medical records, a prospective newborn study, a telephone survey of new mothers, and an office survey were used to investigate the current incidence of circumcision in Utah, the reasons governing parental decisions regarding circumcision, immediate and later complications of circumcision, and genital problems occurring in uncircumcised boys.

Of 15,905 boys born in 16 of 34 Utah hospitals during the period 1977–1979, 13,498 (84.9%) were circumcised. Differences in rates among hospitals generally reflected ethnic background, with white children being circumcised more often than those of other ethnic groups. The most common reason given by parents for circumcision was cleanliness and health, followed by social custom or matter of routine (Table 1). Of parents participating in the newborn study, 67% said that they were counseled regarding the procedure, whereas only 7% of those in the telephone survey recalled such counseling. Complications occurred in 14 (4%) of 361 circumcisions (Table 2), including hemorrhage, surgical complications requiring later revision, infection, and use of a too small Plastibell ring. All complications were treated successfully. Later complications developed in 30 (13%) of 230 circumcised children, the most common of which was foreskin adhesion; 3 children required surgical revision. Only 17 (12%)

TABLE 1.—Parents' Reasons for Circumcision

Reason	Number*	Per Cent
Hygiene	159	69
Social custom, routine	48	21
Circumcised father	39	17
Physical appearance	33	14
No reason	32	14
Decreased infection	14	6
Religion	12	5
Doctor's advice	7	3
Decreased cancer	6	3

*Many parents gave more than one reason.
(Courtesy of Metcalf, T.J., et al.: Clin. Pediatr. (Phila.) 22:575–579, August 1983.)

TABLE 2.—Complications of Circumcision

Neonatal (n = 361)	No.	%	Later (n = 230)	No.	%
Hemorrhage	6	(2)	Foreskin adhesions	18	(8)
Infection	4	(1)	Poor hygiene	6	(3)
Surgical	3	(1)	Meatitis	3	(1)
Bell too small	1	(0.3)	Surgical revision	3	(1)
Total	14	(4)	Total	30	13

(Courtesy of Metcalf, T.J., et al.: Clin. Pediatr. (Phila.) 22:575–579, August 1983.)

of the 142 boys in the office study were not circumcised. The mothers of 2 of these children reported the complication of foreskin adhesion; there were no reports of hygienic problems or infection.

Although the results support the contention that routine neonatal circumcision be discontinued, the physician, if able to dissuade parents from having their infants circumcised, must provide adequate information regarding hygiene and the slow, natural separation of the foreskin from the glans.

▶ For more on circumcision go back to Chapter 1, "The Newborn." For even more on circumcision, read the editorial by Hugh Thompson, "The Value of Neonatal Circumcision: An Unanswered and Perhaps Unanswerable Question" (*Am. J. Dis. Child.* 137:939, 1983). For still more—but certainly not the last word—see the letter by Joseph Ichter and the response by George Little in *Pediatrics* (73:110, 1984). If you have any questions, please do not hesitate to contact Doctor Ichter at (717) 763-3334.—F.A.O.

Fetal Cystic Hygroma: Cause and Natural History
Frank A. Chervenak, Glenn Isaacson, Karin J. Blakemore, W. Roy Breg, John

C. Hobbins, Richard L. Berkowitz, Marge Tortora, Kara Mayden, and Maurice J. Mahoney (Yale–New Haven Med. Center)

N. Engl. J. Med. 309:822–825, Oct. 6, 1983   19–8

Fifteen cases of fetal cystic hygroma, a congenital malformation of the lymphatic system, were diagnosed by ultrasound during a 3-year period. All ultrasound studies were performed for obstetric indications, not because of a family history of a congenital anomaly. Fetal age at time of diagnosis was 18 to 29 weeks.

Fetal cystic hygromas appear ultrasonically as single or multilocular fluid-filled cavities in the posterolateral part of the neck that are not contiguous with the CNS. They probably arise from failure of the lymphatic and venous systems to communicate (Fig 19–2). In theory, if the jugular lymph sacs and jugular veins then connect or an alternative route of lymphatic drainage develops before intrauterine death, the cystic hygromas may regress and peripheral edema may resolve. Webbing of the neck and puffiness of the hands and feet, which are characteristic postnatal features of Turner's syndrome, would result. This series of embryologic events and phenotypic features makes up the jugular-lymphatic obstruction sequence (Fig 19–3).

Of the 15 fetuses studied, 13 were hydropic at the time of diagnosis; 7 of these died in utero, 1 died soon after birth, and 5 were electively aborted (2 of these 5 fetuses had bradycardia). Of the 2 fetuses without hydrops, 1 was electively aborted and the other died of congestive heart failure during the neonatal period. Eleven fetuses (73%) had karyotypes consistent with a diagnosis of Turner's syndrome, and an additional fetus had a 46 XY karyotype and female genitalia without gonads. Three fetuses had 46 XX karyotypes, and 2 of these had multiple malformations.

When a hygroma is detected during fetal life, careful sonographic examination of the entire fetus for skin edema, ascites, pleural and pericardial

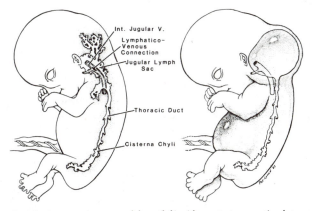

Fig 19–2.—Lymphatic system in a normal fetus *(left)* with a patent connection between the jugular lymph sac and the internal jugular vein and lymphatic system in a fetus with a cystic hygroma and hydrops from a failed lymphaticovenous connection *(right)*. (Courtesy of Chervenak, F.A., et al.: N. Engl. J. Med. 309:822–825, Oct. 6, 1983. Reprinted by permission of the New England Journal of Medicine.)

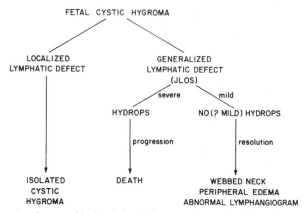

FETAL CYSTIC HYGROMA

LOCALIZED
LYMPHATIC DEFECT

GENERALIZED
LYMPHATIC DEFECT
(JLOS)

severe   mild

HYDROPS   NO (? MILD) HYDROPS

progression   resolution

ISOLATED   DEATH   WEBBED NECK
CYSTIC   PERIPHERAL EDEMA
HYGROMA   ABNORMAL LYMPHANGIOGRAM

Fig 19–3.—Natural course of fetal nuchal cystic hygroma. A generalized lymphatic defect results from the jugular lymphatic-obstruction sequence *(JLOS)*. (Courtesy of Chervenak, F.A., et al.: N. Engl. J. Med. 309:822–825, Oct. 6, 1983. Reprinted by permission of the New England Journal of Medicine.)

effusions, and cardiac or renal anomalies is indicated. Prognosis is poor in the presence of hydrops and uncertain in its absence. Determination of karyotype is important for genetic counseling. Amniocentesis should be attempted. Turner's syndrome and other chromosomal aneuploidies usually have a low risk of recurrence in subsequent pregnancies, but single-gene disorders often carry a high recurrence risk. Future pregnancies should be monitored with ultrasound and possibly with fetal karyotyping.

Iatrogenic Risks and Financial Costs of Hospitalizing Febrile Infants

Catherine DeAngelis, Alain Joffe, Modena Wilson, and English Willis (Johns Hopkins Univ.)
Am. J. Dis. Child. 137:1146–1149, December 1983   19–9

The iatrogenic and financial costs that arise from hospitalizing febrile infants aged 60 days or younger were identified, by diagnostic categories, by using a computer record system of such cases evaluated in a 3-year period.

A total of 191 febrile infants (197 admissions) were evaluated. Seven charts could not be located and 184 infants (190 admissions) were finally included in the study. An additional 106 febrile infants were managed as outpatients and were excluded. Thirty-seven admissions (19.5%) resulted in 48 separate complications (Table 1). Six (12.5%) occurred in infants who probably did not require hospitalization for therapy. Twenty-four (50%) resulted from intravenous therapy. In addition to these complications 26 diagnostic misadventures were identified, including attempts to procure body fluids for analysis, repeating diagnostic tests when unnecessary, following up contaminated cultures, not following up abnormal diagnostic test results, and keeping infants in a hospital unnecessarily to await consultation.

TABLE 1.—COMPLICATIONS BY DIAGNOSTIC CATEGORY

Diagnoses*	No. of Complications	No. of Admissions With Complications
Bacterial meningitis	6	5
Other bacterial infections	13	11
Otitis media	2	2
Aseptic meningitis	9	8
Otitis media and other diagnoses	0	0
Other bacterial infections and aseptic meningitis	2	1
Otitis media and aseptic meningitis	3	1
Other bacterial infections	2	1
Others-NR	6	6
Others-R	5	5
Total	**48**	**40**

*Others-NR = infants with no reason for admission other than fever; others-R = infants with reasons for admission in addition to fever.

(Courtesy of DeAngelis, C., et al.: Am. J. Dis. Child. 137:1146–1149, December 1983; copyright 1983, American Medical Association.)

TABLE 2.—LENGTH OF HOSPITALIZATION BY SELECTED DIAGNOSTIC CATEGORIES

Diagnoses*	Days	
	Mean	Range
Bacterial meningitis	19.0	15-28
Other bacterial infections	8.4	1-24
Otitis media	6.2	2-12
Aseptic meningitis	6.2	3-16
Others-NR	5.3	2-13
Others-R	7.4	5-26

*Others-NR = infants with no reason for admission other than fever; others-R = infants with reasons for admission in addition to fever.

(Courtesy of DeAngelis, C., et al.: Am. J. Dis. Child. 137:1146–1149, December 1983; copyright 1983, American Medical Association.)

Average length of hospitalization for all infants was 7 days (range, 1 to 28 days). Length of stay for selected diagnostic categories is given in Table 2. For the 73 infants who probably did not require hospitalization, average length of stay was 5.3 days.

Average cost of hospitalization per infant for 1979–1980 was $2,130. On the average, 25.6% of bill was for diagnostic studies and 8.3% for pediatricians' fees. Antibiotics were administered intravenously to 81.1% of infants, including 67% of 73 infants who, in retrospect, did not require hospitalization for treatment.

Admission of febrile infants, whose outpatient evaluation does not indicate illness requiring inpatient treatment, is often rationalized on the basis that hospitalization will be brief. However, the study shows that 87 (97.9%) of 89 infants with no obvious bacterial illness and negative cultures stayed longer than 3 days. Of 197 infants evaluated during a 3-year period, only 1 may have had a potentially life-threatening illness that was missed on outpatient evaluation. It is believed that these data on complications and diagnostic misadventures represent a conservative estimate of what actually occurred in the hospital.

▶ The institution of diagnosis-related categories (DRGs) may force a reexamination of this policy of routine admission of all febrile infants. A more useful approach was suggested by a review of the problem presented by Ron Dagan and associates (*Pediatr. Res.* 18:272A, 1984) at the 1984 Society for Pediatric Research meeting. The purpose of their prospective study was to test the ability of simple, objective criteria to identify infants at low risk for bacterial disease. A total of 168 febrile infants were studied; 85% were younger than age 60 days. An etiologic agent for the infection was identified in 72% of the infants.

There were 105 infants considered to be at low risk for bacterial disease by the following criteria: (1) normal neonatal history; (2) no evidence of soft tissue, skeletal, or ear infection; (3) white blood cell count 5,000–15,000, with less than 1,500 bands/cu mm; and (4) normal urinalysis. A group of 63 infants did not meet these criteria and 17 (27%) were found to have bacterial disease. Among the 105 infants who met the criteria, none was found to have bacterial disease and an infecting virus was identified in 70% of the patients. You can't do better than that. I hope someone quickly confirms this study, because it could result in an enormous reduction in the rate of hospitalization and the use of antibiotics.—F.A.O.

Prospective Assessment of Recurrence Risk in Sudden Infant Death Syndrome Siblings
Lorentz M. Irgens, Rolv Skjaerven, and Donald R. Peterson
J. Pediatr. 104:349–351, March 1984   19–10

Few data are available from which to estimate the risk of sudden infant death syndrome (SIDS) in a subsequent child. Data from the Medical Birth Registry of Norway were used to calculate mortality rates in siblings born subsequent to SIDS deaths. The incidence of SIDS deaths in a population of 826,162 children was 1.3/1,000. Of 712 children born immediately after an index SIDS case, 4 died of SIDS, for an incidence of 5.6/1,000 (Table 1). The incidence of SIDS in all 1,043 children born after an index case was 4.8/1,000. Total postperinatal death rates in subsequent siblings were 11.2/1,000 in the next siblings and 10.5/1,000 in all subsequent siblings, compared with a total postperinatal death rate in Norway of 4.3/1,000.

The present results are compared with those of other studies in Table 2. The current recurrence rate is lower than previously reported rates, but the overall incidence of SIDS in Norway also is lower than the rates reported in other studies. The risk of recurrence of SIDS for all subsequent siblings appears low enough to be encouraging from a counseling view-

TABLE 1.—Postperinatal Deaths in Total and Sudden Infant Death Syndrome (SIDS) Deaths in Sibships by Previous Occurrence of SIDS in the Sibship

Category of risk	Number of live births surviving 1 week	All postperinatal deaths			SIDS deaths		
		Number of deaths	Rate per 1000	Relative risk	Number of deaths	Rate per 1000	Relative risk
No previous SIDS case	825,119	3,571	4.3	1.0	1,054	1.3	1.0
Next subsequent sibling	712	8	11.2	2.6	4	5.6	4.4
All subsequent siblings	1,043	11	10.5	2.4	5	4.8	3.7

(Courtesy of Irgens, L.M., et al.: J. Pediatr. 104:349–351, March 1984.)

TABLE 2.—Comparison of Estimates of Sibling Risk to Sudden Infant Death Syndrome (SIDS) Incidence

Author	SIDS/sibs	SIDS/1000 sibs	95% Confidence limits*		Empirical SIDS risk	Sib risk relative to empirical
Froggatt	4/360	11.1	2.8	28.3	3.0	3.7
	6/360	16.7	6.1	36.4		7.4
Peterson	11/567	19.0	9.5	34.7	2.0†	9.5
Beal	6/302	20.0	7.3	43.4	2.0	10.0
Irgens	5/1043	4.8	1.5	11.2	1.3	3.7

*Confidence limits for the expected value of a Poisson distribution. In Beyer, W.H., ed.: *Handbook of Tables for Probability and Statistics.* Chemical Rubber Co., Cleveland, 1966, p. 191.
†Assumed.
(Courtesy of Irgens, L.M., et al.: J. Pediatr. 104:349–351, March 1984.)

point. Further studies are needed to determine whether the relatively low recurrence rate found in Norway is applicable to other countries.

▶ This certainly puts the problem in a more positive perspective for the troubled parent. Yes, the risk of SIDS for a subsequent sibling is 4 to 5 times greater than for the usual infant, but it is still only 5 chances in 1,000. This fact should be borne in mind when one attempts to demonstrate any benefit from home monitoring. One thousand infants must be monitored possibly to save 5.

Another cause for SIDS was added this past year to the ever-expanding list: apnea as the sole manifestation of cord compression or occult hindbrain malformation (Fremion, A. S., et al.: *J. Pediatr.* 104:398, 1984; Pauli, R. M., et al.: ibid., p. 342; and Tomaszek, D. E., et al.: *Ann. Emerg. Med.* 13:136, 1984).—F.A.O.

Home Monitoring for Central Apnea
M. Mackay, F. A. Abreu, E. Silva, U. M. MacFadyen, A. Williams, and H. Simpson (Univ. of Leicester)
Arch. Dis. Child 59:136–142, February 1984   19–11

A review was done of experience with 64 infants thought to be at increased risk of sudden infant death syndrome (SIDS), who were monitored at home for central apnea. Forty were siblings of SIDS victims. Thirty-five of them were monitored from age 1 week, usually after being discharged home. Twenty-four infants had had a "near miss" episode at a median age of 6 weeks. Two who presented as "near misses" were siblings of SIDS victims, and 1 infant in the sibling group had had a near miss episode. In the near miss group, monitoring began at ages 10 to 11 weeks on average. Both the capacitance pad type of monitor and the "volume" capsule were used.

The details of monitoring are given in the table. Thirty-four of the 40 SIDS siblings had had a total of 573 alarms for apnea by age 6 months. Stimulation by shaking was done 32 times and bag and mask resuscitation once. Twenty-two of the near miss infants had 335 alarms for apnea by age 6 months. Shaking was carried out 38 times and bag and mask resuscitation once. The median duration of home monitoring was 45 weeks for the SIDS siblings and 34 weeks for the near miss infants. No infant died. Monitor problems were not uncommon. In both groups, alarms were likelier to occur when respiratory infection was present. Monitoring appeared to have helped relieve parental anxiety and restore confidence during a stressful period.

Home monitoring for central apnea is practical, but it requires considerable commitment and expertise. Infants at increased risk of SIDS cannot

DETAILS OF HOME MONITORING			
	'Near miss'	*SIDS siblings*	*P*
Type of monitor			
RE134	20 (83)	24 (60)	
MR10	4 (17)	13 (33)	
Both	0 (0)	3 (7)	
No in group	24	40	
Age monitor issued (weeks)			
Mean (SD)	10·8±7·5	5·5±8·7	
Median	8·5	1·0	
Range	3–34	0–35	
No in group	24	40	
Duration of monitoring (weeks)			
Mean (±SD)	34·7±10·0	43·7±14·4	
Median	34·0	45·5	
Range	8–87	12–70	
No in group	24	40	
Alarms per patient per month	4·2	3·6	NS
No in group	22	34	
Action in response to alarms			
Number of alarms:			
None	252 (75)	498 (87)	
Flick toes	44 (13)	42 (7)	NS
Shaking	38 (11)	32 (6)	
Bag and mask resuscitation	1 (<1)	1 (<1)	
Total	335	573	
No in group	22	34	
Monitor problems	5 (23)	15 (44)	NS
No in group	22	34	

(Courtesy of MacKay, M., et al.: Arch. Dis. Child. 59:136–142, February 1984.)

yet be identified precisely. Any objective benefit from home monitoring remains unproved. Decisions should be based on the estimated risk, parental anxieties and attitudes, availability of a back-up service, and the degree of support that can be provided at home by a health visitor or trained nurse.

▶ No controls—no conclusions. This is a descriptive study, certainly a step in the right direction. The monitor enthusiasts as well as the reluctant prescribers must acknowledge that there is still no hard evidence as to benefit of monitors or, in fact, who needs them (Simpson, H.: *Arch. Dis. Child.* 58:469, 1983).— F.A.O.

QUAC: A Modest Proposal for Optimal Use of CT Scanning Equipment
Michael H. Reid and Arthur B. Dublin (Univ. of California at Davis)
AJR 142:845–846, April 1984   19–12

Current estimates suggest that 1,500–2,000 body CT examinations annually per CT scanner are an appropriate patient load, but budgetary restraints and increasing costs can be expected to lead to heavier use. The authors propose a new approach, quantity uniaxial compositomography (QUAC), to multiple simultaneous patient examinations as a means of increasing the efficiency of CT. Use of this method is illustrated in Figure 19–4. Occasionally, 5 children might be accommodated at the same time.

As many as 4,000 examinations per year could be done using a single CT scanner, and 8,000 children or even more could be examined. The resultant cost savings would be substantial. Special "batch" rates could be offered to groups of patients fortunate enough to have the same disease, or at least the same insurance carrier. Multi-institutional sharing of a single

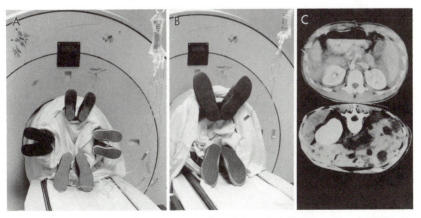

Fig 19–4.—Quantity uniaxial compositomography technique. **A,** 4 children positioned in CT gantry aperture. **B,** 2 adults positioned for simultaneous examination. **C,** resulting image (*bottom,* liver cysts; *top,* ruptured spleen [not related to patient positioning within the gantry]). (Courtesy of Reid, M.H., and Dublin, A.B.: AJR 142:845–846, April 1984.)

scanning facility is another possibility, with the different patient slots (positions) assigned to various hospitals. Scanners having large, padded apertures with low-friction Teflon coating would facilitate patient positioning. A hydraulic-powered ram could be used for patient packing if necessary. The use of QUAC will insure the elimination of air-tissue artifacts due to incomplete filling of the gantry aperture. Also, the recording of multiple patient examinations on the same film can provide some normal anatomical control.

▶ This is your reward for reading right to the end. The best satirical article of the past year! If adopted, this proposal is guaranteed to cut costs. The next step in economy is to redefine a semiprivate accommodation as "two in a bed."—F.A.O.

Review Articles of Interest to the Pediatrician

The Newborn

Cassady G.: Transcutaneous monitoring in infants. *J. Pediatr.* 103:837, 1983.

Committee on Drugs, American Academy of Pediatrics: Neonatal drug withdrawal. *Pediatrics* 72:895, 1983.

Donn S.M., et al.: Neonatal hyperammonemia. *Pediatr. Rev.* 5:203, 1983.

Drummond W.H.: Persistent pulmonary hypertension of the neonate (persistent fetal circulation syndrome). *Adv. Pediatr.* 30:61, 1984.

Ellison P.H.: Neonatal follow-up studies: The predictive value of neurologic abnormalities in the first year of life. *Pediatrics Update, 1984,* Ed. 187.

Fox W.W., et al.: Persistent pulmonary hypertension in the neonate. *J. Pediatr.* 103:505, 1983.

Hathaway W.E.: Neonatal hyperviscosity. *Pediatrics* 72:567, 1983.

Jobe A.: Respiratory distress syndrome: New therapeutic approaches to a complex pathophysiology. *Adv. Pediatr.* 30:93, 1984.

Lucey J.F., et al.: Reexamination of the role of oxygen in retrolental fibroplasia. *Pediatrics* 73:82, 1983.

Monset-Couchard M.: Bronchopulmonary dysplasia. *Pediatrics Update, 1984,* Ed. 145.

Mueller S.M.: Physiologic considerations concerning neonatal intracranial hemorrhage. *Pediatrics Update, 1984,* Ed. 167.

Myers G.J., et al.: Neonatal seizures. *Pediatr. Rev.* 5:67, 1983.

Singer L.P., et al.: Neonatal nutrition. *Pediatrics Update, 1984,* Ed. 111.

Stockman J.A., III: The anemia of prematurity and the decision when to transfuse. *Adv. Pediatr.* 30:191, 1984.

Watchko J.F.: Decision making on critically ill infants by parents. *Am. J. Dis. Child.* 137:795, 1983.

Weinstein R.A., et al.: Isolation guidelines for obstetric patients and newborn infants. *Am. J. Obstet. Gynecol.* 146:353, 1983.

Wolfe R.R.: Heart disease in infants of diabetic mothers. *Pediatrics Update, 1984,* Ed. 175.

Infectious Disease and Immunity

Bale J.T., Jr.: Human cytomegalovirus infection and disorders of the nervous system. *Arch. Neurol.* 41:310, 1984.

Banner W., Jr.: Vancomycin in perspective. *Am. J. Dis. Child.* 138:14, 1984.

Barkin R.M.: Facial and periorbital cellulitis in children. *J. Emerg. Med.* 1:195, 1984.

Clark J.H., et al.: Spontaneous bacterial peritonitis. *J. Pediatr.* 104:495, 1984.

Committee on Infectious Disease, American Academy of Pediatrics: Expanded guidelines for use of varicella-zoster immune globulin. *Pediatrics* 72:886, 1983.

DeVivo D.C.: The diagnosis and management of Reye syndrome. *Pediatrics Update, 1984,* Ed. 231.

Doughty R.A.: Lyme disease. *Pediatr. Rev.* 6:20, 1984.

Gershon A.A.: Immunizations for viral diseases: Past, present, and future. *Pediatrics Update, 1984,* Ed. 253.

Goldman J.N., et al.: The genetics of antibody production: Clinical implications. *JAMA* 251:774, 1984.

Koppe J.G.: Toxoplasmosis in the fetus and newborn. *Pediatrics Update, 1984,* Ed. 133.

Long S.S.: Approach to the febrile patient with no obvious focus of infection. *Pediatr. Rev.* 5:305, 1984.

Merigan T.C.: Human interferon as a therapeutic agent: Current status. *N. Engl. J. Med.* 308:1530, 1983.

Nelson J.D.: A primer for pediatricians on new cephalosporin antibiotics. *Am. J. Dis. Child.* 137:1041, 1983.

Rubenstein A.: Acquired immunodeficiency syndrome in infants. *Am. J. Dis. Child.* 137:825, 1983.

Speck W.: Acquired immunodeficiency syndrome. *J. Pediatr.* 103:161, 1983.

Sullivan J.L.: Epstein-Barr virus and the X-linked lymphoproliferative syndrome. *Adv. Pediatr.* 30:365, 1984.

Whitley R.J., et al.: Therapy for herpesvirus infections in childhood. *Pediatrics Update, 1984,* Ed. 215.

Wilfert C.M., et al.: Enteroviruses and meningitis. *Pediatr. Infect. Dis.* 2:333, 1983.

Wright J.M., et al.: A review of the oral manifestations of infections in pediatric patients. *Pediatr. Infect. Dis.* 3:80, 1984.

Allergy and Dermatology

Bahna S.L., et al.: Diagnosis and management of milk allergy. *Ann. Allergy* 51:574, 1983.

Berman B.A.: Cromolyn: Past, present, and future. *Pediatr. Clin. North Am.* 30:915, 1983.

Casale T.B., et al.: Mast cells and asthma: The role of mast cell mediators in the pathogenesis of allergic asthma. *Ann. Allergy* 1:2, 1983.

Esterly N.B.: Infantile acropustulosis and granuloma gluteale infantum. *Pediatr. Rev.* 5:59, 1983.

Hanifin J.M.: Atopic dermatitis. *J. Allergy Clin. Immunol.* 73:211, 1984.

Honig P.J.: Diaper dermatitis: Factors to consider in diagnosis and treatment. *Postgrad. Med.* 74:79, 1983.

Krowchuk D.P., et al.: Current status of the identification and management of tinea capitis. *Pediatrics* 72:625, 1983.

Matsuoka L.Y.: Acne. *J. Pediatr.* 103:849, 1983.

Norman P.S.: Review of nasal therapy: Update. *J. Allergy Clin. Immunol.* 72:421, 1983.

Rachelefsky G.S., et al.: Revisited: Aerosol corticosteroids in the treatment of childhood asthma. *Pediatrics* 72:130, 1983.

Stiell I.G., et al.: Adrenergic agents in acute asthma. Valuable new alternatives. *Ann. Emerg. Med.* 12:493, 1983.

Weiss R.A., et al: Diagnostic tests and clinical subsets in systemic lupus erythematosus. *Ann. Allergy* 51:135, 1983.

Dentistry and Otolaryngology

Amstey M.S., Insel R.A., Pichichero M.E.: Neonatal passive immunization by maternal vaccination. *Obstet. Gynecol.* 63:105, 1984.

Beare A.S.: Upper respiratory tract infections. *Practitioner* 227:953, 1983.

Centers for Disease Control: Erosion of dental enamel in improperly chlorinated swimming pools. *Morbidity Mortality Weekly Rep.* 32:361, 1983.

Chretien J., Holland W.: Acute respiratory infections in children: A global public health problem. *N. Engl. J. Med.* 310:982, 1984.

Drake-Lee, A.B., Webber P.A.: Adenotonsillectomy: Current debate. *Practitioner* 227:929, 1983.

Goldhagen J.L.: Croup: Pathogenesis and management. *J. Emerg. Med.* 1:3, 1983.

Grodin M.A.: Epiglottitis. *J. Emerg. Med.* 1:12, 1983.

Hall C.B., Breese B.B.: Does penicillin make Johnny's strep throat better? *Pediatr. Infect. Dis.* 3:7, 1984.

Hansen J.G., Schmidt H., Bitsch N.: Sore throat: Principles of diagnosis and management. *Practitioner* 227:937, 1983.

Henry, R.: Moist air in the treatment of laryngotracheitis. *Arch. Dis. Child.* 58:577, 1983.

Lilholdt T.: The significance of middle ear pressure and the results of a controlled study of ventilation tubes. *Dan. Med. Bull.* 30:408, 1983.

Myer C.M., Cotton R.T.: Nasal obstruction in the pediatric patient. *Pediatrics* 72:766, 1983.

Norman P.S.: Review of nasal therapy: Update. *J. Allergy Clin. Immunol.* 72:421, 1983.

Preece N.A.: Are the number of teeth any help in assessing development? *Arch. Dis. Child.* 58:849, 1983.

Schiff M.: Tympanosclerosis: Clinical implications of the failure of pathogenesis. *Ann. Otol. Rhinol. Laryngol.* 92:635, 1983.

Sheiham A.: Sugars and dental decay. *Lancet* 1:282, 1983.

Sidley C.G., Friedman M.: The avulsed tooth. *J. Dent. Assoc. S. Afr.* 38:441, 1983.

Spuance J.S., Bluestone C.D.: Medical management of the chronic draining ear. *Laryngoscope* 93:661, 1983.

Stool S.E., Bluestone C.D.: Studies in otitis media: Pittsburgh Otitis Media Research Center progress report, 1982. *Ann. Otol. Rhinol. Laryngol.* S107:92, 1983.

Winter G.B.: Fluorides and the prevention of caries. *Arch. Dis. Child.* 58:485, 1983.

Wright, R.A., Scholes E.: Streptococcal disease control in an ambulatory practice: Explicit criteria for throat cultures. *West. J. Med.* 140:409, 1984.

The Respiratory Tract

Brasher R.E.: Hyperventilation syndrome. *Lung* 161:257, 1983.

Casale T.B., Marom Z.: Mast cells and asthma: The role of mast cell mediators in the pathogenesis of allergic asthma. *Ann. Allergy* 1:2, 1983.

Ceder O.: Cystic fibrosis. *Acta Paediatr. Scand.*, Suppl. 309, 1983.

Green L.W., Goldstein R.A., Parker S.R.: Self-management of childhood asthma. *J. Allergy Clin. Immunol.* 72:Suppl. 3, 1983.

Hetzel M.R.: Pitfalls in the diagnosis of asthma. *Postgrad. Med. J.* 59:739, 1983.

Katz R.M.: Asthma and aports. *Ann. Allergy* 51:153, 1983.

Krzanowski J.J., Szentivanyi A.: Reflections on some aspects of current research in asthma. *J. Allergy Clin. Immunol.* 72:433, 1983.

Murphy S., Florman, A.L.: Lung defenses against infection: A clinical correlation. *Pediatrics* 72:1, 1983.

Mygind N., Nielsen M.H., Pedersen M.: Kartagener's syndrome and abnormal cilia. *Eur. J. Respir. Dis.* 64:Suppl. 127, 1983.

Rachelefsky G.S., Siegel S.C.: Revisited: Aerosol corticosteroids in the treatment of childhood asthma. *Pediatrics* 72:130, 1983.

Silverman M.: Bronchodilators for wheezy infants? *Arch. Dis. Child.* 59:84, 1984.

Tercier J.A.: Bronchiolitis: A clinical review. *J. Emerg. Med.* 1:119, 1983.

Welliver R.C.: Upper respiratory infections in asthma. *J. Allergy Clin. Immunol.* 72:341, 1983.

The Gastrointestinal Tract

Bachman, B.A.: Gastroesophageal reflux: Simple measures often suffice. *Postgrad. Med.* 74:133, 1983.

Bellman N.H., Hall S.N.: Etiology of Reye's syndrome. *Arch. Dis. Child.* 58:670, 1983.

Bhagwat A.G., et al.: Will the real Indian childhood cirrhosis please stand up? *Cleve. Clin. Q.* 50:323, 1983.

Committee on Nutrition: The use of whole cow's milk in infancy. *Pediatrics* 72:253, 1983.

Consensus Report: National Institutes of Health Consensus Development Conference Statement: Liver Transplantation. *Hepatology* 4:107S, 1984.

DeVio D.C.: How common is Reye's syndrome? *N. Engl. J. Med.* 309:179, 1983.

DuPont H., et al.: Traveler's diarrhea: New insights. *Scand. J. Gastroenterol.* 18:Suppl. 84, 1983.

Editorial comment: Management of gastroesophageal reflux. *Lancet* 1:1054, 1984.

Editor's comment: Bleeding ulcers: Scope for improvement? *Lancet* 1:715, 1984.

Goldman L.T., Weigert J.M.: Corrosive substance ingestion: A review. *Am. J. Gastroenterol.* 79:85, 1984.

Lebenthal E., Rossi T.N.: Intractable diarrhea of infancy: An alternative treatment strategy. *Postgrad. Med.* 74:153, 1983.

Lemanske R.F., Atkins F.M., Metcalfe D.D.: Gastrointestinal mast cells in health and disease: Part I. *J. Pediatr.* 103:177, 1983.

————Part II. *J. Pediatr.* 103:343, 1983.

Maddrey W.VC.: Hepatic vein thrombosis (Budd-Chiari syndrome). *Hepatology* 4:44S, 1984.

Mowe A.P.: Reye's syndrome: Twenty years on. *Br. Med. J.* 286:1999, 1983.

Newcomer A.D., McGill D.B.: Clinical importance of lactase deficiency. *N. Engl. J. Med.* 310:42, 1984.

Nord K.S.: Peptic ulcer disease in children and adolescents: Evolving dilemmas. *J. Pediatr. Gastroenterol. Nutr.* 2:397, 1983.

Rotbart H.A., Levin M.J.: How contagious is necrotizing enterocolitis? *Pediatr. Infect. Dis.* 2:406, 1983.

Rumack B.H., Rumack C.M.: Disk battery ingestion. *JAMA* 249:2509, 1983.

Russell P.S.: Some immunological considerations in liver transplantation. *Hepatology* 4:79S, 1984.

Sach G.: Pump blockers and ulcer disease. *N. Engl. J. Med.* 310:785, 1984.

Schenker S.: Medical treatment versus transplantation in liver disorders. *Hepatology* 4:102S, 1984.

Schmid R.: Issues in liver transplantation. *Hepatology* 4:1S, 1984.

Simon G.L., Gorbach S.L.: Intestinal flora in health and disease. *Gastroenterology* 86:174, 1984.

Starzl T.E., et al.: Donors for liver transplantation. *Pediatrics* 71:856, 1983.

Sternlieb I.: Wilson's disease: Implications for liver transplants. *Hepatology* 4:15S, 1984.

Swedberg J., Steiner J.F.: Oral rehydration therapy in diarrhea. *Postgrad. Med.* 74:335, 1983.

Tolia V., Dubois R.S.: Peptic ulcer disease in children and adolescents: A 10-year experience. *Clin. Pediatr.* 22:665, 1983.

Van Thiel D.H., et al.: Medical aspects of liver transplantation. *Hepatology* 4:79S, 1984.

Winton A.S.W., Singh M.N.: Rumination in pediatric populations: A behavioral analysis. *J. Am. Acad. Child Psychiatry* 3:269, 1983.

The Genitourinary Tract

Abuelo J.G.: The diagnosis of hematuria. *Arch. Intern. Med.* 143:967, 1983.

Alon U., Chan J.C.M.: Calcium and vitamin D homeostasis in the nephrotic syndrome: Current status. *Nephron* 36:1, 1984.

Berg G., Berg R.: Castration complex: Evidence from men operated for hypospadias. *Acta Psychiatr. Scand.* 68:143, 1983.

Duckett J.W.: Vesicourethral reflux: A "conservative" analysis. *Am. J. Kidney Dis.* 3:139, 1983.

Editorial comment: Who shall be dialyzed? *Lancet* 1:717, 1984.

Hayslett J.P.: Role of platelets in glomerulonephritis. *N. Engl. J. Med.* 310:1457, 1984.

Kramer S.A.: Cryptorchidism: Current state of the art in diagnosis and treatment. *Cont. Education*, p. 737, August, 1983.

Lyon R.P., Marshall S., Scott M.P.: Varicocele in youth. *West. J. Med.* 138:832, 1983.

May H.J., Colligan R.C., Schwartz M.S.: Childhood enuresis: Important points in assessment, trends, and treatment. *Postgrad. Med.* 74:111, 1983.

Nussbaum A.R., Lebowitz R.L.: Interlabial masses in little girls: Review and imaging recommendations. *Am. J. Radiol.* 141:65, 1983.

Spitz L.: Maldescent of the testis. *Arch. Dis. Child.* 58:847, 1983.

Thompson H.C.: The value of neonatal circumcision. *Am. J. Dis. Child.* 137:939, 1983.

Woodruff M.F.A., van Root J.J.: Possible implications of the effect of blood transfusion on allograft survival. *Lancet* 1:1201, 1983.

The Heart and Blood Vessels

Berry C.L.: Kawasaki's disease. *Pediatr. Cardiol.* 4:233, 1983.

Dietz W.H.: Childhood obesity: Susceptibility, cause, and management: *J. Pediatr.* 103:676, 1983.

Editorial comment: Infective endocarditis. *Lancet* 1:603, 1984.

Editorial comment: Is reduction of blood cholesterol effective? *Lancet* 1:317, 1984.

Greenwood R.D.: Cardiovascular malformations associated with extracardiac anomalies and formation syndromes: Patterns for diagnosis. *Clin. Pediatr.* 23:145, 1984.

Laragh J.H.: Hypertension: Twenty-five-year update. *Lab. Manag.* 22:23, 1984.

Oliver M.F.: Should we not forget about the mass control of coronary risk factors? *Lancet* 2:37, 1983.

Parrish M., Graham T.P.: Radionuclide angiography in children. *J. Pediatr.* 104:165, 1984.

Perloff J.K.: Adults with surgery-treated congenital heart disease: Sequelae and residua. *JAMA* 250:2033, 1983.

Porter C.J., Garson A., Gillette P.C.: Verapamil: An effective calcium blocking agent for pediatric patients. *Pediatrics* 71:748, 1983.

Selzer A.: The present status of prosthetic cardiac valves. *Arch. Intern. Med.* 143:1965, 1983.

Wilkinson J.L.: Management of paroxysmal tachycardia. *Arch. Dis. Child.* 58:945, 1983.

Wu D.: Supraventricular tachycardias. *JAMA* 249:3357, 1983.

Blood

Alter B.: Historical review of national initiatives for sickle cell disease. *Am J. Pediatr. Hematol. Oncol.* 5:378, 1983.

Benz E.J.: Molecular genetics of the sickling syndromes: Evolution of new strategies for improved diagnosis. *Am. J. Pediatr Hematol. Oncol.* 6:59, 1984.

Brown A.E.: Neutropenia, fever, and infection. *Am. J. Med.* 76:421, 1984.

Burns T.R., Saleem A.: Idiopathic thrombocytopenic purpura. *Am. J. Med.* 75:1001, 1983.

Editorial comment: The bleeding time and the hematocrit. *Lancet* 1:997, 1984.

Editorial comment: Bone marrow aplasia and parvovirus. *Lancet* 2:21, 1983.

Editorial comment: The cause of AIDS? *Lancet* 1:1053, 1984.

Editorial comment: Danazol for severe disease. *JAMA* 249:3279, 1983.

Editorial comment: Graft-versus-host disease after marrow transplantation. *Lancet* 1:491, 1984.

Editorial comment: High-dose chelation therapy in thalassemia. *Lancet* 1:373, 1984.

Editorial comment: Molecular genetics for the clinician. *Lancet* 1:257, 1984.

Editorial comment: New ways to boost factor VIII in hemophilia: DDAVP for mild hemophilia A and von Willebrand's disease. *JAMA* 249:3278, 1983.

Hathaway W.E.: Neonatal hyperviscosity. *Pediatrics* 72:567, 1983.

————The use of antiplatelet agents in pediatric hypercoagulable states. *Am. J. Dis. Child.* 189:301, 1984.

Humbert J.R., Moore L.L.: Iron deficiency and infection: A dilemma. *J. Pediatr. Gastroenterol. Nutr.* 2:403, 1983.

Kadota R.P., Smithson, W.A.: Bone marrow transplantation for diseases of childhood. *Mayo Clin. Proc.* 59:171, 1984.

Marder V.J.: Molecular bad actors and thrombosis. *N. Engl. J. Med.* 310:588, 1984.

Powars D., Overturf G.D., Wilkins J.: Commentary: Infections in sickle and SC disease. *J. Pediatr.* 103:242, 1983.

Rosse W.F.: Whatever happened to vinca-loaded platelets? *N. Engl. J. Med.* 310:1051, 1984.

Scott R.B.: Prenatal diagnosis of hemoglobinopathies. *Am. J. Pediatr. Hematol. Oncol.* 5:346, 1983.

Shumack K.H., Rock G.A.: Therapeutic plasma exchange. *N. Engl. J. Med.* 310:762, 1984.

Smith J.A.: Management of sickle cell disease: Progress during the last 10 years. *Am. J. Pediatr. Hematol. Oncol.* 5:360, 1983.

Speck W.T.: Acquired immune deficiency syndrome. *J. Pediatr.* 103:161, 1983.

Spruce W.E.: Bone marrow transplantation: II. Use for aplastic anemia, hereditary diseases, and hemoglobinopathies. *Am. J. Pediatr. Hematol. Oncol.* 5:295, 1983.

————III. Major problems and future directions. *Am. J. Pediatr. Hematol. Oncol.* 5:301, 1983.

Steinberg M.H., Hubbel R.P.: Clinical diversity of sickle cell anemia: Genetic and cellular modulation of disease severity. *Am. J. Hematol.* 14:405, 1983.

Weller P.F.: Eosinophilia. *J. Allergy Clin. Immunol.* 73:1, 1984.

Williams T.E.: Legal issues and ethical dilemmas surrounding bone marrow transplantation in children. *Am. J. Pediatr. Hematol. Oncol.* 6:83, 1984.

Oncology

Chessells J.M.: Childhood acute lymphoblastic leukemia: The late effects of treatment. *Br. J. Haematol.* 53:369, 1983.

Committee on Infectious Diseases, American Academy of Pediatrics: Expanded guidelines for use of varicella-zoster immune globulin. *Pediatrics* 72:886, 1983.

Editorial comment: Edible carcinogens. *Lancet* 1:87, 1984.

Fanaroff A.A.: Ultrasound studies during pregnancy. *J. Pediatr.* 103:406, 1983.

Gold J.W.M.: Opportunistic fungal infections in patients with neoplastic disease. *Am. J. Med.* 76:458, 1984.

Greene B.G., Adler S.S., Knospe W.H.: Bone marrow transplantation in leukemia. *Postgrad Med.* 74:123, 1983.

Herzog L.W.: Lymphadenopathy of the head and neck in infants and children. *Clin. Pediatr.* 22:485, 1983.

Klastersky J.: Empiric treatment of infections in neutropenic patients with cancer. *Rev. Infect. Dis.* 5:S21, 1983.

Land C.E., McKay F.W., Machado S.G.: Childhood leukemia and fallout from the Nevada nuclear test. *Science* 223:139, 1984.

Martin A.O.: Can ultrasound cause genetic damage? *J. Clin. Ultrasound* 12:11, 1984.

Miller G.: Epstein-Barr virus: Immortalization and replication. *N. Engl. J. Med.* 310:1255, 1984.

Murphree A.L., Benedict W.F.: Retinoblastoma: Clues to human oncogenesis. *Science* 223:1028, 1984.

Phillips H.H.: Clinical approach to the diagnosis and treatment of retinoblastoma. *J. Am. Osteopath. Assoc.* 82:782, 1983.

Pifer L.L.: *Pediatr. Infect. Dis.* 2:177, 1983.

Pizzo P.A., et al.: Approaching the controversies in antibacterial management of cancer patients. *Am. J. Med.* 76:436, 1984.

Shalet S.M.: Disorders of the endocrine system due to radiation and cytotoxic chemotherapy. *Clin. Endocrinol.* 18:637, 1983.

Sullivan J.L., et al.: X-linked lymphoproliferative syndrome. *J. Clin. Invest.* 71:765, 1983.

Willett W.C., MacMahn B.: Diet and cancer: An overview. *N. Engl. J. Med.* 310:633, 1984.

Endocrinology

Balkin M.S.: Precocious puberty: Evaluation and new treatment. *Female Patient* 8:23, 1983.

Barnes N.: Excessive growth. *Arch. Dis. Child.* 58:845, 1984.

Bistritzer T., et al.: Hemoglobin A_1 and pancreatic beta cell function in cystic fibrosis. *Isr. J. Med. Sci.* 19:600, 1983.

Broughard B.H.: Control and monitoring for the child with insulin-dependent diabetes mellitus. *Am. J. Dis. Child.* 137:787, 1983.

Daughady W.H.: Cushing's disease and vasophilic microadenomas. *N. Engl. J. Med.* 310:919, 1984.

Fisher D.A.: Second International Conference on Neonatal Thyroid Screening: Progress Report. *J. Pediatr.* 103:653, 1983.

Gerich J.E.: The role of growth hormone in diabetes mellitus. *N. Engl. J. Med.* 310:848, 1984.

Goldstein D.E.: Is glycosylated hemoglobin clinically useful? *N. Engl. J. Med.* 310:384, 1984.

Grew R.S., et al.: Facilitating patient understanding in the treatment of growth delay. *Clin. Pediatr.* 22:685, 1983.

Hetzel B.S.: Iodine deficiency disorders and their eradication. *Lancet* 2:1126, 1983.

Hulse A.: Congenital hypothyroidism and neurological development. *J. Child Psychol. Psychiatry* 24:629, 1983.

Kaplan S.A.: The insulin receptor. *J. Pediatr.* 104:327, 1984.

Kappy M.S., Stein G.S., Stein J.L.: Recombinant DNA and endocrine therapy in children. *Am. J. Dis. Child.* 137:685, 1983.

Rosenthal S.R., et al.: Growth failure and inflammatory bowel disease: Approach to treatment of a complicated adolescent problem. *Pediatrics* 72:481, 1983.

Schneider A.J.: Starting insulin therapy in children with newly diagnosed diabetes. *Am. J. Dis. Child.* 137:782, 1983.

Singer T.: Abnormal sex differentiation. *J. Pediatr.* 104:1, 1984.

Tamborlane W.V., Sherwin R.S.: Diabetes—Controlling complications: New strategies and insights. *J. Pediatr.* 102:805, 1983.

Underwood L.E.: Growth hormone in the treatment of children with short stature. *Pediatrics* 72:891, 1983.

Zoler M.L.: Probing the causes of type I diabetes. *Geriatrics* 38:121, 1983.

Nutrition and Metabolism

Brouhard B.H.: Control and monitoring for the child with insulin-dependent diabetes mellitus. *Am. J. Dis. Child.* 137:787, 1983.

Brown K.: Chronic protracted diarrhea of infancy: A nutritional disease. *Pediatrics* 72:786, 1983.

Chesney R.W.: Metabolic bone disease. *Pediatr. Rev.* 5:227, 1984.

Committee on Nutrition, American Academy of Pediatrics: Soy-protein formulas: Recommendations for use in infant feeding. *Pediatrics* 72:359, 1983.

Committee on Drugs, American Academy of Pediatrics: The transfer of drugs and other chemicals into human breast milk. *Pediatrics* 72:375, 1983.

Dietz W.H., Jr.: Childhood obesity. *J. Pediatr.* 103:676, 1983.

Kaplan S.A.: The insulin receptor. *J. Pediatr.* 104:327, 1984.

Laurence R.A.: Infant nutrition. *Pediatr. Rev.* 5:133, 1983.

Nichols B.L., et al.: Nutritional physiology in pregnancy and lactation. *Adv. Pediatr.* 30:473, 1984.

Reeves J.D., et al.: Iron deficiency in health and disease. *Adv. Pediatr.* 30:281, 1984.

Riely C.A.: Wilson's disease. *Pediatr. Rev.* 5:217, 1983.

Schneider A.J.: Starting insulin therapy in children with newly diagnosed diabetes. *Am. J. Dis. Child.* 137:782, 1983.

Stegink L.D.: Amino acids in pediatric parenteral nutrition. *Am. J. Dis. Child.* 137:1008, 1983.

Susskind R., et al.: Assessment of nutritional status of children. *Pediatr. Rev.* 5:195, 1983

Tsang R.C.: The quandry of vitamin D in the newborn infant. *Lancet* 1:1370, 1983.

The Musculoskeletal System

Ansell, V.M.: Arthritis in young children. *Br. Med. J.* 286:1917, 1983.

———, Swann M.: The management of chronic arthritis of children. *J. Bone Joint Surg.* [Br.] 65–B:536, 1983.

Baum J.: Treatment of juvenile arthritis. *Hosp. Pract.* 118:121, 1983.

Cambras R.A., et al.: Limb lengthening in children. *Orthopedics* 7:468, 1984.

Coccia P.F.: Cells that resorb bone. *N. Engl. J. Med.* 310:456, 1984.

Committee on Research, American Academy of Pediatrics: Reducing the toll of injuries in childhood requires support for a focused research effort. *Pediatrica* 72:736, 1983.

Editorial note: The viral etiology of rheumatoid arthritis. *Lancet* 1:772, 1984.

Epps C.H., Jr.: Current concepts review: Proximal femoral focal deficiency. *J. Bone Joint Surg. [Am.]* 65–A:687, 1983.

Freischlag J.: Weight loss, body composition, and health of high school wrestlers. *Physician Sportsmed.* 12:121, January 1984.

Gillespie R., Torode I.P.: Classification and management of congenital abnormalities of the femur. *J. Bone Joint Surg. [Br.]* 65–B:557, 1983.

Hensey O.J., et al.: Juvenile diskitis. *Arch. Dis. Child.* 58:983, 1983.

Lamb D.W.: Upper limb displasia. *J. R. Coll. Surg. Edinb.* 28:203, 1983.

Lehman W.B.: Pediatric orthopedic update: Decision-making in Legg-Calve-Perthes disease. *Orthop. Rev.* 13:55, 1984.

Nade S.: Acute septic arthritis in infancy and childhood. *J. Bone Joint Surg. [Br.]* 65–B:234, 1983.

Rosen J.F., Chesney R.W.: Circulating calcitriol concentrations in health and disease. *J. Pediatr.* 103:1, 1983.

Runyan D.K.: Preparticipation examination of the young athlete. *Clin. Pediatr.* 22:674, 1983.

Stewart V.L., Herling P., Dalinka M.K.: Calcification in soft tissues. *JAMA* 250:78, 1983.

Sty J.R., Starschak R.J., Hubbard A.M.: Radionuclide evaluation in childhood injuries. *Sem. Nucl. Med.* 13:258, 1983.

Weiss R.A., et al.: Diagnostic tests and clinical subsets in systemic lupus erythematosus. *Ann. Allergy* 51:135, 1983.

Wilson M.G.: Genetics of common orthopedic and genital malformations. *Contemp. Orthop.* 8:61, 1984.

Ophthalmology

Ball D.M., et al.: Kawasaki syndrome in the United States. *Am. J. Dis. Child.* 137:211, 1983.

Bankes J.L.K.: Do unnecessary spectacles make the eyes worse? *Arch. Dis. Child.* 58:766, 1983.

Editor's comment: Delayed visual maturation. *Lancet* 1:1158, 1984.

Harcourt R.B.: Detection and management of squint. *Arch. Dis. Child.* 58:675, 1983.

Heller M.: Chlamydial infections. *Ann. Emerg. Med.* 13:170, 1984.

Hyvärinen L., Lindstedt E.: Early visual development, normal and abnormal. Proceedings of a Symposium held at the Resource Center for Visually Handicapped Children, Tomtebodaskolan, Solna, Sweden. *Acta Ophthalmol.*, Suppl. 157, 1983.

Lang J.: The two-pencil test for testing stereopsis. *Klin. Monatsbl. Augenheilkd.* 182:576, 1983.

Ludington-Hoe S.M.: What can newborns really see? *Am. J. Nurs.* 83:1286, 1983.

Nelson L.B., et al.: Developmental aspects in the assessment of visual function in young children. *Pediatrics* 73:375, 1984.

Pfister R.R.: Chemical injuries of the eye. *Ophthalmology* 90:1246, 1983.

Neurology and Psychiatry

Fishman M.A.: Multiple sclerosis and related diseases in childhood. *Pediatrics Update, 1984.* Ed. 203.

Gross M.: Anorexia nervosa: An overview. *Cleve. Clin. Q.* 50:371, 1983.

Kay J., et al.: Hematologic and immunologic abnormalities in anorexia nervosa. *South. Med. J.* 76:1008, 1983.

McComb J.G.: Recent research into the nature of cerebrospinal fluid formation and absorption. *J. Neurosurg.* 59:369, 1983.

Metzger R.L., et al.: Use of visual training for reading disabilities. *Pediatrics* 73:824, 1984.

Myers G.J., et al.: Neonatal seizures. *Pediatr. Rev.* 5:67, 1983.

Riikonen R.: Infantile spasms: Modern practical aspects. *Acta Paediatr.* 73:1, 1984.

Russman B.S.: Early intervention for the biologically handicapped infant and young child: Is is of value? *Pediatr. Rev.* 5:51, 1983.

Shaywitz S.E., et al.: Pharmacotherapy of attention deficit disorder. *Pediatrics Update, 1984.* Ed. 43.

Steinhausen H.-C., et al.: Follow-up studies of anorexia nervosa: A review of research findings. *Psychol. Med.* 13:239, 1983.

Taft L.T. : Pediatric management of the physically handicapped child. *Adv. Pediatr.* 30:13, 1984.

Wallace S.J.: Febrile convulsions: Their significance for later intellectual development and behavior. *J. Child Psychol. Psychiatry* 25:15, 1984.

Zuckerman B.S., et al.: Specific learning disability and dyslexia: A language-based model. *Adv. Pediatr.* 30:249, 1984.

Child Development

Lobato D.: Siblings of handicapped children: A review. *J. Autism Develop. Disord.* 13:347, 1983.

Perrin E.C.: Children's understanding of illness. *Pediatrics Update, 1984.* Ed. 293.

Winton A.S.W., et al.: Rumination in pediatric populations: a behavioral analysis. *J. Am. Acad. Child Psychiatry* 22:269, 1983.

Zigler E., et al.: Discerning the future of early childhood intervention. *Am. Psychol.* 38:894, 1983.

Adolescent Medicine

Beardslee W.R., et al.: Adolescents and the threat of nuclear war: The evolution of a perspective. *Yale J. Biol. Med.* 56:79, 1983.

Boeck M.A., et al.: Eating disorders in adolescence. *Pediatrics Update, 1984.* Ed. 63.

Golden N., et al.: An overview of the etiology, diagnosis, and management of anorexia nervosa. *Clin. Pediatr.* 23:209, 1984.

Goldstein S., et al.: The physiology of puberty. *Pediatrics Update, 1984.* Ed. 63.

Macdonald D.I.: Drugs, drinking, and adolescence. *Am. J. Dis. Child.* 138:117, 1984.

Rapp C.E., Jr.: The adolescent patient. *Ann. Intern. Med.* 99:52, 1983.

Therapeutics and Toxicology

Berlin C.A., Jr.: Advances in pediatric pharmacology and toxicology. *Adv. Pediatr.* 30:221, 1984.

Committee on Drugs, American Academy of Pediatrics: Neonatal drug withdrawal. *Pediatrics* 72:895, 1983.

Committee on Drugs, American Academy of Pediatrics: Ethanol in liquid preparations intended for children. *Pediatrics* 73:405, 1984.

Dershewitz R.A., et al.: Childhood household safety. *Am. J. Dis. Child.* 138:85, 1984.

Gladtke E.: Use of antipyretic analgesics in the pediatric patient. *Am. J. Med.* 75(Suppl.):121, 1983.

Goldman L.P., et al.: Corrosive substance ingestion: A review. *Am. J. Gastroenterol.* 79:85, 1984.

Heit W.F.W.: Hematologic effects of antipyretic analgesics. *Amer. J. Med.* 75(Suppl.):65, 1983.

Johnson C., et al.: Psychopharmacological treatment of anorexia and bulemia: Review and synthesis. *J. Nerv. Ment. Dis.* 171:524, 1983.

Lacouture P.G., et al.: Acute isopropyl alcohol intoxication. *Am. J. Med.* 75:680, 1983.

Nelson J.D.: A primer for pediatricians on new cephalosporin antibiotics. *Am. J. Dis. Child.* 137:1041, 1983.

Prescott L.F., et al.: Drug interactions affecting analgesic toxicity. *Am. J. Med.* 75(Suppl.):113, 1983.

Rumack B.H.: Jimsonweed abuse. *Pediatr. Rev.* 5:141, 1983.

Schwartz R.H.: Marijuana and toxicity. *Pediatrics* 73:455, 1984.

Shann F.: Continuous drug infusions in children: A table for simplifying calculations. *Crit. Care Med.* 11:462, 1984.

Temple A.R.: Review of comparative antipyretic activity in children. *Am. J. Med.* 75(Suppl.):38, 1983.

Weiss S.T., et al.: The health effects of involuntary smoking. *Am. Rev. Respir. Dis.* 128:933, 1983.

Miscellaneous

Brady J.P., et al.: Sudden infant death syndrome: The physician's dilemma. *Adv. Pediatr.* 30:635, 1984.

Brown G.W.: Discriminant analyses. *Am. J. Dis. Child.* 138:395, 1984.

Holder A.R.: Parents, courts, and refusal of treatment. *J. Pediatr.* 103:515, 1983.

Kangarloo H.: Abdominal ultrasound in pediatrics. *Pediatrics Update, 1984.* Ed. 339.

McBride J.T.: Infantile apnea. *Pediatr. Rev.* 5:275, 1984.

Nudelman R., et al.: C-reactive protein in pediatrics. *Adv. Pediatr.* 30:517, 1984.

Trunkey D.D.: Trauma. *Sci. Am.* 249:28, 1983.

Subject Index

A

Abdomen
  pain in varicella in
    immunocompromised children, 103
Abnormalities (*see* Anomalies)
ABO hemolytic disease
  hyperbilirubinemia complicating, in
    newborn, 20
Abortion
  during adolescence, risks of, 532
Abuse
  dwarfism, growth of intelligence in, 500
Acid infusion
  intraesophageal, in asthma during sleep,
    485
Acne
  erythromycin vs. clindamycin in, 171
  vulgaris, irradiation for, thyroid
    abnormalities after, 399
ACTH
  in seizures, 493
Adenocarcinoma
  genital clear cell, 391
Adenosine deaminase
  erythrocyte, elevated in hypoplastic
    anemia, 332
Adolescence
  abortion during, risks of, 532
  adrenal hyperplasia and 21-hydroxylase
    deficiency during, 406
  chest pain during, 536
  differences between boys and girls in
    context of their families, 534
  fatherhood during, stresses of, 530
  powerlifting during, medical history in,
    465
  pregnancy during, incidence, 528
  reexamining the concept of adolescence,
    534
  smokeless tobacco use during, oral
    tissue alterations with, 181
Adolescent mother
  birth weight of infant of, 527
Adrenal
  hyperplasia, and 21-hydroxylase
    deficiency, during adolescence, 406
Adrenoleukodystrophy
  cerebrohepatorenal syndrome and, in
    newborn, 284
Aerosol, 214 ff.
  bag in bronchodilator administration in
    asthma, 216
  in bronchoconstriction, with tube
    spacer, 214

Age
  -related changes in T and B lymphocyte
    subpopulations, 131
AIDS, 144
Air leak
  pulmonary, in premature on mechanical
    ventilation, 49
Airflow
  nasal resistance to, menthol in, 191
Alcohol syndrome
  fetal, liver fibrosis in, 245
Allergic
  form of Meadow's syndrome, 160
Allergy, 156 ff.
  cat vs. dog, in atopic children, 160
  food, migraine as, 156
  penicillin, skin testing, 159
Alpha$_1$-antitrypsin deficiency (*see*
    Antitrypsin deficiency)
Aminophylline
  individualized dosing, 542
Amoxicillin
  in maxillary sinusitis, 198
Ampicillin in meningitis, 73 ff.
  bacterial, 75
  Hemophilus influenzae type B, 73
Amyloid-related serum protein
  indicating lung infection in cystic
    fibrosis, 237
Anemia
  of acute inflammation, 337
  classification improvement, 340
  hypoplastic, erythrocyte adenosine
    deaminase elevation in, 332
  sickle cell, *Hemophilus influenzae*
    septicemia in, 350
Angiotensin
  -renin system, after captopril in
    hypertension, 287
Aniridia
  study of anterior segment in, 473
Anomalies
  congenital, in cryptorchid boys, 298
  urinary tract, with supernumerary
    nipples, 291
Anorexia nervosa
  management and outcome, 502
Antenatal diagnosis
  in α_1-antitrypsin deficiency with liver
    disease, 254
Anterior segment
  study in aniridia, 473
Antibody(ies)
  antinuclear antibody tests, positive, 448
  autoantibodies to SS-A/Ro in congenital
    heart block, 309

Index to Authors